Controversies in the Management of Keratoconus

Adel Barbara
Editor

Controversies in the Management of Keratoconus

Springer

Editor
Adel Barbara
Medical Director of IVISION
Refractive Surgery and Keratoconus Treatment Center
Haifa
Israel

ISBN 978-3-319-98031-7 ISBN 978-3-319-98032-4 (eBook)
https://doi.org/10.1007/978-3-319-98032-4

Library of Congress Control Number: 2018962165

This Springer imprint is published by the registered company Springer Nature Switzerland AG
The registered company address is: Gewerbestrasse 11, 6330 Cham, Switzerland

I dedicate this book to every one who utilizes science for the welfare and progress of humanity, to every one who gets up in the morning and lightens a candle in order to reduce the darkness of inequality and suppression, to every one who tries to make this world better for human beings regardless of their color, race, nationality, and religion.

Adel Barbara

Foreword

Following his excellent and comprehensive book on keratoconus, *Textbook on Keratoconus: New Insights*, Dr. Adel Barbara has once again come up with a timely textbook on a thought-provoking topic – *Controversies in the Management of Keratoconus*.

With the explosion of new treatment options and large potential combinations of collagen corneal cross-linking (CXL) with other treatment modalities, there is controversy as to the most appropriate manner in which to combine CXL with other currently accepted treatment modalities.

This book is extremely comprehensive, covering more than 30 chapters by renowned experts in the field, and treatment modalities which are covered are "epi-on vs epi-off," accelerated treatments, customized CXL, and the pros and cons of phakic IOLs combined with CXL.

The book also covers other pertinent topics which relate to assessing treatment outcomes such as the definition of progression in keratoconus, the question if keratoconus is an inflammatory disease, and the significance of the demarcation line after CXL.

It also includes alternative technologies to CXL, additional means to improve visual acuity (VA) after intracorneal ring segments (ICRS), a chapter on photorefractive keratectomy (PRK) in keratoconus (KC), and a chapter by Dr. Barbara on how to navigate through the controversies. Interestingly, there is also a chapter on biomechanics in KC and one on ICRS.

Interesting, relevant, and controversial topics which any physician, interested in using cross-linking, would find stimulating include: collagen cross-linking Dresden protocol (why to stick to it), customized collagen corneal cross-linking for the treatment of keratoconus, beyond the Dresden protocol, optimization of cross-linking, and collagen corneal cross-linking for the treatment of keratoconus in the pediatric group. Other topics include alternative methods for halting the progression of keratoconus, photorefractive keratectomy for the treatment of keratoconus and forme fruste keratoconus, Athens protocol for the treatment of keratoconus, photorefractive keratectomy combined with CXL (why not?), intrastromal corneal rings for the treatment of keratoconus (do they halt the progression of the disease), why to implant intrastromal corneal rings in keratoconus? and how to improve vision after successful intracorneal rings (ICRS).

It also includes phakic lenses for the treatment of keratoconus (why yes and why not), PKP versus DALK, the best approach for CXL from the biomechanical point of view, and toric IOLs in cataract surgery of KC patients.

Once again, Dr. Barbara has hit a home run in providing a book co-authored by leading experts in the field. Any doctor dealing with KC would find this book very valuable, and those patients treated by cross-linking are sure to benefit and will hopefully see optimized outcomes following CXL treatments.

Yaron Rabinowitz, MD
Ophthalmology Research
Cedars-Sinai Medical Centers,
Beverly Hills, CA, USA

Contents

Introduction

Why a book on controversies in the management of keratoconus (KC)? Simply because there are still controversies in every topic that deals with KC, whether it is the epidemiology, diagnosis, pathology, or management of the disease.

KC is classically defined as a noninflammatory corneal disease; this definition is questioned, and the presence of higher rates inflammatory mediators in the tear film of KC patients supports the inflammatory contribution to the development of KC. Eye rubbing is advocated as causative and aggravating factor in keratoconus; the mechanism is mechanical and inflammatory, and some researchers believe that stopping eye rubbing will stop keratoconus formation and progression altogether; this theory is questioned.

Epidemiology of the diseases attracts controversies; higher incidence and prevalence have largely been attributed to advances in imaging and detection, partly driven by the boom in refractive surgery. Are we witnessing a true increase in the incidence of keratoconus? Is it always a bilateral disease? What are the roles of genetics, ethnicity, geography, and the environmental factors, and what are the factors that contribute to the development and progression of KC? What is the role of ultraviolet light exposure, eye rubbing, contact lenses wear, and allergic and atopic eye diseases?

Until two decades ago, there were two treatment modalities only for keratoconus: the first is rigid gas-permeable contact lenses (CLs), and when this fails, then penetrating keratoplasty (PKP) was offered as the ultimate solution for the disease. Very simple, two choices, no more.

Since then, huge advancements were introduced to this field in terms of diagnosis and treatment. In the diagnostic field, new corneal topography and tomography devices which enable earlier detection of the disease are available not only in the advanced centers for refractive surgery but also in general ophthalmic clinics and even in high street opticians. In the treatment field, new treatment modalities have emerged such as collagen corneal cross-linking (CXL) for arresting the progression of the disease, intracorneal ring segments (ICRS) for vision improvement, photorefractive keratectomy either alone or combined with CXL for corneal remolding and vision improvement, and phakic intraocular lenses (pIOLs) mainly toric pIOLs to correct ametropia due to KC. Lamellar keratoplasty such as deep anterior lamellar keratoplasty (DALK) is replacing PKP as the primary corneal grafting technique with better safety profile. Furthermore, we are witnessing innovations and improvements in the design of CLs such as soft keratoconus lenses and hybrid, scleral, and semi-scleral CLs. The availability of these techniques improves quality of life and also increases choice and patients expectations.

These advances made KC a new subspecialty which attracts a lot of interest among ophthalmologists. There is an impressive increase in the number of publications on KC, and for the past 6 years, there is a special journal dedicated solely to keratoconus and ectatic corneal diseases: the *International Journal for Keratoconus and Ectatic Corneal Diseases*.

Disagreements among experts exist in all fields of keratoconus management; this involves the diagnostic criteria, the definition of progression, when and how to perform CXL, and when to use ICRS. Many experts are enthusiastic about this treatment modality, while others are reluctant to implant corneal rings. Some are in favor for PRK whether or not it is combined with CXL, and others are against PRK in KC. The same applies to phakic IOLs.

All these treatments may be combined simultaneously or sequentially, but what treatments are to be combined and when and how? Again, there is no agreement among experts regarding some treatments, and when agreement exists, there is still controversy on the sequence.

CXL is accepted and adopted by the ophthalmic community as a mean of halting KC progression; however, there is no agreement on the definition of progression, and as a result, this affects the indication for treatment and the evaluation of outcomes. If the decision to perform CXL has been made, what type of CXL, namely, the classical Dresden protocol, epi-on CXL, accelerated CXL, pulsed accelerated CXL, or Cretan protocol CXL, is to be performed?

We should adapt our treatment according to the patient's situation, needs, and expectations. These expectations should be understood and addressed accordingly; otherwise, "successful" treatment is perceived as failures.

This book addresses these controversies and aims to provide the reader with the appropriate clues, knowledge, and ability to navigate through these controversies.

Adel Barbara, MD, FRCOphth
Medical Director of IVISION
Refractive Surgery and Keratoconus Treatment Center
Haifa, Israel

Chapter 1
Epidemiology of Keratoconus

Ramez Barbara, A. M. J. Turnbull, A. Malem, D. F. Anderson, P. Hossain, A. Konstantopoulos, and Adel Barbara

1.1 Incidence and Prevalence

Healthcare planners and strategists require knowledge of the epidemiological burden of a disease in order to determine the nature of services required. Estimates of the prevalence of keratoconus have ranged from 0.3 per 100,000 (0.0003%) in Russia [1] to 3300 per 100,000 (3.3%) in Lebanon [2] and Iran [3]. Taken in isolation however, figures for either prevalence or incidence fail to illustrate important regional and ethnic variations, or the methodology of how these estimates were arrived at.

Early screening studies, based on findings with older diagnostic modalities, had a high false negative rate. More recent studies using corneal topography provide more sensitive estimates of prevalence/incidence [4], which have steadily increased over the last few years. Furthermore, cases previously thought to be unilateral have frequently been shown with modern imaging to be bilateral, with one eye at an earlier sub-clinical stage. It is now accepted that truly unilateral keratoconus does

R. Barbara (✉) · A. M. J. Turnbull · D. F. Anderson · A. Konstantopoulos
Southampton Eye Unit, University Hospitals Southampton, Southampton, UK
e-mail: andyt@doctors.org.uk; david@andersoneyecare.co.uk

A. Malem
Ophthalmology Department, Royal Hampshire County Hospital, Winchester, UK
e-mail: andrew.malem@cantab.net

P. Hossain
Southampton Eye Unit, University Hospitals Southampton, Southampton, UK

Clinical Experimental Sciences, Faculty of Medicine, University of Southampton, Southampton, UK
e-mail: P.N.Hossain@soton.ac.uk

A. Barbara
Medical Director of IVISION, Refractive Surgery and Keratoconus Treatment Center, Haifa, Israel

A. Barbara (ed.), *Controversies in the Management of Keratoconus*,
https://doi.org/10.1007/978-3-319-98032-4_1

not exist [5], although it may present unilaterally in the context of asymmetric environmental factors such as eye rubbing [5–7].

There are important methodological differences between hospital or clinic based reports and population-based studies, as explained by Gordon-Shaag et al. [4]. Prevalence is underestimated by hospital-based studies, as they fail to include those being managed in a non-hospital setting, or patients with asymptomatic disease who have not been diagnosed. Population-based studies are the gold-standard, but they too can be hampered by selection bias [8]. Tables 1.1 and 1.2, reproduced from Gordon-Shaag et al. [4], summarize some of the key hospital-based and population-based studies of keratoconus epidemiology, demonstrating dramatic geographic variations.

Since Gordon-Shaag's review in 2015, a Dutch study has been performed in conjunction with a health insurance company that insures 31% (4.4 million) of the Dutch population [9]. In this study, annual incidence was estimated at 13.3 per 100,000 with a prevalence of 265 per 100,000 (0.27%). Mean age at diagnosis was 28.3 years and the lifetime risk of requiring a corneal transplant was 12%.

Whilst the heterogeneous methodology of prevalence studies limits direct comparison between studies, estimates of prevalence have increased over the last few decades. This was highlighted by McMonnies who reviewed several studies, including one from 2003 [10] employing Atlas anterior corneal topography, biomicroscopy and ultrasound pachymetry that found a keratoconus prevalence of 0.9% in patients presenting for laser vision correction i.e. four times the upper range of estimate of prevalence prior to 1966 [11]. A 2010 study in Yemen [12] using TMS-2 topography, biomicroscopy and pachymetry found a combined keratoconus/forme-fruste keratoconus prevalence in keratorefractive surgery candidates of 5.8% i.e. 25 times greater than the mean prior to 1966 [11]. These studies are likely to overestimate the true prevalence of keratoconus due to selection bias, given that the disease is strongly associated with myopia and these were patients presenting for laser vision correction [11]. Nonetheless, the point regarding increasing prevalence is well made.

Middle Eastern and central Asian ethnicity is considered a risk factor for keratoconus [13], with the highest prevalence estimates (3.3%) coming from Lebanon [2] and Iran [3]. Studies have reported a prevalence of 2.3% in India [13], 2.34% among Arab students in Israel [8] and 2.5% in Iran [14]. A prevalence of 3.18% was recorded in a population-based study of Israeli Arabs [9], consistent with other studies from the Middle East [2, 8, 14, 16]. The concordance of results supports a true prevalence in these countries of similar magnitude [14].

A large retrospective longitudinal cohort study conducted in the USA investigating the sociodemographic and systemic associations of keratoconus evaluated 16,053 patients with keratoconus and matched them to a healthy control group [17]. Black and Latino patients were 57% and 43% respectively more likely to develop keratoconus than Caucasians. Asian-Americans were 39% less likely than Caucasians to have keratoconus. There was no correlation between disease prevalence and education or income, but rural communities had a 20% lower rate of the disease. Diabetes also appeared to be protective, with diabetic patients having a 20–50% lower risk of having keratoconus [17].

Table 1.1 Hospital/clinic based epidemiological studies of KC (Gordon-Shaag et al. BioMed Research International 2015 – reproduced with kind permission from authors)

Author	Location	Age in years	Sample size	Incidence/100,000	Prevalence/100,000	Method
Tanabe et al. (1985)	Muroran, Japan	10–60	2601-P		9	Keratometry
Kennedy et al. (1986)	Minnesota, USA	12–77	64-P	2	54.5	Keratometry + retinoscopy
Ihalainen (1986)	Finland	15–70	294-P	1.5	30	Keratometry + retinoscopy
Gorskova and Sevost'ianov (1998)	Urals, Russia				0.2–0.4	Keratometry
Pearson et al. (2000)	Midlands, UK	10–44	382-P	4.5-W	57	Keratometry + retinoscopy
				19.6-A	229	
Ota et al. (2002)	Tokyo, Japan		325-P	9		Keratometry?
Georgiou et al. (2004)	Yorkshire, UK		74-P	3.3-W		Clinical examination
				25-A		
Assiri et al. (2005)	Asir, Saudi Arabia	8–28	125-P	20		Keratometry
Nielsen et al. (2007)	Denmark		NA	1.3	86	Clinical indices + topography
Ljubic (2009)	Skope, Macedonia		2254		6.8	Keratometry
Ziaei et al. (2012)	Yazd, Iran	25.7 ± 9	536	22.3 (221)		Topography

A Asian (Indian, Pakistani, and. Bangladeshi), *W* white, *K* patient, *NA* not available

Table 1.2 Population based epidemiological studies of KC (Gordon-Shaag et al. BioMed Research International 2015 – reproduced with kind permission from authors)

Author	Location	Age in years (mean)	Sample size	Prevalence/100,000 (cases)	Method	Sampling method
Hofstetter (1959)	Indianapolis, USA	1–79	13,345	120 (16)	Placido disc[a]	Rural volunteers
Santiago et al. (1995)	France	18–22	670	1190	Topography	Army recruits
Jonas et al. (2009)	Maharashtra, India	>30 (49.4 ± 13.4)	4667	2300 (128)	Keratometry[a]	Rural volunteers (8 villages)
Millodot et al. (2011)	Jerusalem, Israel	18–54 (24.41 5.7)	991	2340 (23)	Topography	Urban volunteers (1 college)
Waked et al. (2012)	Beirut, Lebanon	22–26	92	3300 (3)	Topography	Urban volunteers (1 college)
Xu et al. (2012)	Beijing, China	50–93 (64.2 ± 9.8)	3166	900 (27)	Optical low coherence reflectometry[a]	Rural + urban volunteers
Hashemi et al. (2013)	Shahrud, Iran	50.83 ± 0.12	4592	760 (35)	Topography	Urban volunteers from random cluster
Hashemi et al. (2013)	Tehran, Iran	14–81 (40.8 ± 17.1)	426	3300 (14)	Topography	Urban volunteers (stratified cluster)
Shneor et al. (2014)	Haifa, Israel	18–60 (25.05 ± 8.83)	314	3180 (10)	Topography	Urban volunteers (1 college)
Hashemi et al. (2014)	Mashhad, Iran	20–34 (26.1 ± 13)	1073	2500 (26)	Topography	Urban volunteers (stratified cluster in 1 university)

[a]The methods for detecting KC used in these studies are now considered inadequate and the results should be interpreted with caution

Similar to prevalence, estimates of annual incidence of keratoconus range widely [18]; Assiri et al. reported an incidence of 20 per 100,000 per year in one Saudi Arabian province [18], although this figure was based only on referrals to a tertiary clinic. In Denmark, a much lower annual incidence has been estimated at 1.3 per 100,000 [19]. While this may point to geographical variation, it seems likely that ethnic and genetic differences may be more relevant. An annual incidence of 25 per 100,000 for people originally from Indian subcontinents compared with 3.3 per 100,000 for Caucasians ($p < 0.001$) was demonstrated in a single catchment area in Yorkshire, England [20]. In a similar study, Pearson et al. [21], demonstrated an annual incidence of keratoconus in Leicester, England of 19.6 per 100,000 and 4.5 per 100,000 in Asian and Caucasian communities respectively.

1.2 Environmental and Genetic Factors; Separate or Synergistic?

The increasing prevalence of keratoconus has largely been attributed to advances in imaging, increased awareness and higher detection rates. However, we may also be witnessing a true increase in the incidence of keratoconus. The aetiology of keratoconus is generally accepted to be a combination of environmental and genetic factors, as well as biomechanical and biochemical disorders [5, 22–24]. There is a wide variation in prevalence across different geographic areas, with peaks of prevalence recorded in the Middle East lending support to the theory of environmental causation. However, varying prevalence among different ethnic groups in the same geographic location also suggests a genetic basis for the disease. As an illustration, Indian, Pakistani and Bangladeshi communities in the United Kingdom have a significantly higher prevalence of keratoconus than the national average [20, 21]. Further evidence of a genetic basis to the disease includes a significant association with consanguinity [25], autosomal dominant and recessive patterns of familial inheritance [15, 26], higher concordance between monozygotic than dizygotic twins [27], and an association with other genetic disorders [28]. A positive family history has been identified in 18% of keratoconic patients in large population studies [29, 30]. In a separate study, 10% of patients with keratoconus had a family history of the disease, compared with just 0.05% of the age-matched control group [31]. Nonetheless, most cases are still deemed sporadic [28].

The association between family history and disease severity is not clear. One study demonstrated that a positive family history reduced disease severity [30], whereas another study found no correlation between the two [29]. In the former, the positive family history was credited with facilitating earlier diagnosis. One study has shown a positive association between family history and disease severity [32].

Several studies have attempted to find a causative gene for keratoconus through linkage analysis. A Finnish study mapped the disease locus of 20 families with autosomal dominant keratoconus and mapped the disease locus to chromosome 16q, suggesting that a causative gene in autosomal dominant keratoconus is located within the 16q22.3–q23.1 chromosomal region [33]. An Australian study of Tasmanian patients performed genome analysis on six patients of undefined genetic relationship and one affected sibling pair. This study identified chromosome 21 as a possible disease locus, with further analysis also suggesting an association at 20q12 [34]. An Italian study found a novel locus for autosomal dominant keratoconus on chromosome 3p14–q13 [35]. A study of families from France, Spain, and Guadeloupe found a locus for isolated familial keratoconus at 2p24 [36].

Geographic variations, but consistently higher prevalence in certain ethnic groups, may be attributable to environmental factors promoting the expression of genetic factors related to ethnicity [11]. The underlying mechanism for this is likely to be epigenetic modifications leading to altered gene expression and phenotype [37]. The most widely implicated environmental stressors are ultraviolet (UV) light exposure and eye-rubbing [11], although exposure to certain toxins and microbes may also play a role [37].

1.3 Ultraviolet Light Exposure

As well as the Middle East, a high prevalence of keratoconus has also been identified in New Zealand [38] and some Pacific island populations [39]. High UV light levels in these areas go some way towards explaining this geographic distribution. It is proposed that UV light increases the production of reactive oxygen species within the cornea [40] and that keratoconic corneas lack the ability to process these [41], leading to oxidative stress, cytotoxicity and corneal thinning [42]. A counter-argument is that corneal collagen cross-linking is induced by UV light, so keratoconus may actually be expected to have a lower prevalence in these areas [43].

Certainly, UV exposure cannot fully explain regional variations in keratoconus prevalence. It has been observed that Asians living in the United Kingdom have nearly eight times higher prevalence of keratoconus than Caucasians [20]. Similarly, keratoconus is more than three times more prevalent in non-Persians (Arabs, Turks and Kurds) living in Tehran (7.9%) than Persians (2.5%) [3]. These findings suggest that non-environmental factors such as genetics are also at play.

1.4 Eye Rubbing and Allergy

The link between eye rubbing and keratoconus was first described in 1956 [44]. While similar rates of eye-rubbing among patients with keratoconus and normal controls have been described [8, 45], the association with eye-rubbing and atopic or allergic eye disease is now accepted [4].

Recurrent epithelial trauma from habitual eye-rubbing leads to stromal remodeling and keratocyte apoptosis, secondary to the release of matrix metalloproteinases 1 and 13, interleukin-1 and tumour necrosis factor-alpha [46–48]. Raised intraocular pressure caused by eye-rubbing has also been cited as a contributory factor [49].

It has been found that patients with keratoconus who rub their eyes, tend to have been rubbing their eyes for a longer period than patients with allergic eye disease but without keratoconus [50]. This could explain why the majority of patients with allergic eye disease fortunately do not develop ectasia. High levels of dust in arid countries may promote a tendency for eye rubbing, providing another potential explanation for the higher prevalence in the Middle East [4].

Reports of asymmetric keratoconus in the context of asymmetric eye-rubbing provide compelling evidence for a causative link [51, 52]. In 1984, Coyle described an 11-year-old boy who could stop his paroxysmal atrial tachycardia by rubbing his left eye, thus eliciting the oculo-cardiac reflex, up to 20 times a day. He initially had a normal ocular examination, but when examined 4 years later he was diagnosed with unilateral keratoconus [7].

The increasing prevalence of keratoconus may be related to a similar rise in atopic/allergic disease in developed countries [53, 54]. In the USA, prevalence has been estimated at 13% for asthma, 17% for atopic dermatitis, and up to 16% for allergic rhinitis [55]. Worldwide prevalence of allergic conjunctivitis has been estimated as up to 25% [56]. Similar to keratoconus, atopy is thought to be caused by epigenetic modifications related to genetic and environmental factors [11]. There is controversy as to whether there is a true association between atopy and keratoconus, and if there is, to what extent this might be. Whilst allergic eye disease causes itch that leads to eye-rubbing, atopy is common in the general population as well as in keratoconics.

Some studies have recorded low correlations between atopy and keratoconus in large series [57–59] but others have reported strong associations [60–62]. Keratoconus was found to be associated with eye rubbing, atopy and family history in a univariate analysis [63]. However, multivariate analysis of the same data revealed eye rubbing as the only significant predictor of disease [63]. More recently, a cross-sectional study by Merdler et al. [64] found an increased prevalence of asthma, allergic rhinitis and the combination of allergic conjunctivitis, chronic blepharitis and vernal keratoconjunctivitis in patients with keratoconus. No association was found between keratoconus and angioedema, urticarial, atopic dermatitis or history of anaphylaxis [64]. While keratoconus seems to be associated with allergic tendencies, it is thought to be more through the promotion of eye-rubbing than related to the atopic process itself [63]. This theory is supported by the fact that keratoconus is associated with other non-atopic conditions where eye-rubbing is a feature (e.g. Leber's congenital amaurosis and Down syndrome) [65].

1.5 Gender

Current evidence suggests that keratoconus does not have a particular gender predilection. Whereas some studies have demonstrated female preponderance [13, 66–68], others have either found a male preponderance [38, 69–72] or no significant difference between genders [73]. The Collaborative Longitudinal Evaluation of Keratoconus (CLEK) study reported similar progression rates in both men and women [74].

1.6 Age

Keratoconus typically presents in the third decade of life [75]. In a Japanese study, HLA antigen association was found to be higher in keratoconics diagnosed under the age of 20 years, in particular HLA-A26, B40, and DR9 antigens [76], suggesting that younger age of onset may be related to different pathophysiology. It is uncommonly diagnosed beyond the age of 35 [4], apart from when patients in whom keratectasia has previously gone undetected present for other reasons, such as for cataract or refractive surgery.

Age of diagnosis is quite different from age of onset, and the latency between the two varies for multiple reasons. Younger age of onset predicts greater severity [77] and faster progression [77]. Early diagnosis has been facilitated by advances in imaging, and this is crucial as corneal collagen cross-linking can now be offered to arrest disease progression. Age of onset is difficult to determine, but symptoms of reduced vision or frequent changes in refraction over several years can often be elicited from the clinical history. Nearly three quarters of patients in a Finnish cohort from 1986, were aged 24 years or below at the first onset of symptoms, with a mean age of 18 years [78]. A mean age of symptom onset of 15.39 years was reported in a Spanish cohort from 1997 [79]. Again, ethnic variations are apparent, with Asians having a significantly lower age (4–5 years less) of first presentation compared with Caucasians [20, 21, 80].

A low prevalence of keratoconus in patients aged over 50 years is somewhat surprising given the chronic nature of the disease [4]. Only 15% of patients in the CLEK study were aged over 49 years [81]. Several explanations have been proposed for this. Some have pointed to associations with conditions that reduce life expectancy, including mitral valve prolapse [82], obesity [83] obstructive sleep apnoea [83, 84] and Down syndrome. However, this theory has been debunked by studies that have shown the mortality rate in keratoconics to be the same as that of the general population [85], or indeed significantly lower [86]. Thus, the relative lack of documented older keratoconics is more likely to represent loss to follow-up after patients have achieved disease stability [86].

1.7 Corneal Hydrops

Keratoconus can be complicated by acute corneal hydrops, whereby a split occurring in Descemet's membrane leads to rapid stromal imbibition of aqueous. This results in acute loss of vision often associated with pain. Spontaneous resolution occurs over weeks to months, but is often complicated by stromal scarring that limits visual prognosis.

A recent UK population based case-control study estimated an annual incidence of acute corneal hydrops of 1.43 per 1000 cases of keratoconus [87]. Mean age of onset was 32 years, with 75% presenting in males. The proportion of South Asian and black patients suffering acute corneal hydrops was significantly higher than the general population. Keratoplasty was ultimately required in 20% of these cases. An earlier study reported that 59.2% of patients with hydrops went on to require keratoplasty, compared to 13.1% of patients without an episode of hydrops [88]. In contrast, a New Zealand study found no difference in rates of keratoplasty between patients with and without a history of hydrops [89]. Risk of corneal graft rejection has been found to be higher in eyes with previous hydrops [88], most likely due to secondary neovascularization.

The following risk factors for developing hydrops, in order of decreasing risk, have been identified in univariate logistic regression analysis: previous hydrops (odds ratio (OR) 40.2), learning difficulties (OR 7.84), minimum keratometry ≥48D (OR 4.91), vernal keratoconjunctivitis (OR 4.08), atopic dermatitis (OR 3.13), black ethnicity (OR 2.98) and asthma (OR 2.70) [87]. Eye rubbing was not reported as a key risk factor in this particular study, but has been identified as a risk factor for hydrops previously [90]. Anterior segment OCT has demonstrated other anatomical predictive factors for hydrops to be epithelial thickening, stromal thinning, hyperreflectivity of Bowman's layer and absence of stromal scarring [91].

1.8 Associations with Other Diseases

Keratoconus has been associated with other syndromic conditions, which has helped improve our understanding of both the epidemiology and pathophysiology of the disease.

1.8.1 Down Syndrome

Patients with Down syndrome have a higher than average prevalence of keratoconus [92]. Prevalence rates of 5.5% [93], 15% [94] and 30% [95] have been reported. In contrast, an Italian study found no keratoconus patients among 157 children with Down syndrome aged 1 month to 18 years [96], and a similar finding was also reported in separate studies of Malaysian and Chinese children [96–98]. It is unclear whether the higher prevalence of keratoconus in some populations of Down syndrome is related to eye rubbing and atopy, or some other phenotypic consequence of the chromosomal abnormality.

1.8.2 Leber's Congenital Amaurosis

Keratoconus is more commonly found with Leber's congenital amaurosis (LCA) than other hereditary blinding diseases [99]. Eye rubbing (the 'oculo-digital sign') was traditionally thought to be the associating factor, but it is now considered more likely to be genetic factors that link keratoconus with LCA [99]. Keratoconus was identified in 26% (5/19 patients) of LCA patients with mutations in aryl hydrocarbon receptor interacting protein-like 1 protein (AIPL1) [100], and others have reported an association with the CRB1 gene [101, 102].

1.8.3 Connective Tissue Disorders

Several connective tissue disorders that have their basis in defective collagen or elastin have been associated with keratoconus.

- **Mitral valve prolapse**
  Mitral valve prolapse is frequently linked with keratoconus. The cross-linking enzyme lysyl oxidase (LOX) is markedly decreased in keratoconus patients [103], and this could explain the association with mitral valve prolapse, via its effects on the extracellular matrix [104]. Prevalence in patients with keratoconus varies between 5.7% and 58% [105–107], while mitral valve prolapse affects between 0.36% and 7% of the general population [108, 109].
- **Ehlers-Danlos syndrome**
  Ehlers-Danlos syndrome (EDS) is a connective tissue disorder, of which there are six subtypes, related to defective structure and function of collagen [110]. In 1975, Robertson found 50% of 44 keratoconus patients to have features of classical EDS (previously types I and II) [111]. Vascular and kyphoscoliotic EDS (previously known as types IV and VI respectively) have ocular manifestations including myopia and blue sclera [110], but keratoconus remains rare with this syndrome [112]. A study by Woodward found that keratoconus patients are five times more likely to have hypermobility of the metacarpo-phalyngeal and wrist joints, a characteristic of EDS [113].
  Conversely, McDermott et al. found just one keratoconus patient when examining the corneal topography of 72 patients with various EDS subtypes [114]. Recent studies have found no definitive keratoconus in EDS patients, however, there was evidence of corneal thinning [115, 116] and steepening [116, 117].
- **Osteogenesis imperfecta**
  Osteogenesis imperfecta is a rare autosomal dominant inherited disease characterised by collagen type I abnormality. It is classically known for its ophthalmic manifestation of blue sclera, but an association with keratoconus in some affected families has also been found [103, 118].
- **Obstructive sleep apnoea**
  Keratoconus has a well-described association with obstructive sleep apnoea (OSA). The causative factor is thought to be floppy eyelid syndrome, which is commonly encountered with OSA and leads to an increased tendency towards eye rubbing [119]. OSA has been reported in 18–24% patients with keratoconus [83, 120, 121], compared with 1–5% of the general population [122]. A separate case-control study showed that patients with keratoconus had nearly twice the risk of developing OSA (according to the Berlin questionnaire) than those

without keratoconus (12.3% versus 6.5%; $p < 0.001$). The patients with keratoconus who were at higher risk of OSA also tended to have more severe keratoconus [32]. The hypothesis for this was a synergistic effect of keratoconus and OSA in causing central corneal thinning, a finding replicated in earlier work by Metin et al. [123].

1.8.4 Thyroid Dysfunction

One study has investigated the link between keratoconus and thyroid dysfunction. Thanos et al. [124] found the prevalence of thyroid gland dysfunction to be higher among patients with keratoconus. Prevalence of hypothyroidism was 23.3% of females and 5.3% of males in the keratoconus group, while prevalence in the general population is 2% and 0.2% respectively [124]. T4 tear levels were found to be higher in the keratoconus patients with and without thyroid gland dysfunction. T4 receptors are found in keratocytes and the authors postulated that T4 might have a role in the pathogenesis of keratectasia. Further work is required to elucidate this possible association.

1.9 Discussion

With the wider availability of corneal topography, our understanding of the epidemiology of keratoconus has improved and it is clear that the incidence and prevalence may have previously been underestimated. Prevalence rates vary widely and are dependent on both geographic and ethnic differences; this variation however has shed light on the underlying pathophysiology.

Early detection should facilitate earlier treatment of the condition, aiming to maintain visual function, reduce the demand for corneal transplantation, improve patients' quality of life and alleviate the economic burden on healthcare services. Disease progression can now be delayed or halted through corneal collagen cross-linking, a true paradigm shift in the management of keratoconus. Consideration should therefore be given to introducing national screening programs at schools or universities to enable the timely detection of keratoconus in asymptomatic individuals.

References

1. Gorskova EN, Sevost'ianov EN. Epidemiology of keratoconus in the Urals. Vestn Oftalmol. 1998;114(4):38–40.
2. Waked N, Fayad A, Fadlallah A, El Rami H. Keratoconus screening in a Lebanese students' population. J Fr Ophtalmol. 2012;35(1):23–9.

3. Hashemi H, Khabazkhoob M, Fotouhi A. Topographic Keratoconus is not rare in an Iranian population: the Tehran eye study. Ophthalmic Epidemiol. 2013;20(6):385–91.
4. Gordon-Shaag A, Millodot M, Shneor E, Liu Y. The genetic and environmental factors for Keratoconus. BioMed Res Int. 2015;2015:19.
5. Gomes JAP, Tan D, Rapuano CJ, Belin MW, Ambrósio R, et al. Global consensus on keratoconus and ectatic diseases. Cornea. 2015;34(4):359–69.
6. Ioannidis AS, Speedwell L, Nischal KK. Unilateral keratoconus in a child with chronic and persistent eye rubbing. Am J Ophthalmol. 2005;139(2):356–7.
7. Coyle JT. Keratoconus and eye rubbing. Am J Ophthalmol. 1984;97:527–8.
8. Millodot M, Shneor E, Albou S, Atlani E, Gordon-Shaag A. Prevalence and associated factors of keratoconus in Jerusalem: a cross-sectional study. Ophthalmic Epidemiol. 2011;18(2):91–7.
9. Godefrooij DA, Wit GA, Uiterwaal CS, Imhof SM, Wisse RP. Age-specific Incidence and prevalence of Keratoconus: a nationwide registration study. Am J Ophthalmol. 2017;175:169–72.
10. Ambrosio R, Klyce S, Wilson S. Corneal topographic and pachymetric screening of keratorefractive patients. Surg. 2003;19:24–9.
11. McMonnies CW. Screening for keratoconus suspects among candidates for refractive surgery. Clin Exp Optom. 2014;97(6):492–8.
12. Bamashmus MA, Saleh MF, Awadalla MA. Reasons for not performing keratorefractive surgery in patients seeking refractive surgery in a hospital-based cohort in "yemen". Middle East Afr J Ophthalmol. 2010;17(4):349–53.
13. Gomes JA, Rapuano CJ, Belin MWARJ. Global consensus on Keratoconus diagnosis. Group of panelists for the global Delphi panel of Keratoconus and ectatic diseases. Cornea. 2015;34(12):e38–9.
14. Hashemi H, Beiranvand A, Khabazkhoob M, Asgari S, Emamian MH, Shariati M, et al. Prevalence of keratoconus in a population-based study in Shahroud. Cornea. 2013;32(11):1441–5.
15. Shneor E, Millodot M, Gordon-Shaag A, Essa M, Anton M, Barbara R, Barbara A. Prevalence of Keratoconus among young Arab students in Israel. Int J Kerat Ect Cor Dis. 2014;3(1):9–14.
16. Hashemi H, Khabazkhoob M, Yazdani N, Ostadimoghaddam H, Norouzirad R, Amanzadeh K, et al. The prevalence of keratoconus in a young population in Mashhad. Iran Ophthalmic Physiol Opt. 2014;34(5):519–27.
17. Woodward MA, Maria A, et al. The association between sociodemographic factors, common systemic diseases, and Keratoconus. Ophthalmology. 2016;12(3):457–465.e2.
18. Assiri AA, Yousuf BI, Quantock AJMP. Incidence and severity of keratoconus in Asir province. Saudi Arabia Br J Ophthalmol. 2005;89:1403–6.
19. Nielsen K, Hjortdal J, Aagaard Nohr E, Ehlers N. Incidence and prevalence of keratoconus in Denmark. Acta Ophthalmol Scand. 2007;85(8):890–2.
20. Georgiou T, Funnell CL, Cassels-Brown AOR. Influence of ethnic origin on the incidence of keratoconus and associated atopic disease in Asians and white patients. Eye. 2004;8:379–83.
21. Pearson AR, Soneji B, Sarvananthan NS-S, JH. Does ethnic origin influence the incidence or severity of keratoconus? Eye. 2000;4(4):625–8.
22. Sugar JMM. What causes keratoconus? Cornea. 2012;31(6):716–9.
23. Edwards M, McGhee C, Dean S. The genetics of keratoconus. Clin Exp Ophthalmol. 2001;29(6):345–51.
24. Barbara A. Textbook on Keratoconus: new Insights. New Delhi: Jaypee Brothers. 2012; p. 3–11.
25. Gordon-Shaag A, Millodot M, Essa M, Garth J, Ghara M, Shneor E. Is consanguinity a risk factor for keratoconus? Optom Vis Sci. 2013;90(5):448–54.
26. Burdon KP, Coster DJ, Charlesworth JC, Mills RA, Laurie KJ, et al. Apparent autosomal dominant keratoconus in a large Australian pedigree accounted for by digenic inheritance of two novel loci. Hum Genet. 2011;124(4):379–86.
27. Tuft SJ, Hassan H, George S, Frazer DG, Willoughby CE, Liskova P. Keratoconus in 18 pairs of twins. Acta Ophthalmol. 2012;90(6):e482–6.

28. Nowak DM, Gajecka M. The genetics of keratoconus. Middle East Afr J Ophthalmol. 2011;18(1):2–6.
29. Szczotka-Flynn L, Slaughter M, McMahon T, Barr J, Edrington T, et al. Disease severity and family history in keratoconus. Br J Ophthalmol. 2008;92(8):1108–11.
30. Jordan CA, Zamri A, Wheeldon C, Patel DV, Johnson R, et al. Computerized corneal tomography and associated features in a large New Zealand keratoconic population. J Cataract Refract Surg. 2011;8:1493–501.
31. Rabinowitz YS. The genetics of keratoconus. Ophthalmol Clin N Am. 2003;16(4):607–20.
32. Naderan M, Rajabi MT, Zarrinbakhsh P, Naderan M, Bakhshi A. Association between family history and Keratoconus severity. Curr Eye Res. 2016;41(11):1414–8.
33. Tyynismaa H, Sistonen P, Tuupanen S, Tervo T, Dammert A. A locus for autosomal dominant Keratoconus: linkage to 16q22.3–q23.1 in Finnish families. Invest Ophthalmol Vis Sci. 2002;43:3160–316.
34. Fullerton J, Paprocki P, Foote S, Mackey D, Williamson R, et al. Identity-by-descent approach to gene localisation in eight individuals affected by keratoconus from north-west Tasmania, Australia. Hum Genet. 2002;110:462.
35. Brancati F, Valente EM, Sarkozy A, Feher J, Castori M, et al. A locus for autosomal dominant keratoconus maps to human chromosome 3p14–q13. J Med Genet. 2004;41:188–92.
36. Hutchings H, Ginisty H, Le Gallo M, Levy D, Stoesser F. Identification of a new locus for isolated familial keratoconus at 2p24. J Med Genet. 2005;42:88–94.
37. Barros SP, Offenbacher S. Epigenetics: connecting environment and genotype to phenotype and disease. J Dent Res. 2011;88(5):400–8.
38. Owens HGG. A profile of keratoconus in New Zealand. Cornea. 2003;22:122–5.
39. Gordon-Shaag A, Millodot M, Shneor E. The epidemiology and etiology of Keratoconus. Int J Keratoconus Ectatic Corneal Dis. 2012;1:7–15.
40. Marchitti SA, Chen Y, Thompson DC, Vasiliou V. Ultraviolet radiation: cellular antioxidant response and the role of ocular aldehyde dehydrogenase enzymes. Eye Contact Lens. 2011;37(4):206–13.
41. Kenney MC, Brown DJ, Rajeev B. Everett Kinsey lecture. The elusive causes of keratoconus: a working hypothesis. CLAO J. 2000;26(1):10–3.
42. Cristina Kenney MBD. The cascade hypothesis of keratoconus. Cont Lens Anterior Eye. 2003;26(3):139–45.
43. Chan ESG. Current status of corneal collagen cross-linking for keratoconus: a review. Clin Exp Optom. 2013 96(2):155–64.
44. Ridley F. Contact lenses in treatment of keratoconus. Br J Ophthalmol. 1956;5:295–304.
45. Weed KH, MacEwen CJ, Giles T, Low J, McGhee CNJ. The Dundee University Scottish Keratoconus study: demographics, corneal signs, associated diseases, and eye rubbing. Eye (Lond). 2008;22(4):534–41.
46. Mackiewicz Z, Määttä M, Stenman M, Konttinen L, Tervo T, Konttinen YT. Collagenolytic proteinases in keratoconus. Cornea. 2006;25(5):603–10.
47. Zhou L, Zhao SZ, Koh SK, Chen L, Vaz C, et al. In-depth analysis of the human tear proteome. J Proteome. 2012;75(13):3877–85.
48. Wilson SE, He YG, Weng J, Li Q, McDowall AW, et al. Epithelial injury induces keratocyte apoptosis: hypothesized role for the interleukin-1 system in the modulation of corneal tissue organization and wound healing. Exp Eye Res. 1996;62(4):325–7.
49. McMonnies CW. Mechanisms of rubbing-related corneal trauma in keratoconus. Cornea. 2009;28(6):607–15.
50. Krachmer JH. Eye rubbing can cause keratoconus. Cornea. 2004;23(6):539–40.
51. Jafri B, Lichter H, Stulting RD. Asymmetric keratoconus attributed to eye rubbing. Cornea. 2004;23(6):560–4.
52. Zadnik K, Steger-May K, Fink BA, Joslin CE, Nichols JJ, et al. Between-eye asymmetry in keratoconus. Cornea. 2002;21(7):671–9.
53. Romagnani S. The increased prevalence of allergy and the hygiene hypothesis: missing immune deviation, reduced immune suppression, or both? Immunology. 2004;112(3):352–63.

54. McMonnies CW. Keratoconus fittings: apical clearance or apical support? Eye Contact Lens. 2004;27(1):15–20.
55. Centre for disease control 2014. https://www.cdc.gov/nchs/fastats/allergies.htm.
56. Cingu A, Cinar Y, Turkcu F, Sahin A, Aris S, et al. Effects of vernal and allergic conjunctivitis on severity of keratoconus. Int J Ophthalmol. 2013;6(3):370–4.
57. Spencer WH. The association of keratoconus with atopic dermatitis. Am J Ophthalmol. 1959;47:332–44.
58. Galin M, Berger R. Atopy and keratoconus. Am J Ophthalmol. 1958;45(6):904–6.
59. Roth HL, Kierland R. The natural history of atopic dermatitis. A 20-year follow-up study. Arch Dermatol. 1964;89:209–14.
60. Davies PD, Lobascher D, Menon JA, Rahi AH, Ruben M. Immunological studies in keratoconus. Trans Ophthalmol Soc U K. 1976;96(1):173–8.
61. Rahi A, Davies P, Ruben M, Lobascher D, Menon J. Keratoconus and coexisting atopic disease. Br J Ophthalmol. 1977;61(12):761–4.
62. Gasset AR, Hinson WAFJ. Keratoconus and atopic diseases. Ann Ophthalmol. 1978;10:991–4.
63. Bawazeer AM, Hodge WG, Lorimer B. Atopy and keratoconus: a multivariate analysis. Br J Ophthalmol. 2000;84(8):834–6.
64. Merdler, et al. Keratoconus and allergic diseases among Israeli adolescents between 2005 and 2013. Cornea. 2015;34(5):525–9.
65. McMonnies CW. Keratoconus, allergy, itch, eye-rubbing and hand-dominance. Clin Exp Optom. 2003;86:376–84.
66. Laqua H. Hereditary diseases in keratoconus. Klin Monatsbl Augenheilkd. 1971;159:609–18.
67. Amsler M. The "forme fruste" of keratoconus. Wien Klin Wochenschr. 1961;73:842–3.
68. Hammerstein W. Keratoconus concurrent in identical twins. Ophthalmology. 1972;165:449–52.
69. Ertan A. Keratoconus clinical findings according to different age and gender groups. Cornea. 2008;27:1109–13.
70. Street DA, Vinokur ET, Waring GO, Pollak SJ, Clements SD. Ack of association between keratoconus, mitral valve prolapse, and joint hypermobility. Ophthalmology. 1991;98:170–6.
71. Fatima T, Acharya MC, Mathur U. Demographic profile and visual rehabilitation of patients with keratoconus attending contact lens clinic at a tertiary eye care centre. Cont Lens Anterior Eye. 2010;33:19–22.
72. Pouliquen Y, Forman MR, Giraud JP. Evaluation of the rapidity of progression of keratoconus by a study of the relationship between age when first detected and age at operation. J Fr Ophtalmol. 1981;4(3):219–21.
73. Kennedy RH, Bourne WM. A 48-year clinical and epidemiologic study of keratoconus. Am J Ophthalmol. 1986;101(3):267–73.
74. Fink BA, Sinnott LT, Wagner H, Friedman C. The influence of gender and hormone status on the severity and progression of keratoconus. Cornea. 2010;29(1):65–72.
75. Galvis V, Sherwin T, Tello A, Merayo J, Barrera R, et al. Keratoconus: an inflammatory disorder? Eye. 2015;29(7):843–59.
76. Adachi W, Mitsuishi Y, Terai K, Nakayama C, Hyakutake Y, et al. The association of HLA with young-onset keratoconus in Japan. Am J Ophthalmol. 2002;133(4):557–9.
77. Caroline P, Andre M, Kinoshita B, Choo J. Etiology, diagnosis, and management of Keratoconus: new thoughts and new understandings. Pacific Univ Coll Optom. 2008:12–5.
78. Ihalainen A. Clinical and epidemiological features of keratoconus genetic and external factors in the pathogenesis of the disease. Acta Ophthalmol Suppl. 1986;178:1–64.
79. Olivares L, Guerrero C, Bermudez J, Jimenez J, Jurado J, et al. Serrano Keratoconus: age of onset and natural history. Optom Vis Sci. 1997;74:147–51.
80. Cozma I, Atherley C, James NJ. Influence of ethnic origin on the incidence of keratoconus and associated atopic disease in Asian and white patients. Eye. 2005;19(8):924–6.
81. Zadnik K, Barr J, Edrington T, Everett D, Jameson M, et al. Baseline findings in the collaborative longitudinal evaluation of Keratoconus (CLEK) study. Invest Ophthalmol Vis Sci. 1998;39:2537–46.

82. Beardsley TL, Foulks GN. An association of keratoconus and mitral valve prolapse. Ophthalmology. 1982;89(1):35–7.
83. Pihlblad MS, Schaefer DP. Eyelid laxity, obesity, and obstructive sleep apnea in keratoconus. Cornea. 2013;32(9):1232–6.
84. Arora R, Gupta D, Goyal JL, Jain P. Results of corneal collagen cross-linking in pediatric patients. J Refract Surg. 2012;28(11):759–62.
85. Moodaley LC, Woodward EG, Liu CS, Buckley RJ. Life expectancy in keratoconus. Br J Ophthalmol. 1992;76(10):590–1.
86. Popiela M, Young-Zvandasara T, Veepanat E, Saunders D. Demographics of older keratoconics in Wales and their mortality rates—where are the older keratoconics? Contact Lens and Anterior Eye. 2016;39(5):365–8.
87. Barsam A, Brennan N, Petrushkin H, Xing W, Qaurtilho A, et al. Case-control study of risk factors for acute corneal hydrops in keratoconus. Br J Ophthalmol. 2017;101(4):499–502.
88. Tuft S, Gregory W, Buckley R. Acute corneal hydrops in Keratoconus. Ophthalmology. 1994;101(10):738–1744.
89. Grewal S, Laibson PR, Cohen EJ, Rapuano CJ. Acute hydrops in the corneal ectasias: associated factors and outcomes. Trans Am Ophthalmol Soc. 1999;97:187–203.
90. Fan Gaskin JC, Good WR, Jordan CA, Patel DV, McGhee C. The Auckland keratoconus study: identifying predictors of acute corneal hydrops in keratoconus. Clin Exp Optom. 2013;96(2):208–13.
91. Fuentes E, Sandali O, Sanharawi M, Basli E, Hamiche T, et al. Anatomic predictive factors of acute corneal hydrops in Keratoconus. Ophthalmology. 2015;122(8):1653–9.
92. Van Splunder J, Stilma JS, Bernsen RM. Prevalence of ocular diagnoses found on screening 1539 adults with intellectual disabilities. Ophthalmology. 2004;111(8):1457–63.
93. Cullen J, Butler HG. Mongolism (Down's syndrome) and Keratoconus. Br J Ophthal. 1963;47:321–30.
94. Shapiro MB, France TD. The ocular features of Down's syndrome. Am J Ophthalmol. 1985;99(6):659–63.
95. Hestnes A, Sand TFK. Ocular findings in Down's syndrome. J Ment Defic Res. 1991;35(3):194–203.
96. Fimiani F, Iovine A, Carelli R, Pansini M, Sebastio G. Incidence of ocular pathologies in Italian children with Down syndrome. Eur J Ophthalmol. 2007;17(5):817–22.
97. García MJ. Outcomes of penetrating keratoplasty in mentally retarded patients with keratoconus. Cornea. 2008;27(9):980–7.
98. Koppen C, Leysen I. Riboflavin/UVA cross-linking for keratoconus in Down syndrome. J Refract Surg. 2010;26(9):623–4.
99. Elder MJ. Leber congenital amaurosis and its association with keratoconus and keratoglobus. J Pediatr Ophthalmol Strabismus. 1994;31(1):38–40.
100. Dharmaraj S, Leroy BP, Sohocki MM, Koenekoop RK, Perrault I, et al. The phenotype of Leber congenital amaurosis in patients with AIPL1 mutations. Arch Ophthalmol. 2004;122(7):1029–37.
101. Ehrenberg M, Pierce EA, Cox GF. CRB1: one gene, many phenotypes. Semin Ophthalmol. 2013;28(5–6):397–405.
102. McMahon TT, Kim LS, Fishman GA, Stone EM, Zhao XC, et al. CRB1 gene mutations are associated with keratoconus in patients with leber congenital amaurosis. Invest Ophthalmol Vis Sci. 2009;50(7):3185–7.
103. Greenfield G, Stein R, Romano A, Goodman RM. Blue sclerae and keratoconus: key features of a distinct heritable disorder of connective tissue. Clin Genet. 1973;4(1):8–16.
104. Dudakova L. The impairment of lysyl oxidase in keratoconus and in keratoconus-associated disorders. J Neural Transm. 2013;120(6):977–82.
105. Ackay E, Akcay M, Uysal BS, Kosekahya P, Aslan AN, et al. Impaired corneal biomechanical properties and the prevalence of keratoconus in mitral valve prolapse. Ophthalmol J. 2014;2014:402193.
106. Lichter H, Loya N, Sagie A, Cohen N, Muzmacher L, et al. Keratoconus and mitral valve prolapse. Am J Ophthalmol. 2000;129(5):667–8.

107. Sharif KW, Casey TA, Coltart J. Prevalence of mitral valve prolapse in keratoconus patients. J R Soc Med. 1992;85(8):446–8.
108. Turker Y, Turker Y, Baltaci D, Basar C, Akkaya M. The prevalence and clinical characteristics of mitral valve prolapse in a large population-based epidemiologic study: the MELEN study. Eur Rev Med Pharmacol Sci. 2015;19(12):2208–12.
109. Savage DD, Garrison RJ, Devereux RB, Castelli WP, Anderson SJ, et al. Mitral valve prolapse in the general population. Epidemiologic features: the Framingham study. Am Heart J. 1983;106(3):571–6.
110. Castori M. Ehlers-danlos syndrome, hypermobility type: an underdiagnosed hereditary connective tissue disorder with mucocutaneous, articular, and systemic manifestations. ISRN Dermatol. 2012;2012:751768.
111. Robertson I. Keratoconus, the Ehlers-Danlos syndrome: a new aspect of keratoconus. Med J Aust. 1975;1:571–3.
112. Cameron JA. Corneal abnormalities in Ehlers-Danlos syndrome type VI. Cornea. 1993;12(1):54–9.
113. Woodward EG. Joint hypermobility in keratoconus. Ophthalmic Physiol Opt. 1990;10:360–2.
114. McDermott ML, Holladay J, Liu D, Puklin JE, Shin DH, et al. Corneal topography in Ehlers-Danlos syndrome. J Cataract Refract Surg. 1998;24(9):1212–5.
115. Pesudovs K. Orbscan mapping in Ehlers-Danlos syndrome. J Cataract Refract Surg. 2004;30(8):1795–8.
116. Villani E, Garoli E, Bassotti A, Magnani F, Tresoldi L, et al. The cornea in classic type ehlers-danlos syndrome: macro and microstructural changes. Invest Ophthalmol Vis Sci. 2013;54:8062–8.
117. Gharbiya M, Moramarco A, Castori M, Parisi F, Celletti C, et al. Ocular features in joint hypermobility syndrome/ehlers-danlos syndrome hypermobility type: a clinical and in vivo confocal microscopy study. Am J Ophthalmol Elsevier Inc. 2012;154(3):593–600.
118. Beckh U, Schönherr U, Naumann GO. Autosomal dominant keratoconus as the chief ocular symptom in Lobstein osteogenesis imperfecta tarda. Klin Monatsbl Augenheilkd. 1995;206(4):268–72.
119. Donnenfeld ED, Perry HD, Gibralter RP, Ingraham HJ, Udell IJ. Keratoconus associated with floppy eyelid syndrome. Ophthalmology. 1991;98(11):1674–8.
120. Gupta P, Stinnett S, Carlson A. Prevalence of sleep apnea in patients with Keratoconus. Cornea. 2012;31(6):595–9.
121. Saidel MA, Paik JY, Garcia C, Russo P, Cao D, et al. Prevalence of sleep apnea syndrome and high-risk characteristics among Keratoconus patients. Cornea. 2012;31(6):600–3.
122. Davies RJ, Stradling JR. The epidemiology of sleep apnoea. Thorax. 1996;51:S65–70.
123. Metin E, Nergiz H, Huseyin C, Erdinc C, Sadullah K, et al. Is there a relationship between sleep apnea and central corneal thickness? Curr Eye Res. 2013;38(11):1104–9.
124. Thanos S, Oellers P, Meyer Z, Horste M, Prokosch V, et al. Role of Thyroxine in the development of Keratoconus. Cornea. 2016;35(10):1338–46.

Chapter 2
Chronic Ocular Inflammation and Keratoconus

Igor Kaiserman and Sara Sella

2.1 Is Inflammation Associated with Keratoconus?

Keratoconus (KC) is a progressive, corneal ectatic disorder characterized by stromal thinning and protrusion resulting in irregular astigmatism and a myopic shift [1, 2]. Conventionally, it has been classified as a degenerative non-inflammatory disease, as the classical signs of inflammation (redness, heat, swelling, and pain) are not apparent in KC [2]. However, the pathophysiology of KC remains poorly understood. Currently, it is considered a multifactorial corneal disorder caused by the complex interaction of environmental factors, such as in atopic eye disease [3–5], eye rubbing [6], contact lenses [7–9] and endogenous factors such as a genetic predisposition [10]. Despite the absence of obvious inflammation, studies have demonstrated inflammatory factors such as matrix metalloproteinases (MMPs) and interleukins in the tears of patients with clinical and subclinical KC [11, 12].

Human cells in our body are constantly replacing themselves without causing progressive degradation. This is due to numerous regenerative processes. The bone system, for example, uses osteoblasts and osteoclast to keep homeostasis. The human cornea has similar mechanisms of self-renewal. This homeostasis could be severely affected by inflammation leading towards more tissue degradation and reduced tissue renewal. Such an imbalance induced by chronic inflammation could easily lead to corneal thinning and eventual result in KC.

I. Kaiserman (✉)
Department of Ophthalmology, Barzilai University Medical Center, Ashkelon, Faculty of Health Science, Ben Gurion University of the Nagev, Beer-Sheba, Israel

S. Sella
Department of Ophthalmology, Meir Medical Center, Kefar-Saba, Israel

A. Barbara (ed.), *Controversies in the Management of Keratoconus*,
https://doi.org/10.1007/978-3-319-98032-4_2

2.1.1 Matrix Metalloproteinases (MMPs) Role in KC Development

MMPs are a family of enzymes capable of degrading various components of the extracellular matrix. Tissue inhibitors of metalloproteinases (TIMPs) play an essential role in regulating the activity of MMPs by binding to them. Changes in MMPs and TIMPs expression are extremely important in corneal wound healing [13]. An imbalance in MMPs/TIMPs might lead to stromal degradation and thinning such as in the development of keratoconus [7, 14].

MMPs are zinc-dependent endopeptidases that include gelatinases (MMP-2 and -9) collagenases (MMP-1, -8, and -13), stromelysins (MMP-3 and -10), and matrilysins (MMP-7 and -26). They are synthesized by corneal epithelial cells and stromal cells, and have long been suspected of having a significant role in KC [11, 15–20] as up-regulation of MMPs in patients with KC is well-documented. In mammals, MMPs play an essential role in degrading extracellular components.

MMP's regulate matrix turnover either directly through collagenolytic activity against collagen types I, II, and III, or by activating downstream MMPs such as MMP-2 [21]. MMP-9 is an essential factor in the healing cornea, an enzyme that participates in the wound healing process that follows experimental mechanical, thermal, or laser injury to the cornea, by degrading the corneal epithelial basement membrane and extracellular matrix. Increase in pro-inflammatory IL-1α and MMP-9 causes delayed tear clearance. The later leads to elevation of the former.

Alfonso et al. [22] found higher concentrations of IL-1α and increased activity of MMP-9 in the tears of patients with ocular rosacea and blepharitis than in control subject. The association of the two diseases has recently been published [23]. Like rosacea, KC patients are known for elevated MMP's in their tear film. It is not unlikely that a chronic state of ocular inflammation and chronically elevated MMPs such as is present in chronic blepharitis could lead to the formation or exacerbation of KC.

2.1.2 Interleukin 1 Role in KC

The Interleukin-1(IL-1) family comprises of two pro-inflammatory cytokines (IL-1α and IL-1β) and the IL-1 receptor antagonist (IL-1 Ra). Although IL-1α and IL-1β are expressed by separate genes, both mediate their effects by binding to the same IL-1 receptor type 1 (IL-1 R) [24]. IL-1Ra regulates IL-1α and IL-1β pro-inflammatory activity by competing with them for binding sites of the receptor IL-1R. Studies performed in France approximately 20 years ago [20, 25] demonstrated that keratocytes from eyes with KC have four times as many IL-1 receptors, a pro-inflammatory cytokine, than keratocytes from normal eyes do [26].

The high IL1 levels present during chronic ocular inflammation together with an increased keratocyte sensitivity to interleukin-1 may lead to gradual loss of keratocytes (apoptosis), and any associated reduction in fibrillogenesis and/or the production of proteoglycans can contribute to loss of stromal mass and progression of KC as suggested by Wilson et al. [27].

2.1.3 Catepsin Role in KC

Cathepsins are proteases that were originally identified in the lysosome, where they participate in housekeeping tasks such as degradation of phagocytosed photoreceptors. The most likely mechanism by which Cathepsins contribute to ocular pathologies is via degradation of the extracellular matrix, and/or regulation of angiogenesis [28].

Markedly increased Catepsin S activity has been observed in the tears of patients with dry eyes especially in Sjögren's syndrome(SS). Proteoglycan 4 (PRG4), also known as lubricin, is an effective boundary lubricant that is naturally present on the ocular surface. Degradation of PRG4 by Catepsin S is a potential mechanism for diminished ocular surface lubrication in SS. Remi et al. suggested that tears supplementation with PRG4 may be beneficial for SS patients [29]. As dry eyes are common in KC patients Cathepsins might also play a role in stromal thinning and KC progression.

2.1.4 Elevated Corneal Temperature and KC

Any friction between the eyelid and the cornea due to rubbing might cause an increase in corneal temperature [29–31]. Collagenase activity could be upregulated during periods of rubbing induced temperature spikes, due to triggering of inflammatory process in the conjunctiva, as well as clinical chemosis and hyperemia [32, 33]. A combination of rubbing-related thermal damage to keratocytes and the indentation of the cornea during rubbing that might involve high localized pressure, enzyme release or heat-related processes could lead, in the long run, to reduced corneal rigidity and KC [30].

2.1.5 Oxidative Stress in KC

KC corneas have elevated levels of reactive oxygen species due to an imbalance in enzyme function [34, 35]. An accumulation of reactive oxygen species can severely damage cells by reacting with proteins, DNA, and membrane phospholipids. Normally, the natural antioxidant enzymes of the cornea eliminate the reactive oxygen species before they damage cells [34, 35]; however, chronic oxidative stress can mediate keratocyte apoptosis, leading to a reduced number of keratocytes and their in ability to repair damaged collagen fibrils.

Despite several reports on the association between the oxidative damage and KC, it still unclear whether these are innate defects of corneal fibroblasts or whether the KC is due to excessive environmental oxidative challenges encountered by these patients [4].

2.2 Chronic Ocular Inflammatory Condition Associated with KC

2.2.1 Atopic Inflammatory State and KC

A high incidence of atopy in KC patients has been documented in the literature [5, 35] and it has been postulated that one cause of KC might be eye rubbing, stimulated by ocular itching or discomfort, resulting from atopic diseases [4]. It also might be related to the high levels of inflammatory factors present in atopy patients [9, 21, 34]. Kaya et al. [36] described thinner corneas with lower cone location in KC eyes with atopy than in eyes without atopy. This suggests that atopic KC patients should be evaluated as a separate entity in the KC disease spectrum. Shajari et al. [37] also compared atopic KC to non-atopic KC and used Kmax as the closest approximation for cone localization. They found no significant difference between groups in their Kmax, they also found that atopic KC patients had significantly higher corneal density compared to non-atopic-KC. The deranged corneal histology found in patients with KC can lead to alterations in densitometry readings caused by complex mechanisms, with size regularity and arrangement of collagen fibrils playing an important role [37]. Not surprisingly, the anterior cornea, which is most affected by ocular surface atopy, is also the most damaged layer in KC with changes to the basal epithelial cell layer, thinning of the epithelial layer, breaks in the Bowman layer, and thickened sub-basal nerve plexus.

2.2.2 Chronic Dry Eyes, Blepharitis and KC

Because the ocular surface signs in KC are indicative of dry eye syndrome (DES), a potential relationship between KC and dry eye is under investigation.

Dry eye is a multifactorial disease that is affected by the relationship between the amounts of tears produced, rate of tear evaporation, goblet cell density, and the presence or absence of inflammation. The discordance between symptoms, clinical signs, and diagnostic test results makes the diagnosis and treatment of this condition challenging [38]. Approximately half of patients with symptoms of dry eye have clinically significant inflammation, with or without the presence of Meibomian gland dysfunction (MGD) [39–41]. Desiccating stress to the ocular surface epithelium activates the mitogen-activated protein kinase (MAPK) and nuclear factor (NF)-κB pathways, which stimulate production of epithelial-derived inflammatory mediators such as interleukin (IL)-1β, tumor necrosis factor (TNF)-α, IL-6, IL-8, and matrix metalloproteinase (MMP)-9 [42–44]. MMP-9 is an ideal biomarker for dry eye associated inflammation since it elevates early, is stimulated by IL-1, TNF-α, IL-6, IL-8, IL-17 [42, 43] catalyzes further development of IL-1 and TNF-α [45] and accumulates as part of a persistent cycle of inflammation. Moreover, MMP-9 destabilizes the tear film and directly contributes to corneal barrier dysfunction by breaking down tight junctions, causing epithelial cell desquamation, and facilitating inflammatory cell migration, which ultimately leads to corneal staining and rapid tear break up times [42, 45, 46]. Moreover, downregulation of MMP-9 expression is associated with improvement in ocular surface epithelia. Further, MMP-9 knockout mice are resistant to developing dry eye [47]. A chronic state of elevated MMPs due to dry eyes could lead to persistent corneal degradation and thinning predisposing to KC.

Carracedo et al. [48] compared patients with and without KC, all had clinical signs and symptoms of dry eye disease. They performed impression cytology combined with scanning laser confocal microscopy to evaluate goblet cell density, mucin cloud height, and goblet cell layer thickness, all parameters showed clinically significant differences between groups. These findings indicate that KC patients have more symptoms of dry eye and greater tear instability, primarily due to the decreased mucin production in their tears, than do healthy patients without KC.

Di-adenosine tetraphosphate (Ap4A), has also been proposed as a potential molecular biomarker for dry eye syndrome. This biomarker is also related to symptomatic patients with and without Sjogren's syndrome. Carracedo et al. found it to be significantly higher in KC compared to normal controls [48].

Either through direct eye rubbing secondary to itching or by treating MGD with massage and warm compresses or other methods that deliver heat to the eye, MGD could be associated with KC. Mostovoy et al. [23] recently published their results of a prospective, comparative, observational study who established the association of blepharitis in general and MGD in particular and KC. According to McMonnies et al. [49], patients whose management involves iatrogenic ocular massage for MGD, should be screened for risk of corneal deformation.

2.3 Chronic Eye Rubbing is Associated with KC

Mechanical trauma, in general, is a well-known cause of inflammation as it causes tissue and blood vessels damage and release of pro-inflammatory factors. Chronic eye rubbing causes repeated mechanical trauma to the cornea inducing a chronic state of inflammation. To make things worse, the inflammatory factors themselves can cause severe eye itching leading to further eye rubbing and the perpetuation of a vicious cycle of trauma, eye itching and inflammation that might culminate in KC formations. Thus, chronic habits of abnormal rubbing (CHAR) are strongly associated with the development of KC [30]. A case control study of 120 subjects with KC involved assessment of potential risk factors, including atopy, family history, eye rubbing, and contact lens wear. The univariate analysis found associations between KC and atopy, family history, and eye rubbing [4]. However, in the multivariate analysis, only eye rubbing remained a significant predictor of KC [4].

Greiner et al. demonstrated that eye rubbing histologically disrupts the epithelium and induces significant alteration in the inflammatory cell infiltration [32, 33]. Mostovy et al. [23] established the association of blepharitis and MGD with keratoconus. As one of the most common causes of eye rubbing in the general population is chronic blepharitis induced itching, the mechanical trauma and inflammation that occurs with blepharitic eye rubbing, may play a role in the pathogenesis of keratoconus.

McMonnies reported a reduction in sheer strength and cone-forming deformation of the cornea that may be a result of rubbing trauma. He described increased corneal temperature, epithelial thinning, increased concentrations of inflammatory mediators in pre-corneal tears, increased enzymatic activity, and slippage between collagen fibrils at the corneal apex in response to persistent eye rubbing [30, 49, 50].

2.3.1 Epithelial Changes Due to Eye Rubbing and Inflammation

The epithelial thickness of normal human corneas was reduced by 18.4%, both centrally and mid-peripherally, after 15 s of rubbing [51]. Rubbing-related epithelial thinning may include cell flattening, as well as displacement from the rubbed area of, for example, cells, extracellular fluid, cytoplasm from any burst cells, and/or mucin [51].

After epithelial damage, such as in eye rubbing or trauma, the healing of corneal epithelial wounds begins with the migration of an epithelial sheet at the wound edge to resurface the defect [50]. Thereafter, there is an increase in epithelial cell proliferation away from the wound edge and in the limbal region [51].

Numerous growth factors, cytokines, morphogens, and ECM proteins, derived from either the epithelium or the underlying stromal layer, have been implicated in the regulation of epithelial cell migration and proliferation after epithelial damage.

Pro-inflammatory factors released during this process might penetrate deep into the stroma and affect the homeostasis of keratocytes and the production of Heparan sulfate (HS). HS is highly modified glycosaminoglycan (GAG) bound to a core protein to form heparan sulfate proteoglycans (HSPGs). Heparan sulfate proteoglycans are vital in many cellular processes ranging from development to adult physiology, as well as in disease, through interactions with various protein ligands [52]. V.J Coulson-Thomas et al. [53] demonstrate the mice lacking HS in the corneal epithelium presented significantly thinner corneas than littermate control mice, which became thinner with time after induction. Corneal epithelial cells require Heparan Sulfate for maintaining corneal homeostasis, and the loss of epithelial HS leads to both impaired wound healing and impaired corneal stratification.

2.3.2 KC Bowman's Breakage, Eye Rubbing and Inflammation

The fine reticular scars of Bowman's membrane tears are a well-known and characteristic feature of KC, and are preceded by visible dehiscence at this level. A simplistic interpretation is that the primary event is rupture of Bowman's layer, whereas scarring is a secondary reaction of the injured tissue. Scarred regions of Bowman's membrane might be the result of rubbing-related trauma. Among 1209 patients enrolled in the Collaborative Longitudinal Evaluation of Keratoconus (CLEK) study [26] 19.7% did not wear contact lenses. Of these, 15% had Bowman's membrane scarring at baseline suggesting that besides mechanical trauma, other mechanisms such as inflammatory MMP's could contribute to Bowman's membrane damage.

2.3.3 Collagen Fibers, Inflammation and Eye Rubbing

One of the mechanisms for the development of KC suggests that the ectasia is due to slippage between collagen fibrils [27]. Loss of lamellae might be related to a mechanism of rearrangement or sliding of the collagen bundles, as the cornea takes a conical shape [27]. Rubbing-related forces that are transverse to fibrils, which are susceptible to slippage and perhaps more so for those that have already started slipping from their normal aligned orientation.

Large differences between control and KC corneas, in regard to the ordered proteoglycans along the collagen fibrils have been reported [28]. Some KC proteoglycans were found to take up less stain than their normal control counterparts. Cathepsins B and G are known to degrade proteoglycans and collagens, and the finding that these enzymes are up-regulated in KC suggests that they may be involved in corneal thinning [29].

2.4 Contact Lens Wear, Chronic Inflammation and KC

Although many KC patients are obligatory rigid gas permeable (RGP) contact lens (CL) wearers, chronic CL utilization can induce severe dry eye and itching, and thus, are at higher risk for rubbing-related trauma, elevated pro-inflammatory factors and MMP's. Carracedo et al. evaluated the effect of RGP contact lenses on the ocular surface and found that Ap4A and symptoms of dry eye were higher in RGP wearers compared to non-wearers [54]. This seems to indicate that factors such as RGP contact lens wear might exacerbate the clinical condition of dry eye [48]. Another study performed by their group evaluated the effect of short-term scleral lens wearing among KC patients with intrastromal corneal rings (ICSR) compared to KC without ICSR, and found that after removal of the scleral lens, the patients' experienced improved symptomatology and improved signs of dry eye, such as osmolarity and Ap4A concentration [48].

Given that the cornea is an avascular tissue, it relies primarily on atmospheric oxygen, from tear film anteriorly and nutrients from the aqueous posteriorly. Hard contact lenses, RGP lenses, are associated with significant drawbacks, including reduced availability of the tear film and oxygen to the corneal epithelium and stroma as well as contact lens direct rubbing of the epithelium. As keratocytes of KCs have inherent oxidative stress sensitivity even at normoxic conditions, they are more susceptible to contact lens induced hypoxia leading to cell stress that can reduce ECM secretion, expression, and deposition. Decreased corneal sensitivity is an alternative mechanism for KC progression among CL wearers [50, 55, 56].

McKay et al. [57] found that hypoxic keratocytes of patients with KC have immediate reduction in collagen I secretion, in addition to increased expression of MMP-1 and MMP-2, which lead to lower Keratocan expression in KC patients both at normoxia and hypoxia. Keratocan knockout in mice has been correlated with thinner corneal structure and disorganized collagen fibril deposition [51], suggesting that the altered Keratocan expression detected in patients with KC might contribute to inherent defects in the ECM assembly that promote corneal structural defects.

References

1. Romero-Jimenez M, Santodomingo-Rubido J, Wolffsohn JS. Keratoconus: a review. Cont Lens Anterior Eye. 2010;33(4):157–66; quiz 205.
2. Wisse RP, Kuiper JJ, Gans R, Imhof S, Radstake TR, Van der Lelij A. Cytokine expression in keratoconus and its corneal microenvironment: a systematic review. Ocul Surf. 2015;13(4):272–83.
3. Toprak I, Kucukatay V, Yildirim C, Kilic-Toprak E, Kilic-Erkek O. Increased systemic oxidative stress in patients with keratoconus. Eye (Lond). 2014;28(3):285–9.
4. Bawazeer AM, Hodge WG, Lorimer B. Atopy and keratoconus: a multivariate analysis. Br J Ophthalmol. 2000;84(8):834–6.
5. Wachtmeister L, Ingemansson SO, Moller E. Atopy and HLA antigens in patients with keratoconus. Acta Ophthalmol (Copenh). 1982;60(1):113–22.
6. Jafri B, Lichter H, Stulting RD. Asymmetric keratoconus attributed to eye rubbing. Cornea. 2004;23(6):560–4.
7. Liu Z, Pflugfelder SC. The effects of long-term contact lens wear on corneal thickness, curvature, and surface regularity. Ophthalmology. 2000;107(1):105–10.
8. Moon JW, Shin KC, Lee HJ, Wee WR, Lee JH, Kim MK. The effect of contact lens wear on the ocular surface changes in keratoconus. Eye Contact Lens. 2006;32(2):96–101.

9. Shetty R, Deshmukh R, Ghosh A, Sethu S, Jayadev C. Altered tear inflammatory profile in Indian keratoconus patients – the 2015 Col Rangachari Award paper. Indian J Ophthalmol. 2017;65(11):1105–8.
10. Fabre EJ, Bureau J, Pouliquen Y, Lorans G. Binding sites for human interleukin 1 alpha, gamma interferon and tumor necrosis factor on cultured fibroblasts of normal cornea and keratoconus. Curr Eye Res. 1991;10(7):585–92.
11. Balasubramanian SA, Mohan S, Pye DC, Willcox MD. Proteases, proteolysis and inflammatory molecules in the tears of people with keratoconus. Acta Ophthalmol. 2012;90(4):e303–9.
12. Lema I, Sobrino T, Duran JA, Brea D, Diez-Feijoo E. Subclinical keratoconus and inflammatory molecules from tears. Br J Ophthalmol. 2009;93(6):820–4.
13. Liu C, Feng P, Li X, Song J, Chen W. Expression of MMP-2, MT1-MMP, and TIMP-2 by cultured rabbit corneal fibroblasts under mechanical stretch. Exp Biol Med. 2014;239:907–12.
14. Smith VA, Matthews F, Majid MA, Cook S. Keratoconus: matrix metalloproteinase-2 activation and TIMP modulation. Biochim Biophys Acta (BBA)-Mol Basis Dis. 2006;1762:431–9.
15. Pannebaker C, Chandler HL, Nichols JJ. Tear proteomics in keratoconus. Mol Vis. 2010;16:1949–57.
16. Lema I, Durán JA, Ruiz C, Díez-Feijoo E, Acera A, Merayo J. Inflammatory response to contact lenses in patients with keratoconus compared with myopic subjects. Cornea. 2008;27(7):758–63.
17. Lema I, Durán JA. Inflammatory molecules in the tears of patients with keratoconus. Ophthalmology. 2005;112(4):654–9.
18. Kolozsvári BL, Petrovski G, Gogolák P, Rajnavölgyi É, Tóth F, Berta A, Fodor M. Association between mediators in the tear fluid and the severity of keratoconus. Ophthalmic Res. 2014;51(1):46–51.
19. Matthews FJ, Cook SD, Majid MA, Dick AD, Smith VA. Changes in the balance of the tissue inhibitor of matrix metalloproteinases (TIMPs)-1 and -3 may promote keratocyte apoptosis in keratoconus. Exp Eye Res. 2007;84(6):1125–34.
20. Fabre E, Bureau J, Pouliquen Y, Lorans G. Binding sites for human interleukin 1 α, gamma interferon and tumor necrosis factor on cultured fibroblasts of normal cornea and keratoconus. Curr Eye Res. 1991;10(7):585–92.
21. Collier SA, Madigan MC, Penfold PL. Expression of membrane-type 1 matrix metalloproteinase (MT1-MMP) and MMP-2 in normal and keratoconus corneas. Curr Eye Res. 2000;21:662–8.
22. Afonso AA, Sobrin L, Monroy DC, Selzer M, Lokeshwar B, Pflugfelder SC. Tear fluid gelatinase B activity correlates with IL-1α concentration and fluorescein clearance in ocular rosacea. Invest Ophthalmol Vis Sci. 1999;40(11):2506–12.
23. Mostovoy D, Vinker S, Mimouni M, Goldich Y, Levartovsky S, Kaiserman I. The association of keratoconus with blepharitis. Clin Exp Optom. 2018;101(3):339–44.
24. Garlanda C, Dinarello CA, Mantovani A. The interleukin-1 family: back to the future. Immunity. 2013;39(6):1003–18.
25. Pouliquen Y, Bureau J, Mirshahi M, Mirshahi S, Assouline M, Lorens G. Keratoconus and inflammatory processes. Bull Soc Belge Ophtalmol. 1995;262:25–8.
26. Galvis V, Sherwin T, Tello A, Merayo J, Barrera R, Acera A. Keratoconus: an inflammatory disorder? Eye. 2015;29(7):843–59.
27. Wilson SE, HE YG, Weng J, Li Q, McDOWALL AW, Vital M, Chwang EL. Epithelial injury induces keratocyte apoptosis: hypothesized role for the interleukin-1 system in the modulation of corneal tissue organization and wound healing. Exp Eye Res. 1996;62(4):325–38.
28. Im E, Kazlauskas A. The role of cathepsins in ocular physiology and pathology. Exp Eye Res. 2007;84:383–8.
29. Regmi SC, Samsom ML, Heynen M, et al. Degradation of proteoglycan 4/lubricin by cathepsin S: potential mechanism for diminished ocular surface lubrication in Sjögren's syndrome. Exp Eye Res. 2017;161:1–9.
30. McMonnies CW. Mechanisms of rubbing-related corneal trauma in keratoconus. Cornea. 2009;28(6):607–15.

31. Naoumidi TL, Pallikaris IG, Naoumidi II, Astyrakakis NI. Conductive keratoplasty: histological study of human corneas. Am J Ophthalmol. 2005;140(6):984–92.
32. Greiner JV, Peace DG, Baird RS, Allansmith MR. Effects of eye rubbing on the conjunctiva as a model of ocular inflammation. Am J Ophthalmol. 1985;100(1):45–50.
33. Greiner JV, Leahy CD, Welter DA, Hearn SL, Weidman TA, Korb DR. Histopathology of the ocular surface after eye rubbing. Cornea. 1997;16:327–32.
34. Kenney MC, Brown DJ. The cascade hypothesis of keratoconus. Contact Lens Anterior Eye. 2003;26(3):139–46.
35. Kenney MC, Chwa M, Atilano SR, Tran A, Carballo M, Saghizadeh M, Vasiliou V, Adachi W, Brown DJ. Increased levels of catalase and cathepsin V/L2 but decreased TIMP-1 in keratoconus corneas: evidence that oxidative stress plays a role in this disorder. Invest Ophthalmol Vis Sci. 2005;46(3):823–32.
36. Kaya V, Karakaya M, Utine CA, et al. Evaluation of the corneal topographic characteristics of keratoconus with orbscan II in patients with and without atopy. Cornea. 2007;26:945–8.
37. Shajari M, Eberhardt E, Müller M, Al Khateeb G, Friderich S, Remy M, Kohnen T. Effects of atopic syndrome on keratoconus. Cornea. 2016;35(11):1416–20.
38. Wilson SE, Stulting RD. Agreement of physician treatment practices with the international task force guidelines for diagnosis and treatment of dry eye disease. Cornea. 2007;26(3):284–9.
39. Lam H, Bleiden L, De Paiva CS, Farley W, Stern ME, Pflugfelder SC. Tear cytokine profiles in dysfunctional tear syndrome. Am J Ophthalmol. 2009;147(2):198–205.
40. Boehm N, Riechardt AI, Wiegand M, Pfeiffer N, Grus FH. Proinflammatory cytokine profiling of tears from dry eye patients by means of antibody microarrays. Invest Ophthalmol Vis Sci. 2011;52(10):7725–30.
41. Sambursky R, Davitt WF III, Friedberg M, Tauber S. Prospective, multicenter, clinical evaluation of point-of-care matrix metalloproteinase-9 test for confirming dry eye disease. Cornea. 2014;33(8):812–8.
42. Corrales RM, Stern ME, De Paiva CS, Welch J, Li DQ, Pflugfelder SC. Desiccating stress stimulates expression of matrix metalloproteinases by the corneal epithelium. Invest Ophthalmol Vis Sci. 2006;47(8):3293–302.
43. Massingale ML, Li X, Vallabhajosyula M, Chen D, Wei Y, Asbell PA. Analysis of inflammatory cytokines in the tears of dry eye patients. Cornea. 2009;28(9):1023–7.
44. De Paiva CS, Corrales RM, Villarreal AL, Farley W, Li DQ, Stern ME, Pflugfelder SC. Apical corneal barrier disruption in experimental murine dry eye is abrogated by methylprednisolone and doxycycline. Invest Ophthalmol Vis Sci. 2006;47(7):2847–56.
45. Chotikavanich S, de Paiva CS, Chen JJ, Bian F, Farley WJ, Pflugfelder SC. Production and activity of matrix metalloproteinase-9 on the ocular surface increase in dysfunctional tear syndrome. Invest Ophthalmol Vis Sci. 2009;50(7):3203–9.
46. Li DQ, Lokeshwar BL, Solomon A, Monroy D, Ji Z, Pflugfelder SC. Regulation of MMP-9 production by human corneal epithelial cells. Exp Eye Res. 2001;73(4):449–59.
47. Pflugfelder SC, de Paiva CS, Tong L, Luo L, Stern ME, Li DQ. Stress-activated protein kinase signaling pathways in dry eye and ocular surface disease. Ocul Surf. 2005;3(4):S–154.
48. Carracedo G, Recchioni A, Alejandre-Alba N, et al. Signs and symptoms of dry eye in keratoconus patients: a pilot study. Curr Eye Res. 2015;40:1088–94.
49. McMonnies CW, Alharbi A, Boneham GC. Epithelial responses to rubbing-related mechanical forces. Cornea. 2010;29(11):1223–31.
50. Wilson SE, Mohan RR, Ambrosio R, Mohan RR. Corneal injury: a relatively pure model of stromal-epithelial interactions in wound healing. Wound Healing:Methods Protocol. 2003;78:67–81.
51. Nagasaki T, Zhao J. Centripetal movement of corneal epithelial cells in the normal adult mouse. Invest Ophthalmol Vis Sci. 2003;44:558–66.
52. Gesteira TF, Coulson-Thomas VJ, Ogata FT, et al. A novel approach for the characterisation of proteoglycans and biosynthetic enzymes in a snail model. Biochim Biophys Acta (BBA)-Proteins Proteomics. 2011;1814:1862–9.

53. Coulson-Thomas VJ, Chang S-H, Yeh L-K, et al. Loss of corneal epithelial heparan sulfate leads to corneal degeneration and impaired wound Healing role of HS in the corneal epithelium. Invest Ophthalmol Vis Sci. 2015;56:3004–14.
54. Carracedo G, Gonzalez-Meijome JM, Martin-Gil A, Carballo J, Pintor J. The influence of rigid gas permeable lens wear on the concentrations of dinucleotides in tears and the effect on dry eye signs and symptoms in keratoconus. Cont Lens Anterior Eye. 2016;39:375–9.
55. Chwa M, Atilano SR, Hertzog D, Zheng H, Langberg J, Kim DW, Kenney MC. Hypersensitive response to oxidative stress in keratoconus corneal fibroblasts. Invest Ophthalmol Vis Sci. 2008;49(10):4361–9.
56. Pastori V, Tavazzi S, Lecchi M. Lactoferrin-loaded contact lenses: eye protection against oxidative stress. Cornea. 2015;34(6):693–7.
57. McKay TB, et al. Acute hypoxia influences collagen and matrix metalloproteinase expression by human keratoconus cells in vitro. Ljubimov AV, editor. PLoS One. 2017;12(4):e0176017. PMC Web 24 Jan. 2018.

Chapter 3
Monitoring of Keratoconus Progression

David Smadja and Mark Krauthammer

3.1 Progression of Ectatic Disease: Current State of Art

Detecting the progressive state at the very beginning of the evolution process is as important as the diagnosis itself, as it may helps to preserve satisfying visual capacities when cross linking procedure is performed early enough, before the cornea deteriorates too much [1–3]. Repeated biomechanical evaluation of the cornea would be the optimal way to detect a progressive tissue weakening over time, but although the available devices hold some promises for this monitoring approach, unfortunately to date, none of them have achieved yet the required level of accuracy and reliability for being considered as a gold standard.

This section is summarizing the current indices proposed to define progression, the accepted key factors for optimizing our monitoring, including the identified risk factors of progression, and new insights in the key parameters we should closely monitor in order to raise the red flag of suspect progression.

3.1.1 Definition of a Progressive State

Progression of ectatic disease remains challenging to define, and therefore explains the diversity of indices presented in the literature to consider a progressive stage. A summary of the current indices is showed in Table 3.1. Recently, a group of experts that aimed to arrive to an acceptable consensus in the management of keratoconus,

D. Smadja (✉)
Anterior Segment and Refractive Surgery Unit, Ophthalmology Department, Shaare Zedek Medical Center, Jerusalem, Israel

M. Krauthammer
Ophthalmology Department, Tel Aviv Sourasky Medical Center, Tel Aviv, Israel

A. Barbara (ed.), *Controversies in the Management of Keratoconus*,
https://doi.org/10.1007/978-3-319-98032-4_3

Table 3.1 Diversity of the criteria used in the literature for defining the progressive state of the ectatic disease

	Kmax ant	Corneal thickness	Cylinder	Visual acuity	MRSE	Other criteria
Dresden Protocol Raiskup-Wolf et al. (2008) [4]	**>1D** in 1 year			Subjective loss of BCVA		
Vinciguerra et al. (2009) [5]	**>1.5D** in 6 months	Thinning **TP > 5%** in 6 months	**>3D** in 6 months		**Myopia >3D** in 6 months	
Hersh et al. (2011) [6]	**>1D** in 2 years		**>1D** in 2 years		**SE >0.5D** in 2 years	
Choi et al. (2012) [7]	**>1.5D** in 1 year					
O'Brart et al. (2011) [8]	**>0.75D** in 18 months		**>0.75D** in 18 months	Worsening **>1 line** in 18 months		
Wittig-Silva et al. (2008) [9]	**>1D** over 6–12 months		**>1D** over 6–12 months		**SE >0.5D** in 6–12 months	
Chatzis et al. (2012) [10]	**>1D** in 1 year					
Hashemi et al. (2013) [11]	**>1D** in 1 year		**>1D** in 1 year	Worsening **>2 lines CDVA** in 12 months	**SE >1D** in 1 year	
Mazzotta et al. (2014) [12]	**>1D** in 6 months	Thinning TP **>10 μm** 6 months		Worsening **>0.5 line UDVA/ CDVA** in 6 months	**SE >0.5D** in 6 months	SAI or IS **>0.5D** in 6 months
Stojanovic et al. (2014) [13]	**>1.5D** in 12 months		**>1D** in 12 months		**Myopia >1D** in 12 months	
Shetty et al. (2015) [14]	**>1D** in 6 months	Thinning **TP >5%** in 6 months			**SE >1D** in 6 months	
Poli et al. (2015) [15]	**>0.75D** in 6 months	Thinning TP **>10 μm** in 6 months		Worsening **>1 line UDVA/ CDVA** In 6 months	**SE >0.5D** in 6 months	
Godefrooij et al. (2016) [16]	**>1D** in 6–12 months					

Legends*:* *AntK* Anterior keratometry, *D* diopters, *MRSE* Manifest refractive spherical equivalent, *OZ* Optical Zone, *TP* Thinnest point, *SAI* Surface Asymmetry Index, *IS* Inferior-superior index, *UDVA* Uncorrected Distance visual acuity, *CDVA* Corrected distance visual acuity

The Global Delphi Panel of Keratoconus and Ectatic Disease have recognized that there was no clear definition of ectasia progression, and so the experts suggested that it should be defined by a reliable change for the worse in two or three of the following parameters: radius of the anterior corneal curvature; radius of the posterior corneal curvature and central corneal thickness; or increase in the rate of change of pachymetry from the periphery to the thinnest point [17]. The experts considered that although KCN progression frequently leads to a worsening in CDVA, a change in both UCDVA and CDVA was not required for documenting progression. In addition, they agreed that specific quantitative data were lacking to determine progression and that such data would most probably be specific to a given device. Interestingly, although multiples diagnostic grading system for ectatic disease have been proposed over the past years, to date, there is still neither correlation nor association between those grading system, and the criteria used to monitor its progression. The oldest one, the Amsler-Krumeich scale, which is still the most commonly used, grades the disease from early (grade 1) to the severe (grade 4) keratoconus, and is only based on anterior keratometric, and corneal thickness measurements, together with refraction and clinical assessment [18]. More recent scales such as proposed by Shabayek et al. [19] and the RETICS classification [20] have added coma aberrations measurement, which reflects the level of corneal asymmetry. However, still none of them has been applied for monitoring the disease progression. As illustrated in Table 3.1, the challenge of defining a progressive state for the ectatic disease remains complete and requires more studies to draw acceptable and widespread guidelines for monitoring ectatic disease. The main reasons lie in part on the disparity of the diagnostic tools for measuring the corneal properties as well as on the lack of knowledge on the kinetic of progression of the disease. Further knowledge might lead to an optimization of the monitoring and guidelines on the frequency of the monitoring in order to better match it to the risk factors of progression such as age, hormonal status, allergy, rubbing, etc. To date, it seems reasonable to follow a keratoconic patient under his third decade every 6 months unless risk factors such as younger age, pregnancy or even warning signs such as recent isolated progression of the coma or posterior steepening are identified, which would require closer monitoring every 3 months.

3.1.2 *Identified Risk Factors of Progression*

Several risk factors have been identified for keratoconus and its progression and summarized in Table 3.2.

- **Mechanical factors**: Surgical weakening by LASIK or even PRK is a well known risk factor of decompensating of ectatic disease, but has also been shown in preoperative normal topographic cornea that undergo a surgical procedure with a weakening beyond the natural corneal threshold of resistance. Our group has recently demonstrated that a PTA (percentage of tissue altered by the surgery) above 40% was considered as the strongest risk factor of ectasia and should

Table 3.2 Summary of the identified risk factors of ectatic corneal disease progression

	Risk factors
Mechanical factors	Surgically-induced weakening (LASIK or PRK) in subclinical or early keratoconus
	Surgically-induced weakening in normal preoperative topographies with PTA >40%
	Persistent and forceful eye rubbing
Genetic factors	Relative with KC in the family (first degree at higher risk)
	Connective tissue disorders (Ehlers-Danlos syndrome)
	Down syndrome
	Leber congenital amaurosis
Age	Younger age: children and adolescent
Corneal features	Advanced KC: Ant K >50D; TP <450 μm; MPE >50 μm; Cyl >1.9D
	"Unilateral" keratoconus diagnosed implies FFKC in the CL eye
	Progression of corneal vertical coma over 3 successive examinations
	Progression of posterior Ks over 3 successive examinations
Hormonal factor	Pregnancy

Legends: *KC* keratoconus, *K* keratometry, *TP* Thinning point, *MPE* maximal posterior elevation, *PTA* Percentage tissue altered, *D* Diopters, *μm* microns, *FFKC* Form Frust Keratoconus, *CL* Contralateral

be carefully taken into account at the preoperative screening stage [21]. Another important and well-recognized risk factor of corneal weakening is the eye rubbing and ultimately the diseases that are associated with eyes rubbing such as chronic inflammation of the ocular surface, ocular allergy, atopy [22]. Eye rubbing has been shown to increase the level of inflammatory mediators in tears (MMP-13, IL-6 and TNF-α) in a normal subjects population. This increase in protease, protease activity and inflammatory mediators in tears may be exacerbated even further during persistent and forceful eye rubbing seen in keratoconus population might in turn contribute to the progression of the disease [23].

- **Genetic factors**: Whereas the etiology of keratoconus remains unknown, several studies suggest that the genetic background plays a significant role in the pathogenesis of the disorder [24]. KC has been associated with a wide range of genetic diseases such as Down syndrome, connective tissue disorders (Ehlers-Danlos syndrome), Leber congenital amaurosis, implying that genes may have a key role in the development of KC [24]. Genetic predisposition has been also well characterized with high prevalence in families with one affected individual and high concordance among monozygotic twins [25]. According to reports in the litterature, the prevalence of familial KC varies from 6% to 53% [24, 26]. The most recent reports by Kymionis et al. found that 53% of clinically unaffected relatives presented abnormal corneal patterns in at least one eye, further indicating an increased frequency of abnormal corneal topographic patterns in relatives of keratoconus patients.
- **Age**: Age has been well documented as a critical risk factor of KC progression as the disease may appears very early in life [27]. As the age increases, corneal

collagen fibrils become thicker, and naturally occurring cross-linking increases stiffness of the tissue (determined by a parameter called the Young's modulus). These natural changes might explain that when KCN presents earlier in life, the patient has a higher risk of progression and the classical finding that the condition usually progresses until the third to fourth decade of life, when it typically halts. Therefore, children and adolescent diagnosed with KC are considered at high risk of KC progression.

- **Corneal features**: Advanced KC with higher corneal curvature (Ant K) and high corneal cylinder over 1.9D have been shown in several studies to be associated with greater speed of progression [17]. Same findings were recently confirmed in pediatrics keratoconus, where eyes with thinnest point inferior to 450 μm, anterior keratometry above 50 D, and posterior elevation above 50 μm at presentation, demonstrated higher rates of progressive corneal thinning [28]. More recently, our group has demonstrated the relevance of other key parameters, the posterior steepest keratometry and the vertical corneal coma in early KC as significant warning sign of anterior keratometric progression [29]. Eyes that demonstrated progression of the anterior keratometry after 1 year, were all found with significantly earlier progression of the posterior keratometry (noted after 6 months) and vertical coma (noted after 3 months), than the anterior keratometry (noted only after 1 year). This finding has been recently supported by another group monitoring keratoconus progression using anterior segment optical coherence tomography [30].
- **Hormonal factors**: Hormonal changes during pregnancy have been reported to potentially affect corneal biomechanics negatively, and may be considered as a potential risk factor for progression of keratoconus [31].

3.2 New Insights in Keratoconus Monitoring

3.2.1 Concept of Suspect Progressive Keratoconus

While anterior segment imaging technologies have vastly improved over the last 10 years, thus providing a thorough analysis of the characteristics of the cornea, including posterior surface representation, thickness distribution profile, corneal total power and corneal wavefront. These parameters have been extensively studied with several different systems and found very useful for improving the sensitivity of early keratoconus detection [3, 32–35]. Whereas the current leading hypothesis is that keratoconus disease may be first detectable at the posterior surface [36, 37], interestingly, this finding still did not impact the way we are monitoring the ectatic disease. Indeed, most of the parameters used for the definition of a progressive KC and ultimately for indicating whereas a cross linking procedure should be recommended or not, are still based on the modifications of anterior surface (anterior keratometry and corneal astigmatism) and corneal thinning [38, 39]. However, in view of these recent findings, it seemed reasonable to question the use of anterior corneal parameters alone as a gold standard to monitor the ectatic process and track the earliest sign of progression. In an attempt to evaluate the kinetic of these various corneal parameters in a cohort of progressive keratoconus, our group of work has recently reported the relevance of tracking the changes of the posterior surface and vertical coma, as they were found to be modified significantly earlier than the anterior keratometry readings [29] (Figs. 3.1, 3.2, 3.3, and 3.4). This finding is actually consistent with the generally accepted approach for detecting keratoconus at their mildest stages, which includes the analysis of the posterior surface and corneal coma. Therefore, these parameters may be relevant warning signs to closely look at when monitoring progressive keratoconus. Cutoff values of posterior surface changes and corneal coma, as well as predicting factors of progression still have to be determined through additional studies with larger cohorts of progressive keratoconus. However, the consistency of findings in early keratoconus detection and progressive keratoconus, along with the improvements of the anterior imaging technology should question our current approach of monitoring the disease and our definition of progressive keratoconus. If a cornea is labeled as "suspect keratoconus" because of an abnormal posterior surface, as a keratoconus should also be labeled as "suspect progressive keratoconus" in any case of successive and consistent modifications of the posterior surface over two or three exams within a 6–9 months period, without modification on the anterior cornea. This way, it could impact how close we would monitor keratoconic patients and ultimately at which stage of its progression we would offered a cross-linking therapy to our patients.

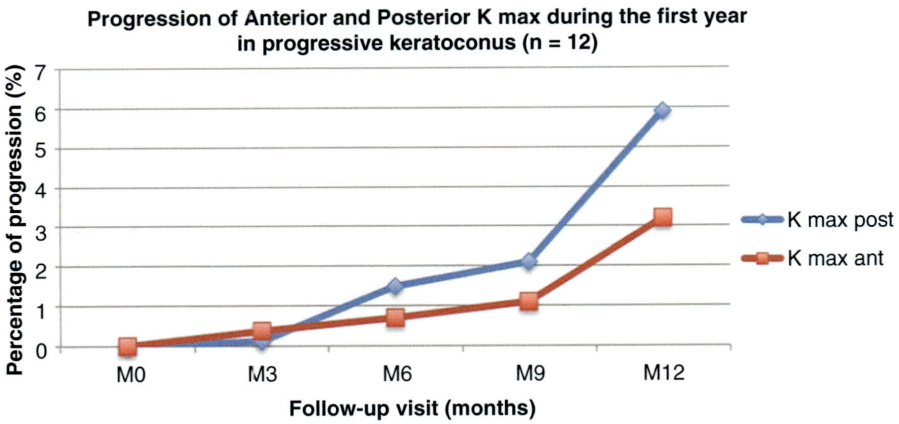

Fig. 3.1 Evolution profile of the anterior maximal keratometry and posterior maximal keratometry in the progressive keratoconus over the 1st year follow-up period

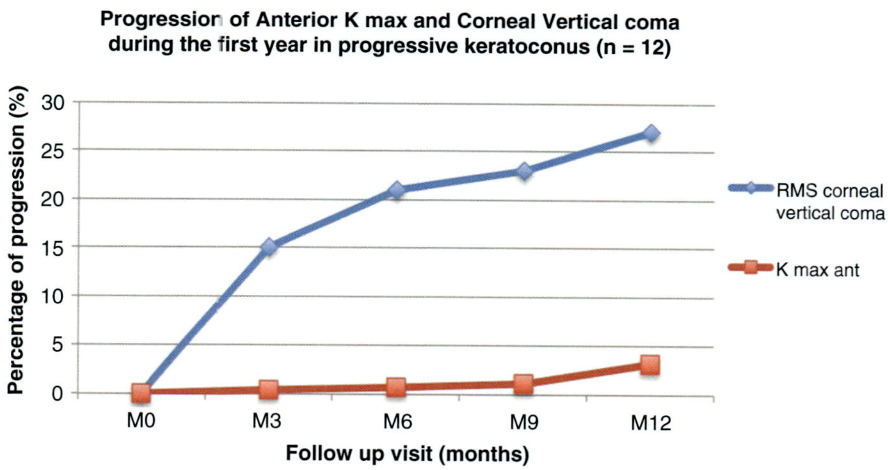

Fig. 3.2 Evolution profile of the anterior maximal keratometry and corneal vertical coma in the progressive keratoconus over the 1st year follow-up period

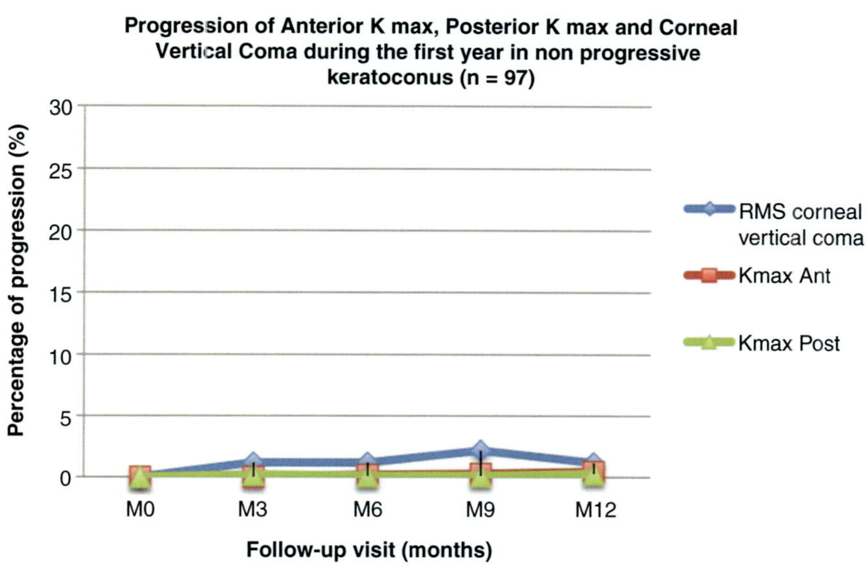

Fig. 3.3 Evolution profile of the anterior maximal keratometry, posterior maximal keratometry and corneal vertical coma in the non-progressive keratoconus over the 1st year follow-up period

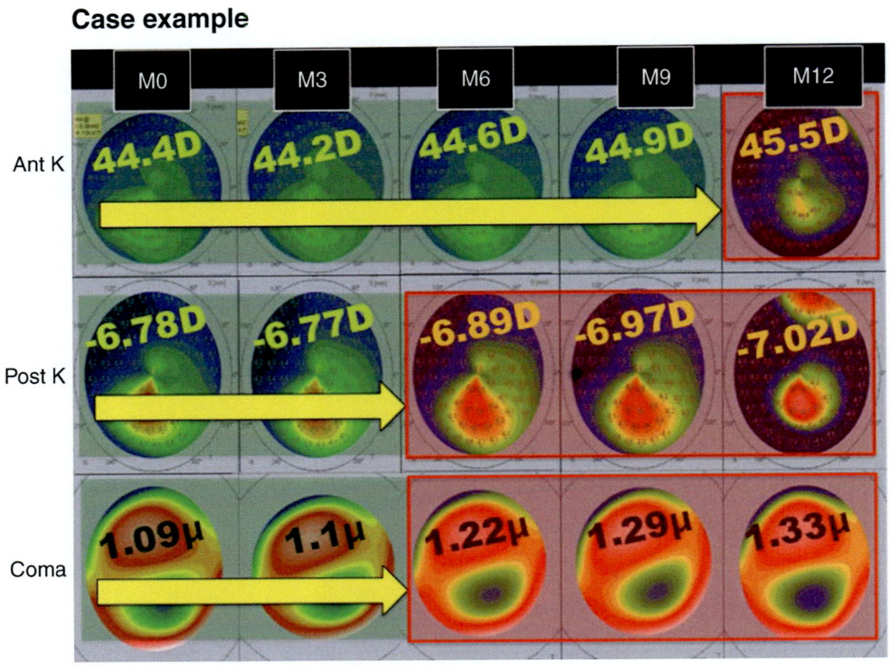

Fig. 3.4 Example of keratoconus monitoring with progression of coma and posterior keratometry detected prior to anterior keratometry modifications

References

1. Wollensak G, Spoerl E, Seiler T. Riboflavin/ultraviolet-A induced collagen crosslinking for the treatment of keratoconus. Am J Ophthalmol. 2003;135:620–7.
2. Bedi R, Touboul D, Pinsard L, Colin J. Refractive and topographic stability of Intacs in eyes with progressive keratoconus: five-year follow-up. J Refract Surg. 2012;28(6):392–6.
3. Kanellopoulos AJ, Asimellis G. Revisiting keratoconus diagnosis and progression classification based on evaluation of corneal asymmetry indices, derived from scheimpflug imaging in keratoconic and suspect cases. Clin Ophthalmol. 2013;7:1539–48.
4. Raiskup-Wolf F, Hoyer A, Spoerl E, Pillunat LE. Collagen crosslinking with riboflavin and ultraviolet-A light in keratoconus: long-term results. J Cataract Refract Surg. 2008;34(5):796–801.
5. Vinciguerra P, Albè E, Trazza S, Seiler T, Epstein D. Intraoperative and postoperative effects of corneal collagen cross-linking on progressive keratoconus. Arch Ophthalmol. 2009;127(10):1258–65.
6. Hersh PS, Greenstein SA, Fry KL. Corneal collagen crosslinking for keratoconus and corneal ectasia: one year results. J Cataract Refract Surg. 2011;37(1):149–60.
7. Choi JA, Kim MS. Progression of keratoconus by longitudinal assessment with corneal topography. Invest Ophthalmol Vis Sci. 2012;53(2):927–35.
8. O'Brart DP, Chan E, Samaras K, Patel P, Shah SP. A randomised, prospective study to investigate the efficacy of riboflavin/ultraviolet A (370 nm) corneal collagen cross-linkage to halt the progression of keratoconus. Br J Ophthalmol. 2011;95(11):1519–24.

9. Wittig-Silva C, Whiting M, Lamoureux E, Lindsay RG, Sullivan LJ. Snibson GR. A randomized controlled trial of corneal collagen cross-linking in progressive keratoconus: preliminary results. J Refract Surg. 2008;24(7):S720–5.
10. Chatzis N, Hafezi F. Progression of keratoconus and efficacy of pediatric [corrected] corneal collagen crosslinking in children and adolescents. J Refract Surg. 2012;28(11):753–8.
11. Hashemi H, Seyedian MA, Miraftab M, Fotouhi A, Asgari S. Corneal collagen cross-linking with riboflavin and ultraviolet a irradiation for keratoconus: long-term results. Ophthalmology. 2013;120(8):1515–20.
12. Mazzotta C, Traversi C, Paradiso AL, Latronico ME, Rechichi M. Pulsed light accelerated crosslinking versus continuous light accelerated crosslinking: one-year results. J Ophthalmol. 2014;2014:604–731.
13. Stojanovic A, Zhou W, Utheim TP. Corneal collagen cross-linking with and without epithelial removal: a contralateral study with 0.5% hypotonic riboflavin solution. Biomed Res Int. 2014;2014:6193–8.
14. Shetty R, Pahuja NK, Nuijts RM, Ajani A, Jayadev C, Sharma C, Nagaraja H. Current protocols of corneal collagen cross-linking: visual, refractive, and tomographic outcomes. Am J Ophthalmol. 2015;160(2):243–9.
15. Poli M, Lefevre A, Auxenfans C, Burillon C. Corneal collagen cross-linking for the treatment of progressive corneal ectasia: 6-Year prospective outcome in a French Population. Am J Ophthalmol. 2015;160(4):654–62.
16. Godefrooij DA, Soeters N, Imhof SM, Wisse RP. Corneal cross-linking for pediatric keratoconus: long-term results. Cornea. 2016;35(7):954–8.
17. Gomes J, Rapuano C, Belin MW, Ambròsio RJ. Disease G of panelist for the global DP of K and E. Global consensus on keratoconus diagnosis. Cornea. 2015;34(12):38–9.
18. Amsler M. Keratocone classique et keratocone fruste, arguments unitaires. Oftalmologica. 1946;111:96–101.
19. Alió JL, Shabayek MH. Corneal higher order aberrations: a method to grade keratoconus. J Refract Surg. 2006;22(6):539–46.
20. Alió JL, Piñero DP, Alesón A, et al. Keratoconus-integrated characterization considering anterior corneal aberrations, internal astigmatism, and corneal biomechanics. J Cataract Refract Surg. 2011;37(3):552–68.
21. Santhiago MR, Smadja D, Gomes BAF, et al. Association between the percent tissue altered and post-laser in situ keratomileusis ectasia in eyes with normal preoperative topography. Am J Ophthalmol. 2014;158(1):87–95.
22. Galvis V, Sherwin T, Tello A, Merayo-Lloves J, Barrera R, Acera A. Keratoconus: an inflammatory disorder? Eye (Lond). 2015;29(7):843–59.
23. Shetty R, Sureka S, Kusumgar P, Sethu S, Sainani K. Allergen-specific exposure associated with high immunoglobulin E and eye rubbing predisposes to progression of keratoconus. Indian J Ophthalmol. 2017;65(5):399–402.
24. Nielsen K, Hjortdal JØ, Pihlmann M, Corydon T. Update on keratoconus genetics. Acta Ophthalmol. 2013;91(2):106–13.
25. Tuft SJ, Hashemi H, George S, Frazer D, Willoughby C, Liskova P. Keratoconus in 18 pairs of twins. Acta Ophthalmol. 2012;90(6):482–6.
26. Kymionis GD, Blazaki S, Tsoulnaras K, Giarmoukakis A, Grentzelos M, Tsilimbaris M. Corneal imaging abnormalities in familial keratoconus. J Refract Surg. 2017;33(1):62–3.
27. Zadnik K, Barr JT, Edrington TB, et al. Baseline findings in the collaborative longitudinal evaluation of keratoconus (CLEK) study. Invest Ophthalmol Vis Sci. 1998;39:2537–46.
28. Hamilton A, Wong S, Carley F, Chaudhry N, Biswas S. Tomographic indices as possible risk factors for progression in pediatric keratoconus. J AAPOS. 2016;20(6):523–6.
29. Tellouck J, Touboul D, Santhiago MR, Tellouck L, Paya C, Smadja D. Evolution of different corneal parameters in progressive keratoconus. Cornea. 2016;35(6):807–13.

30. Fujimoto H, Maeda N, Shintani A, et al. Quantitative evaluation of the natural progression of keratoconus using three-dimensional optical coherence tomography. Invest Ophthalmol Vis Sci. 2016;57(9):169–75.
31. Bligihan K, Hondur A, Sul S, Ozturk S. Pregnancy-induced progression of keratoconus. Cornea. 2011;30(9):991–4.
32. Smadja D, Touboul D, Cohen A, et al. Detection of subclinical keratoconus using an automated decision tree classification. Am J Ophthalmol. 2013;156(2):237–46.
33. Saad A, Gatinel D. Topographic and tomographic properties of forme fruste keratoconus corneas. Invest Ophthalmol Vis Sci. 2010;51(11):5546–55.
34. Ambrósio R, Caiado ALC, P F, et al. Novel pachymetric parameters based on corneal tomography for diagnosing keratoconus. J Refract Surg. 2011;27(10):753–8.
35. Bühren J, Kook D, Yoon G, Kohnen T. Detection of subclinical keratoconus by using corneal anterior and posterior surface aberrations and thickness spatial profiles. Invest Ophthalmol Vis Sci. 2010;51(7):3424–32. https://doi.org/10.1167/iovs.09-4960.
36. Smadja D, Santhiago MR, Mello GR, Krueger RR, Colin J, Touboul D. Influence of the reference surface shape for discriminating between normal corneas, subclinical keratoconus and keratoconus. J Refract Surg. 2013;29(4):274–81.
37. Khachikian SS, Belin MW. Posterior elevation in keratoconus. Ophthalmology. 2009;116(4):816–7.
38. Brown SE, Simmasalam R, Antonova N, Gadaria N, Asbell PA. Progression in keratoconus and the effect of corneal cross-linking on progression. Eye Contact Lens. 2014;40(6):331–8.
39. Belin MW. Tomographic parameters for the detection of keratoconus: suggestions for screening and treatment parameters. Eye Contact Lens. 2014;40(6):326–30.

Chapter 4
Epithelium-Off Corneal Cross-Linking

Frederik Raiskup

4.1 Standard: "Dresden Protocol"

Corneal crosslinking (CXL) is performed in an outpatient setting. Thirty minutes in advance, a systemic analgosedation can be administered. Some surgeons use Pilocarpin 2% eye drops in order to reduce potential thermal and photochemical effects of UVA-radiation on the retina and the lens.

The procedure is performed under sterile conditions in an operating room. After topical anesthesia, an eye lid retractor is inserted and the epithelium is removed with a diameter of 8 mm so that riboflavin can penetrate into the corneal stroma leading to a high UVA-absorption.

Riboflavin 0.1% is a photosensitizer which is instilled every 2 min for 30 min, ensuring maximum penetration into the cornea. During this riboflavin application is the eyelid retractor removed. Before UV-irradiation, the surgeon checks the appearance of riboflavin in the anterior chamber via slit lamp with blue filter. Corneal thickness is measured (ultrasonic pachymetry) immediately after the epithelium removal (in order to decide which kind of riboflavin solution should be used: isoosmolar or hypoosmolar) and before irradiation in order to ensure that the corneal thickness is above 400 μm and endothelium remains protected from UV-light. A special UV-sensor is used in order to detect intensity of irradiation before the procedure. An area of 8 mm of central cornea is irradiated with UV-light of a wave length of 370 nm and intensity of 3 mW/cm^2. The irradiation lasts 30 min and riboflavin is applied every 5 min.

Local antibiotics and lubricants are applied after the CXL and a soft contact lens is applied till the epithelium is fully restored. The systemic use of analgesics is possible. After epithelial closure, topical steroids are prescribed for a duration of

F. Raiskup (✉)
Department of Ophthalmology, Cornea and Refractive Surgery Unit,
C. G. Carus University Hospital, Dresden, Germany
e-mail: frederik.raiskup@uniklinikum-dresden.de

A. Barbara (ed.), *Controversies in the Management of Keratoconus*,
https://doi.org/10.1007/978-3-319-98032-4_4

3 weeks. Patients are followed-up every day till the reepithelialization process is completed and after 1, 3, 6, 12 months and every year. Fitting of new rigid contact lenses is recommended about 6–8 months after the procedure [1, 2].

4.2 Accelerated CXL

One major disadvantage of this standard CXL procedure so far is the long total treatment time of 1 h, therefore, in order to increase patient's comfort and the surgeon's work-flow in a clinical practice, a shorter CXL procedure would be desirable.

According to the photochemical law of reciprocity (Bunsen-Roscoe law), the same photochemical effect can be achieved with reduced illumination time and correspondingly increased irradiation intensity, meaning that 3-min irradiation at 30 mW/cm^2, 5-min irradiation at 18.0 mW/cm^2, and 10-min irradiation at 9.0 mW/cm^2 should provide the same effect obtained with a 30-min irradiation at 3.0 mW/cm^2, all delivering 5.4 J/cm^2 of fluence [3]. The biomechanical effect has been shown to be the same with same fluence and shortened treatment duration [4], but decreases with higher radiation energy and less radiation time with even no effect at a cut-off of 45 mW/cm^2 respectively [5, 6]. Hafezi et al. observed even more pronounced decreased stiffening effect with increasing UV-A intensity. Young's modulus at 10% strain showed significant differences between 3 mW/cm^2 and used higher UV-A intensities (9 mW/cm^2 and 18 mW/cm^2). The biomechanical effect of CXL decreased significantly when using high irradiance and short irradiation time settings. These results confirmed authors' hypothesis that intrastromal oxygen diffusion capacity and increased oxygen consumption associated with higher irradiances may be a limiting factor leading to reduced treatment efficiency [5].

The Bunsen-Roscoe law does not apply in full for CXL, because not only Riboflavin and UV-radiation but also oxygen plays an important role in this process. Oxygen must penetrate in a sufficient concentration into the corneal stroma in order to create free oxygen radicals [6, 7].

4.3 Medical History

An exact medical history is crucial for differentiation of low and high risk keratoconus patients. High risk patients need a more frequent follow-up in order to detect early progression of the disease. For low risk patients a follow-up once a year seems to be sufficient. The following parameters are essential for division into the two groups: age, sex, sport and other leisure-time activities (e.g. body-building, heavy weight lifting, yoga, playing high resistance wind instruments etc.), pregnancy, regular medical intake (contraceptives, anabolics, steroids), allergy, atopy, thyroid gland dysfunction (TGD), diabetes mellitus and smoking habits.

In our experience (which is similar as the one of an Italian study group) in adolescent patients (up to 18 years) with keratoconus there is a clear dominance of male sex (M/F 4/1) [8].

In the group of children and adolescent patients, mostly male, keratoconus seems to be very aggressive with rapid progression compared to the older age groups [9]. Also patients with a history of atopy are in a risk of more rapid keratoconus progression not only because of the atopy itself but also due to regular intake of steroids. Another experimental study showed a change in biomechanical corneal properties in terms of decrease of corneal stiffness due to steroid exposure in vitro [10].

Regular systemic intake of steroids for example in patients with chronic systemic inflammatory diseases or estrogens (hormonal contraception) or anabolic steroids (body-building) seems to induce the progression of the ectasia in susceptible corneas [11].

There seems to be a negative influence of pregnancy due to changes in hormone levels on corneal biomechanical properties. Pregnant women with keratoconus should be examined more frequently and in case of keratoconus progression, CXL should be performed after the delivery [12, 13].

Hormonal changes affecting corneal biomechanics and topography during pregnancy could be also thyroid related. Dysthyroidism may directly influence corneal biomechanics and represents a clinically relevant factor that need further investigation [14].

We do not perform CXL in pregnant women, because of possible postoperative complications such as infections or corneal melting and consecutive necessity of systemic medical intake and surgery requiring general anesthesia. Female patients with keratoconus should be informed, that a pregnancy due to hormonal changes, especially estrogens, could lead to a progression of the disease [15].

In patients with TGD was found higher prevalence of keratoconus (13.6%), than in general population (about 2%). The tear thyroxine (T4) level and imunohistochemical staining of keratocyte receptors (T4Rs) were also higher in keratoconus group compared with controls. These data of Swiss investigators implicated a crucial role of T4 in KC pathophysiology, which is most likely mediated by T4Rs [16].

There are several sports, hobbies and physical activities leading to a repeated long-standing elevation of intraocular pressure (IOP), for example during weight lifting (up to 30 mmHg), yoga (e.g. inverted body position: mean elevation of 36 mmHg), playing high-resistance wind instruments (elevation up to 44 mmHg), which might be a risk factor for progression in predisposed ectatic corneas [17, 18].

There is another very important risk factor for keratoconus and its progression acknowledged by the Group of Panelists for the Global Delphi Panel of Keratoconus and Ectatic Diseases, thus eye rubbing. Chronic eye rubbing (IOP elevation up to 400 mmHg) could result in the progressive deformation and thinning of the corneal wall, that is a hallmark of the ectatic process [18]. This fact is also the reason why the Global Consensus on Keratoconus and Ectatic Diseases places in its algorithm of the keratoconus therapy "Advice NO eye rubbing" on the first place [19].

In contrast to previously described circumstances, there are systemic diseases such as diabetes mellitus or certain habits for example smoking, which induce a natural cross-linking in different human tissues. In these patients a mild or none progression is expected, thus frequent examinations are not necessary.

The "protective" effect of diabetes could be explained via the induction of cross-links in the corneal stroma preventing from a weakening of the cornea [20, 21].

Smoking is also negatively associated with keratoconus progression. A strengthening effect for smokers was shown in skin and blood vessels [22, 23].

Smoke contains toxic substances inducing chemical cross-linking of the cornea. Nevertheless, due to its numerous negative effects on health, smoking should not be recommended as a prevention for keratoconus patients [24].

4.4 Evidence of Progression

Not every ectatic cornea needs to be crosslinked. A record of progression of the disease indicates CXL, which was the case in every of the above mentioned clinical trials, whereas the parameters for the definition of progression were slightly different. In Dresden, progression is defined according to an increase in Kmax at the apex of the cone of about 1 D within 1 year, decrease in BCVA, or frequent need for new contact lens fitting more than once within 2 years because of refraction changes [2]. Vinciguerra defined progression of keratoconus as changes in myopia and/or astigmatism of >3 D within the last 6 months, a mean change of central K-value of >1.5 D in three consecutive corneal topographic measurements within 6 months or a mean decrease in central corneal thickness >5% in three consecutive tomographic measurements within 6 months [25].

FDA study group in US performed CXL when one or more of the following changes within 24 months were reported: (a) increase of maximum K-value of >1 D, (b) increase of >1D in astigmatism, (c) increase of >0.5 D in spherical equivalent (SE). Exclusion criteria were a history of corneal surgery and/or ocular surface pathology, pachymetric values less than 300 μm, pregnancy and current breastfeeding [26].

A new keratoconus classification/staging system utilizes current tomographic data and reflects better anatomical and functional changes seen in keratoconus. This keratoconus staging incorporates anterior and posterior curvature (ARC and PRC), thinnest pachymetric values, and distance visual acuity. These parameters, especially PRC and measurements based on the thinnest point, rather than apical measurements are supposed to be better reproducible in repeated measurements in order to determine objectively significant progression of the ectatic process [27, 28].

4.5 Clinical Studies

The last decade has brought a dramatic change in the management of corneal ectatic diseases. New treatment modalities such as corneal crosslinking (CXL) have moved the timing of intervention to much earlier in the disease process. No longer are we delaying invasive treatment until there is significant loss of vision. CXL is currently available and is performed by the majority of the panelists for the Global Delphi Panel of Keratoconus and Ectatic Diseases (83%) for keratoconus, using a variety of techniques. The panelists who do not have current access to CXL were willing to use this technique once it becomes available [19].

After years of experimental studies, it was the first clinical pilot study on CXL that was conducted in Dresden and published by Wollensak in 2003. This prospective, non-randomized study with follow-up time up to 4 years analyzed results of 23 eyes of 22 patients. The study found in all eyes cessation of the progression of keratoconus and in 70% of the eyes was recorded even decrease of keratometry readings with mild improvement of corrected visual acuity in 65% [1].

Meanwhile was the effectiveness and safety of the procedure for treatment of keratoconus demonstrated in various clinical trials in Europe, Australia and the US. In 2008, Dresden group reported results of a retrospective study of 241 eyes in 130 patients with a follow-up of 6 years after CXL. This analysis confirmed that CXL leads to a significant decrease in keratometric values at the apex of the cone, reduction of astigmatism and improvement of best corrected visual acuity [29].

Durability, stability and safety of this procedure could be demonstrated in a 10-year-follow-up as well, that was published by the same group in 2015 [2].

The first randomized controlled trial was initiated by Wittig-Silva et al. in Australia. This prospective study found similar results compared to those from Dresden [30].

The study was conducted in Melbourne in 2006 including refractive, topographic and clinical results of 46 eyes with progressive keratoconus after CXL. There was another control group of 48 eyes with a follow-up of 3 years. The standard protocol for CXL was used. The eyes in the control group showed both a statistically significant increase in Kmax and astigmatism and a decrease in BCVA. In contrast to this, the CXL-group revealed a statistically significant decrease of Kmax and an improvement of corrected and uncorrected visual acuity.

The 1-year results of a multicenter, prospective, randomized clinical trial revealed, according to FDA guidelines, an improvement of corrected and uncorrected visual acuity, Kmax, and mean K-values [26].

Another prospective study in the UK showed a significant and continuous improvement of topographic and wave front parameters with a follow-up of 5 years. Stability was achieved up to 7 years after CXL [31].

A prospective randomized trial in an Asian population with progressive keratoconus showed a statistical significant improvement of uncorrected VA and decrease in K-values in the treated group compared to control group [32].

A multicenter, prospective, randomized, double-blind clinical trial initiated in 2008 in Germany investigated efficacy and safety of CXL in patients with progressive keratoconus. 29 eyes were included in treatment and control group, respectively. Follow-up was 3 years. Results confirmed efficacy of CXL, but 4 out of 15 eyes in the treatment group showed an increase in K-values. Eleven eyes in the treatment and six eyes in a control group did not show any further progression. In the treatment group, a decrease in Kmax-value of 0.35 ± 0.58 D per year was recorded. The control group revealed a significant increase of 0.11 ± 0.61 D [33]. All these studies have been conducted according to the standard "Dresden protocol".

The effect of conventional (standard) versus accelerated CXL has been estimated also by visualization of the demarcation line in the depth of corneal stroma which is in accelerated CXL procedure not as deep as in conventional process [34–39].

Kymionis et al. determined in a prospective comparative interventional case series study corneal stroma demarcation line after standard and high-intensity CXL by anterior segment optical coherence tomography (AS OCT). As a high intensity CXL their used 9 mW/cm^2 for 10 min. The demarcation line was significantly deeper after the standard treatment than after a 10-min procedure [40].

The same group performed similar measurements using a very high intensity of 18 mW/cm^2 of UV-A for a 5-min CXL procedure in patients with progressive keratoconus. The mean corneal stromal demarcation line was at the depth of 223 ± 32 μm (range 159–265 μm), that was shallower then measured in the standard protocol [41].

The change in these measurements appears in use of modified accelerated protocol providing higher total energy dose of 7.5 J/cm^2. Greek investigators observed similar demarcation line depth using 9 mW/cm^2 for 14 min or 18 mW/cm^2 for 7 min without recording of any statistically significant change in mean endothelial cell density [34, 39].

Focusing on the safety of the high-intensity CXL showed Kymionis' group that using 9 mW/cm^2 of irradiance for 10 min did not cause any significant changes in endothelial cell density, any intraoperative or early postoperative complications and none of the patients lost a line of CDVA 3 months after the procedure [42].

A short-term prospective randomized clinical trial comparing accelerated (18 mW/cm^2) and standard protocol (3 mW/cm^2) showed no statistical significant difference in uncorrected and corrected distance visual acuities 6 months postoperatively. The mean decrease in Kmax and mean K was also not statistically significantly different between the two groups. The similar results were in the mean decrease of the endothelial cell count [43].

Recent study comparing conventional Dresden protocol with modified accelerated protocol with higher total energy dose of 6.6 J/cm^2 (30 mW/cm^2 applied for 3 min 40 s) showed a smaller topographic flattening effect in the group of accelerated CXL than did the group of standard protocol [44].

4.6 Complications

The clinical trials mentioned above could show, that CXL is effective in halting of keratectasia progression and stabilizes corneal architecture. None of these studies evaluated potential complications and failure rate of the procedure. CXL is technically easy to perform; but pain and reduced visual acuity after epithelial debridement within first postoperative days are common side effects, which are completely resolved after a few days when reepithelialization is completed. There are reports on corneal infections and melting with consecutive corneal perforation as sequelae of persistent epithelial defect and/or applying of therapeutic contact lenses [45–48].

Koller et al. investigated failure rate after CXL within the first postoperative year and analyzed 117 eyes of 99 patients with primary keratectasia [49].

Progression of keratectasia was recorded by Scheimpflug images over a period of 6 months (range: 6 months −2 years). Progression was assumed when Kmax value increased more than 1 D. The fellow eye was treated not earlier than 6 months after the first one.

Only eyes with mild to moderate keratoconus were included (Kmax <65 dpt, CCT >400 μm). Complication rate was defined as percentage of eyes losing two or more lines of BCVA in 1 year. Failure rate was defined as percentage of eyes with an increase of Kmax of more than 1 D. Ninety percent of patients completed follow-up of 1 year. Complication rate was 2.9% and failure rate 7.6%. Age above 35 years and preoperative BCVA better than 20/25 were identified as risk factors for complications.

If the age of 35 years had been defined as upper age limit for inclusion, complication rate would have been 1.04%. There was no clear cause sufficiently explaining the loss of visual acuity. A high preoperative Kmax-value was a negative predictor for failure. If Kmax of 58 D would have been the upper limit for inclusion instead of 65 D, failure rate would have decreased to 2.8%.

In 2.8% of eyes there were stromal scars and in 7.6% of eyes could be observed sterile infiltrates. The results of Koller's study suggested, that modification of inclusion criteria for CXL could minimize complication and failure rate respectively. Consequently, patients should be carefully counseled about individual risk factors, prognosis and potential postoperative complications of this procedure. Furthermore, they should be advised about postoperative behavior reducing the risk of microbial keratitis.

Kymionis et al. reported about a case where CXL induced herpes keratitis with iritis even if there was no history of herpes infection previously [45].

Typical changes after CXL is occurrence of corneal haze. It has been observed that the depth of the crosslinked stromal tissue can be estimated detected by visualizing of stromal demarcation line [50] or evaluating of haze via slit lamp finding [49].

Herrmann et al. reported a case with temporary subepithelial haze after CXL which completely resolved within a few months [51].

Mazotta et al. investigated stromal haze using in vivo confocal microscopy, demonstrating that it occurred 2–3 months after CXL with no improvement after topical steroid treatment. Confocal microscopy revealed a tighter fibrillary matrix, which was even more intense in patients with advanced stages of keratoconus. Preoperative confocal analysis of patients younger than 20 years revealed hyperactive keratocytes nuclei in the anterior stroma up to a depth of 80 μm. Patients above 20 years showed dark, reticular microstriae. This group also showed preoperative Vogt striae, which could be a risk factor for development of corneal haze after CXL [52, 53].

A multicenter, prospective randomized study investigated the natural development of CXL-associated haze using Scheimpflug-Imaging (densitometry) and slit-lamp evaluation of patients with keratoconus und iatrogenic induced ectasia. There was an objective quantification of the time course of haze formation. They found the maximum haze after 1 month after CXL with a consecutive plateau after 3 months and a significant decrease between the 3rd and 12th month. Changes of haze structure were not correlated to postoperative results [54].

Dresden group investigated retrospectively the development of stromal scaring after CXL [55].

The cohort comprised 163 eyes of 127 patients with keratoconus stage 1–3 according to Amsler-Krumeich scale. One year after CXL, 8.6% of eyes developed significant stromal scaring. Eyes with scaring revealed higher Kmax-value at the apex (mean 71.1 ± 13.2 D) and thinnest central corneal thickness (mean: 420.0 ± 33.9 μm). We therefore assume that the risk of scar formation is increased in patients with advanced keratoconus due to reduced CCT and a higher corneal curvature.

Another complication after CXL is loss of endothelial cells. Kymionis et al. treated 14 eyes of 12 patients with a mean CCT of 373.92 ± 22.92 μm after removal of epithelium. After 1 year there was a significant decrease in endothelial cell count from 2733 ± 180 cells/mm^2 to 2441 ± 400 cells/mm^2 [56].

They applied 0.1% riboflavin and 20% dextran solution. This combination could possibly cause intraoperative decrease of corneal thickness and increased thinning of the already thinned corneas. Reports of other investigators using similar procedure of CXL in patients with thin corneas did not record CCT after removal of epithelium [57, 58].

Corneal melting is another possible complication after CXL. There was a case described of a young patient, that within 1 day after CXL developed significant stromal haze, endothelial precipitates and cells in anterior chamber. Reepithelialization was very slow and progressive corneal thinning resulted in descemetocoele with spontaneous rupture 2 months after procedure [59].

Consequently, a careful and regular examination after CXL is essential. Patients with delayed reepithelialization could benefit from amnion membrane transplantation or the use of serum eye drops in order to support epithelialization preventing corneal perforation.

Another keratoconus patient suffered from corneal melting 1 week after CXL because of uncontrolled use of diclofenac and proparacaine eye drops [60].

Faschinger et al. reported a case of patient with Down syndrome and keratoconus with thin corneas without signs of progression who underwent CXL on both eyes. This patient developed corneal melting and perforation in both eyes 1 and 4 weeks after procedure and had to undergo urgent penetrating keratoplasty [61].

Critically analyzing, these cases arise questions, whether patients without significant ectasia progression and potential postoperative risk factors such as eye rubbing, uncontrolled application of eye drops due to incompliance and thin corneas are good candidates for CXL? Eberwein et al. reported a case of a 45-year-old patient with a history of severe atopy and keratoconus, who developed corneal melting due to herpes simplex infection after CXL and deep anterior keratoplasty. In the course of this case a penetrating keratoplasty and intensive immunosuppressive and antiviral therapy were necessary to restore the ocular surface [62].

We are of the opinion, that patients with a history of atopy belong to a high risk group concerning postoperative complications after CXL, especially regarding postoperative corneal healing, delayed epithelialization and higher susceptibility to infections.

There was a one case described from Australia, reporting a poly-microbial keratitis occurring 1 day after CXL. This patient admitted to clean his therapeutic contact lens in his mouth before re-inserting it into the eye again [48].

All the mentioned complications and irreversible damage should force us to careful preoperative examination and thorough recording of patient's medical history. We should guarantee that patients are good candidates for CXL, fulfill all the inclusion criteria and that we shall be able to examine them regularly after the procedure.

4.7 Conclusion

Almost 20 years ago, has been corneal crosslinking with riboflavin and UVA light proposed as a therapeutic procedure improving biomechanical properties in corneal ectatic diseases. Until that time, could the available conservative and surgical therapeutic options only improve refractive effect of keratoconus, whereas they had no impact on its progression. Corneal graft, an invasive surgical procedure, was the only definite therapeutic choice solving negative consequences of this corneal pathology – still, with possible intra- and postoperative complications limiting the outcomes in the long run.

Although systematic reviews and meta-analysis grade the evidence of the effect of CXL therapy in cases of progressive keratoconus from some well-known reasons (trial design, no comparator, large drop-out rate, incomplete reporting, etc.) as "low" [63, 64], there are many clinical trials proving that this procedure can stop progression of corneal ectasia with a low complication rate. Apart from clinical aspects, there are several economic and psychosocial advantages of this procedure. CXL can be performed in an outpatient setting, it is minimal invasive, cost-efficient and with a manageable minimal stress for the patient [2, 19, 26, 30–32, 65–68].

References

1. Wollensak G, Spoerl E, Seiler T. Riboflavin/ultraviolet-a-induced collagen crosslinking for the treatment of keratoconus. Am J Ophthalmol. 2003;135:620–7.
2. Raiskup F, Theuring A, Pillunat LE, et al. Corneal collagen crosslinking with riboflavin and ultraviolet-A light in progressive keratoconus: ten-year results. J Cataract Refract Surg. 2015;41:41–6.
3. Schumacher S, Oeftiger L, Mrochen M. Equivalence of biomechanical changes induced by rapid and standard corneal cross-linking, using riboflavin and ultraviolet radiation. Invest Ophthalmol Vis Sci. 2011;52:9048–52. https://doi.org/10.1167/iovs.11-7818.
4. Krueger RR, Herekar S, Spoerl E. First proposed efficacy study of high versus standard irradiance and fractionated riboflavin/ultraviolet a cross-linking with equivalent energy exposure. Eye Contact Lens. 2014;40:353–7. https://doi.org/10.1097/icl.0000000000000095.

5. Hammer A, Richoz O, Arba Mosquera S, et al. Corneal biomechanical properties at different corneal cross-linking (CXL) irradiances. Invest Ophthalmol Vis Sci. 2014;55:2881–4. https://doi.org/10.1167/iovs.13-13748.
6. Wernli J, Schumacher S, Spoerl E, et al. The efficacy of corneal cross-linking shows a sudden decrease with very high intensity UV light and short treatment time. Invest Ophthalmol Vis Sci. 2013;54:1176–80. https://doi.org/10.1167/iovs.12-11409.
7. Richoz O, Hammer A, Tabibian D, et al. The biomechanical effect of corneal collagen cross-linking (CXL) with riboflavin and UV-A is oxygen dependent. Transl Vision Sci Technol. 2013;2:6. https://doi.org/10.1167/tvst.2.7.6.
8. Caporossi A, Mazzotta C, Baiocchi S, et al. Age-related long-term functional results after riboflavin UV A corneal cross-linking. J Ophthalmol. 2011;2011:608041. https://doi.org/10.1155/2011/608041.
9. Chatzis N, Hafezi F. Progression of keratoconus and efficacy of pediatric corrected corneal collagen cross-linking in children and adolescents. J Refract Surg (Thorofare, NJ: 1995). 2012;28:753–8. https://doi.org/10.3928/1081597x-20121011-01.
10. Spoerl E, Zubaty V, Terai N, et al. Influence of high-dose cortisol on the biomechanics of incubated porcine corneal strips. J Refract Surg. 2009;25:S794–8. https://doi.org/10.3928/1081597x-20090813-06.
11. Spoerl E, Zubaty V, Raiskup-Wolf F, et al. Oestrogen-induced changes in biomechanics in the cornea as a possible reason for keratectasia. Br J Ophthalmol. 2007;91:1547–50. https://doi.org/10.1136/bjo.2007.124388.
12. Bilgihan K, Hondur A, Sul S, et al. Pregnancy-induced progression of keratoconus. Cornea. 2011;30:991–4. https://doi.org/10.1097/ICO.0b013e3182068adc.
13. Gatzioufas Z, Panos GD, Gkaragkani E, et al. Recurrence of keratoconus after deep anterior lamellar keratoplasty following pregnancy. Int J Ophthalmol. 2017;10:1011–3. https://doi.org/10.18240/ijo.2017.06.28.
14. Tabibian D, Tejada BMD, Gatzioufas Z, et al. Pregnancy-induced changes in corneal biomechanics and topography are thyroid hormone related. Am J Ophthalmol. 2017; https://doi.org/10.1016/j.ajo.2017.10.001.
15. Hafezi F, Iseli HP. Pregnancy-related exacerbation of iatrogenic keratectasia despite corneal collagen crosslinking. J Cataract Refract Surg. 2008;34:1219–21. https://doi.org/10.1016/j.jcrs.2008.02.036.
16. Thanos S, Oellers P, Meyer Zu Horste M, et al. Role of thyroxine in the development of keratoconus. Cornea. 2016;35:1338–46. https://doi.org/10.1097/ico.0000000000000988.
17. Kappmeyer K, Lanzl IM. Intra-ocular pressure during and after playing high and low resistance wind instruments. Ophthalmologe. 2010;107:41–6.
18. McMonnies CW. The possible significance of the baropathic nature of keratectasias. Clin Exp Optom. 2013;96:197–200.
19. Gomes JAP, Tan D, Rapuano CJ, et al. Global consensus on keratoconus and ectatic diseases. Cornea. 2015;34:359–69. https://doi.org/10.1097/ico.0000000000000408.
20. Kuo IC, Broman A, Pirouzmanesh A, et al. Is there an association between diabetes and keratoconus? Ophthalmology. 2006;113:184–90. https://doi.org/10.1016/j.ophtha.2005.10.009.
21. Seiler T, Huhle S, Spoerl E, et al. Manifest diabetes and keratoconus: a retrospective case-control study. Graefes Arch Clin Exp Ophthalmol. 2000;238:822–5.
22. Morita A. Tobacco smoke causes premature skin aging. J Dermatol Sci. 2007;48:169–75. https://doi.org/10.1016/j.jdermsci.2007.06.015.
23. Mahmud A, Feely J. Effect of smoking on arterial stiffness and pulse pressure amplification. Hypertension (Dallas, Tex: 1979). 2003;41:183–7.
24. Spoerl E, Raiskup-Wolf F, Kuhlisch E, et al. Cigarette smoking is negatively associated with keratoconus. J Refract Surg. 2008;24:S737–40.
25. Vinciguerra P, Albe E, Trazza S, et al. Refractive, topographic, tomographic, and aberrometric analysis of keratoconic eyes undergoing corneal cross-linking. Ophthalmology. 2009;116:369–78. https://doi.org/10.1016/j.ophtha.2008.09.048.

26. Hersh PS, Greenstein SA, Fry KL. Corneal collagen crosslinking for keratoconus and corneal ectasia: one-year results. J Cataract Refract Surg. 2011;37:149–60.
27. Duncan JK, Belin MW, Borgstrom M. Assessing progression of keratoconus: novel tomographic determinants. Eye Vision (London, England). 2016;3:6. https://doi.org/10.1186/s40662-016-0038-6.
28. Belin MW, Duncan JK. Keratoconus: the ABCD grading system. Klin Monatsbl Augenheilkd. 2016;233:701–7. https://doi.org/10.1055/s-0042-100626.
29. Raiskup-Wolf F, Hoyer A, Spoerl E, et al. Collagen crosslinking with riboflavin and ultraviolet-A light in keratoconus: long-term results. J Cataract Refract Surg. 2008;34:796–801.
30. Wittig-Silva C, Chan E, Islam FM, et al. A randomized, controlled trial of corneal collagen cross-linking in progressive keratoconus: three-year results. Ophthalmology. 2014;121:812–21.
31. O'Brart DP, Patel P, Lascaratos G, et al. Corneal cross-linking to halt the progression of keratoconus and corneal ectasia: seven-year follow-up. Am J Ophthalmol. 2015;160:1154–63.
32. Sharma N, Suri K, Sehra SV, et al. Collagen cross-linking in keratoconus in Asian eyes: visual, refractive and confocal microscopy outcomes in a prospective randomized controlled trial. Int Ophthalmol. 2015;35:827–32. https://doi.org/10.1007/s10792-015-0054-x.
33. Lang SJ, Messmer EM, Geerling G, et al. Prospective, randomized, double-blind trial to investigate the efficacy and safety of corneal cross-linking to halt the progression of keratoconus. BMC Ophthalmol. 2015;15:78.
34. Kymionis GD, Tsoulnaras KI, Liakopoulos DA, et al. Corneal stromal demarcation line depth following standard and a modified high intensity corneal cross-linking protocol. J Refract Surg (Thorofare, NJ: 1995). 2016;32:218–22. https://doi.org/10.3928/1081597x-20160216-01.
35. Ozgurhan EB, Akcay BIS, Kurt T, et al. Accelerated corneal collagen cross-linking in thin keratoconic corneas. J Refract Surg (Thorofare, NJ: 1995). 2015;31:386–90. https://doi.org/10.3928/1081597x-20150521-11.
36. Ng ALK, Chan TCY, Lai JSM, et al. Comparison of the central and peripheral corneal stromal demarcation line depth in conventional versus accelerated collagen cross-linking. Cornea. 2015;34:1432–6. https://doi.org/10.1097/ico.0000000000000626.
37. Tomita M, Mita M, Huseynova T. Accelerated versus conventional corneal collagen crosslinking. J Cataract Refract Surg. 2014;40:1013–20. https://doi.org/10.1016/j.jcrs.2013.12.012.
38. Ozgurhan EB, Sezgin Akcay BI, Yildirim Y, et al. Evaluation of corneal stromal demarcation line after two different protocols of accelerated corneal collagen cross-linking procedures using anterior segment optical coherence tomography and confocal microscopy. J Ophthalmol. 2014;2014:981893. https://doi.org/10.1155/2014/981893.
39. Kymionis GD, Tsoulnaras KI, Grentzelos MA, et al. Evaluation of corneal stromal demarcation line depth following standard and a modified-accelerated collagen cross-linking protocol. Am J Ophthalmol. 2014;158:671–675.e671. https://doi.org/10.1016/j.ajo.2014.07.005.
40. Kymionis GD, Tsoulnaras KI, Grentzelos MA, et al. Corneal stroma demarcation line after standard and high-intensity collagen crosslinking determined with anterior segment optical coherence tomography. J Cataract Refract Surg. 2014;40:736–40. https://doi.org/10.1016/j.jcrs.2013.10.029.
41. Kymionis GD, Tsoulnaras KI, Liakopoulos DA, et al. Corneal stromal demarcation line determined with anterior segment optical coherence tomography following a very high intensity corneal collagen cross-linking protocol. Cornea. 2015;34:664–7. https://doi.org/10.1097/ico.0000000000000427.
42. Kymionis GD, Grentzelos MA, Kankariya VP, et al. Safety of high-intensity corneal collagen crosslinking. J Cataract Refract Surg. 2014;40:1337–40. https://doi.org/10.1016/j.jcrs.2013.11.041.
43. Hashemi H, Fotouhi A, Miraftab M, et al. Short-term comparison of accelerated and standard methods of corneal collagen crosslinking. J Cataract Refract Surg. 2015;41:533–40. https://doi.org/10.1016/j.jcrs.2014.07.030.

44. Choi M, Kim J, Kim EK, et al. Comparison of the conventional dresden protocol and accelerated protocol with higher ultraviolet intensity in corneal collagen cross-linking for keratoconus. Cornea. 2017;36:523–9. https://doi.org/10.1097/ico.0000000000001165.
45. Kymionis GD, Portaliou DM, Bouzoukis DI, et al. Herpetic keratitis with iritis after corneal crosslinking with riboflavin and ultraviolet A for keratoconus. J Cataract Refract Surg. 2007;33:1982–4. https://doi.org/10.1016/j.jcrs.2007.06.036.
46. Pollhammer M, Cursiefen C. Bacterial keratitis early after corneal crosslinking with riboflavin and ultraviolet-A. J Cataract Refract Surg. 2009;35:588–9. https://doi.org/10.1016/j.jcrs.2008.09.029.
47. Rama P, Di Matteo F, Matuska S, et al. Acanthamoeba keratitis with perforation after corneal crosslinking and bandage contact lens use. J Cataract Refract Surg. 2009;35:788–91. https://doi.org/10.1016/j.jcrs.2008.09.035.
48. Zamora KV, Males JJ. Polymicrobial keratitis after a collagen cross-linking procedure with postoperative use of a contact lens: a case report. Cornea. 2009;28:474–6. https://doi.org/10.1097/ICO.0b013e31818d381a.
49. Koller T, Mrochen M, Seiler T. Complication and failure rates after corneal crosslinking. J Cataract Refract Surg. 2009;35:1358–62.
50. Seiler T, Hafezi F. Corneal cross-linking-induced stromal demarcation line. Cornea. 2006;25:1057–9. https://doi.org/10.1097/01.ico.0000225720.38748.58.
51. Herrmann CI, Hammer T, Duncker GI. Hazeformation (corneal scarring) after cross-linking therapy in keratoconus. Ophthalmologe. 2008;105:485–7.
52. Mazzotta C, Traversi C, Baiocchi S, et al. Corneal healing after riboflavin ultraviolet-A collagen cross-linking determined by confocal laser scanning microscopy in vivo: early and late modifications. Am J Ophthalmol. 2008;146:527–33. https://doi.org/10.1016/j.ajo.2008.05.042.
53. Mazzotta C, Balestrazzi A, Baiocchi S, et al. Stromal haze after combined riboflavin-UVA corneal collagen cross-linking in keratoconus: in vivo confocal microscopic evaluation. Clin Exp Ophthalmol. 2007;35:580–2.
54. Greenstein SA, Fry KL, Bhatt J, et al. Natural history of corneal haze after collagen crosslinking for keratoconus and corneal ectasia: Scheimpflug and biomicroscopic analysis. J Cataract Refract Surg. 2010;36:2105–14.
55. Raiskup F, Hoyer A, Spoerl E. Permanent corneal haze after riboflavin-UVA-induced cross-linking in keratoconus. J Refract Surg. 2009;25:S824–8.
56. Kymionis GD, Portaliou DM, Diakonis VF, et al. Corneal collagen cross-linking with riboflavin and ultraviolet-A irradiation in patients with thin corneas. Am J Ophthalmol. 2012;153:24–8. https://doi.org/10.1016/j.ajo.2011.05.036.
57. Gokhale NS. Corneal endothelial damage after collagen cross-linking treatment. Cornea. 2011;30:1495–8. https://doi.org/10.1097/ICO.0b013e31820687f7.
58. Bagga B, Pahuja S, Murthy S, et al. Endothelial failure after collagen cross-linking with riboflavin and UV-A: case report with literature review. Cornea. 2012;31:1197–200. https://doi.org/10.1097/ICO.0b013e31823cbeb1.
59. Labiris G, Kaloghianni E, Koukoula S, et al. Corneal melting after collagen cross-linking for keratoconus: a case report. J Med Case Rep. 2011;5:152. https://doi.org/10.1186/1752-1947-5-152.
60. Gokhale NS, Vemuganti GK. Diclofenac-induced acute corneal melt after collagen crosslinking for keratoconus. Cornea. 2010;29:117–9. https://doi.org/10.1097/ICO.0b013e3181a06c31.
61. Faschinger C, Kleinert R, Wedrich A. Corneal melting in both eyes after simultaneous corneal cross-linking in a patient with keratoconus and Down syndrome. Ophthalmologe. 2010;107:951–2, 954–5.
62. Eberwein P, Auw-Hadrich C, Birnbaum F, et al. Corneal melting after cross-linking and deep lamellar keratoplasty in a keratoconus patient. Klin Monatsbl Augenheilkd. 2008;225:96–8. https://doi.org/10.1055/s-2008-1027128.

63. Craig JA, Mahon J, Yellowlees A, et al. Epithelium-off photochemical corneal collagen cross-linkage using riboflavin and ultraviolet a for keratoconus and keratectasia: a systematic review and meta-analysis. Ocul Surf. 2014;12:202–14. https://doi.org/10.1016/j.jtos.2014.05.002.
64. Pron G, Ieraci L, Kaulback K. Collagen cross-linking using riboflavin and ultraviolet-a for corneal thinning disorders: an evidence-based analysis. Ont Health Technol Assess Ser. 2011;11:1–89.
65. Sandvik GF, Thorsrud A, Raen M, et al. Does corneal collagen cross-linking reduce the need for keratoplasties in patients with keratoconus? Cornea. 2015;34:991–5.
66. Godefrooij DA, Gans R, Imhof SM, et al. Nationwide reduction in the number of corneal transplantations for keratoconus following the implementation of cross-linking. Acta Ophthalmol. 2016;94:675–8.
67. Rebenitsch RL, Kymes SM, Walline JJ, et al. The lifetime economic burden of keratoconus: a decision analysis using a markov model. Am J Ophthalmol. 2011;151:768–73.e762. https://doi.org/10.1016/j.ajo.2010.10.034.
68. Salmon HA, Chalk D, Stein K, et al. Cost effectiveness of collagen crosslinking for progressive keratoconus in the UK NHS. Eye (London, England). 2015;29:1504–11.

Chapter 5
Epithelium-On Corneal Cross-Linking

David P. S. O'Brart

5.1 Synopsis

This chapter reviews the published literature on epithelium-on (trans-epithelial) Riboflavin and Ultraviolet A (UVA) 370 nanometre (nm) light corneal collagen cross-linking (TE-CXL). Importance has been placed on seminal publications, systemic reviews, meta-analyses and randomized controlled clinical trials. Where such evidence was not available, cohort studies, case controlled studies and case series with follow-up greater than 12 months were examined.

Studies with epithelium-off corneal collagen cross-linking (SCXL) show it to be capable of arresting the progression of ectatic corneal disorders. In addition, most studies report significant improvements in visual, keratometric and topographic measurements. TE-CXL investigations suggest some efficacy but often less than with SCXL, with fewer reported improvements in keratometric parameters and increased rates of treatment failure. Long-term data (over 5 years) on TE-CXL are as yet unavailable. Sight-threatening complications of TE-CXL are rare and typically reported to be less frequent that those with SCXL.

Although studies of TE-CXL generally support its efficacy they indicate that it is often less than with SCXL. However, TE-CXL may allow for safer procedures with less patient discomfort. Refinements in TE-CXL using new Riboflavin formulations and modified iontophoretic protocols to increase Riboflavin stromal concentrations, together with refinements in UVA dosing with pulsing and supplement oxygen show promise in improved efficacy but require further investigation and refinement.

D. P. S. O'Brart (✉)
King's College, London and Guy's and St. Thomas' NHS Foundation Trust, Department of Ophthalmology, St. Thomas' Hospital, London, UK
e-mail: davidobrart@aol.com

A. Barbara (ed.), *Controversies in the Management of Keratoconus*,
https://doi.org/10.1007/978-3-319-98032-4_5

5.2 Background

5.2.1 Historical Aspects

It is more than two decades since Seiler and Spoerl at the University of Dresden postulated the concept of cross linking the cornea to treat Keratoconus and other corneal ectasias [1–4]. Cross-linking occurs physiologically with aging in biological tissues via enzymatic pathways such as Transglutaminase and Lysyl Oxidase. Seiler and Spoerl theorized that the generation of oxygen free radicals created by the photo-chemical interaction of Riboflavin (vitamin B2) and Ultraviolet A (UVA) 370 nm light might activate the Lysyl Oxidase pathway resulting in cross-linking of the macro-molecules within the stroma, thereby improving its biomechanical strength to halt ectasia progression [1–4]. Despite the knowledge that UVA can at high enough dosage be both cytotoxic and mutagenic, they also theorized that as well as acting as a photo-sensitizer, Riboflavin would prevent injury to the corneal endothelium, by absorbing most UVA radiation within the anterior stroma allowing non-toxic levels only to reach internal ocular structures [1–4].

5.3 The Photochemistry of CXL

Whilst the occurrence of Lysine-based cross-links in the CXL process was hypothesised by Seiler and Spoerl [1–4], they have not been found chemically after CXL. McCall et al. documented that CXL was inhibited by blocking of carbonyl groups with 2,4-dinitrophenylhydrazide/hydroxylamine but still transpired when amine groups were blocked with acetic anhydride/ethyl acetimidate. From these observations, they postulated that CXL was not probably occurring via the Lysyl Oxidase pathway but other mechanisms, including imidazolone formation, which can attach to molecules, such as histidine, to form new covalent bonds, the triggering of endogenous populations of carbonyl groups in the extra cellular matrix (allysine, hydroxyallysine) to form cross-links there, and/or the degradation of the riboflavin molecule itself, releasing 2,3-butanedione, which can react with the endogenous carbonyl groups of proteins [5].

The majority of research on Riboflavin photo-chemical reactions has been undertaken in food products. Such reactions have been reported to be associated with the creation of singlet oxygen radicals [6–8], with the cross-linking reactions reported to involve tyrosine residues [9, 10], glycation end products [11] as well as alterations in secondary and tertiary protein structures [12]. McCall et al. in their in vitro study of Rabbit and Shark corneas discussed above [5], found that Riboflavin/UVA CXL was inhibited by azide, which blocks singlet oxygen reactions [7, 8, 13], and promoted by deuterium oxide (D_2O), which prolongs the half-life of oxygen free radicals [13]. Such findings confirm the importance of singlet oxygen to the CXL process. This central role of oxygen was reinforced by Richoz et al. [14] who treated ex-vivo porcine corneas under two different atmospheres: one with oxygen at 21% and the other at less than 0.1%. They reported that under normal atmospheric oxygen levels, CXL was successful, with a resultant increase in corneal extensiometry following treatment. This increase in biomechanics did not happen in corneas undergoing CXL treatment in a low-oxygen atmosphere and untreated controls [14].

Despite such results, exact the role of oxygen in the Riboflavin/UVA CXL process, although important, is still unclear. Kamaev et al. measured oxygen consumption in the stroma during CXL and discovered very brisk oxygen depletion within 10–15 s of 3 mW/cm^2 UVA exposure. They proposed that aerobic conditions, allowing a type II photo-chemical reaction, are only present during the first seconds after UVA exposure and hypothesized that the majority of the Riboflavin/UVA CXL process might be initiated by excited Riboflavin triplets, with singlet oxygen playing only a transitory role [15]. They observed that sodium azide, used in the study by McCall, also impairs the action of excited Riboflavin triplets, as well as oxygen singlets [15, 16]. It is of note that, Kato et al., found that both azide and another singlet oxygen quencher, 1,4-diazabicyclo(2,2,2)octane, did not prevent Riboflavin photodynamic cross-linking of collagen [7]. They also noted that these photochemical cross-linking changes were associated with loss of tyrosine and histidine residues within the collagen molecules and that this tyrosine deficit could be inhibited by oxygen [7]. They recorded that dityrosine formation was seen with the loss of tyrosine and proposed that photodynamic modification of tyrosine may contribute to the riboflavin-sensitized CXL through the formation of dityrosine [7]. In a recent study looking at the effects of Riboflavin concentration on the efficacy of CXL using a pepsin digestion model in porcine eyes, O'Brart et al. reported a dose response curve with higher concentrations of riboflavin, up to 0.3%, achieving greater efficacy in terms of total mass of tissue cross-linked [17]. This was under taken in an accelerated CXL model without supplemental oxygen, where oxygen depletion in the stromal tissues would have occurred in seconds, and suggests that whilst aerobic type II reactions are important in CXL, perhaps in initiating the process, given the increased efficacy of CXL with increased Riboflavin concentrations type I anaerobic mechanisms may play a more important role than we have previously appreciated [17].

In addition to the uncertainty regarding the precise chemical interactions, and the interplay between aerobic and anaerobic photo-chemical mechanisms, involved in Riboflavin/UVA CXL, the location of the cross-links at the molecular level is uncertain. Certainly, cross-links cannot be formed between the collagen fibrils themselves, as the distance between individual fibrils is too large for any intramolecular bond to be possible. Hayes et al. [18] in a series of experiments to investigate stromal ultra-structure after CXL using X-ray scattering, hydrodynamic behaviour and enzyme digestion in ungulate and human ex-vivo corneas, hypothesized that it was likely that the cross links were occurring on the surface of the collagen fibrils, rather than within them, and in the glycosaminoglycan protein network adjacent to the fibrils [18].

5.4 Clinical Studies of Epithelium-Off CXL (SCXL)

Riboflavin is a hydrophilic molecule, with poor lipid solubility. As such it is unable to pass through intact epithelial tight junctions and lipid membranes. In pre-clinical studies, Spoerl et al. confirmed the necessity to fully debride the corneal epithelium to allow adequate Riboflavin absorption within the underlying stroma [1–3]. They reported no alterations in the biomechanical properties of corneal tissue when CXL was performed with the overlying epithelium intact [1–3]. For this reason in all the initial clinical studies an epithelium off CXL (SCXL) technique was employed.

The first published clinical investigation of CXL was not to address corneal ectasias, but to prevent corneal melting [19]. The Dresden group postulated that the ability of CXL not only to improve corneal biomechanics but also to resist enzymatic digestion to proteases might be of benefit in such cases [1–3]. They reported positive outcomes with SCXL successfully halting melting in a case series of three out of four eyes [19]. In 2003 Wollensak, Speorl and Seiler published the first prospective case series of eyes treated with SCXL for Keratoconus [4]. In 23 eyes they documented stabilization of ectasia in all cases with up to 5 years follow-up, with an improvement in corneal topography in 70% of eyes, with an average reduction in maximum keratometry (Kmax) of 2.0 diopters (D) and spherical equivalent refractive error (SEQ) of 1.0D. Endothelial counts were unaltered, with no loss of transparency or functionality of the cornea or lens [4]. Since this seminal publication, multiple prospective, cohort case series of SCXL with up to 24 months follow-up [20–31], including case series of paediatric patients [32, 33] and advanced keratoconus [34] have been published by other research groups throughout the world. These studies have corroborated the initial results of Wollensak et al.. with stabilization of keratoconus in the vast majority of treated eyes, with only rarely documented sight-threatening complications and many observations of statically significant improvements in visual performance, topographic indices and higher order aberrations [20–34]. With regards to SCXL in the management of other corneal ectasias, prospective case series in iatrogenic post-laser refractive surgery ectasia have recorded stability of topography and improvements in vision with up to 5 year follow-up [35–38]. Similarly, favourable outcomes have been seen in case series of SCXL in Pellucid Marginal Degeneration [39–41].

Subsequent randomized, controlled studies have supported the efficacy of SCXL for the management of progressive corneal ectasias. In 2011, O'Brart et al. in a bilateral study reported stabilization in SCXL treated eyes with significant improvements in corrected distance visual acuity (CDVA), topographic keratometry, cone apex power and higher order aberrations, while progression was documented in 14% of untreated contralateral eyes over an 18 month follow-up period [42]. Wittig-Silva et al. in 48 untreated control eyes and 46 SCXL treated eyes with 3 year follow-up documented a significant increase in Kmax and refractive cylinder with a reduction in uncorrected distance visual acuity (UDVA) in untreated control eyes, while treated eyes showed a reduction in Kmax and improvement in UDVA and CDVA [43, 44]. Similarly, Hersh, Greenstein and Chang et al. documented significant improvements in UDVA, CDVA, topography and higher order aberrations in 66 eyes with keratoconus and 38 with iatrogenic ectasia with 12 month follow-up [31, 45, 46] and Lang et al. reported a significant differences between treated and untreated control eyes, with corneal refractive power reducing in SCXL treated and increasing in control cases over 36 months follow-up [47]. Seyedian et al. in their randomized, bilateral, controlled study also found a significant difference in Kmax and CDVA at 12 months between treatment groups, which improved in SCXL treated and worsened in contra-lateral untreated eyes [48], while Sharma et al. in a randomized trial with a control sham treatment (Riboflavin administration with no UVA exposure), demonstrated an improvement in SCXL treated eyes in UDVA, refractive cylindrical correction and Kmax while the sham control group showed no such changes [49]. Most recently, Hersh et al. have published two multi-centre, randomized prospective studies comparing SCXL with a sham control treatment, where eyes received riboflavin on an intact epithelium. Both studies, one with 205 Keratoconic patients and the other with 179 patients with iatrogenic ectasia showed improvements in Kmax, UDVA and CDVA in SCXL treated cases at 12 months and worsening of these parameters in sham control treatments [50, 51]. Four recently published meta-analyses, including one study just concerned with iatrogenic ectasia after refractive surgery, have confirmed the consistent improvements in visual performance and the reduction in keratometry values seen in these various randomized clinical trials discussed above. They support the use of SCXL in as a therapeutic intervention to stabilize keratoconus and iatrogenic ectasia, whilst stating that further follow-up studies are necessary to determine the longevity of efficacy [52–55].

In terms of the long-term efficacy of SCXL there is indeed a paucity of data especially with follow-up over 5 years. Keratoconus typically presents during teenage years and then evolves at an unpredictable rate for approximately two decades, becoming stable, probably as a consequence of age-related physiological cross-linking [56–58]. The rate of molecular turnover of collagen and the ECM within the corneal stroma is as yet undetermined. Given these considerations, the duration of effectiveness of CXL and the necessity to repeat the procedure is unknown and continued follow-up of treated case are a necessity and needs to be discussed with patients pre-operatively. In terms of long-term follow-up studies, Raiskup-Wolf et al. in 33 eyes al documented stabilization of ectasia with reduction of keratometry and improvements in vision 3 years after SCXL [59]. Caporossi et al. reported stability in 44 eyes after 4 years, with a reduction in keratometry, coma and improvements in visual parameters [60] and O'Brart et al. found stabilization of ectasia in 100% of a series of 29 eyes after SCXL, with increasing improvements in refractive, visual, keratometric parameters and higher order aberrations over 5 years [61]. Similarly, Hashemi et al. reported cessation of ectasia progression in a series of 40 eyes, with progressive improvements in corneal elevation measurements over 5 years [62] and in a series of 40 eyes of 40 paediatric patients aged between 10 and 18 years, Uçakhan et al. found no ectasia progression with improvements in UCVA and CDVA and reduction in Kmax with, in similarity to other studies, continued improvements in topographic indices with continued follow-up [63].

Of the few studies reporting follow-up of SCXL beyond 5 years, Poli et al. in 36 eyes found no ectasia progression 6 years after SCXL and no late sight-threatening complications [64] and with a follow-up of 10 years, Theuring and Raiskup et al. in 34 eyes reported significant improvements in vision and keratometry with progression in only 6% of cases [65, 66]. Similarly, O'Brart et al. in 36 eyes of 36 patients documented no ectasia progression in treated eyes 7 years after SCXL with continuing improvements in visual, topographic and corneal wave-front parameters and no late sight-threatening complications [67]. They noted that at 7 year follow-up, 24% of untreated fellow eyes had progressed (increase in Kmax >1.0D) and underwent SCXL [67]. This documented progression in fellow untreated eyes, they suggested implied that the improvements in visual and topographic parameters in treated eyes with long-term follow up were not due to physiological age-related changes but to the SCXL itself. Most recently there have been two papers documenting encouraging long-term results of up to 10 years after SCXL in paediatric case series, where Keratoconus can typically progress rapidly. Zotta et al. in 20 eyes of 10 patients with an average follow-up of 7.5 years reported stabilization and significant improvements of UDVA, CDVA and all topographic indices [68], while Mazzotta et al. in 62 eyes of 47 paediatric Keratoconic patients found that at 10 years after SCXL significant improvements in UDVA and CDVA were evident with ectatic stability in nearly 80% of cases [69].

Such long-term data from different independent investigators supports the efficacy and safety of SCXL with up to a decade of follow-up. Continued follow-up will determine the need if any to repeat the procedure and elucidate how long and to what degree eyes might continue with improvement in visual and topographic parameters even years after SCXL. Mazzotta et al. in their paediatric series postulated that a 24% regression rate 10 years after SCXL might be expected in patients who were aged 15 years and younger [69]. This recurrence rate would be expected to be less in older individuals due to natural age-related cross-linking. Indeed, the recurrence of keratoconus following keratoplasty, which classically, albeit rarely, occurs 10–20 years following surgery [70], suggests that turnover of corneal collagen and ECM may be measured in decades and that CXL might be effective for at least this length of time if not longer given physiological cross-linking changes with age discussed above.

5.5 Epithelium-On Cross-Linking (TECXL)

5.5.1 *Background*

Riboflavin is a water soluble vitamin with poor lipid solubility and therefore is unable to pass easily through the tight junctions and lipid membranes of an intact epithelial barrier. Hayes et al. [71–73] in a series of ex-vivo porcine and rabbit eye laboratory studies, utilizing spectrophotometry to indirectly measure corneal

Riboflavin concentrations, confirmed the need to remove the epithelium to achieve sufficient stromal Riboflavin absorption which had been first documented by Speorl et al. [1–3]. Riboflavin 0.1% instillation with TE-CXL techniques such as multiple administration of topical anaesthetics (Tetracaine 1%), superficial epithelial trauma, pre-drop application of 20% alcohol solution and grid pattern full-thickness epithelial removal were all found to be insufficient to attain homogeneous Riboflavin stromal absorption at concentrations similar to that achieved by the epithelium-off SCXL technique [71–73].

Utilizing 2-photon fluorescence microscopy to directly assess Riboflavin stromal concentrations, Gore, O'Brart et al. have confirmed the results of these studies and need to remove the epithelium prior to CXL to achieve homogeneous and effective Riboflavin stromal absorption [74–76]. This group tested all the currently commercially available TE-CXL Riboflavin solutions and protocols, including those with so-called chemical enhancers, such as Benzalkonium Chloride (BAC), Trometamol (Tris-(hydroxymethyl)aminometane), Sodium Ethylenediaminetetraacetic acid (EDTA) and d-Alpha-tocopheryl poly(ethylene glycol) 1000 succinate (Vitamin E-TPGS), as well as TE-CXL utilizing iontophoresis. With all tested currently commercially available TE-CXL protocols, stromal absorption appeared to be limited compared to SCXL [75, 76]. The most efficacious were Mediocross TE (0.25% Riboflavin with 0.01% BAC, Peschke Meditrade GmbH Germany) which achieved, compared to SCXL with 0.1% Riboflavin, only 40–50% uptake and only in the first 100 um of the stroma and Ricrolin +0.1% (Riboflavin 0.1% with Troetamol, Sooft Italia SPA Italy) with iontophoresis 1 milliamp (mA) for 5 min which achieved just 30% of epithelium off concentrations for depths up to 150 um [76].

However, despite the difficultly of achieving adequate stromal Riboflavin absorption through the intact corneal epithelium, there is still great interest from investigators throughout the world in undertaking TE-CXL. This because TE-CXL has several perceived advantages over SCXL. It can be assumed that performing CXL with an intact epithelium, would considerably lessen post-operative pain and discomfort as well as hasten visual recovery and importantly in these eyes with irregular astigmatism allow early return to contact lens wear. In addition, it is likely to reduce sight-threatening risks such as post-operative infectious and non-infectious keratitis, lessen the dangers of corneal scarring, by decreasing epithelial/stromal cytokine interaction, and minimize potential endothelial damage, by having a greater overall corneal thickness and limiting peri-operative stromal dehydration and thinning. Currently, published research has been focussed on a number of methodologies. These include partial mechanical disruption [77], the use of chemical enhancement of epithelial permeability by using multiple applications of topical anaesthesia [78], reduced solution osmolarity [79], the addition of chemical additives to the Riboflavin solution such as Trometamol [80], EDTA [80], BAC and Sodium Chloride [81] and alternative drug delivery technologies such as iontophoresis [82].

5.5.2 Partial Mechanical Epithelial Disruption

Partial Mechanical Epithelial Disruption has been undertaken using superficial scratches or specially designed surgical instruments [77, 83]. Rechichi et al. used an epithelial disruptor to pot-mark the epithelial surface (Daya disruptor, Duckworth and Kent Ltd, England) in 28 patients and reported an improvements in vision and to a partial extent refraction and keratometry at 12 months [83]. Hashemi et al. in a series of 40 eyes employed a technique with three to four vertical strips of complete debridement with intact islands of epithelium between and documented significant improvements in CDVA and anterior and posterior corneal elevation at 5 years but no changes in Kmax or refraction [62]. While such results are encouraging, two recent comparative studies have shown more ambiguous results. Hashemi et al. in a retrospective, comparative study of 80 eyes in 65 patients [84] and Razmjoo et al. in a bilateral study of 44 eyes of 22 patients [85], illustrated that while visual outcomes in terms especially CDVA might be improved with partial disruption, enhancements in topographic indices were superior with SCXL. Such limited outcomes of CXL with partial mechanical disruption compared to SCXL are supported by the laboratory studies of Samaras and Hayes et al. [71, 72] where using standard Riboflavin solutions with 20% dextran, although partial epithelial disruption improved Riboflavin absorption, uptake was only significant below the areas of complete epithelial debridement resulting in non-homogeneous stromal absorption. Given the dose repose curve of CXL recently reported by O'Brart et al. [17] with increasing concentrations of Riboflavin solutions, it is not unreasonable to suppose, that the efficacy of the procedure might be reduced with non-homogeneous absorption, with clinically effective CXL only taking place in the areas of complete epithelial debridement where stromal concentrations of riboflavin are adequate. It is of note that in his study, Tariq et al., documented limited Riboflavin stromal absorption, even using a combination of partial mechanical de-bridement and a Riboflavin solution with chemical enhancers (Ricrolin TE ®, Riboflavin 0.1% with trometamol and sodium EDTA (Sooft Italia SPA, Italy)) compared to complete epithelial debridement [73]. Undoubtedly, long-term comparative studies are required to compare these two methodologies in terms of stability of outcomes and cessation of progression of ectasia, before partial disruption can be considered as efficacious as the gold standard total epithelium off technique.

5.5.3 Chemical Enhancers to Increase Epithelial Permeability for TE-CXL

The use of chemicals such as BAC, Trometamol, EDTA, and Vitamin E-TGPS amongst other substances in Riboflavin solutions to increase epithelial permeability by disrupting epithelial tight junctions has been postulated. BAC a cationic surfactant, is a common preservative used in topical ophthalmic medications and is known to disrupt epithelial tight junctions, as well in high dose and prolonged administration result in epithelial cytotoxicity [86]. Similarly, Trometamol $(HOCH_2)_3CNH_2$ or "Tris" is an organic compound which is extensively utilized as a component of buffer solutions and has been shown to increase the permeability of cell membranes [87]. EDTA which is an aminopolycarboxylic acid is widely used in medicine and industry as a chelating agent and has been shown to disrupt epithelial tight junctions and the integrity of lipid cellular membranes [88], while Vitamin E-TPGS is an anti-oxidant surfactant used to increase the adsorption of drugs through biological barriers [89].

The first published clinical studies of TE-CXL employed the multiple administrations of topical aneasthetics to enhance epithelial permeability [78, 90]. Chan et al. documented an enhanced clinical effect of intra-stromal ring segment insertion when combined with TE-CXL using this methodology [78]. However, little has been published on their technique since and laboratory studies using spectrophotometry, as discussed above, have demonstrated poor stromal Riboflavin penetration with this methodology [71].

Filippello et al. using Ricrolin TE (Riboflavin 0.1% with trometamol and sodium EDTA) (Sooft Italia SPA, Italy) [80], in a prospective case series, reported rapid visual recovery with little post-operative pain and outcomes in terms of reduction in Kmax comparable to epithelium-off CXL at 12 months albeit with a shallower demarcation line [80]. Using the same formulation, Salman et al. in 22 eyes of paediatric patients, found a 2.0D decrease in keratometry, improved vision and no progression at 12 months in treated eyes with a worsening of topographic parameters in untreated control eyes [91], while Magli et al. in a retrospective comparative study found little differences in outcomes compared to standard epithelial off CXL [92]. However, conflicting results with this formulation for TE-CXL have been reported suggesting limited efficacy. Buzonetti et al. in 13 eyes found that although CDVA had improved following surgery, keratometry and higher order aberrations were seen to have worsened at 12 months [93], and Caporossi et al. recorded progression of ectasia, especially in paediatric cases and had to retreat 50% of such cases at 24 months, suggesting little efficacy with the use of Trometamol and EDTA as chemical enhancers for TE-CXL [94]. Limited outcomes might be expected given the findings of laboratory studies with photospectometry and 2-photon fluorescent microscopy which identify limited trans-epithelial stromal riboflavin absorption with Ricrolin TE [71–76].

Despite positive results in laboratory studies [81], the use of combinations of Riboflavin solutions with BAC, sodium chloride and multiple administrations of topical aneasthetics to enhance epithelial permeability, have in published outcomes in clinical trials have been more ambiguous [90, 95, 96]. Leccisotti et al. in a prospective, paired-eye study in 51 patients, with the eye with more severe keratoconus being treated and the fellow remaining untreated eye to act as a control, reported an improvement in CDVA, refraction and keratometry in treated eyes compared to controls, but with less effect than that reported with SCXL [95], while Koppen et al. in 53 eyes of 38 patients, documented improvements in CDVA, but progression of Kmax and worsening of pachymetry at 12 months [96].

More recently, Gatzioufas et al. documented a high treatment failure rate in TE-CXL using Mediocross TE (Riboflavin 0.25% with BAC 0.01%, Peschke Meditrade GmbH Germany). Not only did 24% of eyes in their series progress, with an increase in Kmax greater than 1.0D at 12 months, which is similar to progression rates in untreated eyes reported in some randomized, prospective studies of SCXL [42, 67], but almost 50% of eyes had epithelial defects on the 1st day due to epithelial toxicity from prolonged BAC application [97]. It is of note that such evidence of epithelial damage with these BAC containing TE-CXL formulations are consistent with the study by Yuksel et al. who found higher pain scores on day 1 and longer epithelialisation times with such TE-CXL treatments [98]. Using ParaCel (Riboflavin 0.25% with BAC, EDTA and Trometamol and VibeX Xtra (riboflavin 0.25%) (Avedro, USA), Akbar et al. in 26 eyes of 26 patients with thin corneas reported significant improvements in UCVA, CDVA, SEQ, refractive astigmatism and Kmax at 12 months [99], while Kir et al. at 2 years using the same TE-CXL formulation in 48 eyes of 48 patients and an extended, accelerated UVA protocol with 45 mW/cm^2, found no changes in visual and topographic indices at 1 and 2 years although thinnest point pachymetry appeared to increase compared to pre-operative values [100]. Further prospective and comparative studies with CXL to test the efficacy of such formulations are indicated, but laboratory investigations discussed above suggest that efficacy might be limited by poor stromal Riboflavin concentrations. Indeed, Gore et al. demonstrated only 54% with Mediocross TE and 21% with ParaCel of the comparable stromal riboflavin concentration seen in SCXL within the superficial stroma [75, 76].

Ostacolo et al. reported positive laboratory outcomes in porcine eyes, with good trans-epithelial absorption in just 15 min of application with a Riboflavin formulation containing Vitamin E-TPGS [89]. Caruso from this same research group, using a trans-epithelial application time of 15 min and low dose UVA energies less than 3 mW/cm^2 for 10 min, has recently reported clinical outcomes in 25 eyes of 19 patients. Postoperatively, the Kmax decreased by -1.01 ± 1.22D at 2 years an improvement of CDVA. He reported no post-operative abrasions and no use or need of post-operative bandage contact lenses or analgesics [101]. Such results are very encouraging and further prospective and comparative studies using Riboflavin/Vitamin E-TPGA formulations are indicated by independent investigators. Interestingly Gore et al. using this formulation found only 15% of the comparative SCXL Riboflavin 0.1% concentration at a stromal depth of 10 um and less than 5% at a depth of 300 um after 30 min of trans-epithelial application [76]. Based on the work by O'Brart, investigating CXL efficacy with differing Riboflavin solution concentrations in an SCXL model, one would expect such low stromal Riboflavin concentrations seen with this formulation to limit the efficacy of CXL [17].

5.5.4 Comparative Studies of TE-CXL with SCXL with Riboflavin Solutions Containing Chemical Enhancers

In terms of comparative studies with SCXL there is a paucity of such publications and similar to the case series discussed above, results are equivocal. Whilst a number have shown little difference between the techniques some indicate better results with SCXL. Rossi et al. in a randomized, albeit small, prospective study of 20 eyes (10 per treatment group), employing TE-CXL with Ricrolin TE reported no differences in outcomes compared to SCXL at 12 months [102]. Nawaz et al. in a non-randomized study of 40 patients using an isotonic Riboflavin solution for TE-CXL, similarly documented no differences in outcomes at 6 months between TE-CXL and SCXL [103]. While Henriquez et al. in a prospective, cohort study of 61 eyes in 51 paediatric patients using Riboflavin 0.25% with BAC found no differences between SCXL and TE-CXL at 12 months [104]. In contrast, Al Fayez et al. in a prospective, randomized study of 70 patients with 3 year follow-up found better results with SCXL, with no progression of ectasia and an average reduction of Kmax of 2.4D in SCXL treated eyes, while 55% of eyes with SCXL demonstrated keratoconic progression and an average increase of Kmax of 1.1D [105]. Likewise, Soeters et al. in a randomized study of 51 eyes and utilizing Ricrolin TE, documented greater reduction of Kmax with CXL, with evidence of progression in 23% of TE-CXL treated eyes at 12 months [106] and Kocak et al. in a retrospective study in 36 eyes showed a greater reduction in cone apex power with SCXL with progression in 65% of TE-CXL treatments at 12 months [107].

Such results demonstrate uncertainty regarding the efficacy compared to SCXL of many currently commercially available TE-CXL methodologies, utilizing Riboflavin solution modifications in terms of osmolarity, concentration and chemical enhancers. As discussed above, while some clinical studies are supportive, many report high rates of treatment failure. In addition, whilst there are at present many different commercially available TE-CXL solutions, there is a great paucity of well-constructed randomized, prospective clinical studies. Indeed, in a recent meta-analysis Li and Wang could only identify the one suitable study for inclusion in their meta-analysis which utilized TE-CXL with chemical enhancers [108]. It is not unreasonable to suppose that some of the poor results seen with TE-CXL and formulations containing chemical enhancers is due to inadequate stromal Riboflavin penetration through the intact hydrophobic epithelial barrier as seen in photo-spectrometry studies and corroborated by 2-photon fluorescence microscopy [76]. As discussed above only 20–50% of the Riboflavin concentration is achieved with the use of such solutions compared to SCXL and this concentration is not homogeneous reducing considerably at increasing stromal depths [76]. In addition in the

2-photon studies, with BAC containing compounds significant epithelial damage was observed after 30 min of solution application time and there appeared to be loading of the epithelium with a considerable amount of Riboflavin with all tested solutions that would produce shielding of the stroma from UVA energy during irradiation [76]. This shielding of UVA reaching the stroma is likely to further limit the efficacy of such TE-CXL on treatments. Finally, in SCXL during UV irradiation, especially with the 30 min at 3 mW/cm^2 Dresden protocol, Riboflavin is regularly reapplied to the stromal surface to replenish Riboflavin that has been lost through photo-bleaching [4, 15], with an TE-CXL technique this is difficult to achieve without loading the epithelium with Riboflavin and further shielding the stroma from the UVA.

5.5.5 *Other Techniques Using Chemical Enhancers: CXL USA Study*

In an as yet unpublished study the CXL study group has reported very encouraging results with TE-CXL using a novel Riboflavin formulation. The exact detail of this formulation has not as yet been fully revealed but it apparently contains Sodium Iodine (personal communication, Dr. Doyle Stulting, CXL 2017 Experts Meeting, Zurich). In a prospective series of 592 eyes with Keratoconus and iatrogenic ectasia, they have reported an improvement in UDVA and CDVA at 1 and 2 years with a significant reduction in Kmax of approximately 0.5D, with no reports of progression (personal communication, Dr. Doyle Stulting, CXL 2017 Experts Meeting, Zurich). As yet there are no published studies in the peer-reviewed literature of this technique, supporting investigations by independent investigators or comparative studies with SCXL to fully assess the efficacy of this technique and support its implementation into clinical practice.

5.5.6 *Iontophoresis for TE-CXL*

In addition to the novel formulations described above, laboratory investigations have shown enhanced trans-epithelial riboflavin absorption with the use of iontophoresis [109–112]. Riboflavin is a suitable molecule for iontophoretic transport as it is small, negatively charged at physiological pH and soluble in water. Cassagne et al. in Rabbit eyes using iontophoresis with a 0.1% Riboflavin solution and 1 milliampere (mA) current for 5 min, reported 50% of the expected stromal concentration of Riboflavin compared to SCXL with similar biomechanical enhancements in both extensiometry measurements and resistance to collagenase digestion between the two treatments [109]. Vinciguerra et al. in both rabbit and human cadaver eyes, found greater riboflavin uptake and increased extensiometry measurements with iontophoretic CXL (iCXL) compared to TE-CXL with chemical enhancers but with less biomechanical changes compared to SCXL treatments [110], while Mastropasqua et al. reported increased stiffening of ex-vivo human corneas using a noncontact air pulse tonometry methodology following iCXL [111]. Finally, Lombardo et al. found comparable stiffness after iCXL to that seen with SCXL using an inflation methodology in ex-vivo human globes [112].

Published clinical studies of iCXL are relatively few and limited in follow-up. Bikbova et al. treated 22 eyes with iCXL, using Riboflavin 0.1% and 1 mA for 10 min with the standard UVA protocol of 3 mw/cm^2 for 30 min and reported a mean reduction of Kmax of 2.0D at 12 months [113]. Vinciguerra et al. published on 20 eyes, which underwent iCXL with Riboflavin 0.1% (Ricrolin +, Sooft Italia SPA, Italy) at 1 mA for 5 min and documented an improvement in CDVA and stable keratometry, higher order aberrations, pachymetry and endothelial counts at 12 months [114]. Li et al. utilizing the same protocol as Vincinguerra, in 15 eyes, documented an improvement in visual and topographic parameters, with a demarcation line with an average depth of 288 um at 6 months [115]. Buzzonetti et al. in 14 paediatric cases utilizing iCXL at 1 mA for 5 min and an accelerated UVA protocol demonstrated an improvement in CDVA and topography with stability of refraction at 15 months but with an average demarcation line depth of only 180 um [116]. Magli et al. documented stability of keratoconus 18 months after iCXL in 13 paediatric patients [117] and Laborante et al. in 15 eyes of 15 patients showed stabilization of vision and topography after iCXL at 6–12 months [118]. More recently, Jia et al. published a larger series of 94 eyes of 75 patients with progressive keratoconus who underwent iCXL with a longer term 24 month follow-up. They documented statistically significant improvements in CDVA and reductions in keratometry at 2 years with a mean reduction of maximum keratometry of over 2.0 diopters [119]. It is note that in this study they used Riboflavin 0.1% in distilled water, with no phosphate buffer to control ph. Such prospective case series are encouraging and suggest some promise for the use of iontophoresis in TE-CXL.

In terms of comparative studies of iCXL versus SCXL a number of investigations have been recently published. Bikbova et al. reported on a randomized, controlled study in a series of 73 eyes treated with standard CXL and 76 eyes iCXL, with Riboflavin 0.1% and iontophoresis with 1 mA for 10 min. At 24 months, there were no differences in visual performance between groups but greater improvements keratometric parameters with SCXL [120]. One eye progressed in the iCXL. Vinciguerra et al. published the outcomes of a comparative, prospective clinical study with 20 eyes in each group and 12 month follow-up, with Ricrolin + (Riboflavin 0.1%, trometamol, phosphate buffer) (Sooft, Italia SPA) and iCXL at 1 mA for 5 min. They documented a significant reduction in Kmax in the SCXL treated eyes of -1.05 ± 1.51D at 12 months, whereas the iCXL group showed little change [121]. Most recently, Lombardo et al. in a prospective randomized controlled trial in 34 eyes reported significant visual and refractive improvements 12 months after iCXL, though the measured improvements in topography were lower than that achieved after SCXL [122]. Such outcome indicate that while efficacy can be realized with current iCXL protocols with Riboflavin 0.1%, results in terms of improvement in topographic indices are better with SCXL.

5.5.7 Future Developments of iCXL

Iontophoresis in commercial protocols is currently being utilized to provide reduced application times of 5–10 min, instead of the usual 30 min epithelium off Riboflavin application time proposed in the original Dresden protocol [4]. In a series of laboratory investigations, O'Brart and colleagues have shown that by increasing Riboflavin concentration from 0.1% to 0.25%, together with increased iontophoresis application times with intervals between iontophoretic applications to allow for Riboflavin to diffuse form the sub-epithelial tissues deeper into the stroma, concentrations of up to 60–80% of that with SCXL applications with Riboflavin 0.1% can be achieved and with a homogeneous distribution throughout the stroma [123–125]. Indeed, this represents twice the concentrations reached with the commercial protocols used in many of the currently published studies [123–125].

Similarly, the same investigators have shown that by using such modified iCXL protocols and extending the ultraviolet dosage, further augmentation of CXL can be achieved. Using a pepsin digestion model, Aldahlawi et al. showed that with an extended iontophoretic 0.25% Riboflavin protocol and an extended UVA dosage of 6.75 joules per centimeter squared (J/cm^2) the CXL process can be augmented achieving the same efficacy in terms of corneal button pepsin digestion times as SCXL and much better outcomes than those using Riboflavin 0.1% and shortened iontophoretic protocols [126].

With such modified iCXL protocols is hoped that results similar to SCXL can be achieved. At present a controlled, randomized, bilateral, prospective studies of such protocols compared to SCXL is currently being undertaken (O'Brart, personal communication, International Standard Randomized Controlled trials Number: 04451470). The results of this study are encouraging. So far 86 eyes have reached 18 month follow-up (43 treated with iCXL CXL and 43 with SCXL). At this time Kmax has reduced by −1.04D ($p < 0.005$) point in the iCXL eyes and by −0.95D ($p < 0.0001$) in the SCXL treated eyes, with documented progression (defined as an increase in Kmax >1.5D) in two eyes (5%) after iCXL and one eye after SCXL. There appear to be no differences in 20 visual, refractive, topographic and tomographic parameters between the two groups at 18 months. Such results are encouraging and suggest that with protocol modifications, iCXL may be an alternative to SCXL. It is of note, however, that even with this TE-CXL methodology, almost 50% of iCXL treated eyes had some post-operative corneal erosions seen on the 1st day after surgery although visual analogue pain scores were generally better with iCXL. Further studies are underway both to further enhance iCXL efficacy to allow it to outperform SCXL by increasing Riboflavin concentrations for iontophoresis beyond 0.25% and by undertaking further limited iontophoresis halfway through UVA irradiation to replace stromal Riboflavin that has been photo-bleached, as well as time to replenish corneal oxygen to pre-irradiation levels. Strategies to improved post-operative comfort and post-operative epithelial integrity with the use of bandage contact lenses, amnion bandages and treatments low UVA irradiation energies are also being undertaken.

5.6 TE-CXL Other Investigative Methodologies

As well as iontophoresis, other methodologies currently postulated to facilitate TE-CXL include the use of ultrasound [127], nano-emulsion systems [128] and the creation of femto second laser intra-stromal pockets [128]. At present these methodologies are either at a pre-clinical investigational stage or at an early clinical stage with no large prospective case series or comparative studies, so it is not possible at present to comment on their merits.

5.7 Summary

Multiple clinical studies of SCXL, especially using the standard UVA irradiation protocol of 3 mW/cm^2 for 30 min have demonstrated efficacy in stabilizing keratoconus and post-refractive surgery ectasia with up to 10 years follow-up. This methodology must at present be regarded as the gold standard. Whilst further randomized, prospective and long-term follow up studies are indicated, it can be expected that with SCXL in the future corneal ectasia can be halted at an early stage and conceivably the necessity for rigid contact lenses and keratoplasty reduced or even circumvented The outcomes of TE-CXL with currently available techniques are somewhat ambiguous. Whilst some investigators have reported results comparable to SCXL, many, including comparative studies, have shown outcomes that are inferior. Newer methodologies including modified iontophoresis using high dose Riboflavin, may in the future hold great promise for TE-CXL and because of improved patient comfort and safety may become the gold standard treatment although clearly further studies are indicated to optimize treatment protocols.

Financial Disclosures Related to Manuscript Professor O'Brart holds non-commercial research grants from Alcon Inc. and Avedro Inc.

He has undertaken paid consultancy work for Alcon Inc. and Sooft Italia SPA in the past 12 months

References

1. Spoerl E, Huhle M, Seiler T. Erhohung der Festigkeit der Horn haut durch Vernetzung. Ophthalmologe. 1997;94(12):902–6.
2. Spoerl E, Huhle M, Seiler T. Induction of cross-links in corneal tissue. Exp Eye Res. 1998;66(1):97–103.
3. Spoerl E, Schreiber J, Hellmund K, et al. Untersuchungen zur Verfestigung der Hornhaut am kaninchen. Ophthalmologe. 2000;97(3):203–6.
4. Wollensak G, Spoerl E, Seiler T. Riboflavin/ultraviolet-A-induced collagen cross-linking for the treatment of kertatoconus. Am J Ophthalmol. 2003;135(5):620–7.

5. McCall AS, Kraft S, Edelhauser HF, et al. Mechanisms of corneal tissue cross-linking in response to treatment with topical riboflavin and long-wavelength ultraviolet radiation (UVA). Invest Ophthalmol Vis Sci. 2010;51(1):129–38.
6. Min DB, Boff JM. Chemistry and reaction of singlet oxygen in foods. Compr Rev Food Sci Food Saf. 2002;1:58–72.
7. Huang R, Choe E, Min DB. Kinetics for singlet oxygen formation by riboflavin photosensitization and the reaction between riboflavin and singlet oxygen. J Food Sci. 2004;69:C726–32.
8. Choe E, Min DB. Chemistry and reactions of reactive oxygen species in foods. Crit Rev Food Sci Nutr. 2006;46:1–22.
9. Kato Y, Uchida K, Kawakishi S. Aggregation of collagen exposed to UVA in the presence of riboflavin: a plausible role of tyrosine modification. Photochem Photobiol. 1994;59(3):343–9.
10. Spikes JD, Shen HR, Kopecková P, Kopecek J. Photodynamic crosslinking of proteins, III: kinetics of the FMN- and rose Bengal-sensitized photooxidation and intermolecular crosslinking of model tyrosine-containing N-(2-hydroxypropyl)methacrylamide copolymers. Photochem Photobiol. 1999;70:130–7.
11. de La Rochette A, Birlouez-Aragon I, Silva E, Morlière P. Advanced glycation endproducts as UVA photosensitizers of tryptophan and ascorbic acid: consequences for the lens. Biochim Biophys Acta. 1621;2003:235–41.
12. Dalsgaard TK, Otzen D, Nielsen JH, Larsen LB. Changes in structures of milk proteins upon photo-oxidation. J Agric Food Chem. 2007;55:10968–76.
13. Wright A, Bubb WA, Hawkins CL, Davies MJ. Singlet oxygen-mediated protein oxidation: evidence for the formation of reactive side chain peroxides on tyrosine residues. Photochem Photobiol. 2002;76:35–46.
14. Richoz O, Hammer A, Tabibian D, Gatzioufas Z, Hafezi F. The biomechanical effect of corneal collagen cross-linking (CXL) with riboflavin and UV-A is oxygen dependent. Transl Vis Sci Technol. 2013;2(7):6. Epub 2013 Dec 11.
15. Kamaev P, Friedman MD, Sherr E, Muller D. Photochemical kinetics of corneal cross-linking with riboflavin. Invest Ophthalmol Vis Sci. 2012;53(4):2360–7.
16. Lu C, Lin W, Wang W, Han Z, Yao S, Lin N. Riboflavin (VB2) photosensitized oxidation of 2′-deoxyguanosine-5′-monophosphate (dGMP) in aqueous solution: a transient intermediates study. Phys Chem Chem Phys. 2000;2:329–34.
17. O'Brart NA, O'Brart DPS, Aldahlawi NH, Hayes S, Meek KM. An investigation of the effects of riboflavin concentration on the efficacy of corneal collagen cross-linking using an enzymatic resistance model in porcine corneas. Invest Ophthalmol Vis Sci. 2018;59:1058–65.
18. Hayes S, Kamma-Lorger CS, Boote C, Young RD, Quantock AJ, Rost A, Khatib Y, Harris J, Yagi N, Terrill N, Meek KM. The effect of riboflavin/UVA collagen cross-linking therapy on the structure and hydrodynamic behaviour of the ungulate and rabbit corneal stroma. PLoS One. 2013;8(1):e52860.
19. Scnitzler E, Sporl E, Seiler T. Crosslinking of the corneal collagen by UV radiation with riboflavin for the mode of treatment melting ulcer of the cornea, first results of four patients. Klin Monatsbl Augenheilkd. 2000;217(3):190–3.
20. Caporossi A, Baiocchi S, Mazzotta C, et al. Parasurgical therapy for keratoconus by riboflavin-ultraviolet type A rays induced cross-linking of the corneal collagen; preliminary refractive results in an Italian study. J Cataract Refract Surg. 2006;32(5):837–45.
21. Vinciguerra P, Albe E, Trazza S, et al. Refractive, topo graphic, tomographic, and abberometric analysis of keratoconic eyes undergoing corneal cross-linking. Ophthalmology. 2009;116(3):369–78.
22. Coskunseven E, Jankov MR 2nd, Hafezi F. Contralateral eye study of corneal collagen cross-linking with riboflavin and UVA radiation in patients with keratoconus. J Refract Surg. 2009;25(4):371–6.
23. Agrawal VB. Corneal collagen cross-linking with riboflavin and ultraviolet – a light for keratoconus: results in Indian eyes. Indian J Ophthalmol. 2009;57(2):111–4.

24. Arbelaez MC, Sekito MB, Vidal C, Choudhury SR. Collagen cross-linking with riboflavin and ultraviolet-A light in keratoconus: one-year results. Oman J Ophthalmol. 2009;2(1):33–8.
25. Vinciguerra P, Albè E, Trazza S, Seiler T, Epstein D. Intraoperative and postoperative effects of corneal collagen cross-linking on progressive keratoconus. Arch Ophthalmol. 2009;127(10):1258–65.
26. Fournié P, Galiacy S, Arné JL, Malecaze F. Corneal collagen cross-linking with ultraviolet-A light and riboflavin for the treatment of progressive keratoconus. J Fr Ophtalmol. 2009;32(1):1–7.
27. Henriquez MA, Izquierdo L Jr, Bernilla C, Zakrzewski PA, Mannis M. Riboflavin/ultraviolet A corneal collagen cross-linking for the treatment of keratoconus: visual outcomes and Scheimpflug analysis. Cornea. 2011;30(3):281–6.
28. Kampik D, Koch M, Kampik K, Geerling G. Corneal riboflavin/UV-A collagen cross-linking (CXL) in keratoconus: two-year results. Klin Monatsbl Augenheilkd. 2011;228(6):525–30.
29. Goldich Y, Marcovich AL, Barkana Y, Mandel Y, Hirsh A, Morad Y, Avni I, Zadok D. Clinical and corneal biomechanical changes after collagen cross-linking with riboflavin and UV irradiation in patients with progressive keratoconus: results after 2 years of follow-up. Cornea. 2012;31(6):609–14.
30. Asri D, Touboul D, Fournié P, Malet F, Garra C, Gallois A, Malecaze F, Colin J. Corneal collagen crosslinking in progressive keratoconus: multicenter results from the French National Reference Center for Keratoconus. J Cataract Refract Surg. 2011;37(12):2137–43.
31. Hersh PS, Greenstein SA, Fry KL. Corneal collagen crosslinking for keratoconus and corneal ectasia: one-year results. J Cataract Refract Surg. 2011;37(1):149–60.
32. Arora R, Gupta D, Goyal JL, Jain P. Results of corneal collagen cross-linking in pediatric patients. J Refract Surg. 2012;28(11):759–62.
33. Vinciguerra P, Albé E, Frueh BE, Trazza S, Epstein D. Two-year corneal cross-linking results in patients younger than 18 years with documented progressive keratoconus. Am J Ophthalmol. 2012;154(3):520–6.
34. Ivarsen A, Hjortdal J. Collagen cross-linking for advanced progressive keratoconus. Cornea. 2013;32(7):903–6.
35. Hafezi F, Kanellopoulos J, Wiltfang R, Seiler T. Corneal collagen crosslinking with riboflavin and ultraviolet A to treat induced keratectasia after laser in situ keratomileusis. J Cataract Refract Surg. 2007;33(12):2035–40.
36. Vinciguerra P, Camesasca FI, Albè E, Trazza S. Corneal collagen cross-linking for ectasia after excimer laser refractive surgery: 1-year results. J Refract Surg. 2010;26(7):486–97.
37. Salgado JP, Khoramnia R, Lohmann CP, Winkler von Mohrenfels C. Corneal collagen cross-linking in post-LASIK keratectasia. Br J Ophthalmol. 2011;95(4):493–7.
38. Richoz O, Mavrakanas N, Pajic B, Hafezi F. Corneal collagen cross-linking for ectasia after LASIK and photorefractive keratectomy: long-term results. Ophthalmology. 2013;120(7):1354–9.
39. Spadea L. Corneal collagen cross-linking with riboflavin and UVA irradiation in pellucid marginal degeneration. J Refract Surg. 2010;26(5):375–7.
40. Hassan Z, Nemeth G, Modis L, Szalai E, Berta A. Collagen cross-linking in the treatment of pellucid marginal degeneration. Indian J Ophthalmol. 2014;62:367–70.
41. Bayraktar S, Cebeci Z, Oray M, Alparslan N. Corneal collagen cross-linking in pellucid marginal degeneration: 2 patients, 4 eyes. Case Rep Ophthalmol Med. 2015;2015:840687.
42. O'Brart DP, Chan E, Samaras K, Patel P, Shah SP. A randomised, prospective study to investigate the efficacy of riboflavin/ultraviolet A (370 nm) corneal collagen cross-linkage to halt the progression of keratoconus. Br J Ophthalmol. 2011;95(11):1519–24.
43. Wittig-Silva C. A randomized controlled trial of corneal collagen cross-linking in progressive keratoconus; preliminary results. J Refract Surg. 2008;24(7):S720–5.
44. Wittig-Silva C, Chan E, Islam FM, Wu T, Whiting M, Snibson GR. A randomized, controlled trial of corneal collagen cross-linking in progressive keratoconus: three-year results. Ophthalmology. 2014;121(4):812–21.

45. Chang CY, Hersh PS. Corneal collagen cross-linking: a review of 1-year outcomes. Eye Contact Lens. 2014;40(6):345–52.
46. Greenstein SA, Fry KL, Hersh PS. Corneal topography indices after corneal collagen crosslinking for keratoconus and corneal ectasia: one-year results. J Cataract Refract Surg. 2011;37(7):1282–90.
47. Lang SJ, Messmer EM, Geerling G, Mackert MJ, Brunner T, Dollak S, Kutchoukov B, Böhringer D, Reinhard T, Maier P. Prospective, randomized, double-blind trial to investigate the efficacy and safety of corneal cross-linking to halt the progression of keratoconus. BMC Ophthalmol. 2015;15:78.
48. Seyedian MA, Aliakbari S, Miraftab M, Hashemi H, Asgari S, Khabazkhoob M. Corneal collagen cross-linking in the treatment of progressive keratoconus: a randomized controlled contralateral eye study. Middle East Afr J Ophthalmol. 2015;22(3):340–5.
49. Sharma N, Suri K, Sehra SV, Titiyal JS, Sinha R, Tandon R, Vajpayee RB. Collagen cross-linking in keratoconus in Asian eyes: visual, refractive and confocal microscopy outcomes in a prospective randomized controlled trial. Int Ophthalmol. 2015;35(6):827–32.
50. Hersh PS, Stulting RD, Muller D, Durrie DS, Rajpal RK, United States Crosslinking Study Group. United States multicenter clinical trial of corneal collagen crosslinking for keratoconus treatment. Ophthalmology. 2017;124(9):1259–70.
51. Hersh PS, Stulting RD, Muller D, Durrie DS, Rajpal RK, U.S. Crosslinking Study Group. U.S. multicenter clinical trial of corneal collagen crosslinking for treatment of corneal ectasia after refractive surgery. Ophthalmology. 2017;124(10):1475–84.
52. Li J, Ji P, Lin X. Efficacy of corneal collagen cross-linking for treatment of keratoconus: a meta-analysis of randomized controlled trials. PLoS One. 2015;10(5):e0127079.
53. Meiri Z, Keren S, Rosenblatt A, Sarig T, Shenhav L, Varssano D. Efficacy of corneal collagen cross-linking for the treatment of keratoconus: a systematic review and meta-analysis. Cornea. 2016;35(3):417–28.
54. Chunyu T, Xiujun P, Zhengjun F, Xia Z, Feihu Z. Corneal collagen cross-linking in keratoconus: a systematic review and meta-analysis. Sci Rep. 2014;4:5652. https://doi.org/10.1038/srep05652.
55. Wan Q, Wang D, Ye H, Tang J, Han Y. A review and meta-analysis of corneal cross-linking for post-laser vision correction ectasia. J Curr Ophthalmol. 2017;29(3):145–53.
56. Krachmer JH, Feder RS, Belin MW. Keratoconus and related non-inflammatory corneal thinning disorders. Surv Ophthalmol. 1984;28:293–322.
57. Rabinowitz YS. Keratoconus. Surv Ophthalmol. 1998;42(4):297–319.
58. Kennedy RH, Bourne WM, Dyer JA. A 48-year clinical and epidemiological study of keratoconus. Am J Ophthalmol. 1986;101(3):267–73.
59. Raiskup-Wolf F, Hoyer A, Spoerl E, Pillunat LE. Collagen cross-linking with riboflavin and ultraviolet A light in keratoconus: long term results. J Cataract Refract Surg. 2008;34(5):796–801.
60. Caporossi A, Mazzotta C, Baiocchi S, Caporossi T. Long-term results of riboflavin ultraviolet a corneal collagen cross-linking for keratoconus in Italy: the Siena eye cross study. Am J Ophthalmol. 2010;149(4):585–93.
61. O'Brart DP, Kwong TQ, Patel P, McDonald RJ, O'Brart NA. Long-term follow-up of riboflavin/ultraviolet A (370 nm) corneal collagen cross-linking to halt the progression of keratoconus. Br J Ophthalmol. 2013;97(4):433–7.
62. Hashemi H, Seyedian MA, Miraftab M, Fotouhi A, Asgari S. Corneal collagen cross-linking with riboflavin and Ultraviolet A irradiation for keratoconus: long-term results. Ophthalmology. 2013;120(8):1515–20.
63. Uçakhan ÖÖ, Bayraktutar BN, Saglik A. Pediatric corneal collagen cross-linking: long-term follow-up of visual, refractive, and topographic outcomes. Cornea. 2016;35(2):162–8.
64. Poli M, Lefevre A, Auxenfans C, Burillon C. Corneal collagen cross-linking for the treatment of progressive corneal ectasia: 6-year prospective outcome in a French population. Am J Ophthalmol. 2015;160(4):654–62.

65. Theuring A, Spoerl E, Pillunat LE, Raiskup F. Corneal collagen cross-linking with riboflavin and ultraviolet-A light in progressive keratoconus. Results after 10-year follow-up. Ophthalmologe. 2015;112(2):140–7.
66. Raiskup F, Theuring A, Pillunat LE, Spoerl E. Corneal collagen crosslinking with riboflavin and ultraviolet-A light in progressive keratoconus: ten-year results. J Cataract Refract Surg. 2015;41(1):41–6.
67. O'Brart DP, Patel P, Lascaratos G, Wagh VK, Tam C, Lee J, O'Brart NA. Corneal cross-linking to halt the progression of keratoconus and corneal ectasia: seven-year follow-up. Am J Ophthalmol. 2015;160(6):1154–63.
68. Zotta PG, Diakonis VF, Kymionis GD, Grentzelos M, Moschou KA. Long-term outcomes of corneal cross-linking for keratoconus in pediatric patients. J AAPOS. 2017;21(5):397–401.
69. Mazzotta C, Traversi C, Baiocchi S, Bagaglia S, Caporossi O, Villano A, Caporossi A. Corneal collagen cross-linking with riboflavin and ultraviolet A light for pediatric keratoconus: ten-year results. Cornea. 2018;37(5):560–6. https://doi.org/10.1097/ICO.0000000000001505.
70. Javadi MA, Motlagh BF, Jafarinasab MR, et al. Outcomes of penetrating keratoplasty in keratoconus. Cornea. 2005;24:941–6.
71. Hayes S, O'Brart DP, Lamdin LS, Doutch J, Samaras K, Meek KM, Marshall J. An investigation into the importance of complete epithelial debridement prior to riboflavin/ultraviolet A (UVA) corneal collagen cross-linkage therapy. J Cat Ref Surg. 2008;34:557–61.
72. Samaras K, O'Brart DPS, Doutch J, Hayes S, Marshall J, Meek K. Effect of epithelial retention and removal on riboflavin absorption in porcine corneas. J Refract Surg. 2009;25(9):771–5.
73. Tariq AA, O'Brart DPS, O'Brart NAL, Meek KM. An investigation of trans-epithelial stromal riboflavin absorption with Ricrolin TE ® (riboflavin 0.1% with trometamol and sodium EDTA) using spectrophotometry. J Cat Ref Surg. 2012;38:884–9.
74. Gore D, Margineanu A, French P, O'Brart D, Dunsby C, Allan D. Two-photon fluorescence microscopy of corneal riboflavin absorption. Invest Ophthamol Vis Sci. 2014;55(4):2476–81.
75. Gore DM, French F, O'Brart D, Dunsby C, Allan BD. Two-photon fluorescence microscopy of corneal riboflavin absorption through an intact epithelium. Invest Ophthamol Vis Sci. 2015;56(2):1191–2.
76. Gore DM, O'Brart D, Dunsby C, French P, Allan BD. Transepithelial riboflavin absorption in an ex-vivo rabbit corneal model. Invest Ophthamol Vis Sci. 2015;56(8):5006–11.
77. Samaras KE, Lake DB. Corneal collagen cross linking: a review. Int Ophthalmol Clin. 2010;50(3):89–100.
78. Chan C, Sharma M, Wachler B. Effect of inferior segment Intacs with and without C3-R on keratoconus. J Cataract Refract Surg. 2007;33(1):75–80.
79. Raiskup F, Pinelli R, Spoerl E. Riboflavin osmolar modification for transepithelial corneal cross-linking. Curr Eye Res. 2012;37(3):234–8.
80. Filippello M, Stagni E, O'Brart D. Trans-epithelial corneal collagen cross-linking: a bilateral, prospective study. J Cat Ref Surg. 2012;38(2):283–91.
81. Kissner A, Spoerl E, Jung R, Spekl K, Pillunat LE, Raiskup F. Pharmacological modification of the epithelial permeability by benzalkonium chloride in UVA/riboflavin corneal collagen cross-linking. Curr Eye Res. 2010;35(8):715–21.
82. Vinciguerra R, Spoerl E, Romano MR, Rosetta P, Vinciguerra P. Comparative stress strain measurements of human corneas after transepithelial UV-A induced cross-linking: impregnation with iontophoresis, different riboflavin solutions and irradiance power. ARVO 2012 Abstract 1518.
83. Rechichi M, Daya S, Scorcia V, Meduri A, Scorcia G. Epithelial-disruption collagen crosslinking for keratoconus: one-year results. J Cataract Refract Surg. 2013;39(8):1171–8.
84. Hashemi H, Miraftab M, Hafezi F, Asgari S. Matched comparison study of total and partial epithelium removal in corneal cross-linking. J Refract Surg. 2015;31(2):110–5.
85. Razmjoo H, Rahimi B, Kharraji M, Koosha N, Peyman A. Corneal haze and visual outcome after collagen crosslinking for keratoconus: a comparison between total epithelium off and partial epithelial removal methods. Adv Biomed Res. 2014;3:221.

86. Chen W, Hu J, Zhang Z, Chen L, Xie H, Dong N, Chen Y, Liu Z. Localization and expression of zonula occludins-1 in the rabbit corneal epithelium following exposure to benzalkonium chloride. PLoS One. 2012;7(7):e40893.
87. Irvin RT, MacAlister TJ, Costerton JW. Tris(hydroxymethyl)aminomethane buffer modification of *Escherichia coli* outer membrane permeability. J Bacteriol. 1981;145(3):1397–403.
88. Rojanasakul Y, Liaw J, Robinson J. Mechanisms of action of some penetration enhancers in the cornea: laser microscopic and electrophysiology studies. Int J Pharm. 1990;66:131–42.
89. Ostacolo C, Caruso C, Tronino D, et al. Enhancement of corneal permeation of riboflavin-5′-phosphate through vitamin E TPGS: a promising approach in corneal trans-epithelial cross linking treatment. Int J Pharm. 2013;440:148–53.
90. Ramselaar JA, Boot JP, van Haeringen NJ, van Best JA, Oosterhuis JA. Corneal epithelial permeability after instillation of ophthalmic solutions containing local anaesthetics and preservatives. Curr Eye Res. 1988;7(9):947–50.
91. Salman AG. Transepithelial corneal collagen crosslinking for progressive keratoconus in a pediatric age group. J Cataract Refract Surg. 2013;39(8):1164–70.
92. Magli A, Forte R, Tortori A, Capasso L, Marsico G, Piozzi E. Epithelium-off corneal collagen cross-linking versus transepithelial cross-linking for pediatric keratoconus. Cornea. 2013;32(5):597–601.
93. Buzzonetti L, Petrocelli G. Transepithelial corneal cross-linking in pediatric patients: early results. J Refract Surg. 2012;28(11):763–7.
94. Caporossi A, Mazzotta C, Paradiso AL, Baiocchi S, Marigliani D, Caporossi T. Transepithelial corneal collagen crosslinking for progressive keratoconus: 24-month clinical results. J Cataract Refract Surg. 2013;39(8):1157–63.
95. Leccisotti A, Islam T. Transepithelial corneal collagen cross-linking in keratoconus. J Refract Surg. 2010;26(12):942–8.
96. Koppen C, Wouters K, Mathysen D, Rozema J, Tassignon MJ. Refractive and topographic results of benzalkonium chloride-assisted transepithelial crosslinking. J Cataract Refract Surg. 2012;38(6):1000–5.
97. Gatzioufas Z, Raiskup F, O'Brart D, Spoerl E, Panos GD, Hafezi F. Transepithelial corneal crosslinking using an enhanced riboflavin solution. J Cataract Refract Surg. 2016;32:372–7.
98. Yuksel E, Novruzlu S, Ozmen MC, Bilgihan K. A study comparing standard and transepithelial collagen cross-linking riboflavin solutions: epithelial findings and pain scores. J Ocul Pharmacol Ther. 2015;31(5):296–302.
99. Akbar B, Intisar-Ul-Haq R, Ishaq M, Arzoo S, Siddique K. Transepithelial corneal cross-linking in treatment of progressive keratoconus: 12 months' clinical results. Pak J Med Sci. 2017;33(3):570–5.
100. Kır MB, Türkyılmaz K, Öner V. Transepithelial high-intensity cross-linking for the treatment of progressive keratoconus: 2-year outcomes. Curr Eye Res. 2017;42(1):28–31.
101. Caruso C, Ostacolo C, Epstein RL, Barbaro G, Troisi S, Capobianco D. Transepithelial corneal cross-linking with vitamin E-enhanced riboflavin solution and abbreviated, low-dose UV-A: 24-month clinical outcomes. Cornea. 2016;35(2):145–50.
102. Rossi S, Orrico A, Santamaria C, Romano V, De Rosa L, Simonelli F, De Rosa G. Standard versus trans-epithelial collagen cross-linking in keratoconus patients suitable for standard collagen cross-linking. Clin Ophthalmol. 2015;9:503–9. https://doi.org/10.2147/OPTH.S73991. eCollection 2015.
103. Nawaz S, Gupta S, Gogia V, Sasikala NK, Panda A. Trans-epithelial versus conventional corneal collagen crosslinking: a randomized trial in keratoconus. Oman J Ophthalmol. 2015;8(1):9–13.
104. Henriquez MA, Rodríguez AM, Izquierdo L Jr. Accelerated epi-on versus standard epi-off corneal collagen cross-linking for progressive keratoconus in pediatric patients. Cornea. 2017;36(12):1503–8.
105. Al Fayez MF, Alfayez S, Alfayez Y. Transepithelial versus epithelium-off corneal collagen cross-linking for progressive keratoconus: a prospective randomized controlled trial. Cornea. 2015;34(Suppl 10):S53–6.

106. Soeters N, Wisse RP, Godefrooij DA, Imhof SM, Tahzib NG. Transepithelial versus epithelium-off corneal cross-linking for the treatment of progressive keratoconus: a randomized controlled trial. Am J Ophthalmol. 2015;159(5):821–8.
107. Kocak I, Aydin A, Kaya F, Koc H. Comparison of transepithelial corneal collagen cross-linking with epithelium-off crosslinking in progressive keratoconus. J Fr Ophtalmol. 2014;37(5):371–6.
108. Li W, Wang B. Efficacy and safety of transepithelial corneal collagen crosslinking surgery versus standard corneal collagen crosslinking surgery for keratoconus: a meta-analysis of randomized controlled trials. BMC Ophthalmol. 2017;17(1):262.
109. Cassagne M, Laurent C, Rodrigues M, Galinier A, Spoerl E, Galiacy SD, Soler V, Fournié P, Malecaze F. Iontophoresis transcorneal delivery technique for transepithelial corneal collagen crosslinking with riboflavin in a rabbit model. Invest Ophthalmol Vis Sci. 2014. pii: iovs.13-12595v1. https://doi.org/10.1167/iovs.13-12595. [Epub ahead of print].
110. Vinciguerra P, Mencucci R, Romano V, Spoerl E, Camesasca FI, Favuzza E, Azzolini C, Mastropasqua R, Vinciguerra R. Imaging mass spectrometry by matrix-assisted laser desorption/ionization and stress-strain measurements in iontophoresis transepithelial corneal collagen cross-linking. Biomed Res Int. 2014;2014:404587. https://doi.org/10.1155/2014/404587. Epub 2014 Sep 2.
111. Mastropasqua L, Lanzini M, Curcio C, Calienno R, Mastropasqua R, Colasante M, Mastropasqua A, Nubile M. Structural modifications and tissue response after standard epi-off and iontophoretic corneal crosslinking with different irradiation procedures. Invest Ophthalmol Vis Sci. 2014;55(4):2526–33.
112. Lombardo M, Serrao S, Rosati M, Ducoli P, Lombardo G. Biomechanical changes in the human cornea after transepithelial corneal crosslinking using iontophoresis. J Cataract Refract Surg. 2014;40(10):1706–15.
113. Bikbova G, Bikbov M. Transepithelial corneal collagen cross-linking by iontophoresis of riboflavin. Acta Ophthalmol. 2014;92(1):e30–4.
114. Vinciguerra P, Randleman JB, Romano V, Legrottaglie EF, Rosetta P, Camesasca FI, Piscopo R, Azzolini C, Vinciguerra R. Transepithelial iontophoresis corneal collagen cross-linking for progressive keratoconus: initial clinical outcomes. J Refract Surg. 2014;30(11):746–53.
115. Li N, Fan Z, Peng X, Pang X, Tian C. Clinical observation of transepithelial corneal collagen cross-linking by lontophoresis of riboflavin in treatment of keratoconus. Eye Sci. 2014;29(3):160–4.
116. Buzzonetti L, Petrocelli G, Valente P, Iarossi G, Ardia R, Petroni S. Iontophoretic transepithelial corneal cross-linking to halt keratoconus in pediatric cases: 15-month follow-up. Cornea. 2015;34(5):512–5.
117. Magli A, Chiariello Vecchio E, Carelli R, Piozzi E, Di Landro F, Troisi S. Pediatric keratoconus and iontophoretic corneal crosslinking: refractive and topographic evidence in patients underwent general and topical anesthesia, 18 months of follow-up. Int Ophthalmol. 2016;36:585–90.
118. Laborante A, Longo C, Mazzilli E, Giardinelli K. Corneal iontophoresis and cross linking: a preliminary report of our experience. Clin Ter. 2015;166(4):e254–6.
119. Jia HZ, Pang X, Fan ZJ, Li N, Li G, Peng XJ. Iontophoresis-assisted corneal crosslinking using 0.1% riboflavin for progressive keratoconus. Int J Ophthalmol. 2017;10(5):717–22.
120. Bikbova G, Bikbov M. Standard corneal collagen crosslinking versus transepithelial iontophoresis-assisted corneal crosslinking, 24 months follow-up: randomized control trial. Acta Ophthalmol. 2016;94(7):e600–6. https://doi.org/10.1111/aos.13032. Epub 2016 Apr 4.
121. Vinciguerra P, Romano V, Rosetta P, Legrottaglie EF, Piscopo R, Fabiani C, Azzolini C, Vinciguerra R. Transepithelial iontophoresis versus standard corneal collagen cross-linking: 1-year results of a prospective clinical study. J Refract Surg. 2016;32(10):672–8.
122. Lombardo M, Giannini D, Lombardo G, Serrao S. Randomized controlled trial comparing transepithelial corneal cross-linking using iontophoresis with the Dresden protocol in progressive keratoconus. Ophthalmology. 2017;124(6):804–12.

123. Hayes S, Morgan S, O'Brart DP, O'Brart N, Meek KM. A study of stromal riboflavin absorption using new and existing delivery protocols for corneal cross-linking. Acta Ophthalmol. 2016;94(2):e109–17.
124. Gore DM, O'Brart D, Dunsby C, French P, Allan BD. A comparison of different corneal iontophoresis protocols for promoting transepithelial riboflavin penetration. Invest Ophthalmol Vis Sci. 2015;56(13):7908–14.
125. Aldahlawi NH, Hayes S, O'Brart DPS, O'Brart NA, Meek KM. An investigation into corneal enzymatic resistance following epithelium-off and epithelium-on corneal cross-linking protocols. Exp Eye Res. 2016;153:141–51.
126. Lamy R, Chan E, Zhang H, Salgaonkar VA, Good SD, Porco TC, Diederich CJ, Stewart JM. Ultrasound-enhanced penetration of topical riboflavin into the corneal stroma. Invest Ophthalmol Vis Sci. 2013;54(8):5908–12.
127. Bottos KM, Oliveira AG, Bersanetti PA, Nogueira RF, Lima-Filho AA, Cardillo JA, Schor P, Chamon W. Corneal absorption of a new riboflavin-nanostructured system for transepithelial collagen cross-linking. PLoS One. 2013;8(6):e66408.
128. Kanellopoulos AJ. Collagen cross-linking in early keratoconus with riboflavin in a femtosecond laser-created pocket: initial clinical results. J Refract Surg. 2009;25(11):1034–7.

Chapter 6
Accelerated Corneal Cross-Linking

Leopoldo Spadea, Rita Napolitano, Emanuele Tonti, and Vittoria De Rosa

6.1 Introduction

Corneal cross-linking (CXL) consists in the induction of a tissue biomechanical alteration, which leads to a stiffening, and strengthening of the ectatic corneal tissue. The treatment involves the use of the riboflavin (Vitamin B2) as a photoinducer, an ultraviolet light source and a photochemical reaction that creates a chemical bond between collagen fibrils. The safety of the ultraviolet light parameters depends on wavelength, irradiance and time of irradiation [1]. According to the original standard Dresden protocol, firstly described by Wollensak et al., the maximum efficacy of tissue stiffening is obtained by using 3 mW/cm^2 of energy for 30 min, which corresponds to a total energy dose (fluence) of 5.4 J/cm^2 [2]. The procedure includes the prior epithelium removal and the application of 0.1% riboflavin solution for 30 min followed by 30 min of UVA irradiation.

The effectiveness and safety of standard CXL has been demonstrated by several clinical trials [3–6], however the long UVA exposure required is considered as a drawback of the procedure since it reduces the patient's comfort and increases the risk of corneal dehydration [7, 8]. To limit these complications, several modifications to standard CXL have been proposed, including the use of higher intensity and shorter duration radiation (accelerated CXL, ACXL). The safety and effectiveness of ACXL is based on the Bunsen-Roscoe law of reciprocity [9], stating that a photochemical effect should be similar as long as total fluence remains constant. That means that with shorter treatment times and higher intensity UV exposure is it possible to obtain the same results. Currently available devices allow to achieve irradiance intensity up to 43 mW/cm^2 thus providing a

L. Spadea (✉) · R. Napolitano · E. Tonti · V. De Rosa
Department of Biotechnology and Medical-Surgical Sciences, "Sapienza" University of Rome, Latina, Italy
e-mail: leopoldo.spadea@uniroma1.it

A. Barbara (ed.), *Controversies in the Management of Keratoconus*,
https://doi.org/10.1007/978-3-319-98032-4_6

radiant exposure of 5.4 J/cm^2 within a total treatment time up to 2 min, which is exactly the same amount of energy of Dresden protocol. Treatment protocols, concerning the relationship between treatment time and UV intensity, are still in evolution.

6.2 Treatment Protocols for Accelerated Corneal Cross-Linking

6.2.1 High Fluency Cross-Linking

The most widely used treatment protocols for ACXL use an irradiation time of 10, 5, or 3 min with an irradiance intensity respectively of 9 mW/cm^2, 18 mW/cm^2 and 30 mW/cm^2, so that the total energy levels achieved are similar to that proposed by the Dresden protocol [10]. However, animal studies demonstrated that the Bunsen and Roscoe reciprocity law is valid only for illumination intensity up to 45 mW/cm^2 and an irradiance time greater than 2 min, since a loss of effectiveness was shown by treatment protocols using an irradiation intensity from 50 mW/cm^2 up to 90 mW/cm^2 [11].

It has also been shown that high irradiation intensity led to an higher increase in corneal densitometry, demonstrating that the energy dose used in AC protocols, plays a role in the CXL-induced postoperative corneal haze. However the increase in corneal density progressively decreased over time and returned completely to the baseline level at 12 months [12].

Clinical results concerning ACXL have been generally positive to date. Kanellopoulos demonstrated a similar efficacy and refractive effect between conventional crosslinking and an accelerated protocol (7 mW/cm^2 for 15 min), with no adverse effects [13]. Several studies reported the achievement of the corneal stability and an improvement in visual acuity following a 10-min irradiation at 9 mW/cm^2 [14–16].

The higher energy and shorter duration of treatment has proven to be a good option for paediatric patients as well [17].

6.2.2 Pulsed Accelerated Cross-Linking

Another treatment modification for ACXL include the pulsed ACXL [18]. It has been evidenced that the corneal cross-linking is an oxygen-dependent reaction since the responsible for the creation of new covalent bonds between collagen fibrils are the reactive oxygen species (ROS) created by irradiation of riboflavin applied on corneal tissue [19]. Hence, pulsing the UV light during crosslinking treatment seems to allow the achievement of an additional oxygen concentration, thus increasing the effectiveness of the procedure. Mazzotta et al. in their comparative study demonstrated that pulsed light treatment give a better functional outcome compared to continuous light procedure, thanks to its better capabilities to penetrate deeper in the corneal stroma [20]. A subsequent study investigating the depth of corneal stromal demarcation line, the transition zone between the anterior cross-linked stroma and the posterior untreated stroma, after continuous and pulsed ACXL, confirmed this outcomes [21, 22].

6.2.3 Transepithelial Accelerated Cross-Linking

Newer techniques, by using different delivery method of riboflavin, allow the diffusion of the photoinducer across an intact corneal epithelium. There are three different methods through which the transepithelium diffusion of the riboflavin is made possible: modifying the epithelium permeability [23], changing the physiochemical propriety of riboflavin molecule [24] and delivering the riboflavin directly into the corneal stroma [25]. The first method involves the use of chemical enhancers, such as benzalkonium chloride (BAK), ethylenediaminetetracetic acid (EDTA) or trometamol (TE), in way to loose intraepithelial tight-junction and facilitate the diffusion of the riboflavin into the stroma. However experimental data have shown that BAK-enhanced CXL, without epithelial debridement, reduced the biomechanical effect by approximately one fifth compared to standard crosslinking [26].

As a negatively charged, water soluble molecule with a low molecular weight (376.40 g/mol), riboflavin is known to be useful for iontophoresis, a non-invasive delivery system via a small electric current [27, 28]. It has been shown that iontophoresis assisted transepithelial CXL is effective in stopping keratoconus progression after 2 years, with an improvement in the visual and topographic parameters. However with regard to a visible demarcation line, it seems to provide a more superficial effect compared to standard procedures [29].

The third delivery method of riboflavin is the intrastromal administration through a femtosecond-laser created corneal pocket. Kanellopoulus theorized that instilling the riboflavin solution directly into the corneal stroma would achieve a greater concentration of the photoinducer in the anterior two-thirds of the cornea. Thus, with the aid of a femtosecond laser, he created an intrastromal pocket at 100-μm corneal depth through which the riboflavin solution was administered. This technique is significantly less painful for patients, however potential risks of the femtosecond laser application (suction, corneal dissection, and potential microbial implantation) should be weighed by the clinician [25].

6.3 Comparison of Accelerated vs Conventional Corneal Cross-Linking

Although various clinical studies demonstrated that the ACXL provided stabilization of corneal ectasia, it is still controversial whether the ability of modified cross-linking to stop progression of keratoconus is equivalent to that of standard procedures. The main drawback of comparative studies between conventional and ACXL is the variety of protocols. Regarding the 9 mW/cm^2 protocols, Cummings et al., found out no differences between standard and accelerated treatment in terms of uncorrected visual acuity, best spectacle-corrected visual acuity and refractive astigmatism. Additionally corneal flattening was found in both protocols, and no adverse events were observed [30]. Sadoughi et al., in another recent randomized intrapatient comparative study, demonstrated analogous results with similar outcomes between groups in terms of functional and topographic values [31]. Kymionis analyzed the depth of the corneal demarcation line, to valuate the extent of the ACXL (9 mW/cm^2) compared to the standard treatment. He observed that it was significantly deeper after a 30-min CXL treatment than after a 10-min CXL procedure [32]. This was also supported by a subsequent study of Ng, who used the same illumination intensity of 9.0 mW/cm^2, demonstrating that the demarcation line was significantly shallower after ACXL compared to that observed in conventional CXL. He postulated that with decreasing duration and increasing intensity of UVA irradiation, the depth and visibility of the demarcation line reduced. This is probably due to the insufficient oxygen diffusion into the cornea, for the raised oxygen consumption required for high intensity CXL [33]. For this reason Kymionis propose a 40% increase in irradiation time using an intensity of 9 mW/cm^2 for 14 min, instead of 10 min. In this way a total energy of 7.5 J/cm^2 was achieved and a similar central demarcation line depth was reported between both ACXL and conventional treatment protocol [34].

As of the 18 mW/cm^2 treatment, a study by Chow et al. find out no statistically significant differences between both treatment modalities. However a more effective topographic flattening was observed with conventional CXL [35]. Similarly, Hashemi et al., in two consecutive studies, showed a comparable outcome and safety profile between conventional and 18 mW/cm^2 ACXL, but better corneal flattening was achieved with the standard method [36, 37].

The 30 mW/cm^2 irradiance for 3 min in all published studies demonstrated to be safe and effective. Tomita et al. reported two separate cohorts with similar accelerated protocols (30 mW/cm^2 for 3 min), but different riboflavin soak times (10 min or 15 min), and they found all measured outcomes were similar to standard protocol [38]. Hashemi et al. reported 15 months follow- up of standard and accelerated (30 mW/cm^2 for 3 min) protocols with similar equivalent outcomes. They also found less decrease in anterior stromal keratocyte density with the accelerated protocol and less disruption of the sub-basal nerve plexus in the accelerated group [39]. Ozgurhan et al. also observed less sub-basal nerve disruption with an accelerated protocol [40]. In a prospective randomized study, Shetty et al. compared the conventional technique with ACXL using an irradiance intensity of 9 mW/cm^2, 18 mW/cm^2 and 30 mW/cm^2 in four different groups of patients. The authors found greater refractive and keratometric efficacy in the 3 mW/cm^2 and 9 mW/cm^2 groups as compared to the higher irradiation protocols and all groups showed a reduction in endothelial cell density [10].

A recent study involving 36 progressive keratoconus patients treated with ACXL, demonstrated a transient toxic effect on the endothelium. More specifically it was found a change in the endothelial cell density, in percentages of hexagonality and coefficient of variation of endothelial cell area, 1 month postoperatively. However a resolution of these changes has been seen during the follow-up period, thus suggesting the reversibility of toxic effect of the treatment [41].

6.4 Conclusion

Cross-linking is still an evolving technology and literature on ACXL is continuously expanding. Both standard procedures and accelerated techniques have been proved to halt progressive keratoconus. In fact, although not all accelerated protocols provide equivalent outcomes, they all seem to be safe and effective. The 9 mW/cm^2 accelerated protocol seems to be more similar to conventional CXL, while the higher irradiance accelerated protocols exhibit less topographical flattening. Regarding the depth of stromal demarcation line, the outcomes of several studies are in favor of the conventional protocol, but it is not proven that the morphological outcome translates into the clinical and functional efficacy. Furthermore the high fluency procedures offer the advantage of reducing the patient discomfort, achieving a more effective time management, and avoiding the excessive corneal dehydration and thinning which can occur during the 30 min of the standard protocol. Hence, thus far, accelerated corneal collagen cross-linking can be considered a safe, quick and efficient procedure for the management of corneal ectatic disorders.

References

1. Remé C, Reinboth J, Clausen M, Hafezi F. Light damage revisited: converging evidence, diverging views? Graefes Arch Clin Exp Ophthalmol. 1996;234(1):2–11.
2. Wollensak G, Spoerl E, Seiler T. Riboflavin/ultraviolet-a-induced collagen crosslinking for the treatment of keratoconus. Am J Ophthalmol. 2003;135:620–7.
3. Hafezi F, Kanellopoulos J, Wiltfang R, Seiler T. Corneal collagen crosslinking with riboflavin and ultraviolet A to treat induced keratectasia after laser in situ keratomileusis. J Cataract Refract Surg. 2007;33(12):2035–40.
4. Caporossi A, Mazzotta C, Baiocchi S. Long-term results of riboflavin ultraviolet a corneal collagen cross-linking for keratoconus in Italy: the Siena Eye Cross Study. Am J Ophthalmol. 2010;149(4):585–93.
5. Vinciguerra P, Albe E, Trazza S. Intraoperative and postoperative effects of corneal collagen cross-linking on progressive keratoconus. Arch Ophthalmol. 2009;127(10):1258–65.

6. Spoerl E, Mrochen M, Sliney D, Trokel S, Seiler T. Safety of UVAriboflavin cross-linking of the cornea. Cornea. 2007;26(4):385–9.
7. Kymionis GD, Kontadakis GA, Hashemi KK. Accelerated versus conventional corneal cross-linking for refractive instability: an update. Curr Opin Ophthalmol. 2017;28(4):343–7.
8. Randleman JB, Khandelwal SS, Hafezi F. Corneal cross-linking. Surv Ophthalmol. 2015;60(6):509–23.
9. Bunsen RW, Roscoe HE. Photochemical researches – part V. On the measurement of the chemical action of direct and diffuse sunlight. Proc R Soc Lond. 1862;12:306–12.
10. Shetty R, Pahuja NK, Nuijts RM, et al. Current protocols of corneal collagen cross-linking: visual, refractive, and tomographic outcomes. Am J Ophthalmol. 2015;160:243–9.
11. Wernli J, Schumacher S, Spoerl E, Mrochen M. The efficacy of corneal cross-linking shows a sudden decrease with very high intensity UV light and short treatment time. Invest Ophthalmol Vis Sci. 2013;54:1176–80.
12. Akkaya TS, Toker E. Changes in corneal density after accelerated corneal collagen cross-linking with different irradiation intensities and energy exposures: 1-year follow-up. Cornea. 2017;36(11):1331–5.
13. Kanellopoulos AJ. Long term results of a prospective randomized bilateral eye comparison trial of higher fluence, shorter duration ultraviolet A radiation, and riboflavin collagen cross linking for progressive keratoconus. Clin Ophthalmol. 2012;6:97–101.
14. Elbaz U, Shen C, Lichtinger A, et al. Accelerated (9-mW/cm^2) corneal collagen crosslinking for keratoconus-A 1-year follow-up. Cornea. 2014;33:769–73.
15. Cınar Y, Cingü AK, Türkcü FM, et al. Comparison of accelerated and conventional corneal collagen cross-linking for progressive keratoconus. Cutan Ocul Toxicol. 2014;33:218–22.
16. Kymionis GD, Grentzelos MA, Kankariya VP, et al. Safety of high-intensity corneal collagen crosslinking. J Cataract Refract Surg. 2014;40:1337–40.
17. Ulusoy DM, Göktaş E, Duru N, et al. Accelerated corneal crosslinking for treatment of progressive keratoconus in pediatric patients. Eur J Ophthalmol. 2017;27:319–25.
18. Sachdev GS, Sachdev M. Recent advances in corneal collagen cross-linking. Indian J Ophthalmol. 2017;65:787–96.
19. Richoz O, Hammer A, Tabibian D, et al. The biomechanical effect of corneal collagen crosslinking (CXL) with riboflavin and UV-A is oxygen dependent. Transl Vis Sci Technol. 2013;2:6.
20. Mazzotta C, Traversi C, Paradiso AL, Latronico ME, Rechichi M. Pulsed light accelerated crosslinking versus continuous light accelerated crosslinking: one-year results. J Ophthalmol. 2014;2014:604731.
21. Spadea L, Tonti E, Vingolo EM. Corneal stromal demarcation line after collagen cross-linking in corneal ectatic diseases: a review of the literature. Clin Ophthalmol. 2016;10:1803–10.
22. Moramarco A, Iovieno A, Sartori A, Fontana L. Corneal stromal demarcation line after accelerated crosslinking using continuous and pulsed light. J Cataract Refract Surg. 2015;41(11):2546–51.
23. Akbar B, Intisar-Ul-Haq R, Ishaq M, Arzoo S, Siddique K. Transepithelial corneal cross-linking in treatment of progressive keratoconus: 12 months' clinical results. Pak J Med Sci. 2017;33(3):570–5.
24. Magli A, Chiariello Vecchio E, Carelli R, Piozzi E, Di Landro F, Troisi S. Pediatric keratoconus and iontophoretic corneal crosslinking: refractive and topographic evidence in patients underwent general and topical anesthesia, 18 months of follow-up. Int Ophthalmol. 2016;36(4):585–90.
25. Kanellopoulos AJ. Collagen cross-linking in early keratoconus with riboflavin in a femtosecond laser-created pocket: initial clinical results. J Refract Surg. 2009;25(11):1034–7.
26. Wollensak G, Iomdina E. Biomechanical and histological changes after corneal crosslinking with and without epithelial debridement. J Cataract Refract Surg. 2009;35(3):540–6.
27. Bikbova G, Bikbov M. Transepithelial corneal collagen cross-linking by iontophoresis of riboflavin. Acta Ophthalmol. 2014;92(1):e30–4.

28. Spadea L, Maraone G, Cagini C. Sliding keratoplasty followed by transepithelial iontophoresis collagen cross-linking for pellucid marginal degeneration. J Refract Surg. 2016;31(19):47–50.
29. Bikbova G, Bikbov M. Standard corneal collagen crosslinking versus transepithelial iontophoresis-assisted corneal crosslinking, 24 months follow-up: randomized control trial. Acta Ophthalmol. 2016;94(7):e600–6.
30. Cummings AB, McQuaid R, Naughton S, Brennan E, Mrochen M. Optimizing corneal cross-linking in the treatment of keratoconus: a comparison of outcomes after standard- and high-intensity protocols. Cornea. 2016;35(6):814–22.
31. Sadoughi MM, Einollahi B, Baradaran-Rafii A, et al. Accelerated versus conventional corneal collagen cross-linking in patients with keratoconus: an intrapatient comparative study. Int Ophthalmol. 2018;38:67–74.
32. Kymionis GD, Tsoulnaras KI, Grentzelos MA, et al. Corneal stroma demarcation line after standard and high intensity collagen crosslinking determined with anterior segment optical coherence tomography. J Cataract Refract Surg. 2014;40:736–40.
33. Ng AL, Chan TC, Lai JS, Cheng AC. Comparison of the central and peripheral corneal stromal demarcation line depth in conventional versus accelerated collagen cross-linking. Cornea. 2015;34(11):1432–6.
34. Kymionis GD, Tsoulnaras KI, Grentzelos MA, et al. Evaluation of corneal stromal demarcation line depth following standard and a modified-accelerated collagen cross-linking protocol. Am J Ophthalmol. 2014;158:671–675.e1.
35. Chow VW, Chan TC, Yu M, Wong VW, Jhanji V. One-year outcomes of conventional and accelerated collagen crosslinking in progressive keratoconus. Sci Rep. 2015;5:14425.
36. Hashemi H, Miraftab M, Seyedian MA, et al. Long-term results of an accelerated corneal cross-linking protocol (18 mW/cm^2) for the treatment of progressive keratoconus. Am J Ophthalmol. 2015;160(6):1164–70.
37. Hashemi H, Fotouhi A, Miraftab M, et al. Short-term comparison of accelerated and standard methods of corneal collagen crosslinking. J Cataract Refract Surg. 2015;41:533–40.
38. Tomita M, Mita M, Huseynova T. Accelerated versus conventional corneal collagen crosslinking. J Cataract Refract Surg. 2014;40:1013–20.
39. Hashemian H, Jabbarvand M, Khodaparast M, Ameli K. Evaluation of corneal changes after conventional versus accelerated corneal cross-linking: a randomized controlled trial. J Refract Surg. 2014;30(12):837–42.
40. Ozgurhan EB, Celik U, Bozkurt E, Demirok A. Evaluation of subbasal nerve morphology and corneal sensation after accelerated corneal collagen cross-linking treatment on keratoconus. Curr Eye Res. 2015;40(5):484–9.
41. Cingu AK, Sogutlu-Sari E, Cınar Y, et al. Transient corneal endothelial changes following accelerated collagen cross-linking for the treatment of progressive keratoconus. Cutan Ocul Toxicol. 2014;33:127–31.

Chapter 7
The Role of Oxygen in Corneal Cross-Linking

Emilio A. Torres Netto, Sabine Kling, and Farhad Hafezi

It has been shown in multiple studies that corneal cross-linking (CXL) successfully stops keratoconus [1] progression and arrests post-surgical corneal ectasia [2]. CXL is based on a photochemical process that involves a chromophore (riboflavin, vitamin B2) and energy (UV-A light) [3]. In 2012, our group identified that in addition oxygen is essential for the CXL process. In a mechanism similar to photodynamic therapy, highly reactive oxygen species are created and lead to the formation of new cross-links in the extracellular matrix. These cross-links increase the mechanical resistance and stability of the tissue [4].

From the biochemical perspective, the free oxygen radicals oxidize the extracellular matrix and lead to the formation of additional bonds on the surface of collagen molecules, as well as between proteoglycan core proteins [5]. If too little oxygen is available in the corneal stroma, then fewer cross-links are formed. In the absence of oxygen, no cross-links occur [6, 7].

E. A. Torres Netto · S. Kling
Laboratory for Ocular Cell Biology, University of Zurich, Zürich, Switzerland
e-mail: emilioatorres@me.com; klings@ee.ethz.ch

F. Hafezi (✉)
Laboratory for Ocular Cell Biology, University of Zurich, Zürich, Switzerland

Roski Eye Institute, University of Southern California, Los Angeles, CA, USA

Department of Ophthalmology, Wenzhou Medical University, Wenzhou, China

Faculty of Medicine, University of Geneva, Geneva, Switzerland
e-mail: farhad@hafezi.ch

A. Barbara (ed.), *Controversies in the Management of Keratoconus*,
https://doi.org/10.1007/978-3-319-98032-4_7

7.1 Reaction Mechanism and Kinetics

The green fluorescence of riboflavin indicates the relaxation from the singlet excited state of riboflavin upon the absorption of the UVA; to a certain extent, intersystem crossing occurs leading to the excitation of the triplet excited state. The latter has a longer live time and therefore allows for chemical reactions such as the generation of reactive oxygen species. It is important to note that the UV energy that is applied during CXL treatment is not sufficient for ionization [8].

Nonetheless, the interaction of the triplet excited sate of riboflavin – either with oxygen or the extracellular matrix – has the potential to create highly reactive oxygen species and radicals that in turn oxidize the extracellular matrix. Here, oxygen modulates two mechanisms of photochemical reactions: type-I and type-II, the latter being the one with the highest oxygen consumption [8]. At high oxygen concentrations, type-I mechanism dominates, while at low oxygen concentrations, type-II mechanism dominates. Up to date it is unclear, if type-I or type-II mechanism is responsible for the increase in corneal stiffness.

7.2 Emergence of New Protocols

Standard epithelium-off CXL with total fluence of 5.4 J/cm^2 and irradiation time of 30 min (Dresden protocol) certainly have the greatest body of evidence in CXL technology and it has been in clinical use for more than 15 years. With the emergence of new LED technologies, protocol modifications to make the procedure shorter have been attempted. In this way, the same fluence could be delivered in less time. However, the Bunson-Roscoe law of reciprocity, which states that an equivalent photochemical effect could be achieved with any combination of intensity and fluence, does only apply for photo damage, but not for the generation of stabilizing cross-links in the context of CXL treatment. Therefore, many of the recently suggested CXL protocol modifications are less effective as they result in lower oxygen availability.

To better understand the potential of new accelerated technologies, in 2014 our group studied the stiffening effect under different irradiation times. When compared to the Dresden protocol, 10 min of irradiation at 9 mW/cm^2 already showed a significant decrease in the stiffening effect, which was even more pronounced at 5 min at 18 mW/cm^2 [9]. Not only laboratory, the clinical results also seem to present the same tendency [10], with mixed results when we observe studies that use faster techniques [11].

In the presence of riboflavin and UV irradiation, there is a fast depletion of the oxygen in the cornea, which lasts for about 10–15 s with fluence of 3 mW/cm^2 and only 2–5 s with fluence of 30 mW/cm^2. In addition, it is known that oxygen replenishment is slow, around 34 min. We believe this dependence on oxygen may explain many unsatisfactory results of new protocols under development.

Similarly, oxygen may be involved with epithelial-preserving techniques (epi-on). The epithelium itself consumes 10 times more oxygen than the stroma, and the epithelium also acts as a barrier to oxygen penetration [8, 12]. Even though trans-sepithelial techniques may improve riboflavin diffusion into the stroma, they do not influence the speed of oxygen diffusion.

Recently, contact lens-assisted cross-linking (caCXL) was proposed to treat thin corneas [13]. The contact lens soaked with riboflavin on the corneal surface would have the role of partial absorption of UV and preserve endothelial viability. On the other hand, at the same time the presence of a contact lens limits the diffusion of oxygen. Depending on the oxygen permeability of the applied contact lens, the availability of oxygen can be reduced by around 50%, which correlates with a reduced stiffening effect by the same percentage [6].

Alternating periods of UV radiation with period without irradiation was also another mode of treatment that emerged. The so-called pulsed CXL was intended to increase oxygen diffusion periodically, during the non-irradiated period, and thereby increase the efficacy of CXL. However, clinical studies have shown that although efficient, it is not superior to traditional CXL [14]. This is because the time required to replenish the oxygen in the cornea is much higher than that of its consumption, so short pulse intervals do not allow the complete restoration of the oxygen to the point of having some clinical advantage.

7.3 Final Messages

In order to be effective, the photochemical process of CXL not only requires irradiation with UV and riboflavin. Oxygen is the third fundamental and necessary element. Therefore, any technique or mechanism that decreases the availability of oxygen in the cornea during CXL potentially reduces the therapeutic stiffening effect. Due to limited intrastromal diffusion and rapid consumption, oxygen may be an important factor that leads to reduced biomechanical efficiency of many new modalities of CXL treatments.

References

1. Wollensak G, Spörl E, Seiler T. Treatment of keratoconus by collagen cross linking. Der Ophthalmologe: Zeitschrift der Deutschen Ophthalmologischen Gesellschaft. 2003;100(1):44–9.
2. Hafezi F, Kanellopoulos J, Wiltfang R, Seiler T. Corneal collagen crosslinking with riboflavin and ultraviolet A to treat induced keratectasia after laser in situ keratomileusis. J Cataract Refract Surg. 2007;33(12):2035–40.
3. Spörl E, Huhle M, Kasper M, Seiler T. Increased rigidity of the cornea caused by intrastromal cross-linking. Der Ophthalmologe: Zeitschrift der Deutschen Ophthalmologischen Gesellschaft. 1997;94(12):902–6.

4. Choi S, Shin JH, Cheong Y, Jin KH, Park HK. Structural and biomechanical effects of photooxidative collagen cross-linking with photosensitizer riboflavin and 370 nm UVA light on human corneoscleral tissues. Microsc Microanal. 2013;1:1–7.
5. Hayes S, Kamma-Lorger CS, Boote C, et al. The effect of riboflavin/UVA collagen cross-linking therapy on the structure and hydrodynamic behaviour of the ungulate and rabbit corneal stroma. PLoS One. 2013;8(1):e52860.
6. Kling S, Richoz O, Hammer A, et al. Increased biomechanical efficacy of corneal cross-linking in thin corneas due to higher oxygen availability. J Refract Surg. 2015;31(12):840–6.
7. Richoz O, Hammer A, Tabibian D, Gatzioufas Z, Hafezi F. The biomechanical effect of corneal collagen cross-linking (CXL) with riboflavin and UV-A is oxygen dependent. Transl Vision Sci Technol. 2013;2(7):6.
8. Kamaev P, Friedman MD, Sherr E, Muller D. Photochemical kinetics of corneal cross-linking with riboflavin. Invest Ophthalmol Vis Sci. 2012;53(4):2360–7.
9. Hammer A, Richoz O, Mosquera S, Tabibian D, Hoogewoud F, Hafezi F. Corneal biomechanical properties at different corneal collagen cross-linking (CXL) Irradiances. Invest Ophthalmol Vis Sci. 2014;55(5):2881–4.
10. Ng AL, Chan TC, Cheng AC. Conventional versus accelerated corneal collagen cross-linking in the treatment of keratoconus. Clin Exp Ophthalmol. 2015;44:8–14.
11. Hashemi H, Miraftab M, Seyedian MA, et al. Long-term results of an accelerated corneal cross-linking protocol 18mW/cm for the treatment of progressive keratoconus. Am J Ophthalmol. 2015;160:1164–70.
12. Freeman RD. Oxygen consumption by the component layers of the cornea. J Physiol. 1972;225(1):15–32.
13. Jacob S, Kumar DA, Agarwal A, Basu S, Sinha P, Agarwal A. Contact lens-assisted collagen cross-linking (CACXL): a new technique for cross-linking thin corneas. J Refract Surg. 2014;30(6):366–72.
14. Mazzotta C, Traversi C, Paradiso AL, Latronico ME, Rechichi M. Pulsed light accelerated crosslinking versus continuous light accelerated crosslinking: one-year results. J Ophthalmol. 2014;2014:604731.

Chapter 8
Beyond the Dresden Protocol: Optimization of Corneal Cross-Linking for Visual Function

Grace Lytle and John Marshall

8.1 Introduction

Keratoconus is a bilateral, asymmetric, non-inflammatory ectatic disorder of the cornea which results in progressive corneal thinning, corneal irregularity, and loss of visual function. The condition is a complex disorder of multifactorial etiology, associated with both genetic and environmental factors. The onset of keratoconus often occurs at puberty and commonly worsens until the fourth decade of life before it becomes relatively stabilized.

Temporary visual rehabilitation is often possible in patients with keratoconus with gas permeable and specialty contact lenses. These lenses mask the irregularity of the cornea and create a smooth refracting surface. However, to enable stable clear vision, tolerable all-day wear, and to avoid corneal scarring, rigid lenses must be properly fit to the corneal curvature. Lens fitting is challenging and time consuming in patients with keratoconus, as the progressive nature of ectasia makes the design of a lens to properly fit the cornea a moving target. Intracorneal ring segments (ICRS) may be surgically implanted to alter corneal curvature and reduce irregularity, however they do not stop progression of the disease, and in some cases, may complicate subsequent contact lens fitting. Therefore, management of keratoconus during the progressive years requires frequent office visits. Beyond the costs associated with managing the disease, the burden of time out of school or work, reduced visual function, and unpredictable disease course may have lifelong impact, as the condition is often at its most progressive during the time that affected patients are engaged in study or beginning their careers. This results in a significant reduction in quality of life, and a substantial lifetime economic burden for affected patients [1].

G. Lytle (✉)
Avedro, Waltham, MA, USA

J. Marshall
Institute of Ophthalmology University College London in association with Moorfields Eye Hospital, London, UK

A. Barbara (ed.), *Controversies in the Management of Keratoconus*,
https://doi.org/10.1007/978-3-319-98032-4_8

As keratoconus advances and the corneal irregularity increases, attempts at visual rehabilitation are less successful. Contact lens tolerance decreases, and best corrected visual acuity is reduced, resulting in penetrating keratoplasty in as many as 20% of patients with keratoconus [2]. Corneal transplantation has inherent risks that could result in permanent loss of vision and significantly impact the patient's quality of life during the surgical recovery phase. Therefore, any therapy to slow the progression of the disease is of substantial benefit, and disease modifying therapy is of greatest benefit if introduced prior to loss of visual function.

The corneal cross-linking procedure (CXL) is a minimally invasive, conservative intervention that offers the opportunity to preserve visual function by slowing or eliminating the development of further corneal irregularity. In an ideal scenario, keratoconus would be detected during routine ocular health screening, enabling diagnosis at the onset of the ectasia and CXL treatment to arrest its continual development before visual function is impaired. Today, keratoconus is more commonly diagnosed following the onset of visual systems, and many patients do not present for CXL treatment until visual function has already been significantly compromised.

Since the first reports of the clinical application of this procedure were published in 2003, CXL has rapidly been adopted as the only therapy to halt the progression of ectasia. In 2015, a global Delphi panel comprised of representatives from each of the four supranational corneal societies – the Asia Cornea Society (Asia), Cornea Society (USA and international), EuCornea (Europe) and PanCornea (Latin America, United States and Canada) – published a consensus report that recognized the importance of incorporating CXL as part of the new standard of care in progressive keratoconus and preserving visual function [3]. Multiple research groups around the world have evaluated and introduced modifications to the original procedure to improve efficiency and reduce treatment time. Further, newer treatment protocols aim to not only halt disease progression, but to restore visual function in those patients who did not receive early intervention before visual quality or contact lens tolerance was lost.

8.2 Conventional Corneal Cross-Linking: The Dresden Protocol

Keratoconus progresses most rapidly during puberty and stabilizes with age. Age-related increases in corneal stiffness result from glycation induced cross-linking that occurs between or within stromal collagen lamellae due to the accumulation of non-enzymatic glycation end products over time. Knox Cartwright et al. describe a twofold increase in corneal stiffness between the ages of 20 and 100 years, demonstrated by a linear decrease in apical cornea displacement in response to change in intraocular pressure equivalent to that which occurs during the cardiac cycle [4]. The conventional cross-linking procedure imparts its effect by stiffening the corneal stromal lamellae, mimicking the age-related cross-linking that naturally occurs in the cornea over time. This strengthens the cornea and stabilizes against further progression of the ectasia [5–9].

There are several methods by which cross-linking can be achieved in collagenous tissues, including the non-enzymatic glycation that occurs with age, from aldehyde actions, and through irradiation with ultraviolet light and a photosensitizer. The first series of experiments to determine whether the induction of crosslinks stiffened the cornea with riboflavin were conducted at Technical University of Dresden, Germany and presented in the seminal paper by Spoerl et al. [10]. Photochemical cross-linking techniques using riboflavin and light of wavelengths near the absorption peaks of riboflavin (365 nm and 436 nm) were compared to UV alone (254 nm) and to the standard chemical cross-linking agents glutaraldehyde and Karnovsky's solution. Both chemical cross-linking and photochemical cross-linking with 365 nm UVA were effective at strengthening porcine corneas, as measured by stress-strain testing of corneal strips. Riboflavin and UVA cross-linked corneal tissue demonstrated increased resistance to enzymatic digestion and altered thermal shrinkage behavior. The toxicity of chemical cross-linkers and the long exposure required of aldehyde sugars made the use of UVA and a riboflavin 5-phosphate photosensitizer the most clinically viable of these techniques. Prior to evaluation in human patients, further laboratory experiments were used to measure the dose response to various stiffening techniques of the cornea [11], and to evaluate the safety of the procedure by studying keratocyte cytotoxicity [12], endothelial cytotoxicity in-vitro [13], endothelial cell damage in-vivo [14], and according to international standards for UV exposure.

The results of the first clinical study of the use of riboflavin-5-phosphate and UVA light cross-linking as a treatment for progressive keratoconus were published in 2003 by a group from the same institution, utilizing a set of treatment parameters derived from this early laboratory work. In all cases treated in this initial study, progression of ectasia was stopped, as measured by change in maximum keratometry value (KMax), and no significant adverse events were noted other than transient stromal edema [15].

The technique introduced by the group at the Technical University of Dresden, termed the Dresden protocol, is performed after removal of the central corneal epithelium. First, the stroma is saturated with 0.1% riboflavin 5-phosphate for 30 min. Then, a broad beam (7–9 mm in diameter) of UVA irradiation at at 3 mW/cm^2 is applied for another 30-min interval, resulting in an energy dose of 5.4 J/cm^2. Additional riboflavin drops are instilled at 2–5 min intervals during the irradiation phase, requiring medical staff to remain with the patient throughout the more than one hour long procedure [15].

The clinical goal of Dresden CXL is to decrease disease progression over time by means of corneal biomechanical strengthening. CXL results in the formation of covalent bonds within the intracellular matrix of the collagen lamellae, effectively stiffening the cornea in the treated zone [7]. Because there is no standard clinical approach to evaluate severity of keratoconus through direct biomechanical measurement, disease severity is conventionally assessed through the degree of steepening and irregularity of the anterior corneal curvature. Therefore, maximum keratometry (Kmax) is often used as a quantitative indicator of keratoconus severity, and change in Kmax over time is frequently used as the primary measure of clinical progression.

Several randomized controlled clinical trials have demonstrated that CXL effectively halts the progression of keratoconus. These studies show statistically significant improvement in KMax [16] or cone apex power [17] in Dresden CXL-treated eyes relative to untreated controls, although progression of KMax of 2.00 D or more has been observed between 0% to 4.3% of Dresden CXL-treated eyes [16–18]. A long term study of patients treated with the Dresden protocol reveals persistence of the treatment effect through a 10 year follow-up time period [19].

Two United States phase III multicenter, prospective, randomized, sham-controlled clinical trials have evaluated the safety and efficacy of corneal cross-linking for progressive keratoconus performed according to the Dresden protocol [20, 21]. A difference of at least 1.0 D in the mean change in maximum keratometry from baseline to 1 year, comparing the treatment and control groups, was chosen as a clinically meaningful endpoint of study success. Thus, either stabilization or improvement in maximum keratometry would indicate a positive effect of the procedure on disease evolution, whereas an increase in maximum keratometry would suggest continued progression. In the CXL treatment groups, the maximum keratometry value decreased by 1.6 diopters (D) from baseline to 1 year (pooled data), whereas keratoconus continued to progress in the control group. The trials demonstrated that the procedure was effective at stabilizing the progression of keratoconus with an excellent safety profile, enabling approval of a riboflavin and UVA delivery device combination product (Fig. 8.1: Avedro KXL) for the treatment of progressive keratoconus by the US Food and Drug Administration (FDA) in April 2016.

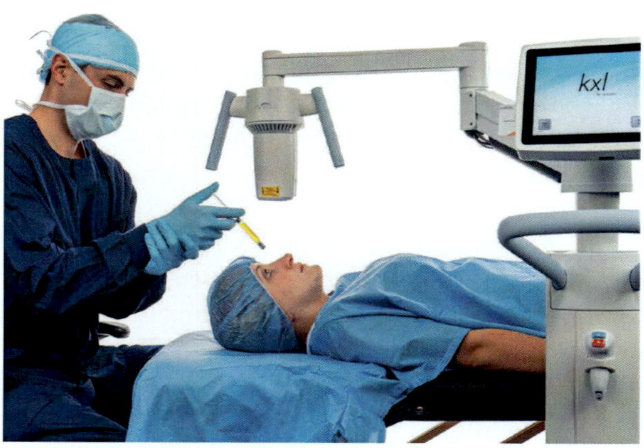

Fig. 8.1 Corneal cross-linking procedure performed with the US FDA approved system (KXL, Avedro)

8.3 Cross-Linking Distribution: Keratoconus Microstructure

Dresden protocol CXL was the first procedure to provide a conservative method of slowing or stopping the progression of ectatic disease, and the introduction of CXL has revolutionized the management of patients with keratoconus. However, while keratoconus is a heterogenous disorder with varied clinical presentation, the conventional approach to CXL uses a single treatment protocol in all eligible cases, regardless of keratoconus severity or degree of visual impairment. The treatment is centered on the cornea, although most cones are eccentric and inferior. While simple to perform, the conventional Dresden protocol is also lengthy, with total treatment time of more than one hour per treated eye. Variations to the original protocol have been introduced to improve procedural efficiency, aiming to reduce treatment time, making the procedure more cost effective and less disruptive to clinical workflow. Additional modifications have been introduced to target disease regression (flattening of steepest keratometry or improved corneal regularization) or improved visual function in addition to stabilization (reduction of optical aberrations or improved contact lens tolerance). These modifications are based on improved understanding of the photochemistry of the procedure and the biomechanical properties of the cornea, which enable personalized application of corneal cross-linking [22].

The clinical CXL procedure using riboflavin in combination with UVA induces extra covalent bonds in the corneal stroma to achieve its stiffening effect [7]. The exact extent of cross-linking that is required to prevent progression of ectasia at any stage of keratoconus has not yet been definitively determined. In considering this, it is helpful to imagine a CXL procedure terminated prematurely. In this scenario, would you expect no stiffening effect, the same effect, or something in between? Likely, your first thought would be to wonder just how prematurely the procedure was terminated- after 20% of UVA dose was delivered, for example, or 80%? We wonder this because we intuitively expect to obtain a partial stiffening effect with partial treatment. Your next thought maybe be to wonder whether a patient with a cornea that is weaker to begin with requires the same degree of stiffening as a patient with a stronger cornea. This exercise helps to remind us that cross-linking is not an "all or nothing" phenomenon, but that the amount and distribution of cross-link bonds formed is the result of a series of photochemical reactions, and therefore it is reasonable to assume that this distribution will vary with modification to the cross-linking protocol. And in fact, when all other factors are held equal, reducing the UVA dose delivered (holding irradiance constant and reducing treatment time), reduces the amount of stiffening obtained [23].

Potential new CXL protocols are often evaluated in laboratory studies by comparing the tissue response to a given treatment to that obtained with the Dresden protocol, using the Dresden results as a relative historical standard. However, the amount of corneal strengthening obtained with the Dresden protocol is not necessarily optimal for every patient, at every stage of keratoconus. The level of strengthening achieved is most likely more than is necessary in some cases, and insufficient in others [24]. In the treatment of ectasia, this has been evidenced by the substantial variability in the degree of corneal flattening that is observed following cross-linking treatment [25], and by a reported failure rate of 1–7.6%, defined as continued progression of Kmax [26–28]. The Dresden protocol may be one step in a continuum of options for cross-linking treatment, and clinical workflow as well as individual patient factors, such as age [29], corneal pachymetry [13], severity of disease state [26], and ability to comply with post-operative instructions [30] may all be considered when determining the optimal treatment approach.

The exact location of the UVA and riboflavin induced cross-links in the corneal stroma is not yet definitively known and may vary based on the rate of cross-link formation. There are several possible molecular sites for UVA and riboflavin induced collagen cross-linking. Intrahelical or interhelical cross-links can form within or between the tropocollagen units that comprise the individual collagen microfibrils. Intermicrofibrillar cross-links can form between adjacent collagen microfibrils that make up the collagen fibrils. The stability (denaturation temperature and resistance against enzymatic degradation) of collagen is mainly determined by its tropocollagen intrahelical and interhelical cross-links, whereas intermicrofibrillar cross-links significantly affect its mechanical properties (tissue shrinkage during fixation, tensile strength, strain at break, and rupture pattern) [31].

Corneal collagen cross-linking increases the corneal resistance to collagenolytic enzymes and increases the temperature threshold for hydrothermal shrinkage. These biomechanical and biochemical properties observed in corneal collagen after UVA-riboflavin cross-linking procedures provide evidence that the cross-linking may occur both within and between the tropocollagen units (interhelically and intrahelically) and between the collagen fibrils (intermicrofibrillar). The interfibrillar bonds are less relevant in normal corneal tissue where most of the collagen lamellae are arranged in parallel sheaths, but may play a significant role in strengthening keratoconic corneal tissue because of the relative disorganization of the collagen fibrils that is observed in the keratoconic cornea compared to normal corneal tissue [7].

The normal cornea has little elasticity and stretches by only about 0.25% in the range of normal intraocular pressure and in its variation with the cardiac cycle [32]. It maintains its reasonably constant curvature due to the tensile strength of the corneal stroma, which is primarily made up of collagen, proteoglycans and water. Triple helixes of protein are bound by interpeptide bonds to form tropocollagen. Multiple tropocollagen units are assembled into microfibrils, which are natively cross-linked into bundles, making up the stromal collagen fibrils. Bands of collagen fibrils form lamellae, running roughly parallel to the plane of the cornea. X-Ray scattering has revealed that throughout most of the central 7 mm of the normal cornea, the collagen lamellae are preferentially arranged in orthogonal sheets, with two thirds of lammellae existing in the preferred orientations, 45° sectors around the horizontal and vertical meridians, with the remaining lamellae running obliquely. In the peripheral cornea, the fibers curve to form a pseudoannulus near the limbus, with increased anchoring lamellae that contribute to greater peripheral thickness [33, 34]. The precise organization of the collagen lamellae, and the spacing between them, is critical to maintain both the strength and the transparency of the cornea. An interconnecting network of proteoglycans maintains this organization.

There are anterior to posterior difference in this lamellar organization, with anterior one third of the cornea most important for maintenance of corneal strength. While the posterior layers are arranged parallel to the corneal surface, the anterior layers are branched and interwoven, inserting into Bowman's membrane. The cornea's mechanical strength is primarily derived from Bowman's membrane and the anterior third of the corneal stroma because the fibers in these layers are the most interwoven [35]. The anterior cornea is resistant to changes in stromal morphology even in extreme hydration states, revealing the importance of this architecture in the maintenance of corneal curvature [36].

While there are still unanswered questions regarding the precise combination of molecular, genetic and environmental factors (such as eye rubbing) contributing to the pathogenesis of keratoconus, the interaction of these factors leads to the loss or slippage of collagen fibrils and changes to the extracellular matrix in the corneal stroma, resulting in a focal weakening of the cornea [37].

The interweaving of collagen lamellae is significantly reduced in the anterior stroma of keratoconus corneas. The normal organization of the lamellae is disrupted in the apical region, with a loss of the usual orthogonal arrangement of the collagen fibrils. This arrangement is shown in Fig. 8.2. In these corneas, cohesive strength between proteoglycan side chains and collagen fibrils is reduced in the region of the cone, allowing the lamellae to slide apart, and may also result in shearing within the lamellae. This disorganization is localized to the cone, with a more normal organization of collagen in the surrounding regions [33]. The result is an asymmetry in thickness and elastic modulus of this one region relative to the surrounding area,

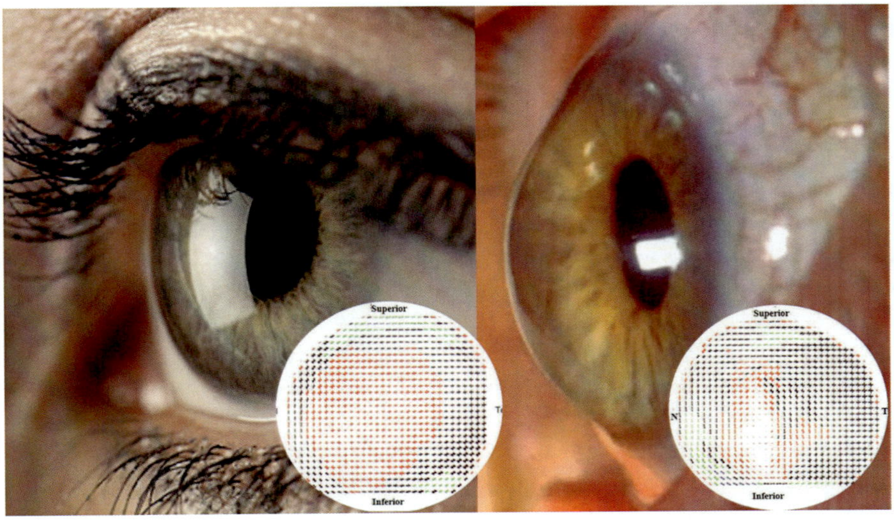

Fig. 8.2 Predominant fibril organization in the normal (left) and keratoconus (right) cornea. (Image Courtesy: John Marshall and Keith Meek)

redistributing the biomechanical forces in the cornea and placing greater strain on the apical region. This weakened region is now susceptible to greater deformation when subjected to the stress of the normal intraocular pressure, leading to further sliding of collagen lamellae, resulting in focal stromal thinning and steepening of the keratoconus cone [38]. The initial focal weakening is therefore amplified in a biomechanical cycle of decompensation, driving disease progression [39].

The differences in collagen arrangement between keratoconus and normal corneas help to elucidate why corneal cross-linking is successful in preventing further progression of ectasia, by increasing the elastic modulus of the cornea and preventing further slippage of collagen lamellae. The differences in anterior to posterior organization of collagen are also helpful in understanding the optimal distribution of induced cross-link bonds in the cornea. The more interwoven anterior one third of the corneal stroma is contributes much of the corneal strength to the normal cornea, and it is in the anterior stroma where lamellar interweaving is significantly reduced in patients with keratoconus, particularly in the apical region. This anterior apical region of the keratoconic stroma is weak and in need of more biomechanical strength than is natively provided by the collagen [37]. As this focal weakening is what drives disease progression, greater stiffening may be needed in the anterior stroma, particularly in the area of the keratoconus cone.

8.4 Corneal Flattening After Conventional CXL

Although the aim of CXL is to induce biomechanical corneal strengthening to slow down or block the progress of the disease (thus preserving visual function), the procedure may also induce flattening of the steepest corneal curvature, resulting in better corneal symmetry that sometimes leads to a refractive improvement (Fig. 8.3. *Change in Corneal Topography at 12 months post-CXL*). In the US phase III multicenter trials of Dresden protocol CXL for treatment of progressive keratoconus, the maximum keratometry value decreased by 2.0 D or more in 31.4% of eyes in the treatment group, and increased by 2.0 D or more in 5.6%. Spectacle corrected distance visual acuity improved by an average of 5.7 logMAR units [21].

In a prospective, randomized, controlled clinical trial, Greenstein et al. assessed the effect of preoperative topographic cone location on 1-year outcomes of corneal cross-linking in 99 eyes (66 keratoconus, 33 ectasia) of 76 patients who underwent corneal cross-linking [25]. The procedure was performed using a 3 mW/cm^2 365 nm UV lamp with a Gaussian beam profile. Subjects were divided into three groups: those with a maximum K located within the central 3-mm optical zone (central cone group), within the 3- to 5-mm optical zone (para-central cone group), and outside the 5-mm (peripheral cone group) optical zone. Cone location was defined by the coordinates of preoperative maximum keratometry (Kmax) using the Pentacam anterior sagittal curvature topography map. It was demonstrated that greater efficacy was achieved in subjects with a central cone location than in subjects with para-central or peripheral cone locations. In the central cone group, Kmax decreased by 2.60±4.50 D ($P < .001$), while statistically significant lesser flattening was

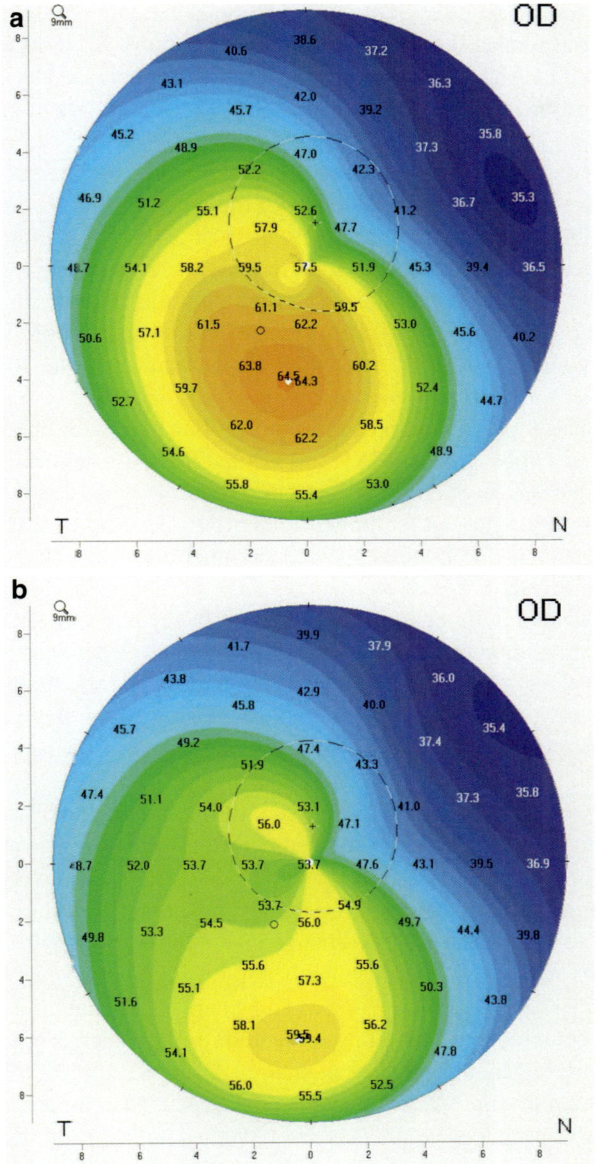

Fig. 8.3 Axial corneal topography map showing flattening of maximum keratometry (KMax) from pre-operative examination (**a**) to 1 year post corneal cross-linking (**b**) for the treatment of progressive keratoconus

observed in the para-central (1.10 ± 2.50 D (P = .02)) and the peripheral cone group (0.40 ± 1.20 D (P = .08)).

In a separate study conducted with the same device (UVX-1000), Tian et al. similarly evaluated the effect of cone location in 64 eyes of 43 keratoconus patients whose highest power of the cornea located in the central 3 mm zone (central cone group) and 24 eyes of 16 keratoconus patients whose highest power located out of the central 3 mm zone (paracentral group). All eyes received standard Dresden CXL. At 2 years postoperatively, Kmax decreased by 5.56 ± 8.31 D in the central group, and lesser flattening of 1.55 ± 2.10 D was observed in the paracentral group [40].

The greater degree of corneal flattening observed in the central keratoconus groups in these studies may be a function of the beam profile of the device used for treatment. Despite a nominal treatment dose of 5.4 J/cm^2 applied in all cases, the effective treatment with this device theoretically resulted in a dose of up to 8.4 J/cm^2 at the apex of cones located in the central position. In treatment of para-central or peripheral cone locations, the effective dose theoretically applied at the apex ranged from 3.7 to 5.9 J/cm^2, dependent upon the location of the corneal apex.

Evaluation of preoperative parameters contributing to greater flattening of maximum keratometry after Dresden CXL reveals that the most important indicator of postoperative success is pre-operative cone location, with the most flattening occurring when the treatment is applied to centrally located cones, and the least flattening effect when the cone is located peripherally [25]. The application of Gaussian beam profile CXL to the center of the cornea in central or peripheral keratoconus provided indirect evidence that the efficacy of cross-linking treatment in achieving stabilization or flattening of Kmax is in part dependent upon the UVA dose applied at the apex of the cone [41]. This finding is consistent with the new understanding of keratoconus microstructure, described in the section above, which has indicated that focal weakening of the cornea is what drives disease progression.

The majority of cross-linking UVA delivery devices commercially available outside of the US today now utilize top hat beam profiles, employing a variety of methods to provide homogenous UVA delivery. UVA delivery devices with cosine beam profiles were introduced to apply more energy in the peripheral cornea than the central cornea, to compensate for the change in curvature from center to periphery. However, to provide benefit, this type of beam profile must be carefully centered and aligned with the apex of the cornea, and maintain alignment throughout the procedure. De-centered application or application to an irregularly shaped cornea may result in misplacement of treatment energy. A simpler approach is the use of a homogenous beam profile with adequate depth of focus to compensate for corneal curvature. An advanced system, the Mosaic (Avedro, Inc.), incorporates active eye tracking with the ability to modify beam shape and energy distribution to fit individual corneal topography, providing the opportunity to apply customized beam profiles accurately.

The finding that CXL results in improved corneal shape in some patients, and that greater flattening occurs when the center of treatment is aligned with the center of the keratoconus cone, highlights the potential to optimize the method of UVA delivery in CXL protocols to target meaningful corneal reshaping in addition to disease stabilization.

8.5 Accelerated CXL

One of the most important advancements in the application of CXL has been the introduction of accelerated CXL. While proven safe and effective, the Dresden protocol requires more than one hour to perform, presenting a challenge to clinical workflow and therefore practice economics. The basic principle of accelerated CXL stems from a fundamental law of photochemistry called the Bunsen-Roscoe Law of Reciprocity. This law states that the photochemical biological effect is proportional to the total energy dose delivered regardless of the applied irradiance and time.

Accelerated cross-linking protocols are used to shorten the total procedure time through the application of higher irradiance UVA. Irradiance refers to the power per area delivered to the surface of the cornea, in units of watts per square centimeter. Dose refers to the energy per area delivered to the surface of the cornea, in units of joules per square centimeter. Dose and irradiance are related by the following equation:

$$\text{Irradiance}\left(\text{W}/\text{cm}^2\right)\times\text{Time}\left(\text{s}\right)=\text{Dose}\left(\text{J}/\text{cm}^2\right)$$

Therefore, while Dresden CXL applies 3 mW/cm^2 irradiance over a period of 30 min to achieve a 5.4 J/cm^2 dose, an equivalent energy dose may be delivered by applying 30 mW/cm^2 irradiance over a period of 3 min. Clinical studies evaluating the efficacy of the application of accelerated CXL according to this principle demonstrate stabilization of keratoconus progression or flattening of KMax [42, 43].

There are other factors beyond the UVA dose that may contribute to the total amount and distribution of cross-links formed in the cornea, and these factors may be influenced by the rate of oxygen consumption by the photochemical reactions that occur during cross-linking [44]. While clinical studies indicate that accelerated CXL is successful in stabilizing keratoconus, several investigators have noted differences in the appearance and depth of the corneal stromal demarcation line that occurs when CXL is performed at different irradiances.

The corneal stromal demarcation line is commonly observed on optical coherence tomography (OCT) in the first 1–3 months after CXL [45, 46]. While this line is not a direct indicator of cross-linking, in vivo confocal microscopy studies after CXL have demonstrated that the depth of the corneal stromal demarcation line is correlated with the depth of keratocyte apoptosis in the cornea. This keratocyte apoptosis occurs in the presence of radicals generated by the photochemical reactions that occur during cross-linking. Therefore, the demarcation line does not represent cross-linking per se, but rather reveals where keratocytes have been disturbed by the cross-linking reactions, visible as backscatter on OCT. The demarcation line depth is used as a convenient clinical proxy for relative (not absolute) treatment depth.

There has been much debate regarding the significance of the depth of this demarcation line, and its relevance to clinical outcomes. Clinical evaluation of the depth of the demarcation line following CXL reveals a trend towards greater depth of this line following the conventional vs accelerated techniques, when UVA dose is held equivalent and continuous irradiation is used [42, 47–49]. Comparative studies of accelerated versus conventional CXL suggest that conventional CXL may result in greater change in corneal curvature, as measured by flattening of KMax relative to baseline, particularly in the first 6 months after cross-linking [50]. However, while differences in the relative magnitude of flattening may exist, the goal of the procedure is to stop progression. When the outcomes of accelerated protocols are evaluated individually, accelerated protocols of duration as short as 3 min have been demonstrated to be effective at halting progression of KMax at follow-up of 12 months [49]. Additionally, it has been suggested that by altering the anterior stroma and maintaining a further distance from the endothelium, accelerated CXL may be a safer option for treatment of thin corneas [49].

This difference in demarcation line depth is likely modulated by oxygen bioavailability within the stroma. Pulsed irradiation protocols are applied to increase the depth of accelerated cross-linking procedures by effectively reducing the rate of oxygen consumption. Clinical studies of pulsed, accelerated cross-linking protocols indicate equivalent safety to continuous exposure protocols but with greater demarcation line depth [51–55]. Similar to comparative studies with conventional cross-linking, these studies reveal greater flattening of KMax following accelerated pulsed irradiation as compared to accelerated continuous irradiation for the same energy dose.

The ability to titrate the depth of the demarcation line by varying irradiance or pulse interval may offer the potential to customize cross-linking treatment for thinner corneas (reducing depth) or to target specific biomechanical changes [56].

8.6 Control of Cross-Linking Distribution: Photochemical Kinetics

The variation in demarcation line depth as a function of irradiation protocol (described above) can be explained by the photochemical kinetic mechanisms that underlie the creation of new bonds during corneal cross-linking procedures. The majority of cross-linking bonds induced by the CXL procedure are generated by reactive oxygen species, predominately hydroxyl radical. When activated with 365-nm UVA, riboflavin acts as a photosensitizer, resulting in reactions with electron donating sites (i.e. amines or amino acids) through mixed Type I – Type II photochemical mechanisms. Type II photochemical mechanisms predominate at the higher oxygen concentration found in the cornea during the first few seconds of irradiation, resulting in the formation of singlet molecular oxygen. While the generation of singlet oxygen results in the formation of cross-link bonds, this mechanism is likely only a minor contributor to the total stiffening effect, because oxygen is diminished within seconds of UVA irradiation and the Type I photochemical mechanisms that are favored at lower oxygen concentrations rapidly take over [44]. The Type I reactions generate the radical form of riboflavin, which creates superoxide radical anion, converts to hydrogen peroxide and finally to hydroxyl radical. Hydroxyl radical then reacts with the donor sites to create most of the induced cross-links [57].

The byproducts of the Type I reactions, particularly a reduced form of riboflavin, undergo additional oxidation chemistry that is not mediated by UVA, but consumes oxygen. The rate of oxygen consumption therefore impacts the cross-linking outcome. When higher irradiance UVA is applied during accelerated CXL, the concentration of reduced riboflavin accumulates at a faster rate, limiting the reactions which form cross-links. Cross-linking occurs in the anterior corneal stroma where oxygen is available, but it does not penetrate as deeply [58].

Intermittently turning the UVA source off during the irradiation period slows the rate of oxygen consumption, enabling replenishment of oxygen. The introduction of this dark period into the ultraviolet light delivery cycle through pulsed irradiation enables conversion of reduced riboflavin back to the radical form. This is the goal of pulsed irradiation procedures. The rate of oxygen diffusion can be increased by a factor of five by increasing the surface concentration of oxygen from atmospheric conditions (approximately 21%) to a highly oxygenated environment (100%). Therefore, the addition of oxygen at the corneal surface significantly increases the availability of oxygen at depth. The addition of supplemental oxygen boosts the efficiency of high irradiance crosslinking [58].

As summarized above, the formation of cross-link bonds is driven by the relative availabilities of riboflavin, UVA, and oxygen. Therefore, modification of UVA irradiance settings enables titration of the distribution of cross-links formed (depth and amount), and enables targeted application of the resultant corneal stiffening. With the ability to target corneal stiffening comes the opportunity to modify biomechanical properties to modify corneal shape and subsequently improve visual function.

8.7 Customized Cross-Linking: Spatially Targeted Cross-Linking Distribution

In addition to varying the depth of cross-linking by modifying parameters such as UVA irradiance, total energy dose and/or pulsing, the lateral distribution of cross-link formation in the cornea may be better controlled through the utilization of customized UVA illumination patterns. Given that keratoconus is the result of a focal weakening of the cornea, it is logical to consider targeting corneal stiffening to this region. A whole eye finite element analysis model developed by Roy et al. has been used to study the theoretical impact of focally stiffening the weakest region of the cornea as compared to the conventional approach of uniformly stiffening the entire central cornea [24]. The results of this work demonstrate greater normalization of the cornea (inferior flattening and superior steepening), presenting the opportunity to combine visual rehabilitation and biomechanical stabilization into a single procedure.

Customized corneal cross-linking, referred to as CuRV, has recently been made possible through the introduction of a UVA delivery system which enables the spatial delivery of cross-linking through user programmable irradiation patterns (Fig. 8.4 – *Mosaic System*). The system can be programmed to deliver personalized treatment patterns based on individual patient tomography using accelerated cross-linking of irradiance 10–45 mW/cm^2, pulsed or continuous irradiation, and treatment doses of up to 15 J/cm^2. When multiple treatment shapes are chosen, all shapes are applied using the same irradiance and pulse interval settings, while the total UVA dose delivered may be selected for each separate shape. UVA irradiation begins across the entire treatment pattern at the initiation of treatment, and each shape disappears once its programmed treatment time is complete.

While conventional cross-linking aims to stabilize against further progression of ectasia by evenly stiffening the central cornea, customized cross-linking aims to preferentially stiffen the keratoconus cone, targeting both stabilization and corneal flattening. Theoretical modeling has indicated that an optimized approach for treatment may include differential stiffening of the weakest region of the cornea. There is currently no clinical diagnostic tool that is widely available to locate the region of biomechanical weakness in an individual patient, and therefore abnormalities in anterior corneal curvature and posterior corneal elevation observed on corneal tomography are used as a proxy to define the cone area [24, 59].

In current treatment protocols for customized cross-linking, a greater total energy dose is applied to the cone area, with an aim of inducing greater stiffness in this region and targeting maximum flattening effect. Additional treatment zones of lower energy are applied to the surrounding area, with an aim of stabilizing the cornea against further progression (Fig. 8.5 – *Example Customized treatment pattern*). Multiple demarcation lines of varying depth are observed in the corneal stroma of eyes treated with these multizone UVA treatment patterns [56]. Evaluation of corneal demarcation line depth in areas of the cornea treated with higher dose UVA (longer irradiation time) versus the areas treated with lower dose within the

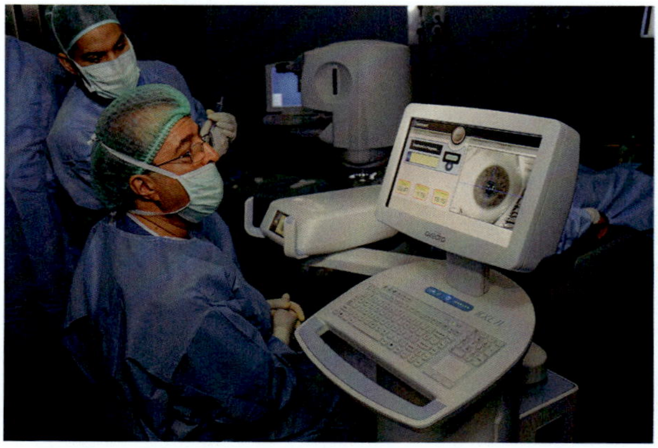

Fig. 8.4 Customized cross-linking procedure performed with the Mosaic system (Avedro)

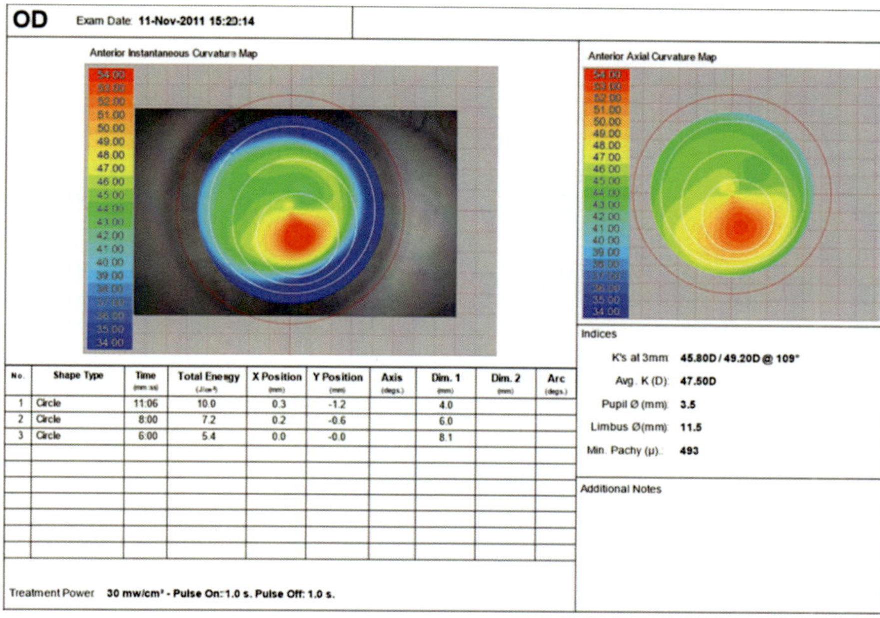

Fig. 8.5 Example UV-A treatment plan for a customized cross-linking procedure for the treatment of keratoconus

same cornea reveals a direct correlation between demarcation line depth and total UVA irradiation time [56, 60]. This variation in demarcation line depth as a function of UVA dose provides indirect evidence that the magnitude of the cross-linking effect can be titrated by varying the total UVA dose applied through varying exposure time at constant irradiance.

Several clinical investigators have compared the efficacy of customized cross-linking with Dresden CXL. Results of these evaluations are shown in Tables 8.1, 8.2a and 8.2b. In one such evaluation conducted by Seiler et al. three concentric circles were applied in each case [59]. Individual patient corneal tomography was evaluated to locate the area of abnormal posterior elevation. This region was used to determine the diameter and centration of each treatment shape. The highest UVA dose (10 J/cm^2) was applied in the inner circle, with diameter defined by the smallest diameter of the posterior float, as defined by the corneal tomography system (Oculyzer, Wavelight, Inc.). The diameter of the outer circle was defined by the largest diameter of the posterior float plus one millimeter, and the diameter of the intermediate circle was set as the average of the two.

In a separate, similar study, Cassange et al. similarly applied a series of two or three superimposed concentric shapes [60]. The posterior elevation map was again used to determine the centration of the inner shape. The diameter of the inner region was chosen such that both the entire area of abnormal posterior elevation and the area of maximum corneal curvature (Kmax) were enclosed within the inner region. The diameter of the second and tertiary treatment zones was

Table 8.1 Summary of publications reporting the application of customized cross-linking for the treatment of keratoconus

		Conventional Control Group			Custom Treatment group							
Reference	Study design	N (eyes)	Irradiance	Dose	N (eyes)	Irradiance	Dose	Shape	Defined by	Inner zone	Middle zone	Outer zone
Nordström et al. (2016)	Prospective, randomized	25	30 mW/cm^2 pulsed [1,1]	5.4 J/cm^2	25	30 mW/cm^2 [1,1]	7.2 J/cm^2; 10 J/cm^2; 15 J/cm^2;	Inferior arcuate	**Anterior axial curvature**	≥52 D	48–52 D	43–47 D
Mazzotta et al. (2016)	Prospective, no control				21	30 mW/cm^2 [1,1]	7.2 J/cm^2; 10 J/cm^2; 15 J/cm^2;	Inferior arcuate and/or circular	**Anterior axial curvature**	≥52 D	48–52 D	43–47 D
Seiler et al. (2016)	Prospective, consecutive control	20	9 mW/cm^2 continuous	5.4 J/cm^2	20	9 mW/cm^2 cw	5.4 J/cm^2; 7.2 J/cm^2; 10 J/cm^2;	Circular	**Posterior float**	Shortest diameter of PF – 0.5mm	Average diameter of outer/inner circles	Maximal diameter of PF + 1.0 mm
Cassagne et al. (2017)	Prospective, retrospective matched control	30	3 mW/cm^2 continuous	5.4 J/cm^2	30	30 mW/cm^2 [1,1]	5.4 J/cm^2; 10 J/cm^2; 15 J/cm^2;	Circular	**Anterior axial curvature & posterior float**	Abnormal posterior elevation and Kmax	Greatest Δ in anterior axial curvature	Abnormal anterior axial curvature
Shetty et al. (2017)	Prospective, randomized	10	9 mW/cm^2 continuous	5.4 J/cm^2	10	9 mW/cm^2 cw	graded- up to 15 J/cm^2	Inferior arcuate	**Anterior axial curvature**	Three stacked arcs, encompass the steepest zone on axial map		
					10		graded- up to 15 J/cm^2	Circular	**Anterior axial curvature**	Five stacked circles, encompass the steepest zone on axial map		
					10		graded- up to 10.8 J/cm^2	Circular	**Anterior tangential curvature**	Five stacked circles, encompass the steepest zone on tangential map		

determined such that transitions between zones occurred at the regions of greatest change in corneal curvature as determined by Pentacam anterior axial curvature. Total energy delivered across the treatment zone ranged from minimum dose of 5.4 J/cm^2 in the outermost treatment zone, and maximum dose of 15 J/cm^2 in the innermost treatment zone.

In both studies, epithelium was debrided over the region designated for UVA treatment prior to the application of riboflavin, and surrounding epithelium was left intact. In the study by Seiler et al. 10 mW/cm^2 continuous irradiance was applied, while in the study by Prof. Malecaze, 30 mW/cm^2 irradiance, pulsed [1,1] was applied. In both cases, CuRV treated eyes were compared to a control group of patients treated with conventional Dresden protocol cross-linking, and statistically significantly greater improvement (flattening of KMax) and greater normalization of corneal shape (reduction of inferior to superior corneal asymmetry) was seen in the customized group relative to the conventional group in both studies at 12 month follow-up. No significant adverse events were observed in either study.

While further studies are needed to elucidate the most optimal treatment pattern design to target maximal visual outcomes following customized cross-linking, clinical studies to date indicate that customized, tomography oriented cross-linking results in significant reduction of corneal irregularity [59–62]. This improved corneal shape leads to improved quality of vision and potentially improved contact lens tolerance. While conventional broad-beam CXL remains a safe and effective treatment to delay or halt progression of corneal ectasia in progressive keratoconus, customized cross-linking represents a new option in personalized medicine, combining disease stabilization with visual rehabilitation.

Table 8.2a Outcomes of the application of customized cross-linking for the treatment of keratoconus

a

		Conventional Control Group				Custom Treatment group			
Reference	Study design	N (eyes)	Δ Kmax	ΔBCVA	ΔUCVA	N (eyes)	Δ Kmax	ΔBCVA	ΔUCVA
Nordström et al. (2016)	Prospective, randomized	25	+0.30 ± 1.33	+0.01 ± 0.29	−0.07 ± 0.16	25	−1.31 ± 1.52	−0.16 ± 0.24	−0.31 ± 0.40
Mazzotta et al. (2016)	Prospective, no control					21	−1.00	−0.1	−0.22
Seiler et al. (2016)	Prospective, consecutive control	20	−0.9 ± 1.3	−0.04 ± 0.14		20	−1.7±2.0	−0.07 ± 0.20	
Cassagne et al. (2017)	Prospective, retrospective matched control	30	0.44 ± 1.61 D	−0.09	−0.06	30	−1.29 ± 2.44 D	−0.06	−0.06
Shetty et al. (2017)	Prospective, randomized	10	−1.707 ± 0.347	−0.055 ± 0.031	−0.254 ± 0.111	10	−1.508 ± 0.255	−0.042 ± 0.036	0.075 ± 0.062
						10	−0.443 ± 0.232	−0.114 ± 0.040	0.043 ± 0.043
						10	−1.308±0.333	−0.067 ± 0.051	0.217 ± 0.122

b

		Conventional Control Group			Custom Treatment group		
Reference	Index	N (eyes)	S	I	N (eyes)	S	I
Nordström et al. 2016	True Net Power in a 1 mm zone centered at point of max irradiation (Pmax) and 1 mm zone 180° from Pmax, at same distance from visual axis (Pmin)	25	−0.07±0.64	+0.03±1.16	25	+1.00±1.22	−0.88±1.02
Seiler et al. 2016	Regularization Index: maximal steepening plus maximal flattening in the difference map compared to pre-op	20	4.1 ± 3.1D		20	5.2 ± 2.7 D	
Cassagne M et al. 2017	S index corresponds to the mean k values from 5 points on the top of the 3 mm diameter circle (crossing the 30°, 60°, 90°, 120° and 150° axes) I index corresponds to the mean keratometry values of 5 points at the bottom of the same circle (crossing 210°, 240°, 270°, 300° and 330° axes)	30	0.580 ± 2.03	0.87 ± 2.369	30	0.063 ± 1.943	−1.017 ± 1.367

8.8 Conclusion

Dresden CXL revolutionized keratoconus management by targeting the underlying corneal instability and successfully stopping or slowing down disease progression. Accelerated, pulsed CXL protocols have enabled shorter treatment times and more precise titration of cross-linking effect, enabling improved clinical workflow and potentially expanding access to the procedure to patients with thinner corneas. Significantly reduced treatment time has resulted in cost savings, making the procedure more acceptable to regulators of national health systems in several countries.

Table 8.2b Customized cross-linking resulted in greater normalization of corneal curvature relative to conventional cross-linking

		Conventional Control Group			Custom Treatment group		
Reference	Index	N (eyes)	S	I	N (eyes)	S	I
Nordström et al. [63]	True Net Power in a 1 mm zone centered at point op max irradiation (Pmax) and 1 mm zone 180° from Pmax. at same distance from visual axis (Pmin)	25	−0.07 ± 064	+0.03 ± 1.16	25	+1.00 ± 1.22	−0.88 ± 1.02
Seiler et al. [59]	Regularization Index: maximal steepening plus maximal flattening in the difference map compared to pre-op	20	4.1 ± 3.1D		20	5.2 ± 2.7 D	
Cassagne et al. [60]	5 index corresponds to the mean k values from S points on the top of the 3 mm diameter circle (crossing the 30°, 60°, 90°, 120° and 150° axes) 1 index corresponds to the mean keratometry values of 5 points at the bottom *of* the same circle (crossing 210°, 240°, 270°, 300° and 330° axes)	30	0.580 ± 2.03	0.87 ± 2.369	30	0.063 ± 1.943	−1 017 ± 1.367

In addition to arresting disease progression and increasing efficacy of CXL procedures, the new generation of customized CXL protocols further normalize the irregular contour of treated corneas and improve patients' visual function.

References

1. Rebenitsch RL, Kymes SM, Walline JJ, Gordon MO. The lifetime economic burden of keratoconus: a decision analysis using a markov model. Am J Ophthalmol. 2011;151(5):768–73.e2. https://doi.org/10.1016/j.ajo.2010.10.034.
2. Rabinowitz YS. Keratoconus. Surv Ophthalmol. 1998;42(4):297–319. https://doi.org/10.1016/S0039-6257(97)00119-7.
3. Gomes JAP, Tan D, Rapuano CJ, et al. Global consensus on keratoconus and ectatic diseases. Cornea. 2015;34(4):359–69.
4. Knox Cartwright NE, Tyrer JR, Marshall J. Age-related differences in the elasticity of the human cornea. Invest Ophthalmol Vis Sci. 2011;52(7):4324–9. https://doi.org/10.1167/iovs.09-4798.
5. Chan E, Snibson GR. Current status of corneal collagen cross-linking for keratoconus: a review. Clin Exp Optom. 2013;17(Figure 2):1–10. https://doi.org/10.1111/cxo.12020.
6. Ashwin PT, McDonnell PJ. Collagen cross-linkage: a comprehensive review and directions for future research. Br J Ophthalmol. 2009;94:965–70.
7. Meek KM, Hayes S. Corneal cross-linking – a review. Ophthalmic Physiol Opt. 2013;33(2):78–93. https://doi.org/10.1111/opo.12032.
8. Raiskup F, Spoerl E Corneal crosslinking with riboflavin and ultraviolet A. I. principles. Ocul Surf. 2013;11(2):65–74. https://doi.org/10.1016/j.jtos.2013.01.002.
9. Knox Cartwright NE, Tyrer JR, Marshall J. In vitro quantification of the stiffening effect of corneal cross-linking in the human cornea using radial shearing speckle pattern interferometry. J Refract Surg. 2012;28(7):503–7. https://doi.org/10.3928/1081597X-20120613-01.
10. Spoerl E, Huhle M, Seiler T. Induction of cross-links in corneal tissue. Exp Eye Res. 1998;66(1):97–103. https://doi.org/10.1006/exer.1997.0410.
11. Spoerl E, Seiler T. Techniques for stiffening the cornea. J Refract Surg. 1999;15:711–3.
12. Wollensak G, Spoerl E, Reber F, Seiler T. Keratocyte cytotoxicity of riboflavin/UVA-treatment in vitro. Eye (Lond). 2004;18(7):718–22. https://doi.org/10.1038/sj.eye.6700751.
13. Wollensak G, Spörl E, Reber F, Pillunat L, Funk R. Corneal endothelial cytotoxicity of riboflavin/UVA treatment in vitro. Ophthalmic Res. 2003;35(6):324–8. https://doi.org/10.1159/000074071.
14. Wollensak G, Spoerl E, Wilsch M, Seiler T. Endothelial cell damage after riboflavin–ultraviolet-A treatment in the rabbit. J Cataract Refract Surg. 2003;29(9):1786–90. https://doi.org/10.1016/S0886-3350(03)00343-2.
15. Wollensak G, Spoerl E, Seiler T. Riboflavin/ultraviolet-A-induced collagen crosslinking for the treatment of keratoconus. Am J Ophthalmol. 2003;135(5):620–7. https://doi.org/10.1016/S0002-9394(02)02220-1.
16. Wittig-Silva C, Chan E, Islam FM, Wu T, Whiting M, Snibson GR. A randomized, controlled trial of corneal collagen cross-linking in progressive keratoconus: three-year results. Ophthalmology. 2014;121(4):812–21. https://doi.org/10.1016/j.ophtha.2013.10.028.
17. O'Brart DPS, Kwong TQ, Patel P, McDonald RJ, O'Brart N. Long-term follow-up of riboflavin/ultraviolet A (370 nm) corneal collagen cross-linking to halt the progression of keratoconus. Br J Ophthalmol. 2013. https://doi.org/10.1136/bjophthalmol-2012-302556.
18. Chang CY, Hersh PS. Corneal collagen cross-linking: a review of 1-year outcomes. Eye Contact Lens. 2014;40(6):345–52. https://doi.org/10.1097/ICL.0000000000000094.

19. Raiskup F, Theuring A, Pillunat LE, Spoerl E. Corneal collagen crosslinking with riboflavin and ultraviolet-A light in progressive keratoconus: 10-year results. J Cataract Refract Surg. 2015;41(1):41–6. https://doi.org/10.1016/j.jcrs.2014.09.033.
20. Hersh PS, Stulting RD, Muller D, et al. U.S. multicenter clinical trial of corneal collagen crosslinking for treatment of corneal ectasia after refractive surgery. Ophthalmology. 2017;124(10):1475–84. https://doi.org/10.1016/j.ophtha.2017.05.036.
21. Hersh PS, Stulting RD, Muller D, et al. United States multicenter clinical trial of corneal collagen crosslinking for keratoconus treatment. Ophthalmology. 2017;124(9):1259–70. https://doi.org/10.1016/j.ophtha.2017.03.052.
22. Lytle G. Advances in the technology of corneal cross-linking for keratoconus. Eye Contact Lens. 2014;0(0):1–7. https://doi.org/10.1097/ICL.0000000000000084.
23. Chai D, Gaster RN, Roizenblatt R, Juhasz T, Brown DJ, Jester JV. Quantitative assessment of UVA-riboflavin corneal cross-linking using nonlinear optical microscopy. Invest Ophthalmol Vis Sci. 2011;52(7):4231–8. https://doi.org/10.1167/iovs.10-7105.
24. Roy AS, Dupps WJ. Patient-specific computational modeling of keratoconus progression and differential responses to collagen cross-linking. Invest Ophthalmol Vis Sci. 2011;52(12):9174–87. https://doi.org/10.1167/iovs.11-7395.
25. Greenstein S, Fry KL, Hersh PS. Effect of topographic cone location on outcomes of corneal collagen cross-linking for keratoconus and corneal ectasia. J Refract Surg. 2012;28(6):397–405. https://doi.org/10.3928/1081597X-20120518-02.
26. Koller T, Mrochen M, Seiler T. Complication and failure rates after corneal crosslinking. J Cataract Refract Surg. 2009;35(8):1358–62. https://doi.org/10.1016/j.jcrs.2009.03.035.
27. Raiskup-Wolf F, Hoyer A, Spoerl E, Pillunat LE. Collagen crosslinking with riboflavin and ultraviolet-A light in keratoconus: long-term results. J Cataract Refract Surg. 2008;34(5):796–801. https://doi.org/10.1016/j.jcrs.2007.12.039.
28. Ivarsen A, Hjortdal J. Collagen cross-linking for advanced progressive keratoconus. Cornea. 2013;0(0):1–4.
29. Vinciguerra R, Romano MR, Camesasca FI, et al. Corneal cross-linking as a treatment for keratoconus: 4-year morphologic and clinical outcomes with respect to patient age. Ophthalmology. 2013;120(5):908–16. https://doi.org/10.1016/j.ophtha.2012.10.023.
30. Buzzonetti L, Petrocelli G. Transepithelial corneal cross-linking in pediatric patients: early results. J Refract Surg. 2012;28(11):763–7. https://doi.org/10.3928/1081597X-20121011-03.
31. Sung H-W, Chang W-H, Ma C-Y, Lee M-H. Crosslinking of biological tissues using genipin and/or carbodiimide. J Biomed Mater Res A. 2003;64(3):427–38. https://doi.org/10.1002/jbm.a.10346.
32. Jaycock PD, Lobo L, Ibrahim J, Tyrer J, Marshall J. Interferometric technique to measure biomechanical changes in the cornea induced by refractive surgery. J Cataract Refract Surg. 2005;31(1):175–84. https://doi.org/10.1016/j.jcrs.2004.10.038.
33. Meek KM, Boote C. The use of X-ray scattering techniques to quantify the orientation and distribution of collagen in the corneal stroma. Prog Retin Eye Res. 2009;28(5):369–92. https://doi.org/10.1016/j.preteyeres.2009.06.005.
34. Lewis PN, White TL, Young RD, Bell JS, Winlove CP, Meek KM. Three-dimensional arrangement of elastic fibers in the human corneal stroma. Exp Eye Res. 2016;146:43–53. https://doi.org/10.1016/j.exer.2015.12.006.
35. Winkler M, Chai D, Kriling S, et al. Nonlinear optical macroscopic assessment of 3-D corneal collagen organization and axial biomechanics. Invest Ophthalmol Vis Sci. 2011;52(12):8818–27. https://doi.org/10.1167/iovs.11-8070.
36. Müller LJ, Pels E, Vrensen GF. The specific architecture of the anterior stroma accounts for maintenance of corneal curvature. Br J Ophthalmol. 2001;85(4):437–43. http://www.pubmedcentral.nih.gov/articlerender.fcgi?artid=1723934&tool=pmcentrez&rendertype=abstract.
37. White TL, Lewis PN, Young RD, et al. Elastic microfibril distribution in the cornea: differences between normal and keratoconic stroma. Exp Eye Res. 2017;159:40–8. https://doi.org/10.1016/j.exer.2017.03.002.

38. Meek KM, Tuft SJ, Huang Y, et al. Changes in collagen orientation and distribution in keratoconus corneas. Invest Ophthalmol Vis Sci. 2005;46(6):1948–56. https://doi.org/10.1167/iovs.04-1253.
39. Roberts CJ, Dupps WJ. Biomechanics of corneal ectasia and biomechanical treatments. J Cataract Refract Surg. 2014;40(6):991–8. https://doi.org/10.1016/j.jcrs.2014.04.013.
40. Tian M, Ma P, Zhou W, Feng J, Mu G. Outcomes of corneal crosslinking for central and paracentral keratoconus. Med (United States). 2017;96(10):e6247. https://doi.org/10.1097/MD.0000000000006247.
41. Koller T, Schumacher S, Fankhauser F, Seiler T. Riboflavin/Ultraviolet a crosslinking of the paracentral cornea. Cornea. 2013;32(2):165–8. https://doi.org/10.1097/ICO.0b013e318269059b.
42. Tomita M, Mita M, Huseynova T. Accelerated versus conventional corneal collagen crosslinking. J Cataract Refract Surg. 2014;40(6):1013–20. https://doi.org/10.1016/j.jcrs.2013.12.012.
43. Mita M, Waring GO, Tomita M. High-irradiance accelerated collagen crosslinking for the treatment of keratoconus: six-month results. J Cataract Refract Surg. 2014;40(6):1032–40. https://doi.org/10.1016/j.jcrs.2013.12.014.
44. Kamaev P, Friedman MD, Sherr E, Muller D. Photochemical kinetics of corneal cross-Linking with riboflavin. Invest Ophthalmol Vis Sci. 2012;53(4):2360–7. https://doi.org/10.1167/iovs.11-9385.
45. Seiler T, Hafezi F. Corneal cross-linking-induced stromal demarcation line. Cornea. 2006;25(9):1057–9. https://doi.org/10.1097/01.ico.0000225720.38748.58.
46. Mazzotta C, Caporossi T, Denaro R, et al. Morphological and functional correlations in riboflavin UV A corneal collagen cross-linking for keratoconus. Acta Ophthalmol. 2012;90:259–65. https://doi.org/10.1111/j.1755-3768.2010.01890.x.
47. Touboul D, Efron N, Smadja D, Praud D, Malet F, Colin J. Corneal confocal microscopy following conventional, transepithelial, and accelerated corneal collagen cross-linking procedures for keratoconus. J Refract Surg. 2012;28(11):769–76. https://doi.org/10.3928/1081597X-20121016-01.
48. Kymionis G, Tsoulnaras K. Corneal stromal demarcation line determined with anterior segment optical coherence tomography following a very high intensity corneal collagen cross. Cornea. 2015;34:664–7.
49. Medeiros CS, Giacomin NT, Bueno RL, Ghanem RC, Moraes HV, Santhiago MR. Accelerated corneal collagen crosslinking: technique, efficacy, safety, and applications. J Cataract Refract Surg. 2016;42(12):1826–35. https://doi.org/10.1016/j.jcrs.2016.11.028.
50. Liu Y, Liu Y, Zhang Y, et al. Systematic review and meta-analysis comparing modified cross-linking and standard cross-linking for progressive keratoconus. Int J Ophthalmol. 2017;10(9):1419–29. https://doi.org/10.18240/ijo.2017.09.15.
51. Mazzotta C, Traversi C, Caragiuli S, Rechichi M. Pulsed vs continuous light accelerated corneal collagen crosslinking: in vivo qualitative investigation by confocal microscopy and corneal OCT. Eye (Lond). 2014;28(10):1179–83. https://doi.org/10.1038/eye.2014.163.
52. Mazzotta C, Traversi C, Paradiso AL, Latronico ME, Rechichi M. Pulsed light accelerated crosslinking versus continuous light accelerated crosslinking: 1-year results. J Ophthalmol. 2014;2014:1–6. https://doi.org/10.1155/2014/604731.
53. Jiang L, Jiang W, Qiu S. Conventional vs. pulsed-light accelerated corneal collagen crosslinking for the treatment of progressive keratoconus: 12-month results from a prospective study. Exp Ther Med. 2017;14:4238–44. https://doi.org/10.3892/etm.2017.5031.
54. Mazzotta C, Baiocchi S, Bagaglia SA, Fruschelli M, Meduri A, Rechichi M. Accelerated 15 mW pulsed-light crosslinking to treat progressive keratoconus: 2-year clinical results. J Cataract Refract Surg. 2017;43(8):1081–8. https://doi.org/10.1016/j.jcrs.2017.05.030.
55. Peyman A, Nouralishahi A, Hafezi F, Kling S, Peyman M. Stromal Demarcation Line in Pulsed Versus Continuous Light Accelerated Corneal Cross-linking for Keratoconus. J Refract Surg. 2016;32(3):206–8. https://doi.org/10.3928/1081597X-20160204-03.

56. Mazzotta C, Moramarco A, Traversi C, Baiocchi S, Iovieno A, Fontana L. Accelerated corneal collagen cross-linking using topography-guided UV-A energy emission: preliminary clinical and morphological outcomes. J Ophthalmol. 2016;2016:1–10. https://doi.org/10.1155/2016/2031031.
57. Scott McCall A, Kraft S, Edelhauser HF, et al. Mechanisms of corneal tissue cross-linking in response to treatment with topical riboflavin and long-wavelength ultraviolet radiation (UVA). Investig Ophthalmol Vis Sci. 2010;51(1):129–38. https://doi.org/10.1167/iovs.09-3738.
58. Muller D, Kamaev P, Friedman M, Sherr E, Eddington W. Accelerated UVA-RF corneal cross-linking through pulsed UVA illumination and oxygen rich environments. Invest Ophthalmol Vis Sci. 2013;54(15):5281.
59. Seiler TG, Fischinger I, Koller T, Zapp D, Frueh BE, Seiler T. Customized corneal cross-linking: one-year results. Am J Ophthalmol. 2016;166:14–21. https://doi.org/10.1016/j.ajo.2016.02.029.
60. Cassagne M, Pierné K, Galiacy SD, Asfaux-Marfaing M-P, Fournié P, Malecaze F. Customized topography-guided corneal collagen cross-linking for keratoconus. J Refract Surg. 2017;33(5):290–7. https://doi.org/10.3928/1081597X-20170201-02.
61. Nordström M, Schiller M, Fredriksson A, Behndig A. Refractive improvements and safety with topography-guided corneal crosslinking for keratoconus: 1-year results. Br J Ophthalmol. 2016; https://doi.org/10.1136/BJOPHTHALMOL-2016-309210.
62. Shetty R, Nethralaya N, Pahuja N, et al. Customized corneal crosslinking using different UVA beam profiles customized corneal crosslinking using different UVA beam profiles. J Refract Surg. 2017;33(10):676–82.
63. Nordström M, Schiller M, Fredriksson A, et al. Refractive improvements and safety with topography-guided corneal crosslinking for keratoconus: 1-year results. Br J Ophthalmol. 2017;101:920–25.

Chapter 9
Biomechanics of Stabilizing the Keratoconic Cornea

Cynthia J. Roberts, G. Martha, and Milton Staub

9.1 Biomechanical Hypothesis of Keratoconus Development and Progression

Understanding the biomechanics of the keratoconic cornea is important in order to predict response to modern biomechanical treatments, as well as response to refractive surgery if a pre-clinical keratoconus patient is subjected to tissue removal after failing pre-operative screening which can occur due to the lack of manifestation of detectable geometric asymmetries in the cornea. What is the first detectable feature of this disease? The keratoconic cornea typically develops asymmetries in curvature and elevation of both the anterior and posterior surfaces, although the asymmetries are often detectable on the posterior surface first due to anterior surface epithelial remodeling which masks developing stromal surface changes [1]. In addition, the pachymetry profile becomes exaggerated as the cornea also thins asymmetrically [2]. These features can all be measured via corneal tomography, which forms the basis of many screening algorithms. However, from a mechanistic perspective, what drives development and progression of corneal asymmetry in keratoconus?

It was first proposed in 2007 that the weakness of the keratoconic cornea is *focal* in nature, and not a generalized weakening, as was believed at the time [3, 4]. This belief was based on early ex vivo strip testing of keratoconic and normal corneas, which showed tissue strips from a keratoconic cornea were weaker than those from a normal cornea [5]. However, this type of analysis would not allow asymmetry to be assessed. Even if only a portion of the strip were weak, the testing would lead to the conclusion that the entire strip was weak. More recent mathematical models based on finite element analysis were constructed to demonstrate keratoconic progression based only on simulated increase in focal weakening [6]. The anterior and

C. J. Roberts (✉) · G. Martha · M. Staub
The Ohio State University, Columbus, OH, USA
e-mail: roberts.8@osu.edu

A. Barbara (ed.), *Controversies in the Management of Keratoconus*,
https://doi.org/10.1007/978-3-319-98032-4_9

posterior surface data of a keratoconic subject were used to construct the model, and then the less involved eye was used to simulate progression by serial increase in focal weakening. The characteristic keratoconic asymmetric curvature pattern was achieved in this eye, demonstrating the biomechanical effect on surface shape of simply reducing the biomechanical properties in a defined region.

The definitive research on focal weakening of the keratoconic cornea was published in 2014 and 2015 [7, 8]. Using Brillouin microscopy to measure depth dependent corneal properties, fresh keratoconic buttons from Deep Anterior Lamellar Keratoplasty (DALK) procedures were measured within the area of steepening from pre-operative tomography, as well as 180° across the central axis of the same graft. In addition, normal donors from Descemet's Stripping Endothelial Keratoplasty (DSEK) procedures were measured using the same technology, but near the center of the cornea. In the keratoconic buttons, the region of pathology was significantly weaker than the normal corneas. However, in the area 180 degrees across the central axis, the corneal properties were not different than the normal corneas. This is strong evidence of focal weakening in disease severe enough to require a lamellar procedure. Brillouin microscopy was also subsequently used to measure a normal subject and a keratoconic subject in vivo, and showed consistent evidence of asymmetric corneal properties in keratoconus (Fig. 9.1).

The proposed biomechanical cycle of decompensation and progression in keratoconus is presented in Fig. 9.2. The primary initiating event is focal weakening that precedes both thinning and steepening. Focal weakening changes the stress distribution, explained in more detail in the next section, leading to focal strain and thinning, which also redistributes the stress. This is followed by increased curvature, which again redistributes the stress, generating a cycle of biomechanical decompensation. What causes the focal weakening that starts this cascade? Eye rubbing is a mechanical trauma which may represent the environmental trigger in a genetically suscepti-

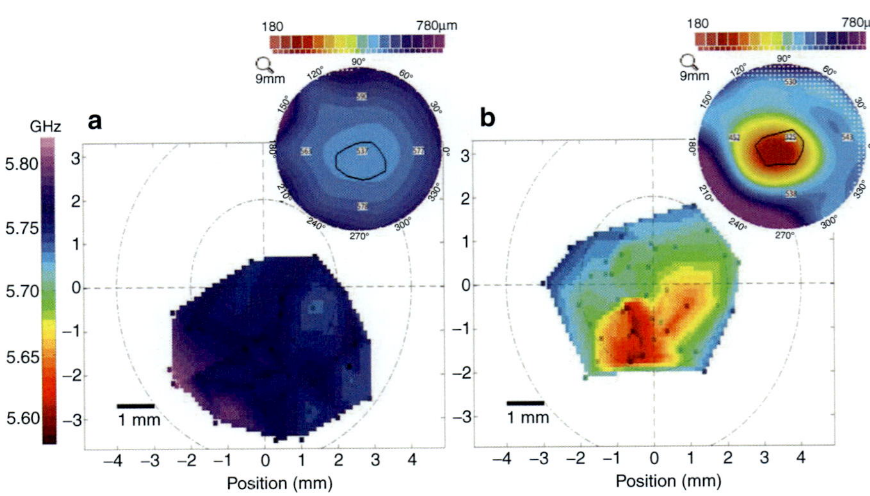

Fig. 9.1 Brillouin microscopy is used to clinically measure a normal subject (**a**) and a keratoconic subject (**b**), showing asymmetry of properties only in the keratoconic subject. (Adapted with permission from Ref. [8])

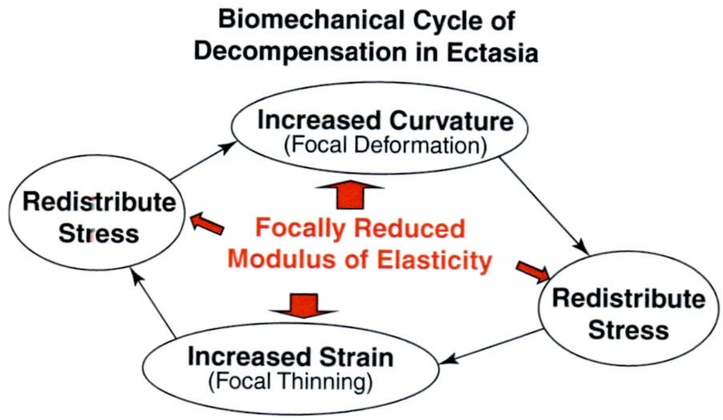

Fig. 9.2 Biomechanical cycle of decompensation in keratoconus, which illustrates the initiating event as a focal reduction in biomechanical properties, which leads to a redistribution of the stress, and subsequent thinning which generates an additional redistribution of stress, followed by a focal increase in curvature which also redistributes the stress. The cycle continues as the asymmetries in biomechanical properties, pachymetry, and curvature progress. (Reprinted with permission from Ref. [4])

ble cornea. Repeated rubbing can lead to focal changes in structure, which is consistent with the asymmetry of the collagen architecture in keratoconus described by Meek et al. [9]. This regional disruption of the normal collagen architecture and corneal structure in keratoconus is also consistent with focal weakening.

9.2 Stress Distribution in the Keratoconic Cornea and Impact on Treatment Response

Stress (σ) is a function of the applied load, which in the cornea is the intraocular pressure (IOP). Strain is stretching or deformation of the cornea under the applied load. The magnitude of the stress vs strain defines the elastic modulus. The greater the stress for a specific strain, the greater the elastic modulus and the stiffer is the cornea. This is illustrated in Fig. 9.3. If there is a regional difference in elastic modulus, then there is a regional difference in strain since the IOP is consistent across the cornea, as shown in Fig. 9.4. The stress in the cornea can be quantified with the formula for Hoop stress:

$$\sigma = P^{*}r/(2t),$$

where P = IOP, r = radius of curvature, and t = thickness

It is clear from the Hoop stress formula that stress is a function of both thickness and curvature with high stress associated with lower thickness and lower curvature (greater radius of curvature). It is often incorrectly assumed that the thinnest point carries the highest stress in keratoconus. However, the thinnest point at higher stress is also the steepest which is a compensatory stress-lowering response. Therefore, as the elastic modulus lowers focally in keratoconus, the strain increases focally, and the cornea thins in this region which generates a stress-lowering steepening to compensate.

When considering how to treat keratoconus, the asymmetry in properties should be considered for an optimal result. In addition, the stress distribution and regional strains can provide guidance. For example, referring to Fig. 9.4, one way to reduce the strain in the focal region would be to increase the elastic modulus. This is the goal of corneal collagen crosslinking. In fact, the measured asymmetry in biomechanical properties in keratoconus means that customized crosslinking, which concentrates the treatment in the area of the pathology, may serve to decrease the asymmetry of properties and provide a more effective result than the global crosslinking of the original standard protocol.

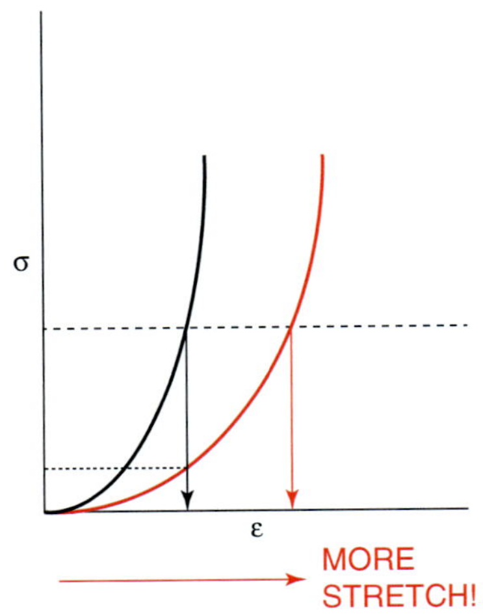

Fig. 9.3 Stress (**σ**) which is a function of load vs strain (**ε**) which is deformation or stretch in the corneal tissue. The black stress-strain curve represents the stiffer cornea since less deformation is associated with the same level of stress at all magnitudes. The red stress-strain curve represents the weaker corneal tissue since the same level of stress is associated with greater strain. (Adapted with permission from Ref. [4])

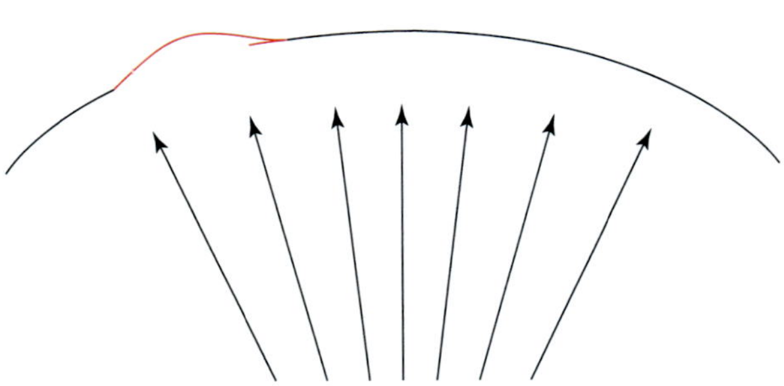

Fig. 9.4 The arrows represent the load produced by intraocular pressure (IOP) across the corneal surface. The black portion of the corneal surface is associated with the black stress-strain curve in Fig. 9.3. The red portion of the corneal surface is associated with the red stress-strain curve in Fig. 9.3, which would stretch to a greater amount under the same load, showing how a focally weak area can initiate the cycle of decompensation. This greater strain leads to subsequent thinning and steepening. (Adapted with permission from Ref. [4])

Intracorneal ring implantation, on the other hand, targets the curvature. It has been reported that properties are not changed by ring insertion [10]. However, by changing the curvature, as seen in Fig. 9.5, the stress distribution is immediately modified which interrupts the biomechanical cycle of decompensation (Fig. 9.6). This new biomechanical environment that is created, allows stabilization of the disease.

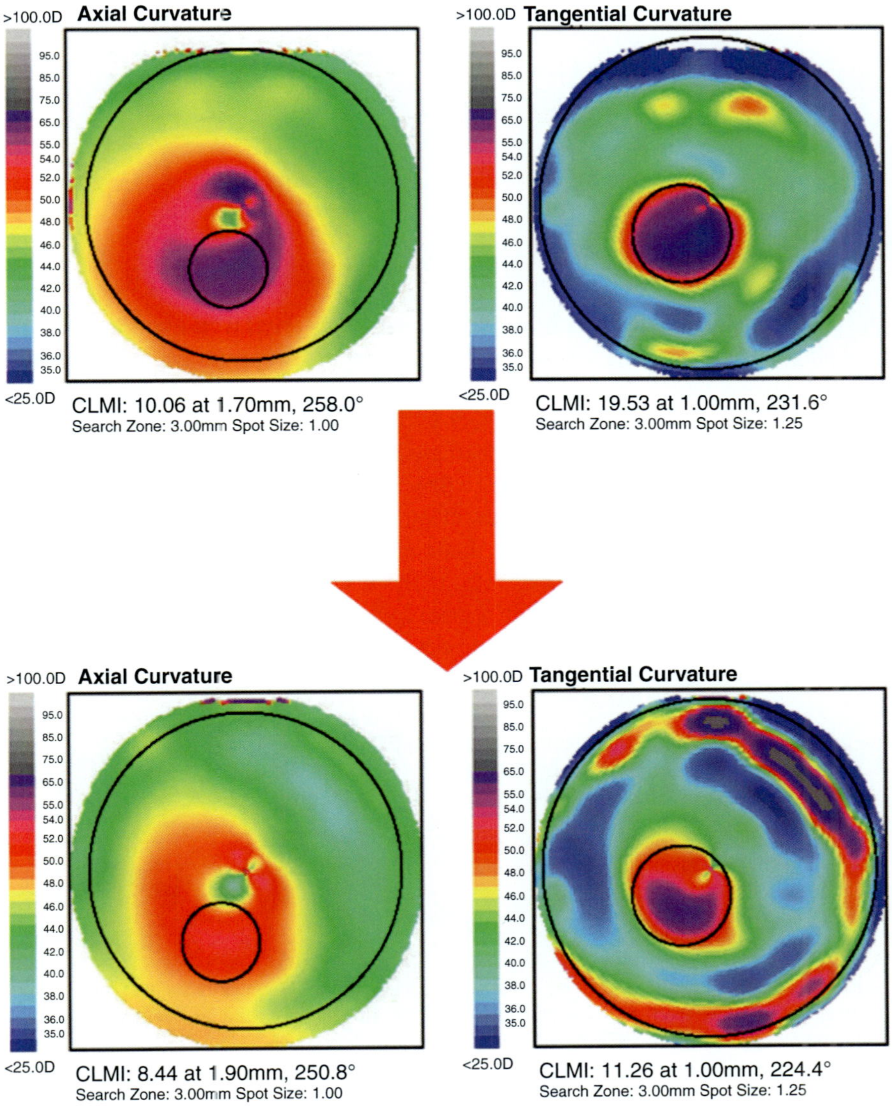

Fig. 9.5 Top row shows the average axial (left) and tangential (right) anterior surface curvature maps of all subjects prior to intracorneal ring placement. The bottom row shows the average corresponding maps of the same subjects after ring insertion. The average tangential map shows steepening over the rings and flattening in the center of the cone. (Adapted with permission from Ref. [10])

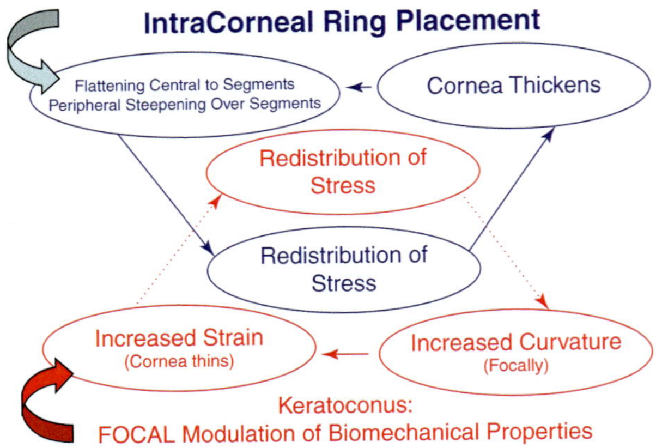

Fig. 9.6 Schematic illustration of how the insertion of intracorneal rings (blue) will interrupt the cycle of decompensation (red) in keratoconus. (Reprinted from Ref. [3])

9.3 Final Thoughts

The primary corneal alteration in keratoconus is likely *focal* weakening in the biomechanical properties. The subsequent asymmetric thinning and steepening are secondary changes which represent a response to the developing asymmetry in the properties. Therefore, one would expect to be able to detect the biomechanical changes prior to the development of decrease in pachymetry and increase in curvature. Recently, it has been reported that a new clinical device that uses an air puff to load the cornea for biomechanical assessment, is able to detect not only keratoconus with obvious geometric asymmetries that can be observed via tomographic mapping [11], but also subclinical cases [12]. In these subclinical cases, biomechanical abnormalities are measured even with normal tomographic parameters. It is expected that as future biomechanical indices are developed, it might be possible to detect biomechanical progression, as well as regression after treatment.

Disclosures Oculus Optikgeräte GmbH, Consultant
Optimeyes, Consultant and Advisory Board
Ziemer Ophthalmic Systems AG, Consultant

References

1. Reinstein DZ, Archer TJ, Gobbe M. Stability of LASIK in topographically suspect keratoconus confirmed non-keratoconic by Artemis VHF digital ultrasound epithelial thickness mapping: 1-year follow-up. J Refract Surg. 2009;25:569–77.
2. Ambrósio R Jr, Klyce SD, Wilson SE. Corneal topographic and pachymetric screening of keratorefractive patients. J Refract Surg. 2003;19:24–9.
3. Roberts CJ. Biomechanics of INTACS in keratoocnus. Chapter 10. In: Ertan A, Colin J, editors. Intracorneal ring segments and alternative treatments for corneal ectatic diseases. Ankara: Kudret Eye Hospital; 2007. p. 157–66.
4. Roberts CJ, Dupps WJ Jr. Biomechanics of corneal ectasia and biomechanical treatments. J Cataract Refract Surg. 2014;40(6):991–8.

5. Andreassen TT, Simonsen AH, Oxlund H. Biomechanical properties of keratoconus and normal corneas. Exp Eye Res 1980. 1980;31:435–41.
6. Sinha Roy A, Dupps WJ. Computational modeling of keratoconus progression and differential responses to collagen crosslinking. Invest Ophthalmol Vis Sci. 2011;52:9174–87.
7. Scarcelli G, Besner S, Pineda R, Yun SH. Biomechanical characterization of keratoconus corneas ex vivo with Brillouin microscopy. Invest Ophthalmol Vis Sci. 2014;55:4490–5.
8. Scarcelli G, Besner S, Pineda R, et al. In vivo biomechanical mapping of normal and keratoconus corneas. JAMA Ophthalmol. 2015;133:480–2.
9. Meek KM, Tuft SJ, Huang Y, Gill PS, Hayes S, Newton RH, Bron AJ. Changes in collagen orientation and distribution in keratoconus corneas. Invest Ophthalmol Vis Sci. 2005;46:1948–56.
10. Dauwe C, Touboul D, Roberts CJ, Mahmoud AM, Kérautret J, Fournier P, Malecaze F, Colin J. Biomechanical and morphological corneal response to placement of intrastromal corneal ring segments for keratoconus. J Cataract Refract Surg. 2009;35:1761–7.
11. Vinciguerra R, Ambrósio R Jr, Elsheikh A, Roberts CJ, Lopes B, Morenghi E, Azzolini C, Vinciguerra P. Dectection of keratoconus with a new biomechanical index. J Refract Surg. 2016;32:803–10.
12. Vinciguerra R, Ambrósio R Jr, Roberts CJ, Azzolini C, Vinciguerra P. Biomechanical characterization of subclinical keratoconus without topographic or tomographic abnormalities. J Refract Surg. 2017;33:399–407.

Chapter 10
Customized Corneal Cross-Linking

Cosimo Mazzotta, Miguel Rechichi, and Marco Ferrise

The term "*Customized Corneal Cross-linking*" (X-CXL) is an umbrella term that denotes a variety of emerging techniques proposed in the recent years for the management of corneal ectasia and other conditions.

Schematically, the three big topics that fall under the X-CXL can be summarized as following (Fig. 10.1):

1. *Accelerated Topography-Guided Corneal Cross-linking* for the treatment of kerectasia and for refractive purposes.
2. *Accelerated Pachymetry-Guided Corneal Cross-linking,* a variation of the standard protocol proposed to shorten the CXL procedure time thus improving the patient's comfort.

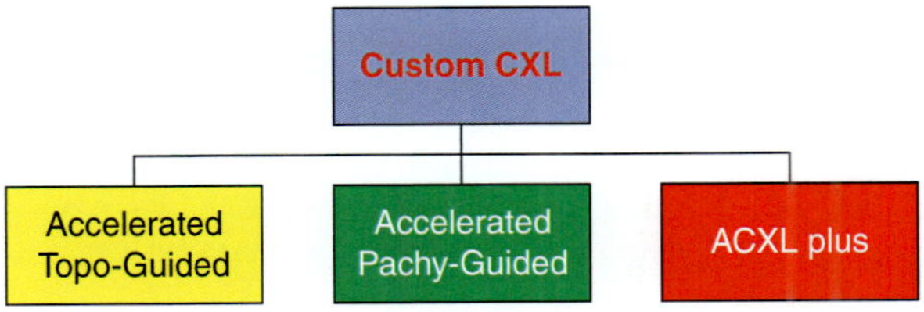

Fig. 10.1 Customized corneal collagen CXL procedures

C. Mazzotta (✉)
Post-Graduate Ophthalmology School, University of Siena, Siena, Italy

Siena Crosslinking Center®, OcuMedical Vision, Siena, Italy

M. Rechichi
Eye Center®, Catanzaro, Italy

Centro Polispecialistico Mediterraneo, Catanzaro, Italy

M. Ferrise
Siena Crosslinking Center®, OcuMedical Vision, Siena, Italy

Centro Polispecialistico Mediterraneo, Catanzaro, Italy

Studio Oculistico Ferrise, Lamezia Terme, Italy

A. Barbara (ed.), *Controversies in the Management of Keratoconus*,
https://doi.org/10.1007/978-3-319-98032-4_10

3. *Accelerated Corneal Cross-linking-Plus*, a combination of corneal cross-linking and refractive surgical techniques for the treatment of corneal ectasia, that adds to the corneal stabilization the benefit of an improvement or empowerment in visual acuity.

10.1 Topography-Guided Corneal Cross-Linking

Riboflavin UV-A corneal cross-linking (CXL) was first developed in Dresden by Wollensak, Seiler and Spoerl and has been widely used to treat both *primary* corneal ectatic disorders, such as Keratoconus (KC), Pellucid Marginal Degeneration (PMD) and *secondary* ectatic disorders like iatrogenic post-refractive procedures (post-Lasik, PRK, RK, Smile) ectasia.

At the base of ectasia is a chronic biomechanical failure that leads to thinning and protrusion of the corneal tissue. KC (word derived from Greek: *Kerato* = Cornea and *Conus* = Cone) is the most common type of ectatic disorder, where the central or paracentral cornea undergoes thinning and steepening resulting in a cone shaped protrusion. The changes are progressive and cause irregular astigmatism and high order aberrations, like coma, which cannot be fully corrected by spectacles, impairing the quality of life of the patients affected by it. The incidence of KC was traditionally considered to be approximately 1 per 2000 in the general population [1], and that number went unchallenged for many years. Recently, the rise in popularity of refractive surgery procedures (Lasik, PRK etc.) and the modernization of the available diagnostic tools (mainly the advent of corneal tomography, both by Scheimpflug camera and by optical coherence tomography of the anterior segment) have revealed, according to some newer studies, that the real incidence of KC is likely higher [2, 3]. Also, in patients of different ethnic origins, exists a significant difference in the relative frequency of KC [4].

KC is a bilateral condition but almost always asymmetrical. It usually has its onset in puberty with progression over a 10–20 years period, with a rate of progression especially high in children [5].

The primary goal in the management of Keratoconus (KC) and other corneal ectatic disorders is to increase corneal rigidity thus halting the progression of the pathology. There is clinical evidence that corneal cross-linking (CXL) is capable to stop the progression of primary and secondary corneal ectasia, and presents a failure rate of approximately 3–10% and a complication rate of 1–13% [6, 7].

CXL has been used to stiffen the keratoconic cornea by instilling riboflavin in combination with exposure to an ultraviolet-A light source, strengthening the biochemical and mechanical properties of the cornea [8].

The current technique of CXL involves an all-over treatment of an 9 mm diameter region of the cornea, even if the characteristic alteration in KC is focal in nature. In fact, it has been postulated that at the origin of KC is a focal biomechanical modification and not a uniform generalized weakening, namely a focal reduction in the tissue elastic modulus, that starts a vicious cycle of biomechanical decompensation driven by asymmetry in the biomechanical properties; the cycle is initiated by asymmetry in the elastic modulus, which causes a corneal thinning, causing a stress increase, which causes the cornea to deform in order to compensate. Biomechanical modelling of the cross-linked cornea made known that for the stabilization of KC could be superfluous to strengthen the entire tissue, in fact similar results could be obtained by treating only the weak parts of the diseased cornea [9]. This reasoning is at the core of the use of Customized CXL for KC, which uses selectively more energy for the weaker area of the corneal tissue and less/no energy in the peripheral stronger areas.

Presently, there is no instrument that can, in the clinical practice, point out to the surgeon the weak areas of the keratoconic cornea by measuring the elastic modulus, so the target of the customized treatment is chosen indirectly by using the traditional parameters of posterior float location and anterior curvature. According to computer simulations, an asymmetric pattern of UV-A irradiation with its center on the ectatic cone provides a greater flattening than conventional treatment [10].

The possibility to differentially cross-link different parts of the cornea was recently introduced by Avedro Company (Avedro, Waltham, MA, USA); this customized procedure, called Photorefractive Intra-stromal Cross-Linking (PiXL), performed using the Avedro's Mosaic® UV-A source, allows to deliver a patterned, topography-guided Accelerated cross-linking to the cornea.

In 2017 Nordström et al. presented an open-label, randomized clinical trial on 50 eyes of 37 patients with progressive keratoconus. The patients included were randomized, and a group received uniform pulsed 1 s on/1 s off pulsed 370 nm UVA irradiation of 30 mW/cm^2 epithelium-off crosslinking with treatment energy of 5.4 J/cm^2 (CXL; n = 25) while the other group received a topography-guided epi-off CXL with asymmetrical treatment zones and variable treatment energies (PiXL, n = 25) using the Avedro KXL II® system (Avedro, Waltham, MA, USA) [11]. Their in vivo findings of a greater potential of PiXL to reshape the cornea compared to uniform broad-beam irradiation CXL seems to be concordant with the previously cited computer simulations by Roy, Dupps et al.

In the first italian multicenter study of customized CXL for treatment of keratoconus [12], Mazzotta, Fontana et al. investigated the 1-year functional and morphological results of Topography-guided ACXL. Topography-guided Accelerated CXL were carried out on 21 eyes with progressive KC by means of the KXL II UV-A illuminator using a 30 mW/cm^2 UV-A power with pulsed-light emission (1 s on/1 s off). Treatments were planned individually based on the preoperative topography data. The 30 mW/cm^2 ACXL treatments presented a different energy dose release correlated to the different corneal curvatures showed by each keratoconus, resulting in a fully customized treatment, Fig. 10.2. The lowest energy dose of 7.2 J/cm^2 was delivered in the flattest peripheral cone area under 48 dioptres (D) of K_{max} (resulting in 8 min of UV-A exposure time). Ectatic areas with maximum corneal curvature over 48 D and under 52 D were treated with an energy dose of 10 J/cm^2 (11 min of total exposure time). The areas of corneal curvature over 52 D were treated by extending the exposure time to 16 min, thus reaching the maximum energy dose of 15 J/cm^2.

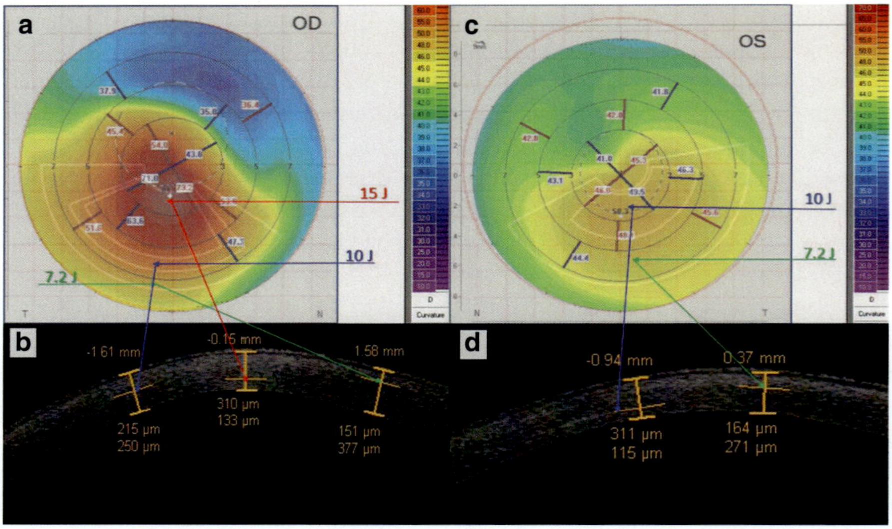

Fig. 10.2 Topography-Guided ACXL treatment programs according to different KC severity. (**a**) Shows a 3-Zone topography guided ACXL treatment planning according to corneal curvatures. Post-operative Corneal Visante® OCT (Zeiss) scans 1 month after treatment, (**b**) revealed a triple demarcation line according to the three different exposure times and energy doses: 7.2 J/cm^2 in the peripheral KC flattest area 48 D and under (depth 151 μm), green arrows (8 min UV-A exposure); 10 J/cm^2 in the intermediate area between 48 and 52 D (depth 215 μm), blue arrows (11 min UV-A exposure); 15 J/cm^2 in the steepest area (depth 310 μm), red arrows (16 min UV-A Exposure). (**c**) Shows a 2-Zone topography guided ACXL treatment with 7.2 (green arrows) and 10 J/cm^2 (blue arrows) E doses treatment planning. OCT scan performed 1 month after treatment, (**d**) revealed a double demarcation line according to the different exposure times and doses delivered according to corneal curvatures, reaching a demarcation line depth of 164 μm in the peripheral area treated with 7.2 J/cm^2 for 8 min of UVA exposure (green arrow) and 311 μm in the steeper paracentral area treated with 10 J/cm^2 for 11 min of UV-A exposure (blue arrow)

At 1-year follow-up, the Italian multicenter (Siena-Reggio Emilia) study showed clinical outcomes on par with conventional broad-beam epi-off CXL, but with a faster improvement in quality of vision and less postoperative glare at 1 month, indicating that topography-guided ACXL reduced the topographic cylinder magnitude better than standard broad-beam CXL and has a potentiality for a better visual rehabilitation other than just stabilizing the ectasia, Fig. 10.3.

10.1.1 PiXL as a Refractive Surgery Procedure

The original purpose of the CXL as described by its creators almost 20 years ago was solely the stabilization of the progression on the kerectasia while sparing corneal tissue. What was noticed during the years was that the tissutal strengthening causes an alteration in the corneal biomechanics which, in the clinical practice, can be observed as a reduction of the corneal curvature [13, 14].

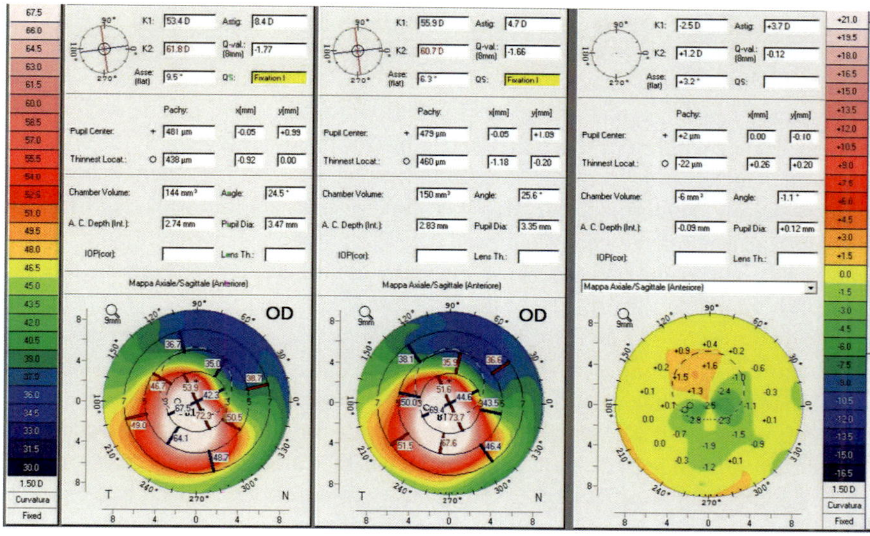

Fig. 10.3 Comparative Pentacam® exams after Topography-Guided ACXL with three zone energy treatment show – 1.8D apex flattening with a compensatory steepening of the flat area in the superior part of the cone, thus improving corneal symmetry and reducing cylinder magnitude by a mean value of −1.4 D ± 0.8

In the recent years it's been proposed that a customized application of CXL on the cornea may be used to selectively stiffen chosen parts of the tissue, thus changing the corneal curvature; this would be done with the purpose to induce specific variations in the *refraction* of the treated eye. Recent studies have confirmed this hypothesis using computational modeling; In fact, smaller diameter simulated treatments centered on the cone provided greater reductions in curvature and high-order aberrations (HOA) than a standard broad-beam CXL pattern [10].

Based on these premises, PiXL has been presented clinically by John Kanellopoulos and used for correction of low-grade refractive errors, such as myopia, astigmatism, hyperopia and even presbyopia. Of course, each procedure needs a custom pattern of UV-A irradiation. The myopic correction is done by applying a central circular pattern of UV-A irradiation [15, 16] resulting in a central corneal flattening. The possibility to have a topography-guided ACXL treatment capable of reducing or eliminating myopia and astigmatism by mean of a non-ablative, non-incisional surgery, presents the potentiality to be a groundbreaking innovation, the biggest point being the absence of removal of stromal tissue that characterizes current refractive surgery procedures. In fact, this preservation of stromal tissue avoids the feared impairment of the biostructural integrity of the cornea that results in a weakening the stroma, and on the contrary this CXL procedure selectively stiffens certains area of the cornea. The astigmatism correction uses a bow-tie pattern, also useful for the management of keratoconus [17]. The hyperopic correction is done by using a peripheral doughnut or annular pattern, that aims to achieve a corneal steepening [18]. The *presbyopic correction* also aims to increase corneal steepening like the hyperopic pattern, since near work needs an increased refractive power; this kind of treatment also increases corneal asphericity and depth of field [19]. One of the current hottest topics regarding PhotoRefractive IntraStromal Cross-Linking is the Epi-Off vs Epi-On debate. Like the conventional CXL, PiXL can be performed with (Epi-Off) or without (transepithelial or Epi-On) the debridement of the corneal epithelium. The advantages of the Epi-On technique are multiple, such as lowered risk of infections, higher post-operative comfort for the patient, lower risk of haze and wound healing related complications [20]. The problem is that epithelium naturally acts as a barrier for UV-A penetration, so by not removing it there is the risk of significantly reducing the efficacy of the CXL treatment [21].

Lim et al. in June 2017 published the 9–12 months outcomes of Epi-On PiXL for the reduction of low myopia on 14 eyes, and reported the safety and effectiveness of this treatment [22]. Since it is a small case study, we need larger clinical studies with longer follow-up to fully comprehend the efficacy of Epi-On PiXL and the stability of the refractive changes. It's known that oxygen is the catalyst of CXL reaction and that the biomechanical effect of CXL are oxygen-dependent, so higher oxygen availability could possibly increase the overall efficacy of riboflavin UV-A CXL treatment [23]. In fact, there is currently at least a clinical trial (named PiXLO2) [24] to evaluate the effectiveness of the PiXL myopic treatment in an high oxygen intraoperative environment without corneal epithelial debridement. The preliminary data of this ongoing Swedish study showed better myopia reducing effects, up to 1 D of supplemental correction, using high oxygen compared to room air with Epi-On PiXL, as discussed in a presentation from the 21st Winter Meeting of the European Society of Cataract and Refractive Surgeons (ESCRS), in Maastricht, Holland [25]. In conclusion, PiXL seems to be a promising addition to the current apparatus of refractive correction options. The patients that could benefit from this treatment are numerous, starting with patients with low refractive errors unwilling to undergo traditional refractive surgery, patients with residual defects after cataract surgery or previous refractive surgery, and patients with borderline suspicious corneal tomography in which a standard refractive surgery procedure may induce a iatrogenic ectasia, like in a forme fruste KC; this last category of patients may as well benefit from the biomechanical corneal strengthening provided by the PiXL.

The PiXL procedure is theoretically still in its embryonic stage; in the coming years, many new improvements have the potentiality be implemented, such as the intraoperative use of supplemental oxygen, the creation of nomograms for all kind of refractive errors, and the evaluation in-vivo of corneal biomechanics.

10.2 Accelerated Corneal Cross-Linking as Base for the New Customized CXL Procedures

After the clinical validation of the conventional Corneal Cross-linking procedure in terms of safety and efficacy [6, 26], one of the strongest priorities of clinical research seems to have been the reduction of treatment times. In fact, the standard protocol times add up to a full hour, between the 30 min required for soaking the stroma with riboflavin and the 30 min of UV-A irradiation.

A reduction of treatment times could in theory present many benefits, ranging from an improved tolerance of the patients, an improved safety of the treatment (shorter procedure times may reduce the risk of intraoperative stromal dehydration, thus providing a more predictable pachimetry), as well as a reduction of operative times for the surgeon. The principle behind accelerated corneal cross-linking resides in photochemistry, more specifically the Bunsen-Roscoe Law of reciprocity. Theoretically this law implies that the standard CXL procedure times could be modified without changes in efficacy, as long as the total irradiation dose stays the same. For example, the same effect as the conventional Dresden protocol of 3 mW/cm^2 for 30 min can be achieved by setting the UV-A power at 9 mW/cm^2 for 10 min, 30 mW/cm^2 for 3 min, 18 mW/cm^2 for 5 min, and 45 mW/cm^2 for 2 min while maintaining a constant energy (fluence) of 5.4 J/cm^2 [27].

Krueger et al. [28] reported in 2014 a preclinical laboratory investigation of accelerated crosslinking on porcine ocular globes; using a 370 nm UV-A source they cross-linked porcine corneas with irradiances of 2, 3, 9, and 15 mW/cm^2 with continous exposure, and with 15 mW/cm^2 with fractionated exposure, alternating 30 s "ON" and 30 s "OFF", for a total dose of 5.4 mJ/cm^2. They subsequently measured corneal stiffness performing extensiometry, and the results showed no statistically significant differences between standard and higher irradiances. Moreover, the results showed no substantial differences between continuous exposure and fractionated exposure. This study seems to indicate that pulsed UV-A delivery should theoretically improve the degree of CXL, especially in conjunction with accelerated treatments during which oxygen is consumed more quickly [29]; the reason behind this is that oxygen, an important factor in the photochemical activation of riboflavin with UV light, can re-diffuse during the pauses of UV-A light exposure thus improving the efficacy of the CXL reaction [12].

The most commonly studied accelerated protocols are the 9 mW/cm^2 Accelerated CXL, the 18 mW/cm^2 Accelerated CXL, the 30 mW/cm^2 Accelerated CXL, the 45 mW/cm^2 Accelerated CXL and the 15 mW/cm^2 Accelerated CXL; the clinical data behind these protocols will be breafly summed up below.

10.2.1 The 9 mW/cm^2 Accelerated CXL

In 2013 Cinar et al. published a study in which they compared the accelerated procedure (9 mW/cm^2) and the conventional procedure (3 mW/cm^2) for the treatment of progressive keratoconus. They highlighted how the refractive and visual results of the two procedures were similar in the short term, but since the accelerated procedure was faster patients were more compliant [30]. The following year, the same authors published a clinical study evaluating the efficiency of accelerated crosslinking at 9 mW/cm^2 in the case of progressive keratoconus, and noted that with the patients treated early there was a significant change in the UDVA, although not in all. Only after 6 months did the CDVA show significant improvement [31]. The same result was observed by Hersh et al. at 6 months [32] while Vinciguerra et al. reported at a year [14]. The improvement in the CDVA could be attributed to changes in the keratometric indexes. Cinar further encountered that the flat keratometry, steep keratometry, average keratometry were significantly reduced 6-months after this procedure. It was noted that the reduction in the Kmax value could be due to an increase in the biomechanical stability of the cornea [31]. Instead, Legare reported a stabilization in the K values. Nonetheless, there are no significant Km and K changes after the 2-year follow-up [33]. In the study of Cinar there were no significant changes in thinnest corneal thickness (TCT) 6 months after 9 mW A-CXL [31]. Kymionis et al. carried out a prospective comparative study to evaluate the depth of the corneal demarcation lines in the two procedures increasing exposure time (9 mW/cm^2 in 14 min instead of 10 min) and standard Dresden Protocol (3 mW/cm^2). They highlighted that the difference in depth of the demarcation line was not statistically significant between the two groups [34]. One of the studies with the broadest follow-ups was carried out by Shetty et al. 18 patients were analysed over 2 years, with an average age of 12.7 years. Their evaluations showed an improvement in visual acuity in terms of average UDVA and average CDVA over 2 years.

Further, there was an improvement of the sphere, the cylinder and the spherical equivalent. As far as the keratometry was concerned, a statically significant flattening of average K 1 and average K 2 at the end of 2 years was observed [35]. Elbaz et al. in a retrospective study 1 year after the accelerated procedure (9 mW/cm^2) concluded that the accelerated procedure is capable of stabilizing corneal parameters, but a larger and longer study with a more complete followup was required to validate it. They reported significant changes in CVDA, cylinder and spherical equivalent, but only a minimal change in the UDVA. All corneal parameters included: Ksteep, Kflat, Km, corneal astigmatism (Kcyl), and maximum curvature of the corneal apex, were stable from 6 to 12 months in all patients [36]. From December 2012 to September 2013 Jain et al. monitored corneal pachimetrical changes during accelerated treatment using isotonic riboflavin with HPMC. In 14 patients with a median age between 19 ± 8, they used pachimetry during the ACXL procedure. An isotonic solution was applied to the cornea after epithelium removal followed by the application of a riboflavin solution for 20 min, and lastly UV-A ray irradiation for 10 min with 9 mW/cm^2. No statistically significant changes of corneal thickness were noted before, during and after the procedure [37]. Pahuja et al. evaluated 33 eyes with a history of keratoconus, and looked at the correlation between the biomechanical results with the molecular operation of correlated ectasia genes. They evaluated visual acuity, keratometry, densitometry and results of corneal deformation after treatment, as well as the association with gene expression of proteins of the extracellular matrix (MMP 9, LOX, TGFβ, TNFα, IL10, IL6, COL A1 e COL IVA 1) using qPCR. They reported that the 9 mW ACXL procedure appears to be secure and provides biomechanical stability. Both keratometry and refraction remained stable after treatment, with a significant improvement of the cylindrical error. Pre-operative levels of the different proteins did not influence the clinical results described [38]. Cross-linking treatment is not only applied in the case of progressive keratoconus. Indeed, Marino et al. applied the 9 mW/cm^2 ACXL procedure to patients with post-LASIK ectasia. Analysing 40 eyes in 24 patients in terms of UDVA, CDVA, central corneal thickness, corneal topography, and endothelial cell density, they reported that the results are secure and efficient in the case of ectasia after a 2-year follow-up. Here, as well, they underlined that a larger group and longer follow-up is necessary to validate this new procedure [39]. In a recent study of Sadoughi et al. [40], the results of the conventional cross- linking (CXL) were compared to 9 mW ACXL in patients with bilateral progressive keratoconus (KC). Fifteen consecutive patients were enrolled with a 12-months follow-up. In each patient, the fellow eyes were randomly assigned to conventional CXL (3 mW/cm^2 for 30 min) or accelerated CXL (9 mW/cm^2 for 10 min) groups. Accelerated CXL with 9 mW/cm^2 for 10 min irradiation had a similar refractive, visual, keratometric and aberrometric result and less adverse effects on the corneal thickness and endothelial cells compared to the conventional method after 12 months of follow-up.

10.2.2 The 18 mW/cm^2 Accelerated CXL

As far as the 18 mW/cm^2/5 min procedure is concerned we can look to the trials of Cingu et al. who evaluated endothelial changes in the ACXL procedure comparing it with the standard procedure. No differences were stressed between the two groups that underwent different protocols, but nonetheless there is a reduction of 500 cell/mm^2 in the first post-operative period after ACXL. From the third to the sixth months the results were similar. Cingu advises that there could be a transient change in human endothelial cells in ACXL. The resolution of these changes during the follow- up indicate a secure recovery [41]. Hashemi et al. [42] evaluated the long and short term effects obtained with the 18 mW/cm^2/5 min ACXL compared to the standard CXL in two randomized studies made up of 31 patients. At 6-months follow-up, the two procedures had stopped the progression of keratoconus in a similar way. UDVA, CDVA, and the spherical equivalent do not show any significant changes between the two groups. In the standard procedure, the thickness of the central cornea results as higher compared to accelerated. The reduction of K max, K average, and average changes in corneal asphericity were not statistically different. Even changes in corneal hysteresis, factors of corneal resistance, and the area under apex were similar. Lastly, reduction in endothelial cells count (ECC) was not statistically significant in both groups [43]. The long-term comparison demonstrated that between the two groups, the results and security profile were similar, but the standard procedure produced higher corneal flattening.

However, both methods have the ability to stop keratoconus progression in a similar way. This affirmation is confirmed evaluating 31 eyes with the accelerated procedure, compared to eyes treated with the standard procedure using the same energy dose of 5.4 J/cm^2. At 18 months from the procedure the group treated with the conventional method presented an improvement in the spherical equivalent, in K-readings, Q Value, improvement of the surface symmetry index and a temporary reduction in corneal thickness, but no significant changes in visual acuity, corneal hysteresis, corneal resistance factor, or endothelial cell density. As far as the group treated with the accelerated procedure was concerned, the corneal thickness was the only parameter that changed in any statically significant way. However, none of these parameters shows a significant difference between the standard and 18 mW/cm^2 ACXL procedures [43]. Chow et al. compared the results of the conventional procedure (3 mW/cm^2; 365-nm ultraviolet-A light, 30 min) with accelerated (18 mW/cm^2; 365-nm ultraviolet-A light, 5 min) in patients with progressive keratoconus. The effect of corneal flattening obtained with conventional CXL was statistically significant compared to that of the 18 mW accelerated procedure after a year follow-up. Except for the corneal thickness that results as thinner, the topographical and clinical parameters were stable in both groups [44]. In this study, there was a significant improvement in the UCVA, BCVA and spherical equivalent in both groups. Previous studies have shown similar functional improvement after CXL [6, 45–49]. This has been attributed to improvement in the regularity of the corneal shape after CXL. From the topographical point of view, there were no clinically significant changes, but a reduction in the keratometry was noted in both the accelerated and the conventional groups. Thus, like other studies demonstrated improvement of the topographical flattening obtainable in more curved corneas. Carrying out an association analysis, Chan et al. found a negative association among the baseline keratometry and the post-operative keratometric values found in the ACXL group. The higher values of maximum baseline keratometry were associated with a greater reduction in the maximum keratometry values. The same negative association was also found in standard procedure cases [50]. One recently published comparative study of four CXL protocols in homogeneous pre-operative keratoconic eyes (steep keratometry between 48.6 and 50.5 D), demonstrated that conventional CXL of 3 mW/cm^2 has a stronger effect on flattening compared to the ACXL protocol of 9, 18 and 30 mW/cm^2 over a year follow-up. This was found in another study with a different selection of patients: that 18 mW/cm^2 concluding that accelerated CXL treatment is not capable of inducing corneal flattening at 1 year in eyes with a base Kmax <58 D, and an average variation of 1.00 ± 1.63 D of Kmax at 1 year. The authors attributed this potential reduction to the biomechanical effect of the 18 mW/cm^2 ACXL treatment [51]. Wernli et al. observed that with 40–45 mW/cm^2 for 2 min an increase in the rigidity equivalent could be reached. For more elevated intensities that go from 50 to 90 mW/cm^2, no statistically significant increase in rigidity could be obtained citing the non-applicability of the Bunsen–Roscoe law of reciprocity for brief, high intensity illumination time [48]. Hammer et al. observed a tendency of the reduction in the Young model with increased irradiation, reaching some statistically significant differences between 18 mW/cm^2 and the controls group. The authors proposed the hypothesis that the intra-stromal capacity of diffusion and the increase in the consumption of oxygen associated with higher irradiation can be a limiting factor, with consequential reduction of the efficiency of the treatment [49]. A reduced depth of postoperative demarcation line was observed with 18 mW/cm^2 ACXL which suggests a reduced effect of treatment compared to conventional CXL treatment [52]. Kymionis et al.

also discovered that a 40% increase in irradiation treatment was needed in the accelerated procedure to obtain a similar demarcation line depth like that obtained in the conventional procedure [53]. Kurt et al. evaluated the results of 18 mW/cm^2 for 5 min ACXL procedure in an 18-month follow-up in patients with progressive keratoconus. Forty-two eyes of 42 patients with an age range from 24 to 36 years were studied. Finding a significant improvement in the UDVA and CDVA, a significant reduction of the Kflat, K steep and K apical curvature (AK), concluding that that the ACXL procedure was effective for the stabilization keratoconus progression during 18-month follow-up [54, 55].

10.2.3 The 30 mW/cm^2 Accelerated CXL

Mazzotta et al. performed a comparative study between 30 mW/cm^2 epithelium-off ACXL with pulsed light (pl-ACXL 8 min UVA exposure) and continuous light (cl-ACXL 4 min UVA exposure). Twenty eyes were treated with a dose of energy used was 7.2 J/cm^2 for both groups, according to Avedro 30 mW first protocol [56]. Through comparative analysis efficiency in the stabilization of the progress of keratoconus was shown for both procedures at a 1-year follow-up. Further, the pulsed light procedure had slightly better results in terms of UCVA, even if a true significant difference was not found between the two treatment modalities. The slight improvement obtained in the UCVA could be attributed to an improvement in K-average values and a reduction of the KC apical curvature (AK). Further, the same study evaluated the effect of the two procedures regarding the degree of ACXL stromal penetration measured by corneal OCT and confocal documenting the demarcation line depth at 1 month. An apoptotic effect was discovered at 215 μm of depth on average in the pl ACXL with 8 min of UVA exposure and at 160 μm of depth on average in the cl ACXL with 4 min of UVA exposure [56, 57]. This was the first study documenting that 30 mW/cm^2 ACXL induced a more superficial cross-linking penetration especially if continuous light irradiation and shorter exposure time is used, opening a new way for the treatment of thin corneas. Moreover, the study demonstrated that pulsing the light intra-operatively the re- uptake of oxygen is induced and the increased exposure time at 8 min influenced a better penetration of the oxidative damage around 200 μm of corneal stroma.

Both procedures reached the anterior part of the corneal stroma up to a depth of 200 μ [56, 58, 59]. The functional improvement of ACXL with pulsed light could be a way to optimize disposition of oxygen, thanks to the on/off cycle of oxygen delivery. In fact, treatments have observed a similar efficiency in keratoconus stabilization in all follow-up periods. Both modalities represent a safe procedure in the short-term evolution of keratoconus stabilization [56, 59]. Even for Mazzotta et al. the efficiency of this technique must be evaluated with longer follow-ups and larger control groups. However, the inferior penetration of these ACXL protocols can be used for CXL customization in different ectatic pathways. Another Italian study performed by Fontana et al. [60] compared the two methods of pulsed and continued light ACXL treatment. They evaluated the stromal demarcation line depth after ACXL with continued light (30 mW/cm^2 for 4 min), and pulsed light (30 mW/cm^2 for 8 min 1 s on – 1 s off) with a total energy dose of 7.2 J/cm^2. A month after the procedure, the stromal corneal demarcation line was measured by two different people using anterior segment optical coherence tomography (AS-OCT). After evaluating 60 patients they concluded that the average demarcation line depth was deeper in the pulsed light group (213 μm) compared to the continuous light group (149.32 μm) showing a statistically significant difference. This study substantially confirmed the findings of Mazzotta et al. concerning a more superficial penetration of 30 mW/cm^2 of ACXL treatment and advantages of pulsed-light treatment increasing depth of demarcation line and ACXL efficiency [56, 59]. Ozgurhan et al. carried out a retrospective study evaluating paediatric patients between 9 and 18 years of age (15.3 ± 2.1 years) treated with the accelerated procedure (30 mW/cm^2) for 24-months follow-up. In this trial as well they concluded that the procedure was capable of stopping the progression of keratoconus without side effects in paediatric patients. Visual acuity, keratometric values and corneal aberrations improved all [61]. Another fundamental aspect evaluated by Ozgurhan et al. in one of their previous works was the effect of 30 mW/cm^2 ACXL in the treatment of keratoconic thin corneas. They treated 34 eyes of 34 patients who had a corneal thickness inferior to 400 μm. UDVA and CDVA, manifested refraction and topography were evaluated at 1–6 and 12-month follow-up. The density of endothelial cells (cell/mm^2) was evaluated pre-and post-operatively at 12 months. Further, they measured the stromal demarcation line with anterior segment OCT 1 month after the procedure. The results show how UDVA, CDVA, average spherical and cylindrical refraction improve, but not in any significant way. They conclude that the accelerated procedure was able to stabilize the progression of keratoconus in thin corneas under 400 μm without a significant loss of endothelial cells (varying from 2726.02 ± 230.21 to 2714.58 ± 218.26 cells/mm^2) during the 12-month follow-up [62]. A 6-month retrospective study by Mita et al. [63] evaluated the efficiency of the 30 mW/cm^2 ACXL procedure at 5.4 J/cm^2 and 3 min of UV-A exposure. They treated 39 eyes in 22 patients with progressive keratoconus by looking at changes in dioptric strength and corneal topography. Per the authors, the 30 mW/cm^2 ACXL procedure at 5.4 J/cm^2 and 3 min of UV-A exposure has the potential to be an effective and efficient way to arrest the progression of keratoconus, and it could also be an efficient therapy option for the treatment of other corneal ectasias. The check-ups were carried out pre-operatively at 1, 3 and 6 months. The changes after the procedure were similar to those of the standard CXL procedure. UDVA and Kmax values showed statistically significant improvement. Regarding the density of endothelial cells, however, there were no significant changes preand post- operatively. These results were encouraging and suggested that 30 mW/cm^2 ACXL could improve corneal steepening, and could prevent the progression of keratoconus and in many cases including the regression of keratoconus. The observed reduction in Kmax values could be the result in improved biomechanical stability of the cornea after accelerated CXL, a result found in numerous studies as well. Even the biomechanical parameters measured with the dynamic bidirectional applanation device (ocular response analyser) did not change after the procedure. Similar results were reported after having used the conventional protocol [64]. In Mita's study the degree of treatment penetration was checked by the Heidelberg Retinal Tomograph II in vivo confocal microscopy, reporting an average was depth approximately at 320 μm, however this data is in contrast will all the repeatable data reported in literature by various European research groups [56, 57, 59, 65, 66]. The typical initial damage of the procedure included the disappearance of stromal keratocytes associated with hyper-reflective extracellular matrix and lacunar stromal oedema, that are all changes similar to those demonstrated for the first time at international level by Mazzotta after the conventional procedure [66]. Another study carried out by Tomita et al. [67] comparing the results obtained through the accelerated procedure (30 mW/cm^2 for 3 min) and the conventional one (3 mW/cm^2 in 30 min) with a 1-year follow-up considered 48 eyes of 39 patients (30 eyes underwent the 30 mW/cm^2 ACXL procedure and 18 underwent the 3 mW/cm^2 conventional procedure). In both procedures, a similar dose of UVA rays (5.4 J/cm^2) was used with the same riboflavin solution and soaking times. Accelerated CXL and conventional CXL both proved safe and efficient. The ACXL, being faster, seemed to be the most advantageous for both patients and surgeons. These authors, too, agreed that an 8–10-year follow-up is needed. There were no statistically significant differences regarding UDVA, CDVA or the spherical equivalent manifested in both procedures. Further, there were no significant changes in the keratometric values measured with the Pentacam, or in the biomechanical response measured with the dynamic bidirectional applanation device ocular response analyser (ORA). There were no differences in pre-and post-operative endothelial cells count in the two procedures.

10.2.4 The 45 mW/cm^2 Accelerated CXL

The study carried out by Sherif et al. at the University of Cairo [68] compared two groups of eyes with mild to moderate keratoconus for 12 months. It was found that the progressive reduction of flat keratometry, steep keratometry and mean keratometry were highlighted in the whole follow-up period in the two groups. The improvement of the keratinometric values were not significant. Visual acuity expressed in BSCVA shows an improvement at both 6 and 12 months, but to validate the procedure there must be more studies done with a longer follow-up and larger group of controls.

10.2.5 The 15 mW/cm^2 Accelerated CXL

Following the aforementioned preclinical study by Krueger et al. [28], in 2017 Mazzotta et al. published a study presenting the 2-year clinical results (both functional and microstructural) of accelerated 15 mW pulsed-light corneal crosslinking to treat progressive keratoconus [69].

After epithelium removal (with Epi-Clear) and 10 min stromal soaking with riboflavin 0.1% hydroxypropyl methylcellulose solution, all 132 eyes (stage II KC by Amsler-krumeich classification) eyes had 15 mW/cm^2 pulsed light epithelium-off accelerated CXL for 6 min of ultraviolet-A (UVA) irradiation (1 s on/1 s off), maintaining a total UVA exposure of 12 min at a fluence of 5.4 J/cm^2. The 2-year follow-up examination included uncorrected (UDVA) and corrected (CDVA) distance visual acuities, Scheimpflug tomography, in vivo confocal microscopy (IVCM), and spectral domain optical coherence tomography (SD-OCT). As demonstrated by Mazzotta in vivo confocal microscopy studies [56, 59, 65, 70–73], by using continuous and pulsed-light UVA emission at 30 mW/cm^2 high irradiance CXL at 5.4 J for 4 and 8 min, the treatment penetration is 200 ± 20 μm and 250 ± 20 μm of corneal stroma respectively. To ensure long-lasting stability of keratoconus and secondary ectasia, the UV-A power setting and exposure time should be targeted to allow a treatment penetration of at least at 250 mm, overcoming the anterior portion of the corneal stroma because the anterior 40% of the central corneal stroma represents the strongest region of the cornea (stiff cornea), whereas the posterior 60% of the stroma is at least 50% weaker [40].

The 15 mW/cm^2 Accelerated pulsed-light "Siena CXL Center protocol®" allows to penetrate at 280 ± 20 μm, resulting an optimal option for both depth and duration of the treatment, and was confirmed to be both clinically safe and effective.

Very recently, Bao et al. published another preclinical study conducted on japanese rabbit eyes using different CXL irradiations, ranging from 3 mW/cm^2 for 30 min to 90 mW/cm^2 for 1 min; the total dose was always 5.4 J/cm^2 [74]. They found that the CXL efficacy consistently decreased with the reduction of the irradiance duration, meaning that the Bunsen-Roscoe law may not be fully applicable in the CXL of corneal tissue. This preclinical data seems to be in contrast with the clinical studies reported above, so the topic still needs more extensive investigation in order to develop customized treatment protocols as a valid substitute to the conventional CXL procedure in treating progressive keratoconus. The optimal "window" of irradiation counterbalancing UV-A power, Exposure Time and to optimize CXL Treatment penetration (apoptosis and demarcation line) seems to be is comprised between 9 and 18 mW/cm^2 maintaining the same fluence of 5.4 J/cm^2. However higher irradiances such as 30 mW with continuous or pulsed light illumination can be used efficiently in the treatment of thin ectatic corneas by targeting the treatment penetration as we will demonstrated with a customized pachymetry guided ACXL nomogram (The M® nomogram).

10.3 Slow-Low Irradiance CXL

The observation that, at the same fluence (Energy dose), the CXL effect decreases using high intensities, is now opening another line of research. In fact, the limiting factor, especially using these accelerated protocols, seems to be the oxygen diffusion, since oxygen is rapidly consumed during CXL, and higher UV intensities cannot compensate for the loss of oxygen diffusion resulting from the shorter times of irradiation; this means that theoretically the UV irradiance could be lowered without decreasing the stiffening effect.Kling and Hafezi recently published a study [75] in which they tested this hypothesis on porcine eyes by comparing a slow-low irradiance CXL setting (1.5 mW/cm^2 for 30 min, with a halved fluence of 2.7 J/cm^2) to the conventional CXL setting at 5.4 J. The results of the study showed no significant differences in the stiffening effect between the slow-low irradiance CXL and the standard CXL protocols; this means that in theory the standard Dresden UV intensity could be lowered by one half without negatively affecting the cross-linking effect, and that even thinner corneas could be treated with CXL, but of course before clinical application can be recommended, in vivo validation studies are required. Moreover, the impact on treatment penetration is studied for the treatment of thin corneas and studies demonstrating the medium-long term stability of the ectatic process are mandatory before to validate the hypothesis.

10.4 Demarcation Line and Accelerated CXL Protocols

The first report in literature on the demarcation line was done by Seiler and Hafezi in 2006 [76].

It is known that the demarcation line indicates a change in the refractive index of the cornea and represents the depth of the cross-linking and the tissue healing response. For this reason it has been used to measure the efficacy of the CXL [52], although an actual correlation with mechanical stiffening still has not been shown. Of course since the line of demarcation is most visible approximately 1–3 months post CXL, the biological processes underlying its formation seems to play a key role.

Conventional CXL almost always creates a demarcation line at a depth of approximately 300 μm [77]. There is some controversy in literature about the demarcation line after different CXL protocols. In fact, some authors found that the demarcation line is less frequent, less uniform and less reflective after accelerated protocols compared to the conventional CXL procedure [78], while others found no significant differences [34]. As seen in Table 10.1, longer irradiation times correlate with deeper demarcation lines, although the reported standard deviations for this measurement are large, revealing variability of as much as 40% in depth of demarcation line depth for nominally equivalent clinical protocols. The findings of this evaluation revealed that inconsistency and variation in surgical procedure, materials and equipment when added up, could lead to variability in the depth of the corneal demarcation line potentially leading to variability in clinical outcomes as well.

Nonetheless, Accelerated CXL offers a great advantage in the management of progressive primary ectasias (Keratoconus, Pellucid Marginal Degeneration), and secondary iatrogenic ectasia (Post-LASIK, post-PRK, post-RK, post-SMILE). Actually, also the thin corneas 400 μm and under can be managed with high fluence accelerated protocols according to customization of treatment depth according to in vivo confocal microscopy studies and OCT evidences published by Mazzotta C, [56, 59, 65, 70–73] UV-A power settings and Exposure time (Fig. 10.4).

Table 10.1 Demarcation lines depths in literature according to various CXL protocols

Protocol				Results		
Presoak, min	UVA Irrad, mW/cm^2	UVA time, min	Dose, J/cm^2	Measured depth, μm	Calculated depth, new model, μm	References
30	3	30 CW	3.4	294.2 ± 51.2	352	Yam (2012)
30	3	30 CW	5,4	350 ± 20	352	Mazzotta (2015)
30	3	30 CW	5.4	341.8 ± 7.02	352	Tsakalis (2016)
30	3	30 CW	5.4	350.78 ± 49-34	352	Kymionis (2013)
30	3	30 CW	S.4	337 ± 46.46	352	Zygoura (2015)
15	30	3 CW	5.4	140.4 ± 39.1	185	Fontana (2014)
30	30	4 CW	7.2	200 ± 20	209	Mazzotta (2015)
30	30	8 pulsed (1 s, 1 s)	7.2	250 ± 20	255	Mazzotta (2015)
15	30	4 CW	7.2	153.85 ±33. II	195	Fontana (2014)
10	30	8 pulsed (1 s, 1 s)	7.2	213 ± 47	239	Fontana (2014)
10	20	12 pulsed (1 s, 1 s)	7.2	233 ± 92	262	Fontana (2014)
20	30	4CW	7.2	160 ± 20	202	Mazzotta (2013, 2014)
20	9	10 CW	54	288.46 ± 42.37	265	Kymionis (2013)
20	18	5 CW	5.4	208.64 ± 18.41	219	Ozgurhan (2014)
30	18	5 CW	*5.4*	240.37 ± 18.89	225	Ozgurhan (2014)
30	18	7 CW	7.56	313.37 ±48.85	245	Bikbova (2016)
30	18	5 CW	5.4	223 ± 32	225	Kymionis (2015)
30	9	14 CW	7.56	322.91 ± 48.28	296	Zygoura (2015)
10	30	4 CW	72	159.88	795	Peyman (2016)
10	30	8 pulsed (1 s 1 s)	7.2	201.11	213	Peyman (2016)

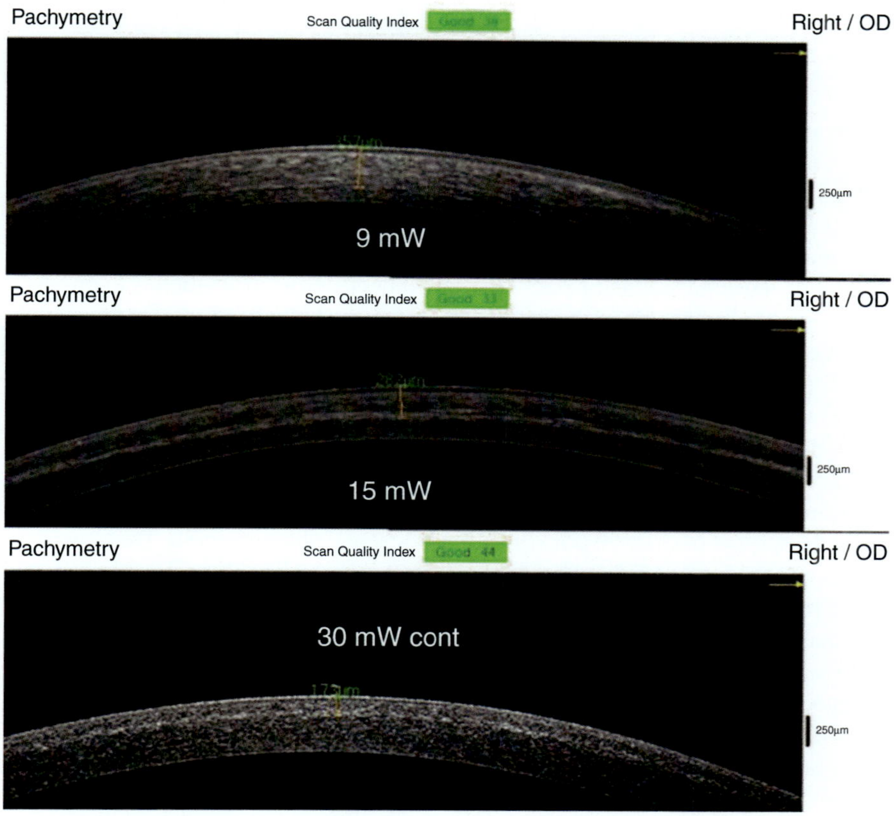

Fig. 10.4 Spectral domain OCT of the cornea (Optovue, Freemont, CA, USA), documenting the different demarcation line depth according to different Accelerated CXL (the M nomogram®)

10.5 ACXL-Plus

As known, the aim of CXL is mainly to induce a corneal stiffening to slow down or arrest the progression of the corneal ectasia, but it also sometimes presents the beneficial collateral effect to positively modify the shape of the cornea, inducing apex flattening and better corneal symmetry, thus sometimes achieving a refractive improvement for the patient. The problem is that these refractive changes are still highly unpredictable, being linked to the biological response of the corneal collagen after UV irradiation. For this reason, lately CXL has been combined with other procedures that have a more predictable and customizable refractive/shape-modifying effect; in fact, sometimes even a successful CXL (in the sense that it achieves an optimal ectasia stabilization) still leads to unsatisfactory results due to the poor visual acuity.

The management modalities that combine CXL to other adjuvant therapies collettively fall under the umbrella term "Corneal collagen cross-linking-Plus" or "ACXL-Plus" [79], and some the main ones will be briefly described below.

10.6 Crosslinking with Combined Surface Laser Ablation: The "STARE XL" Protocol

The treatment of corneas with keratoconus using excimer laser machine was historically considered not appropriate because of further corneal thinning and possible weakening of corneal microstructure followed by iatrogenic ectasia worsening. Recent advances in technology led to development of topography-guided and wavefront-guided treatments that changed the quality of laser treatment introducing the concept of "customized treatments". The target of customized ablation is to improve the quality of visual acuity reducing the lower and the higher-order aberrations with partial or total treatment of corneal irregular astigmatism.

In literature several approaches have been described combining different corneal collagen crosslinking and refractive surgery protocols performed at the same time (same-day) or in two surgical steps [80, 81].

The thinnest corneal thickness (measured with epithelium) considered for residual stromal bed in these papers varied from 300 to 450 μm. The common opinion of the Authors is to consider 50 μm as maximum stromal ablation depth. The benefit of combined CXL plus refractive surgery (CXL Plus procedure) is to directly reshape (regularize) the ectatic cornea and reinforce the reshaped cornea with CXL procedure that will further flatten the cornea in the following months.

To achieve this goal, two Italian researchers, Dr. C. Mazzotta and Dr. M. Rechichi developed an adjustable personalized protocol called "STARE-XL" (Selective Trans-epithelial Ablation for Regularization of Ectasia and simultaneous Cross-linking).

The protocol consisted of a combination of transepithelial topo-guided ablation treatment with Amaris Laser Platform (Schwind Eye tech-Solution) and Accelerated CXL performed with Avedro's (Waltham, MA) KXL I cross-linker.

The inclusion criteria for patient selection were: Age ≥21 years, Mild Ectasia (Stage I-II), necessity of visual quality improvement, HRGP lens Intolerance or altered fitting, CDVA ≤20/40 or ≤0.6 Snellen Lines, K average ≤48 Diopters or K maximum ≤55 Diopters, Optical Thinnest Point pachymetry: 400 μm ≥T-PTK (minimum 350 stromal), maximum stromal ablation ≤50 μm, minimum residual stromal bed ≥350 μm. The exclusion criteria were: Ocular Infections, History of Interstitial Keratitis, HSV or other autoimmune diseases, presence of corneal scars.

The procedure is performed in two separate steps:

First Step: Excimer Laser Corneal Regularization Laser Platform: Schwind Amaris platform linked with Anterior segment Scheimpflug Tomography with integrated placido topography and pupillometry (Sirius, CSO, Florence, Italy). We start from subjective refraction before consider topography- based Trans-epithelial All Surface Laser Ablation (T – ASLA). The procedure consists of Single step corneal topo-guided TRANS-PRK 7 mm optical zone (OZ) plus 0.6 mm transition zone (TZ) for central cone or 6.5 OZ plus TZ 0.5 mm for peripheral cone. Treatment strategy for CENTRAL Kc >50% within 3 mm on posterior elevation map: high negative Q factor with high myopic refractive error. Trans-PRK with planning of partial refractive correction is influenced by pachymetry and spherical equivalent value. We can apply a partial refractive correction planning spherical refraction between −2 or zero and focusing on irregular astigmatism we will preserve the asphericity reducing the Q value to a less negative value. The most suitable patients for this treatment are those with spherical equivalent <5 D and pachymetry over 450 μm. Treatment strategy for PERIPHERAL Kc >50% out of 3 mm on posterior elevation tangential map, have less negative or positive Q value and lower myopia. These are the most complex case. The risk is to induce a significant negative Q value, resulting a myopic shift. In order to compensate this overshot we can apply a refractive correction planning zero as spherical refraction and focusing just on irregular astigmatism and coma aberration, correcting 50% of subjective cylinder refraction keeping always max ablation under 50 μm. The algorithm for laser epithelium removal of Amaris consists in ablation of 55 μm in the center that gradually reach 65 μm at the edge of optical zone. The epithelium removal is trimmed on each case computing the thickness of central cornea and a paracentral point that is calculated half-way between OZ boundary and center. In the keratoconic cornea the epithelium is normally thinner on the cone apex acting as masking agent smoothing the elevation irregularities. We have to consider this important finding because if conventional thickness value in paracentral zone are computed in the planning the ablation in keratoconic cornea we will always ablate much more stromal tissue on the steeper corneal meridian respect to the flatter one. Anyway often the refraction and the corneal asymmetry will improve per se because more stromal tissue will be removed around the corneal apex flattening. To limit the stromal ablation under the cone apex in the STARE-X protocol we computed in the algorithm the central thickness value and the paracentral value corresponding to the thinnest point located on the cone apex, creating a customized epithelium removal ablation. More than this the depth saving mode is always used. This is useful because the limited cylinder correction will be shifted toward the peripheral and thicker cornea. The target is to reduce stromal ablation under the cone during epithelium removal preserving always a RST ≥350 μm. Previous studies showed an average thinning of 10–13 μm at 1.2 mm from corneal vertex between normal and keratoconic eyes. This means that a 60 μm epithelial ablation in the apex zone will remove about 15–18 μm of stromal tissue. This is a crucial information to be considered especially if we plan a further topo-guided stromal regularization to not exceed the ablation depth target.

Second Step: Customized Accelerated Collagen Crosslinking The target RST planned before laser excimer corneal ablation will guide decision about UV-A irradiation power and dose that will be adopted for crosslinking just after the first step.69 The protocol includes the Siena CXL Center Protocol with 15 mW pulsed light UV-A irradiation (12 min, 15 mw/cm^2, 5.4 J Fluence) if the RST is >400 μm and pulsed UVA irradiation (6 min, pulsed-light 1:1 – 30 mw/cm^2, 5.4 J dose energy) if the RST <400 μm. The beam is carefully centered on posterior elevation cone for all the treatment. The Riboflavin solution used in both treatment groups is composed of dextran- free riboflavin 0.1% with hydroxyl, propyl, methyl, and cellulose (VibeX Rapid, Avedro Inc., Waltham, MS, USA), with 10 min of corneal soaking. After treatment, eyes are dressed by a soft contact lens bandage for 3–4 days and medicated with antibiotic, non-steroidal anti-inflammatory and lubricants eye drops four times/day. The application of these protocols will produce a demarcation line between 250 and 280 μm that is ideal for a cornea with a RST >350 μm.

Figures 10.5 and 10.6 shows 1 years results of 30 keratoconic eyes treated with STARE-X protocol divided in two groups: group 1 (G1) was 15 central cones (apex within 3 mm from corneal vertex), group 2 (G2) was peripheral cone (apex outside

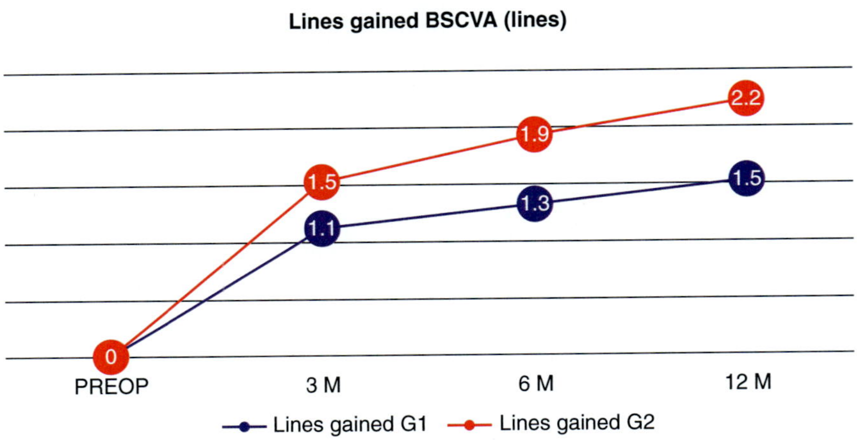

Fig. 10.5 G1 Central cones. G2 Peripheral cones. G2 group gained an average of 0.7 lines more than G1 1 year after STARE XL protocol

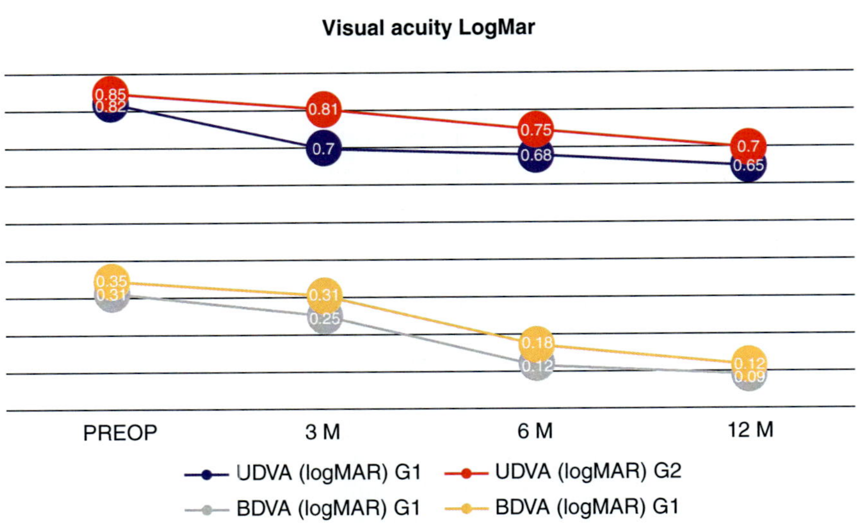

Fig. 10.6 Visual acuity. G1 group gained a better final visual acuity but G2 had the more recently improvement

3 mm from corneal vertex). A marked improvement in UDVA and BDVA was observed in both group. A better improvement in lines gained was observed in G2 nevertheless the G1 was better in terms of visual acuity.

10.7 Intracorneal Rings with Corneal Cross-Linking

The intrastromal ring implant in the deep layers of the stroma in the paracentral area of the cornea was originally developed as a method for surgical correction of high degree myopia and myopic astigmatism thanks to its ability to change refraction in the central zone of the cornea due to its peripheral-only effect [82, 83].

After surgery, a flattening effect takes place not only in the central zone of the cornea, but there is also a reduction in curvature in the peripheral area [84]. Varying the length of the implant, its height and position in the tunnel in respect to the optical centre of the cornea and the ectasic zone, it is possible to prearrange refraction modification.

The rings were first proposed for treating keratoconus in 1995 by Paulo Ferrara [85]. They were made of PMMA, they had a triangular cross-sectional shape with different internal and external diameters, 6.2 mm, and 5.6 mm respectively. The length of the implant at 60° has a base thickness of 600 μm, a radius of curvature of 2.5 mm, whereas the height varies from 150 to 350 μm with a pace of 50 μm. The first surgeries were carried out in patients with keratoconus who could not tolerate rigid gas permeable contact lenses, and in candidates with penetrating keratoplasty. The recommendations for the surgery were for a transparent cornea with a central thickness of at least 400 μm, and an endothelial cell density (ECD) of >1800 cells/mm^2. The ring implants were inserted mechanically with local topical anaesthesia. In all cases, two segments were implanted on both sides from the curved meridian, 5–7 mm from the centre of the cornea to avoid creating peripheral vision obstacles. The depth of the insertion was 50–80% of corneal thickness in the implant zone.

In clinical practice, today there are different possible modifications of the segments (in height, length, curvature radius and shape in the cross-section), and multiple options both in the depth of the implant and the number of segments, as well as in the position of the corneal incision on the strong or weak meridian. The efficiency of the ICRS implant in primary keratoconus eyes is advanced and clear-cut. In most cases a stable result is reached with a small decrease of risk of further progression of the disease, significant reduction of the degree of irregular astigmatism, and an increase of visual acuity with or without contact lenses [86–90].

Presently, in the case of progressive keratoconus the ring implants are used in conjunction with Riboflavin UVA- crosslinking, in both single or multiple procedures. In the combined treatment, regardless of surgery time, UDVA and CDVA, the average spherical equivalent and keratometric data are significantly better than monotherapy. Current data from various studies demonstrate that in the case of progressive keratoconus, the combined treatment is more efficient: the first phase is the rings implant, the second the execution of UVA- crosslinking with a 6-month interval between the two allowing an improvement in the clinical-functional data and contemporary increase in the rigidity of the cornea, stabilizing ectasia progression. When the combined treatment is carried out, but in inverted sequence (Phase 1 – crosslinking, Phase 2 – ICRS implant), the density and rigidity of the corneal tissue is increased due to the CXL effect, for this the ICRS implant is unable to completely change the corneal curvature and therefore optimize visual acuity. The use of ICRS-only offers outstanding functional results. The rings significantly contribute to the flattening of the anterior surface of the cornea and in the optical zone, tending towards an improvement in visual acuity and refraction. The ICRS implant can be used independently when we are facing a refractive stationary keratoconus, but must be used together if we are working on a progressive disease. The application of rings is limited to those keratoconic eyes with poor spectacles CDVA, not suitable or intolerant to contact lenses.

10.8 Pseudo-phakic IOLs (Toric and Non-toric) in Ectasia Treatment

The first implants of the toric IOL to correct high ametropia in the keratoconus were carried out during the phacoemulsification of the cataract after penetrating keratoplasty. Comparing the results of the implant of these toric lenses with that of spherical ones, better results are observed, thanks to the capacity of simultaneous correction of the spherical and cylindrical components of the refractive error [82, 91]. Presently, cataract surgery, indeed phacoemulsification, with the toric IOL is considered an effective and secure correction of ametropia in keratoconus patients. Nonetheless, patient selection for this kind of surgery is complex, because compared to the general population, the cataract in thick keratoconus is diagnosed at a young age and the rehabilitation of the patients requires special attention. At the same time, it is necessary to consider not only the age of the patient, but also their activity, and the status of the other eye. On the other hand, the correct strategy of treatment is necessary: begin with the correction of the ametropia due to ectasia or cataract treatment.

The main criteria for choosing a PHACO + Toric IOL in patients with KC are the following: Cataract diagnosis, stable KC, patients after intrastromal ring implant and or CXL, absence of opacity in the central zone of the cornea.Today, to calculate optic strength of the toric IOL various techniques and formulas are used. At the same time, there are two principal classes of formula: empirical (of regression) SRK II, and the third-generation mixed formulas (Holladay, SRK/T, Hoffer Q, Haigis). Despite the great variety of formulas to calculate toric IOL optic strength, there is still high difficulty for the calculation of keratoconus patients and the biometric surprise is often present in the postoperative requiring IOL exchange. The keratometric parameters cannot be trusted due to their variability, which is based on from whence and how the measurement came, and for the fact that the visual axis in keratoconus eyes as well as others with ectasias is not located on the corneal apex but towards the cone. Further, the software used for the toric IOL optic strength calculation is calibrated and controlled on eyes without keratoconus, and with a regular astigmatism where the corneal apex coincides with the visual axis. Therefore, the keratometric data used for the calculations of toric IOL are generally inaccurate. Further, factors like irregular astigmatism, aberrations, etc. can notably influence refractive results after the intervention [92, 93].

10.9 Phakic IOLs (Toric and Non-toric) in Keratoconus Management

Currently, one of the most promising and rapidly developing methods of correction of high ametropia is the implantation of a toric IOL in phakic eyes. Today this kind of intraocular correction is becoming ever more popular among surgeons who perform surgical correction of high myopia and myopic astigmatism. From their point of view, the precision, predictability, stability of visual function, as well as short rehabilitation time provides a significant increase in quality of life and quick recovery of operated patients [83, 94].

With the development and improvement of modern methods to treat keratoconus (Riboflavin UVA Cross-linking and ICRS), the toric pIOL implant is used most frequently as a final stage in the algorithm of keratectasia treatment. Nonetheless, with the latest clinical data it seems that the pIOL can trigger the onset of side effects like cataracts, oval pupils, the loss of corneal endothelial cells, induced astigmatism, secondary glaucoma, iridocyclitis, etc.

According to the literature, the most used models of toric pIOL to correct residual ametropia in keratoconic eyes are the posterior chamber "Visian™ Toric-ICL" (STAAR) of biocompatible collamer (collagen plus acrylic) and the anterior chamber toric Artiflex/Veryflex foldable lenses of silicone with PMMA aptic. These lenses can be used after ICRS implants, after ACXL or in combination in triple or multiple procedures.

The essential condition for correct residual ametropia is a stabilization of keratoconus for at least 1 year. As far as the recommendations for the combined treatment go the paradigm is always "cornea first" (ICRS, CXL, CXL Plus All Surface Laser minimal Aablation for corneal regularization, pIOLs), this treatment remains reserved for very selected clinical cases of keratoconus. Thus, the ICRS can approximately correct 7.0D with an improvement in CDVA; CXL can further reduce 2.0D of corneal irregularity with an improvement in flat, steep, and mean K values; and pIOL can decrease the spherical component up to 20.0D and cylindrical up to 6 D increasing the UCVA. Very recently, our research group published on the Journal of Refractive Surgery a new Epi-ON CXL method that uses enhanced fluence and pulsed light to increase iontophoresis CXL efficacy closer to standard CXL [95]. This technique can be associated with all the above-mentioned adjuvant therapies. Since the epithelium is spared, this new technique have the advantage of eliminating wound-related complications, of maintaining an adequate ocular surface homeostasis and of preserving the integrity of the subepithelial nerve plexus.

References

1. Rabinowitz YS. Keratoconus. Surv Ophthalmol. 1998;42:297–319.
2. Godefrooij DA, de Wit GA, Uiterwaal CS, et al. Age-specific incidence and prevalence of keratoconus: a nationwide registration study. Am J Ophthalmol. 2017;175:169–72.
3. Ambrosio R Jr, Klyce SD, Wilson SE. Corneal topographic and pachymetric screening of keratorefractive patients. J Refract Surg. 2003;19:24–9.
4. Pearson AR, Soneji B, et al. Does ethnic origin influence the incidence or severity of keratoconus? Eye (Lond). 2000;14:625–8.
5. Chatzis N, Hafezi F. Progression of keratoconus and efficacy of pediatric corneal collagen cross-linking in children and adolescents. J Refract Surg (Thorofare, N.J.: 1995). 2012;28:753–8. https://doi.org/10.3928/1081597X-20121011-01.
6. Caporossi A, Mazzotta C, Baiocchi S, Caporossi T. Long-term results of riboflavin ultraviolet a corneal collagen cross-linking for keratoconus in Italy: the Siena eye cross study. Am J Ophthalmol. 2010;149(4):585–93.
7. Koller T, Mrochen M, Seiler T. Complication and failure rates after corneal crosslinking. J Cataract Refract Surg. 2009;35(8):1358–62.
8. Wollensak G, Spoerl E, Seiler T. Riboflavin/ultraviolet-A–induced collagen crosslinking for the treatment of keratoconus. Am J Ophthalmol. 2003;135:620–7.
9. Roberts CJ, Dupps WJ Jr. Biomechanics of corneal ectasia and biomechanical treatments. J Cataract Refract Surg. 2014;40(6):991–8.
10. Roy AS, Dupps WJ Jr. Patient-specific computational modeling of keratoconus progression and differential responses to collagen cross-linking. Invest Ophthalmol Vis Sci. 2011;52:9174–87.
11. Nordström M, Schiller M, Fredriksson A, et al. Refractive improvements and safety with topography-guided corneal crosslinking for keratoconus: 1-year results. Br J Ophthalmol. 2017;101:920–5.
12. Mazzotta C, Moramarco A, Traversi C, Baiocchi S, Iovieno A, Fontana L. Accelerated corneal collagen cross-linking using topography-guided UV-A energy emission: preliminary clinical and morphological outcomes. J Ophthalmol. 2016; Article ID 2031031. 10 pages.
13. Meek KM, Hayes S. Corneal cross-linking—a review. Ophthalmic Physiol Opt. 2013;33:78–93.
14. Vinciguerra P, Albe E, Trazza S, et al. Refractive, topographic, tomographic, and aberrometric analysis of keratoconic eyes undergoing corneal cross-linking. Ophthalmology. 2009;116:369–78.
15. Kanellopoulos AJ. Novel myopic refractive correction with transepithelial very high-fl uence collagen cross-linking applied in a customized pattern: early clinical results of a feasibility study. Clin Ophthalmol. 2014;8:697–702.
16. Holden BA, Fricke TR, Wilson DA, Jong M, Naidoo KS, Sankaridurg P, Wong TY, Naduvilath TJ, Resnikoff S. Global prevalence of myopia and high myopia and temporal trends from 2000 through 2050. Ophthalmology. 2016;123:1036–42.
17. Kanellopoulos AJ, Dupps WJ, Seven I, Asimellis G. Toric topographically customized transepithelial, pulsed, very high-fl uence, higher energy and higher riboflavin concentration collagen cross-linking in keratoconus. Case Rep Ophthalmol. 2014;5(2):172–80.
18. Kanellopoulos AJ, Asimellis G. Hyperopic correction: clinical validation with epithelium-on and epithelium-off protocols, using variable fl uence and topographically customized collagen corneal crosslinking. Clin Ophthalmol. 2014;8:2425–33.
19. Kanellopoulos J, Asimellis G. Presbyopic PiXL crosslinking. Curr Ophthalmol Rep. 2015. https://doi.org/10.1007/s40135-014-0060-6.
20. Nawaz S, Gupta S, Gogia V, Sasikala NK, Panda A. Trans-epithelial versus Conventional corneal collagen cross-linking: a randomized trial in keratoconus. Oman J Ophthalmol. 2015;8(1):9–13.
21. Scarcelli G, Kling S, Quijano E, Pineda R, Marcos S, Yun SH. Brillouin microscopy of collagen crosslinking: noncontact depth-dependent analysis of corneal elastic modulus. Invest Ophthalmol Vis Sci. 2013;54:1418–25.

22. Lim WK, et al. Epithelium-on photorefractive intrastromal cross-linking (PiXL) for reduction of low myopia. Clin Ophthalmol. 2017;11:1205–11. https://doi.org/10.2147/opth.s137712.
23. Richoz O, Hammer A, Tabibian D, Gatzioufas Z, Hafezi F. The biomechanical effect of corneal collagen cross-linking (CXL) with riboflavin and UV-A is oxygen dependent. Trans Vis Sci Technol. 2013;2(7):6.
24. https://clinicaltrials.gov/ct2/show/NCT03197272. Accessed 27 Jan 2018.
25. https://www.eyeworld.org/high-oxygen-enhances-epi-pixl-efficacy. Accessed 27 Jan 2018.
26. O'Brart DPS, Patel P, Lascaratos G, Wagh VK, Tam C, Lee J, O'Brart NA. Keratoconus and corneal ectasia: seven-year follow-up. Am J Ophthalmol. 2015;160:1154–63. 3.
27. Schumacher S, Oeftiger L, Mrochen M. Equivalence of biomechanical changes induced by rapid and standard corneal cross-linking using riboflavin and ultraviolet radiation. Invest Ophthalmol Vis Sci. 2011;52:9048–52.
28. Krueger RR, Herekar S, Spoerl E. First proposed efficacy study of high versus standard irradiance and fractionated riboflavin/ultraviolet A cross-linking with equivalent energy exposure. Eye Contact Lens. 2014;40:353–7.
29. Kling S, Richoz O, Hammer A, Tabibian D, Jacob S, Agarwal A, Hafezi F. Increased biomechanical efficacy of corneal cross-linking in thin corneas due to higher oxygen availability. J Refract Surg. 2015;31:840–6.
30. Cınar Y, Cingü AK, Türkcü FM, Çınar T, Yüksel H, Özkurt ZG, Çaça I. Comparison of accelerated and conventional corneal collagen cross-linking for progressive keratoconus. Cutan Ocul Toxicol. 2014;33(3):218–22.
31. Cınar Y, Cingü AK, Turkcu FM, Yüksel H, Sahin A, Yıldırım A, Caca I. Accelerated corneal collagen cross-linking for progressive keratoconus. Cutan Ocul Toxicol. 2014;33(2):168–71.
32. Hersh PS, Greenstein SA, Fry KL. Corneal collagen crosslinking for keratoconus and corneal ectasia: one-year results. J Cataract Refract Surg. 2011;37:149–60.
33. Legare ME, Iovieno A, Yeung SN, et al. Corneal collagen cross-linking using riboflavin and ultraviolet A for the treatment of mild to moderate keratoconus: 2-year follow-up. J Ophthalmol. 2013;48:63–8.
34. Kymionis GD, Tsoulnaras KI, Grentzelos MA, Liakopoulos DA, Tsakalis NG, Blazaki SV, Paraskevopoulos TA, Tsilimbaris MK. Evaluation of corneal stromal demarcation line depth following standard and a modified-accelerated collagen cross-linking protocol. Am J Ophthalmol. 2014;158(4):671–5.
35. Shetty R, Nagaraja H, Jayadev C, Pahuja NK, Kurian Kummelil M, Nuijts RM. Accelerated corneal collagen cross-linking in pediatric patients: two-year follow-up results. Biomed Res Int. 2014;2014:894095.
36. Elbaz U, Shen C, Lichtinger A, Zauberman NA, Goldich Y, Chan CC, Slomovic AR, Rootman DS. Accelerated (9-mW/cm2) corneal collagen crosslinking for keratoconus-A 1-year follow up. Cornea. 2014;33(8):769–73.
37. Jain V, Gazali Z, Bidayi R. Isotonic riboflavin and HPMC with accelerated cross-linking protocol. Cornea. 2014;33(9):910–3.
38. Pahuja N, Kumar NR, Francis M, Shanbagh S, Shetty R, Ghosh A, Roy AS. Correlation of clinical biomechanical outcomes of accelerated crosslinking (9 mW/cm^2 in 10 minutes) in keratoconus with molecular expression of ectasia-related genes. Curr Eye Res. 2016;41(11):1419–23.
39. Marino GK, Torricelli AA, Giacomin N, Santhiago MR, Espindola R, Netto MV. Accelerated corneal collagen crosslinking for postoperative LASIK ectasia: two-year outcomes. J Refract Surg. 2015;31(6):380–4.
40. Sadoughi MM, Einollahi B, Baradaran-Rafii A, Roshandel D, Hasani H, Nazeri M. Accelerated versus conventional corneal collagen cross-linking in patients with keratoconus: an intrapatient comparative study. Int Ophthalmol. 2018;38(1):67–74.
41. Cingü AK, Sogutlu-Sari E, Cınar Y, Sahin M, Türkçü FM, Yüksel H, Sahin A, Caça I. Transient corneal endothelial changes following accelerated collagen cross-linking for the treatment of progressive keratoconus. Cutan Ocul Toxicol. 2014;33(2):127–31.
42. Hashemi H, Fotouhi A, Miraftab M, Bahrmandy H, Seyedian MA, Amanzadeh K, Heidarian S, Nikbin H, Asgari S. Short-term comparison of accelerated and standard methods of corneal collagen crosslinking. J Cataract Refract Surg. 2015;41(3):533–40.

43. Hashemi H, Miraftab M, Seyedian MA, Hafezi F, Bahrmandy H, Heidarian S, Amanzadeh K, Nikbin H, Fotouhi A, Asgari S. Long-term results of an accelerated corneal cross- linking protocol (18 mW/cm²) for the treatment of progressive keratoconus. Am J Ophthalmol. 2015;160(6):1164–70.
44. Chow VW, Chan TC, Yu M, Wong VW, Jhanji V. One year outcomes of conventional and accelerated collagen crosslinking in progressive keratoconus. Sci Rep. 2015;5:14425.
45. Asri D, Touboul D, Fournié P, Malet F, Garra C, Gallois A, Malecaze F, Colin J. Corneal collagen crosslinking in progressive keratoconus: multicenter results from the French National Reference Center for keratoconus. J Cataract Refract Surg. 2011;37(12):2137–43.
46. Kanellopoulos AJ. Long term results of a prospective randomized bilateral eye comparison trial of higher fluence, shorter duration ultraviolet A radiation, and riboflavin collagen cross linking for progressive keratoconus. Clin Ophthalmol. 2012;6:97–101.
47. Gatzioufas Z, Richoz O, Brugnoli E, Hafezi F. Safety profile of high-fluence corneal collagen cross-linking for progressive keratoconus: preliminary results from a prospective cohort study. J Refract Surg. 2013;29(12):846–8.
48. Wernli J, Schumacher S, Spoerl E, Mrochen M. The efficacy of corneal cross-linking shows a sudden decrease with very high intensity UV light and short treatment time. Invest Ophthalmol Vis Sci. 2013;54(2):1176–80.
49. Hammer A, Richoz O, Arba Mosquera S, Tabibian D, Hoogewoud F, Hafezi F. Corneal biomechanical properties at different corneal cross-linking (CXL) irradiances. Invest Ophthalmol Vis Sci. 2014;55(5):2881–4.
50. Chan TC, Chow VW, Jhanji V, Wong VW. Different topographic response between mild to moderate and advanced keratoconus after accelerated collagen cross-linking. Cornea. 2015;34(8):922–7.
51. Shetty R, Pahuja NK, Nuijts RM, Ajani A, Jayadev C, Sharma C, Nagaraja H. Current protocols of corneal collagen crosslinking—visual, refractive and tomographic outcomes. Am J Ophthalmol. 2015;160(2):243–9.
52. Kymionis GD, Tsoulnaras KI, Grentzelos MA, Plaka AD, Mikropoulos DG, Liakopoulos DA, Tsakalis NG, Pallikaris IG. Corneal stroma demarcation line after standard and high- intensity collagen crosslinking determined with anterior segment optical coherence tomography. J Cataract Refract Surg. 2014;40(5):736–40.
53. Kymionis GD, Grentzelos MA, Plaka AD, Tsoulnaras KI, Diakonis VF, Liakopoulos DA, Kankariya VP, Pallikaris AI. Correlation of the corneal collagen cross-linking demarcation line using confocal microscopy and anterior segment optical coherence tomography in keratoconic patients. Am J Ophthalmol. 2014;157(1):110–5.
54. Kurt T, Ozgurhan EB, Yildirim Y, Akcay BI, Cosar MG, Bozkurt E, Taskapili M. Accelerated (18mW/cm²) corneal cross-linking for progressive keratoconus: 18-month results. J Ocul Pharmacol Ther. 2016;32(4):186–91.
55. Razmjoo H, Peyman A, Rahimi A, Modrek HJ. Cornea collagen cross-linking for keratoconus: a comparison between accelerated and conventional methods. Adv Biomed Res. 2017;6:10.
56. Mazzotta C, Traversi C, Paradiso AL, Latronico ME, Rechichi M. Pulsed light accelerated crosslinking versus continuous light accelerated crosslinking: one-year results. J Ophthalmol. 2014;2014:604731.
57. Touboul D, Efron N, Smadja D, et al. Corneal confocal microscopy following conventional, transepithelial, and accelerated corneal collagen cross-linking procedures for keratoconus. J Refract Surg (Thorofare, N.J.: 1995). 2012;28(11):769–76.
58. Merwald H, Klosner G, Kokesch C, Der-Petrossian M, Hönigsmann H, Trautinger F. UVA-induced oxidative damage and cytotoxicity depend on the mode of exposure. J Photochem Photobiol B. 2005;79(3):197–207.
59. Mazzotta C, Traversi C, Caragiuli S, Rechichi M. Pulsed vs continuous light accelerated corneal collagen crosslinking: in vivo qualitative investigation by confocal microscopy and corneal OCT. Eye (Lond). 2014;28(10):1179–83.
60. Moramarco A, Iovieno A, Sartori A, Fontana L. Corneal stromal demarcation line after accelerated crosslinking using continuous and pulsed light. J Cataract Refract Surg. 2015;41(11):2546–51.

61. Ozgurhan EB, Kara N, Cankaya KI, Kurt T, Demirok A. Accelerated corneal cross-linking in pediatric patients with keratoconus: 24-month outcomes. J Refract Surg. 2014;30(12):843–9.
62. Ozgurhan EB, Akcay BI, Kurt T, Yildirim Y, Demirok A. Accelerated corneal collagen cross linking in thin keratoconic corneas. J Refract Surg. 2015;31(6):386–90.
63. Mita M, Waring GO 4th, Tomita M. High-irradiance accelerated collagen crosslinking for the treatment of keratoconus: six-month results. J Cataract Refract Surg. 2014;40(6):1032–40.
64. Spoerl E, Terai N, Scholz F, Raiskup F, Pillunat LE. Detection of biomechanical changes after corneal cross-linking using ocular response analyzer software. J Refract Surg. 2011;27:452–7.
65. Mazzotta C, Traversi C, Baiocchi S, et al. Corneal healing after riboflavin ultraviolet-A collagen cross-linking determined by confocal laser scanning microscopy in vivo: early and late modifications. Am J Ophthalmol. 2008;146:527–33.
66. Mazzotta C, Caporossi T, Denaro R, Bovone C, Sparano C, Paradiso A, Baiocchi S, Caporossi A. Morphological and functional correlations in riboflavin UV A corneal collagen crosslinking for keratoconus. Acta Ophthalmol. 2012;90:259–65.
67. Tomita M, Mita M, Huseynova T. Accelerated versus conventional corneal collagen crosslinking. J Cataract Refract Surg. 2014;40(6):1013–20.
68. Sherif AM. Accelerated versus conventional corneal collagen cross-linking in the treatment of mild keratoconus: a comparative study. Clin Ophthalmol. 2014;8:1435–40.
69. Mazzotta C, Baiocchi S, Simone AB, Fruschelli M, Alessandro M, Rechichi M. Accelerated 15 mW pulsed-light crosslinking in treatment of progressive keratoconus: two year clinical results. J Cataract Refract Surg. 2017;43:1081.
70. Mazzotta C, Hafezi F, Kymionis G, Caragiuli S, Jacob S, Traversi C, Barabino S, Randleman B. In vivo confocal microscopy after corneal collagen cross-linking. Ocul Surf. 2015;13(4):298–314.
71. Mazzotta C, Balestrazzi A, Traversi C, et al. Treatment of progressive keratoconus by riboflavin- UVA-induced cross-linking of corneal collagen: ultrastructural analysis by Heidelberg Retinal Tomograph II in vivo confocal microscopy in humans. Cornea. 2007;26(4):390–7.
72. Mazzotta C, Paradiso AL, Baiocchi S, Caragiuli S, Caporossi A. Qualitative investigation of corneal changes after accelerated corneal collagen cross-linking (A-CXL) by in vivo confocal microscopy and corneal OCT. J Clin Exp Ophthalmol. 2013;4:313.
73. Caporossi A, Mazzotta C, Baiocchi S, Caporossi T, Paradiso AL. Transepithelial corneal collagen crosslinking for keratoconus: qualitative investigation by in vivo HRT II confocal analysis. Eur J Ophthalmol. 2012;22(Suppl 7):S81–8.
74. Bao F, et al. Changes in corneal biomechanical properties with different corneal cross-linking irradiances. J Refract Surg. 2018;34:51–8.
75. Kling S, Hafezi F. Biomechanical stiffening: slow low-irradiance corneal crosslinking versus the standard Dresden protocol. J Cataract Refract Surg. 2017;43:975–9. https://doi.org/10.1016/j.jcrs.2017.04.041.
76. Seiler T, Hafezi F. Corneal cross-linking-induced stromal demarcation line. Cornea. 2006;25:1057–9.
77. Kymionis GD, Grentzelos MA, Plaka AD, et al. Evaluation of the corneal collagen crosslinking demarcation line profile using anterior segment optical coherence tomography. Cornea. 2013;32:907–10.
78. Bouheraoua N, Jouve L, El Sanharawi M, et al. Optical coherence tomography and confocal microscopy following three different protocols of corneal collagen-crosslinking in keratoconus. Invest Ophthalmol Vis Sci. 2014;55:7601–9.
79. Kymionis GD. Corneal collagen cross linking-Plus. Open Ophthalmol J. 2011;5:10.
80. Kymionis GD, Grentzelos MA, Kankariya VP, Pallikaris IG. Combined transepithelial phototherapeutic keratectomy and corneal collagen crosslinking for ectatic disorders: Cretan protocol. J Cataract Refract Surg. 2013;39:1939.
81. Kymionis GD, Grentzelos MA, Portaliou DM, Kankariya VP, Randleman JB. Corneal collagen cross-linking (CXL) combined with refractive procedures for the treatment of corneal ectatic disorders: CXL plus. J Refract Surg. 2014;30(8):566–76.

82. Alfonso JF, Fernandez-Vega L, Lisa C, Fernandes P, Gonzalez-Meijome JM, Montes-Mico R. Collagen copolymer toric posterior chamber phakic intraocular lens in eyes with keratoconus. J Cataract Refract Surg. 2010;36(6):906–16. 43.
83. Alio JL. Advances in phakic intraocular lenses: indications, efficacy, safety, and new designs. Curr Opin Ophthalmol. 2004;15(4):350–7.
84. Burris TE, Ayer CT, Evensen DA, Davenport JM. Effects of Instrastromal corneal ring size and thickness on corneal flattening in human eyes. Refract Corneal Surg. 1991;7(1):46–50.
85. de Ferrara A, Cunha P. Tecnica cirurgica para correçao de miopia; Anel corneano intra- estromal. Rev Bras Oftalmol. 1995;54:577–88.
86. Baiocchi S, Mazzotta C, Cerretani D, Caporossi T, Caporossi A. Corneal crosslinking: riboflavin concentration in corneal stroma exposed with and without epithelium. J Cataract Refract Surg. 2009;35(5):893–9.
87. Belin MW, Khachikian SS, Ambrosio R Jr. Elevation based corneal tomography. 2nd ed. New Delhi: Jaypee-Highlights Medical Publishers, Inc; 2011.
88. Colin J. Intacs safe and viable long-term treatment for keratoconus. Eurotimes. 2009;16.
89. Samimi S, Leger F, Touboul D, Colin J. Histopathological findings after intracorneal ring segment implantation in keratoconic human corneas. J Cataract Refract Surg. 2007;33(2):247–53.
90. Sansanayudh W, Bahar I, Kumar NL, Shehadeh-Mashour R, Ritenour R, Singal N, Rootman DS. Intrastromal corneal ring segment SK implantation for moderate to severe keratoconus. J Cataract Refract Surg. 2010;36(1):110–3. 19.
91. Alio JL, Agdeppa MC, Pongo VC, El Kady B. Microincision cataract surgery with toric intraocular lens implantation for correcting moderate and high astigmatism: pilot study. J Cataract Refract Surg. 2010;36(1):44–52.
92. Parikakis EA, Chatziralli IP, Peponis VG, David G, Chalkiadakis S, Mitropoulos PG. Toric intraocular lens implantation for correction of astigmatism in cataract patients with corneal ectasia. Case Rep Ophthalmol. 2013;4:219–28.
93. Lee SJ, Kwon HS, Koh IH. Sequential intrastromal corneal ring implantation and cataract surgery in a severe keratoconus patient with cataract. Korean J Ophthalmol. 2012;26(3):226–9.
94. Hoffmann PC, Auel S, Hutz WW. Results of higher power toric intraocular lens implantation. J Cataract Refract Surg. 2011;37(8):1411–8.
95. Mazzotta C, Bagaglia S, Vinciguerra R, Ferrise M, Vinciguerra P. Enhanced-fluence pulsed-light iontophoresis corneal cross-linking: 1-year morphological and clinical results. J Refract Surg. 2018;34(7):438–44.

Chapter 11
The Logic Behind Customized Corneal Crosslinking

Theo G. Seiler and Tobias Koller

11.1 Theoretical Background

Keratoconus is a disease that may have several causes. Today, one of the most important reasons for keratoconus is eye-rubbing that is mediated through allergic diseases [1, 2]. Family histories and the occurance of keratoconus in siblings advocate for a genetic background of keratoconus which may or may not be mediated through the allergic component [3]. Subclinical inflammations were also in discussion about the causes of keratoconus [4]. Because unilateral keratoconus seems to be a rare situation it was also believed that if it is a genetic disease at all, it would affect the entire cornea and not only parts of it.

A few years ago, a new approach came into discussion, mainly proposed by the Cleveland/Ohio-group around Dupps and Roberts. They claimed that not necessarily the entire cornea needs to have a reduced stiffness but already a localized weakening of the cornea may induce a keratoconus and supported this idea by means of finite-element-modelling and assumed a localized reduction of the elastic modulus of various degrees [5]. A weakening of the elastic modulus by 10% had nearly no impact, but implying 30% and up to 45% weakening a nice keratoconus shape of the cornea resulted. Although this idea was at first glance convincing there were still some questions remaining: (1) the weakest point of the normal cornea is clearly the thinnest point which is in most cases in the center of the cornea. Why do keratoconus

T. G. Seiler (✉)
Universitätsklinik für Augenheilkunde, Inselspital Bern, Bern, Switzerland

Wellman Center for Photomedicine – Massachusetts General Hospital, Harvard Medical School, Boston, MA, USA

Institut für Refraktive und Ophthalmo-Chirurgie (IROC), Zürich, Switzerland
e-mail: theo@seiler.tv; https://www.iroc.ch/

T. Koller
Institut für Refraktive und Ophthalmo-Chirurgie (IROC), Zürich, Switzerland

A. Barbara (ed.), *Controversies in the Management of Keratoconus*,
https://doi.org/10.1007/978-3-319-98032-4_11

corneas then show an eccentric bulging forward-effect which happens in majority of the cases? Central keratoconus is a rare disease which occurs only in a small portion of all keratoconus-cases. (2) The assumption that the elastic modulus is focally reduced is not very reasonable because the turnover of the cornea is mediated by keratocytes and the distribution of the keratocytes is homogeneous.

Most of our doubts were overruled by Brillouin spectroscopy measurements in keratoconus corneas, in which a transplantation (DALK or PKP) was performed [6]. Brillouin spectroscopy measures the bulk modulus M of a cornea which is different from the well-known elastic modulus E representing the surface parallel component of the elastic tensor. Although measuring not the usual elasticity of the cornea this bulk modulus M represents a measure for stiffness and the Boston group demonstrated nicely that in the cone region the bulk modulus was significantly lower compared to the periphery (opposite to the cone region). So it is not only the thinning of the cone region that makes the cornea locally weak but also the elastic moduli decrease in the cone region which can be interpreted as focal weakening of the cornea.

By interpreting these findings, the idea came up to strengthen the cornea focally as a prevention for keratoconus progression. If keratoconus is a local disease the treatment should be also local!

11.2 Technical Requirements and Limitations

If we reduce the area of treatment to the weak part of the cornea we first have to decide where the weakest point of the cornea is located: is it the point of K_{max}, the thinnest point, or the locus of the maximal posterior float?

The case that is shown in Fig. 11.1, an iatrogenic keratectasia after LASIK with an inferior steepening that was progressive, illustrates the difference of these three points. Here the distance between the thinnest point, the point of K_{max} and the point of maximal float is more than 2 mm. The answer of this question for the weakest point was, again, answered by Brillouin spectroscopy which was performed in a clinical environment at IROC in Zürich, in 2017. Brillouin spectroscopy defined the weakest point clearly close to the maximum of the posterior float (Fig. 11.1). This decision is also plausible because the epithelium modulates the anterior surface by the XYZ-strategy: epithelial thickness is greater over flat areas and thinner over steep areas.

The next questions that had to be answered was the areal distribution of the ultraviolet radiation assuming that we had homogeneous riboflavin distribution in the corneal stroma. For standard keratoconus we decided to use concentric circular areas with diameters depending on the dimensions of posterior float ranging from 2 mm to 7 mm. The common center of the three circles was located over the maximum of the posterior float. In pellucid marginal degeneration cases the posterior float is not circular anymore and has rather elliptical shapes and that is why in a second approach three concentric ring segments were used.

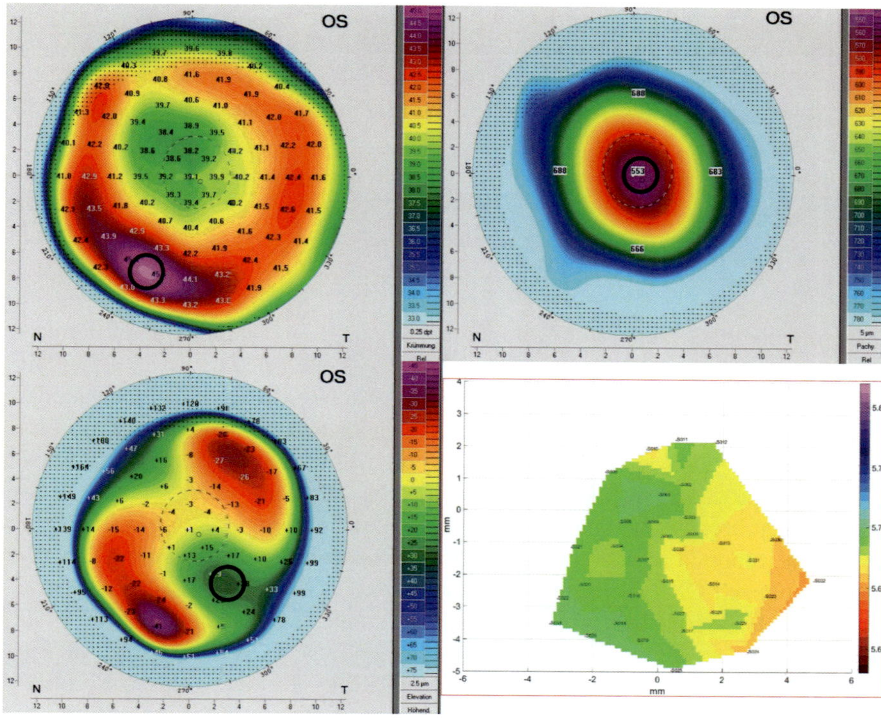

Fig. 11.1 Anterior curvature (top left), pachymetry (top right), posterior float with an 8 mm approximated sphere (bottom left) and Brillouin frequency shift map (bottom right) of a patient suffering from a progressive iatrogenic post-LASIK ectasia. Black circles are indicating the maxima of each map. The maximal posterior float has the best overlap with the weakest point obtained from Brillouin spectroscopy

Although some studies used 15 J/cm^2 as the total radiant exposure we perform customized CXL with an upper limit of 10 J/cm^2. The reason is a recommendation of the committee for safety of non-ionizing radiation of the European community that reported an upper limit of such radiation at 360 nm to be 1 J/cm^2 to prevent thermal cataractogenesis [7]. From earlier experiments we know that approximately 90% of the 360 nm radiation is absorbed by the riboflavin within the corneal stroma, so that we can go up to 10 J/cm^2 as total dose when looking for crosslinking in the cornea [8].

It is well known from several publications that the efficiency of CXL decreases with increasing irradiances [9, 10]. Therefore, we recommend using irradiances not greater than 18 mW/cm^2. As a consequence, to complete full irradiation pattern in customized crosslinking, it may take up to 20 min which makes eye-tracking device mandatory.

The Avedro System Mosaic fulfills all these requirements and the location of the centers of the irradiation areas can be imported digitally but also Pentacam-files can be imported.

The surgical part consists of a manual epithelial debridement within the irradiation area followed by the imbibition using 0.1% riboflavin with 1.1% HPMC for 10 min or 30 min if 20% dextran is used as the osmotic agent [11]. When a sufficient corneal pachymetry is assured (>400 μm) the irradiation using the predesigned pattern can be initiated.

11.3 Clinical Experience

In the international literature there are currently three publications on customized crosslinking. The first data on customized CXL was published in 2016 [12] and the results were confirmed in two subsequent studies in 2017 [13, 14]. All three studies used a prospective design comparing results of customized CXL with standard CXL according to the Dresden protocol. The first clinical benefit derived by customization of the procedure is a shorter epithelial healing time resulting in a safety improvement because the vulnerable phase for infections and melting is shortened. Seiler et al. reported an average time until the closure of the epithelium of 2.6 days after customized CXL compared to 3.2 days after standard CXL. Similar to standard CXL, demarcation lines are also visible 1 month after customized CXL in the majority of the treated eyes. But in contrast to standard CXL, demarcation lines after customized CXL were not surface-parallel but showed "Gaussian-profile": deep in cone area, more shallow towards the peripheral, non-ectatic part of the cornea as depicted in Fig. 11.2. During the first postoperative year, the Toulouse study group [14] analyzed corneal nerve density and keratocyte apoptosis by means of confocal microscopy. A significant lower apoptosis rate is reported outside the cone as well as a higher nerve density. This might serve as another good reason why patients who experienced both procedures describe the customized treatment as more comfortable. Topographical results after one year show a superior behavior of customized CXL over standard CXL. A typical case in depicted in Fig. 11.2. K_{max} and also K_{steep} experienced a significant higher reduction after customized CXL compared to standard CXL with average regression rates of K_{max} between −1.1 D and −1.7 D in customized CXL. When analyzing the distribution of flattening after both procedures, a flattening of ≥1 D is observed in 40% of eyes treated with standard CXL and in 60% of eyes treated with customized CXL. This difference of 50% is remarkable. However, not only the ratio of patients experiencing a flattening is increased but also the chance of achieving strong flattening is increased. In standard CXL only 10% of the treated eyes flatten ≥3 D, whereas in customized CXL this strong flattening is observed in more than 20% of eyes treated.

It is not only the flattening that makes the shape of the keratoconus cornea better, but parallel to the flattening the steepening of the originally flat areas may occur (Fig. 11.2). This results in a regularization of the highly aberrated keratoconus cornea and, therefore, a regularization index was coined that includes the flattening and the steepening effect [12]. This regularization index was significantly better after customized CXL compared to standard CXL.

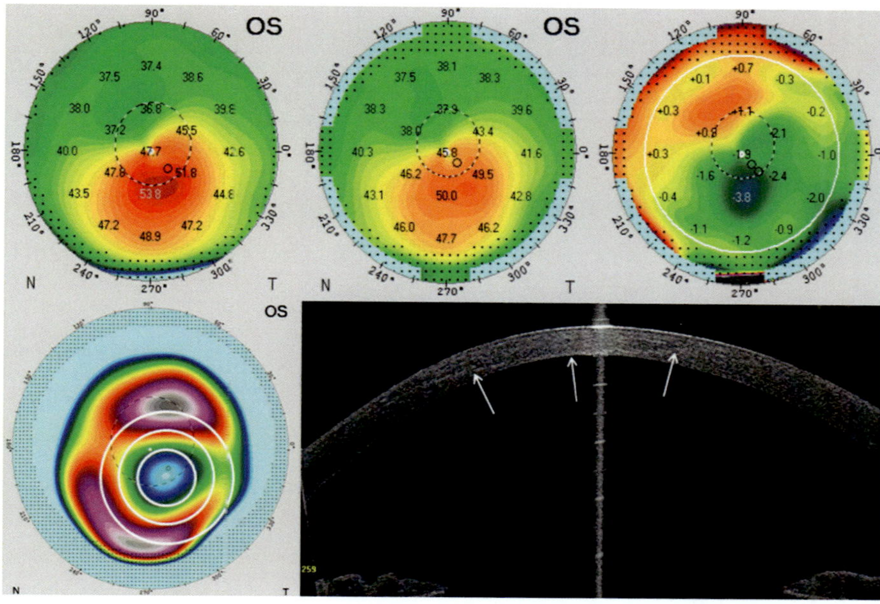

Fig. 11.2 Typical evolution of a patient treated with customized corneal crosslinking with preoperative axial curvature (top left), axial curvature at the 12-month follow-up (top middle), difference map in axial curvature (top right), preoperative posterior float with an 8 mm approximated sphere and the irradiation pattern (bottom left), demarcation line at the 1-month follow-up emphasized with arrows (bottom right). ΔK_{max} is 3.6 diopters (D); regularization index RI is 5.3 D

In summary, customization of CXL increases the safety of the procedure and enhances the outcome resulting in higher qualitative and quantitative flattening. Although these 1-year results are promising for the treatment of keratoconus, longer follow-up are not yet available and a final assessment of the procedure can currently not be made.

References

1. Krachmer JH. Eye rubbing can cause keratoconus. Cornea. 2004;23:539–40.
2. Sugar J, Macsai MS. What causes keratoconus? Cornea. 2012;31:716–9.
3. Valgaeren H, Koppen C, Van Camp G. A new perspective on the genetics of keratoconus: why have we not been more successful? Ophthalmic Genet. 2017;7:1–17.
4. Galvis V, Sherwin T, Tello A, et al. Keratoconus: an inflammatory disorder? Eye (Lond). 2015;29:843–59.
5. Roberts CJ, Dupps WJ Jr. Biomechanics of corneal ectasia and biomechanical treatments. J Cataract Refract Surg. 2014;40:991–8.
6. Scarcelli G, Besner S, Pineda R, et al. Biomechanical characterization of keratoconus corneas ex vivo with Brillouin microscopy. Invest Ophthalmol Vis Sci. 2014;55:4490–5.
7. The International Commission on Non-Ionizing Radiation Protection. Health Physics. 2013;105(3):271–95.

8. Seiler TG, Fischinger I, Senfft T, et al. Intrastromal application of riboflavin for corneal cross-linking. Invest Ophthalmol Vis Sci. 2014;55:4261–5.
9. Hammer A, Richoz O, Arba Mosquera S, et al. Corneal biomechanical properties at different corneal cross-linking (CXL) irradiances. Invest Ophthalmol Vis Sci. 2014;55:2881–1884.
10. Wernli J, Schumacher S, Spoerl E, et al. The efficacy of corneal cross-linking shows a sudden decrease with very high intensity UV light and short treatment time. Invest Ophthalmol Vis Sci. 2013;54:1176–80.
11. Ehmke T, Seiler TG, Fischinger I, et al. Comparison of Corneal Riboflavin Gradients Using Dextran and HPMC Solutions. J Refract Surg. 2016;32:798–802.
12. Seiler TG, Fischinger I, Koller T, et al. Customized Corneal Cross-linking: One-Year Results. Am J Ophthalmol. 2016;166:14–21.
13. Nordström M, Schiller M, Fredriksson A, et al. Refractive improvements and safety with topography-guided corneal crosslinking for keratoconus: 1-year results. Br J Ophthalmol. 2017;101:920–5.
14. Cassagne M, Pierné K, Galiacy SD, et al. Customized Topography-Guided Corneal Collagen Cross-linking for Keratoconus. J Refract Surg. 2017;33:290–7.

Chapter 12
Demarcation Line in Corneal Collagen Crosslinking and Its Clinical and Topographic Significance

David P. Piñero Llorens

12.1 Concept of Demarcation Line in Corneal Collagen Crosslinking (CXL)

Corneal collagen cross-linking (CXL) is a surgical treatment used to increase corneal strength and to stabilize the ectatic cornea [1]. The first protocol described (conventional protocol, C-CXL) was based on the application of riboflavin and ultraviolet (UV) radiation after epithelium removal in order to improve the level of penetration of riboflavin and the depth of the treatment effect [1]. Several studies have confirmed the efficacy and safety of this procedure [2–9], even in the long term (10 years after CXL) [10, 11]. However, in the last years, a variety of protocols have been suggested to reduce operative time, increase patient comfort and minimize the incidence of complications, such as infectious keratitis and stromal haze [12–20]. Accelerated CXL (A-CXL) [12, 13, 15, 17–20] and transepithelial CXL with iontophoresis (I-CXL) [14, 16, 18] are two protocols developed with the aim of avoiding epitelial debridement and the potential complications associated to this procedure. In spite of some reports showing the potential stabilization of ectatic conditions with these two procedures, it is still controversial the level of penetration achieved with these techniques and consequently the potentially lower stabilizing effect achieved [18]. Indeed, experimental studies have confirmed the lower level of riboflavin penetration achieved when the treatment is applied without debridation of the epithelium [21].

One sign used to characterize the level of penetration achieved with CXL in the clinical practice is the demarcation line [12–20]. This sign was first described as a

D. P. Piñero Llorens (✉)
Department of Optics, Pharmacology and Anatomy, University of Alicante, Alicante, Spain

Department of Ophthalmology (OFTALMAR), Vithas Medimar International Hospital, Alicante, Spain
e-mail: david.pinyero@gcloud.ua.es

A. Barbara (ed.), *Controversies in the Management of Keratoconus*,
https://doi.org/10.1007/978-3-319-98032-4_12

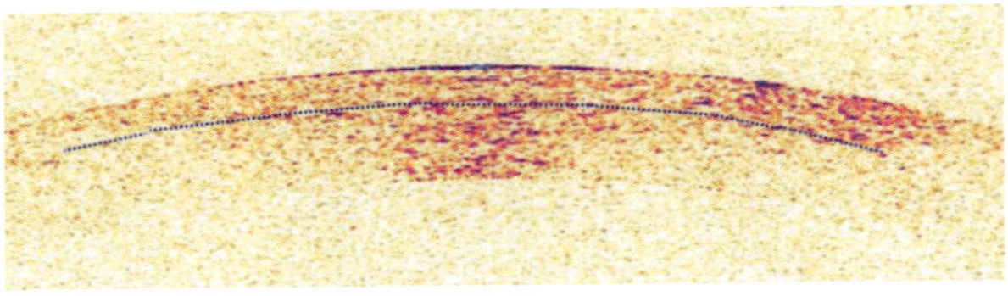

Fig. 12.1 Corneal scan obtained by optical coherence tomography (OCT) (OCT 3D-1000, Topcon) immediately after accelerated corneal collagen crosslinking (A-CXL). The demarcation line is remarked with a blue dot line

thin line detectable on slit lamp examination 2 weeks after C-CXL [20]. Afterwards, the demarcation line has been shown to be also detectable using confocal microscopy and anterior segment optical coherence tomography (AS-OCT) (Fig. 12.1) [12–20]. The depth of this acelular zone has been associated with the level of effectiveness of the CXL treatment [12–20]. However, there no studies showing the relationship between the depth of this line and the real changes induced in the mechanical properties of the cornea with the treatment [22]. Considering that the mechanical strength of the anterior corneal stroma is significantly higher than that of the posterior corneal stroma and that intraocular pressure (IOP) can differ significantly between healthy individuals, there should be a variable depth threshold of CXL treatment for achieving a biomechanical stabilization of the corneal structure [22]. Therefore, the clinical importance of the corneal demarcation line depth may be considered as relative [22].

12.2 Determination of the Demarcation Line After CXL

There is a lack of a standardized descriptive method of calculating the corneal stromal demarcation line and therefore comparison between studies should be done with caution [23]. Indeed, the difference between studies in the stromal demarcation line depth measured can be substantial considering the significant variation in axial resolution between imaging devices [23]. To this date, three different technologies have been used for measuring the depth of the demarcation line: Scheimpflug imaging [23], AS-OCT [12–20, 23] and in vivo confocal microscopy [16, 18, 19, 23]. With AS-OCT, the demarcation line can be detected by using the enhanced corneal high-resolution mode of the device and after this it can be measured manually by using a caliper or automatically with the LASIK flap tool [23]. With Scheimpflug imaging, the procedure to obtain the measurement is more complicated. Thorsud and colleagues [23] defined the following procedure to be applied in the clinical practice:

1. Selection of the image closest to the horizontal meridian
2. Use of the maximum zoom at the center of the cornea

3. Placement of a line at the center of the cornea between the anterior and posterior surface perpendicular to the corneal surface
4. After this, placement of a rule at 90° on this line and drawing of a new line in the transition zone from the anterior hyperreflective area to the posterior normal cornea.
5. Measurement of the distance between the anterior surface and this transition zone, being this considered as the depth of the demarcation line [23].

These same authors [23] also described a second procedure based on the digital analysis of the Scheimpflug image obtained. Specifically, in this method, the Scheimpflug image closest to the horizontal meridian is exported as a bitmap file (.bmp). This image is analyzed with the ImageJ software, using the line tool to create a line parallel and adjacent to the central line. Using the "Set Scale" function, the central corneal thickness provided by the Scheimpflug device is entered. After this, the "Plot Profile" tool is used and then "List" functions and these intensity plot values (arbitrary units) from the entire cornea are exported. Using Excel software, the intensity against the depth can be plotted to visualize the intensity profile. An increase of two intensity levels or more from the posterior part in two sequential values can be considered as a cutoff value representing the intensity change associated to the depth of the CXL treatment [23].

Concerning confocal microscopy, different approaches have been defined for determining the depth of the demarcation line depending on how the images obtained are analyzed [14, 16, 18, 23]. One approach consists on the determination of the depth at which the keratocytes are poorly defined. If several images satisfy this criterion, the median depth of the pictures can be calculated. Another method for determining the demarcation line is to detect the depth associated to an increase in intensity by five brightness units or more after two sequential pictures [23].

Thorsud and coauthors [23] demonstrated that Scheimpflug images were inaccurate for measuring the CXL demarcation line depth. Likewise, these same authors demonstrated that the two confocal microscopy approaches and OCT outcomes were correlated, with only OCT and confocal microscopy analysis considering intensity increase depths being in the same level of measurement [23]. Similarly, Bouheraoua and colleagues [18] did not find statistically significant differences in the measurement of the demarcation line depth after C-CXL, A-CXL and I-CXL using either OCT or confocal microscopy.

12.3 Demarcation Line After Different Procedures of CXL

Most of studies evaluate the demarcation line depth in the center of the cornea, ignoring the effect in the mid-peripheral cornea. It has been demonstrated that the C-CXL depth 3 mm away from the center decreases on average 65% of the central depth (range: 52–73%) [24]. Polymerization theory predicts this decay, however,

Table 12.1 Summary of the main outcomes reported in terms of demarcation line after CXL in keratoconus in different studies

Author (year)	Eyes	CXL method (postop period)	Demarcation line depth (% eyes in which is visible)	Measuring device
Jia et al. (2017) [14]	94	I-CXL (1 month)	298.95 ± 51.97 μm (83.1%)	OCT
Mazzotta et al. (2017) [13]	132	A-CXL (pulsed light) (1 month)	± 32 μm	OCT
Malhotra et al. (2017) [25]	12	CL-CXL dextran-based rioboflavin	235.33 ± 64.87 μm	OCT
	9	CL-CXL HPMC-based riboflavin (both 1 month)	308.22 ± 84.19 μm	
Bikbova and Bikbov (2016) [16]	73	C-CXL (14 days)	292 ± 14 μm (100%)	OCT/CM
	76	I-CXL (14 days)	176 ± 16 μm (100%)	
Piñero et al. (2016) [15]	21	A-CXL (1 day)	202.72 ± 19.99 μm	OCT
Moramarco et al. (2015) [17]	30	A-CXL (continuous light) (1 month)	149.32 ± 36.03 μm	OCT
	40	A-CXL (pulsed light) (1 month)	213.00 ± 47.38 μm	
Bouheraoua et al. (2014) [18]	15	C-CXL (1 month)	302.8 ± 74.6 μm (93.0%)	OCT/CM
	15	A-CXL (1 month)	184.2 ± 38.9 μm (87.5%)	
	15	I-CXL (1 month)	212.0 ± 36.5 μm 47.7%)	
Mazzotta et al. (2014) [19]	10	A-CXL (pulsed light)	180 μm (range 180–210)/200 μm (190–210)	OCT/CM
	10	A-CXL (continuous light)	160 μm (range 140–180)/160 μm (150–180)	
Tomita et al. (2014) [20]	30	A-CXL (1 month)	294.38 ± 60.57 μm	OCT
	18	C-CXL (1 month)	380.78 ± 54.99 μm	
Kymionis et al. (2014) [19]	9	C-CXL (1 month)	350.78 ± 49.34 μm	OCT
	12	A-CXL (1 month)	288.46 ± 42.37 μm	

Abbreviation: *C-CXL* conventional crosslinking, *I-CXL* transepithelial crosslinking with iontophoresis, *A-CXL* accelerated crosslinking, *OCT* optical coherence tomography, *CM* confocal microscopy, *CL-CXL* contact-lens assisted crosslinking, *HPMC* hydroxypropyl methylcellulose

underestimates the effect [24]. Therefore, more studies evaluating this issue are still necessary. Concerning measures in the center of the cornea, Table 12.1 shows a summary of the main outcomes reported after CXL in different studies [12, 20, 25–27]. As shown, a significant variability has been reported between studies evaluating the demarcation line after CXL, even when using the same protocol [12, 20, 25–27]. Possibly, these differences between studies may be explained in part by the discrepancies among them in terms of sample size, severity of the keratoconus cases included, clinical methods used, and follow-up. In any case, a general trend that can be observed is the significantly higher depth of the demarcation line obtained with C-CXL compared to other epi-on procedures. This is consistent with the results obtained in experimental studies [22]. Another important issue to remark from all these studies is that the demarcation line is not visible in most of patients more than 1 month after surgery [14, 16, 18].

12.4 Correlation Between Demarcation Line Depth and Clinical Outcomes

Although the demarcation line depth is a parameter evaluated in a lot of articles on CXL outcomes [12–20], there are no studies demonstrating the real relationship between this depth and the CXL effect achieved. Indeed, Bouheraoua et al. [18] demonstrated in a comparative study between C-CXL, A-CXL and I-CXL that there were no significant correlations of the CXL demarcation line depth with the change achieved postoperatively (6 months) in corrected distance visual acuity, maximum keratometry and central corneal thickness. Malhotra et al. [25] did not find strong and significant correlations between baseline clinical data and the demarcation line depth observed after contact lens-assisted CXL using dextran-based and hydroxypropyl methylcellulose-based riboflavin.

Chow and colleagues [28] reported a case series of early postoperative complications following A-CXL in keratoconus. From 11 patients undergoing surgery, 7 eyes (64%) developed complications in the first week postoperatively. Early transient stromal haze was seen in eyes with epithelial complications. Anterior segment optical coherence tomography showed a faint demarcation line in six eyes (55%) with epithelial complications. According to this, it is not still clear if a clear delimitation of the demarcation line may be a sign revealing that previous epithelial complications occurred. This should be investigated in future studies.

In conclusion, more studies are still necessary to confirm if there is a direct relationship between the depth of the demarcation line and the CXL effect achieved in terms of changes in the mechanical properties of the cornea. To this date, with the available scientific evidence, it cannot be stated that a lower depth of the demarcation line is associated to a lower effect of the CXL treatment or a higher potential of corneal instability in the future.

References

1. Wollensak G, Spoerl E, Seiler T. Riboflavin/ultraviolet-a-induced collagen crosslinking for the treatment of keratoconus. Am J Ophthalmol. 2003;135:620–7.
2. Wisse RP, Gadiot S, Soeters N, Godefrooij DA, Imhof SM, van der Lelij A. Higher-order aberrations 1 year after corneal collagen crosslinking for keratoconus and their independent effect on visual acuity. J Cataract Refract Surg. 2016;42:1046–52.
3. Sadoughi MM, Feizi S, Delfazayebaher S, Baradaran-Rafii A, Einollahi B, Shahabi C. Corneal changes after collagen crosslinking for keratoconus using dual Scheimpflug imaging. J Ophthalmic Vis Res. 2015;10:358–63.

4. Khattak A, Nakhli FR, Cheema HR. Corneal collagen crosslinking for progressive keratoconus in Saudi Arabia: One-year controlled clinical trial analysis. Saudi J Ophthalmol. 2015;29:249–54.
5. De Bernardo M, Capasso L, Lanza M, Tortori A, Iaccarino S, Cennamo M, Borrelli M, Rosa N. Long-term results of corneal collagen crosslinking for progressive keratoconus. J Optom. 2015;8:180–6.
6. Sedaghat M, Bagheri M, Ghavami S, Bamdad S. Changes in corneal topography and biomechanical properties after collagen crosslinking for keratoconus: 1-year results. Middle East Afr J Ophthalmol. 2015;22:212–9.
7. Steinberg J, Ahmadiyar M, Rost A, Frings A, Filev F, Katz T, Linke SJ. Anterior and posterior corneal changes after crosslinking for keratoconus. Optom Vis Sci. 2014;91:178–86.
8. Ghanem RC, Santhiago MR, Berti T, Netto MV, Ghanem VC. Topographic, corneal wavefront, and refractive outcomes 2 years after collagen crosslinking for progressive keratoconus. Cornea. 2014;33:43–8.
9. Sloot F, Soeters N, van der Valk R, Tahzib NG. Effective corneal collagen crosslinking in advanced cases of progressive keratoconus. J Cataract Refract Surg. 2013;39:1141–5.
10. Mazzotta C, Traversi C, Baiocchi S, Bagaglia S, Caporossi O, Villano A, Caporossi A. Corneal collagen cross-linking with riboflavin and ultraviolet A light for pediatric keratoconus: ten-year results. Cornea. 2018;37:560–6.
11. Raiskup F, Theuring A, Pillunat LE, Spoerl E. Corneal collagen crosslinking with riboflavin and ultraviolet-A light in progressive keratoconus: ten-year results. J Cataract Refract Surg. 2015;41:41–6.
12. Artola A, Piñero DP, Ruiz-Fortes P, Soto-Negro R, Pérez-Cambrodí RJ. Clinical outcomes at one year following keratoconus treatment with accelerated transepithelial cross-linking. Int J Ophthalmol. 2017;10:652–5.
13. Mazzotta C, Baiocchi S, Bagaglia SA, Fruschelli M, Meduri A, Rechichi M. Accelerated 15 mW pulsed-light crosslinking to treat progressive keratoconus: two-year clinical results. J Cataract Refract Surg. 2017;43:1081–8.
14. Jia HZ, Pang X, Fan ZJ, Li N, Li G, Peng XJ. Iontophoresis-assisted corneal crosslinking using 0.1% riboflavin for progressive keratoconus. Int J Ophthalmol. 2017;10:717–22.
15. Piñero DP, Artola A, Ruiz-Fortes P, Soto-Negro R, Pérez-Cambrodi RJ. Clinical outcomes at 1 year following corneal ectasia treatment with accelerated transepithelial cross-linking. Int J Kerat Ect Cor Dis. 2016;5:93–8.
16. Bikbova G, Bikbov M. Standard corneal collagen crosslinking versus transepithelial iontophoresis-assisted corneal crosslinking, 24 months follow-up: randomized control trial. Acta Ophthalmol. 2016;94:e600–6.
17. Moramarco A, Iovieno A, Sartori A, Fontana L. Corneal stromal demarcation line after accelerated crosslinking using continuous and pulsed light. J Cataract Refract Surg. 2015;41:2546–51.
18. Bouheraoua N, Jouve L, El Sanharawi M, Sandali O, Temstet C, Loriaut P, Basli E, Borderie V, Laroche L. Optical coherence tomography and confocal microscopy following three different protocols of corneal collagen-crosslinking in keratoconus. Invest Ophthalmol Vis Sci. 2014;55:7601–9.
19. Mazzotta C, Traversi C, Caragiuli S, Rechichi M. Pulsed vs continuous light accelerated corneal collagen crosslinking: in vivo qualitative investigation by confocal microscopy and corneal OCT. Eye. 2014;28:1179–83.
20. Tomita M, Mita M, Huseynova T. Accelerated versus conventional corneal collagen crosslinking. J Cataract Refract Surg. 2014;40:1013–20.
21. Wollensak G, Iomdina E. Biomechanical and histological changes after corneal crosslinking with and without epithelial debridement. J Cataract Refract Surg. 2009;35:540–6.
22. Gatzioufas Z, Balidis M, Kozeis N. Is the corneal stromal demarcation line depth a true indicator of corneal collagen crosslinking efficacy? J Cataract Refract Surg. 2016;42:804.

23. Thorsud A, Sandvik GF, Hagem AM, Drolsum L. Measuring the depth of crosslinking demarcation line in vivo: comparison of methods and devices. J Cataract Refract Surg. 2017;43:255–62.
24. Koller T, Schumacher S, Fankhauser F 2nd, Seiler T. Riboflavin/ultraviolet a crosslinking of the paracentral cornea. Cornea. 2013;32:165–8.
25. Malhotra C, Jain AK, Gupta A, Ram J, Ramatchandirane B, Dhingra D, Sachdeva K, Kumar A. Demarcation line depth after contact lens-assisted corneal crosslinking for progressive keratoconus: comparison of dextran-based and hydroxypropyl methylcellulose-based riboflavin solutions. J Cataract Refract Surg. 2017;43:1263–70.
26. Kymionis GD, Tsoulnaras KI, Grentzelos MA, Plaka AD, Mikropoulos DG, Liakopoulos DA, Tsakalis NG, Pallikaris IG. Corneal stroma demarcation line after standard and high-intensity collagen crosslinking determined with anterior segment optical coherence tomography. J Cataract Refract Surg. 2014;40:736–40.
27. Tomita M, Yoshida Y, Yamamoto Y, Mita M, Waring G IV. In vivo confocal laser microscopy of morphologic changer after simultaneous LASIK and accelerated collagen crosslinking for myopia: one-year results. J Cataract Refract Surg. 2014;40:981–90.
28. Chow SSW, Chan TCY, Wong IYH, Fan MCY, Lai JSM, Ng ALK. Early epithelial complications of accelerated trans-epithelial corneal crosslinking in treatment of keratoconus: a case series. Int Ophthalmol. 2017. https://doi.org/10.1007/s10792-017-0734-9. [Epub ahead of print].

Chapter 13
Corneal Cross Linking in Pediatric Keratoconus

Vasilios F. Diakonis and Mohammad Shehadeh

13.1 Introduction

Keratoconus is a non-inflammatory corneal biomechanical weakening, which results in progressive corneal thinning and steepening [1]. The corneal macrostructural morphological changes induce myopia, irregular astigmatism and high order aberrations which lead to variable impairment of vision [2]. The ametropia introduced may be managed initially (when the corneal surface irregularity is minor) with spectacles and when the corneal surface becomes highly irregular visual rehabilitation is achieved with rigid contact lenses. Keratoconus in most patients initiates in a young age and is usually diagnosed during adolescence. The main reasons for the underdiagnoses of keratoconus in its early stages is the ability to rehabilitate vision using spectacles, which does not raise concerns initially and rather the need or rapid change of spectacle prescription in young patients during their developing years is considered physiologic. Furthermore, younger patients are usually unable to assess their visual performance and identify visual impairment; most likely their parents, guardians or teachers are the first to notice their visual disturbance especially in cases of advanced keratoconus [3].

The diagnosis of keratoconus in pediatric patients is considered a negative prognostic factor for its progression, due to the lack of the age related corneal crosslinking which occurs naturally as the cornea ages. Thereby, early diagnosis and appropriate management is paramount in this sensitive age group, as poor visual performance may significantly affect the social and academic life of these patients [4].

V. F. Diakonis (✉)
The Eye Institute of West Florida, Largo, FL, USA

M. Shehadeh
An-Najah National University Hospital, Faculty of Medicine and Health Sciences, An-Najah National University, Nablus, West Bank, Palestine

A. Barbara (ed.), *Controversies in the Management of Keratoconus*,
https://doi.org/10.1007/978-3-319-98032-4_13

Corneal crosslinking (CXL) has been widely used in adults over the past 15 years, demonstrating success in halting or delaying the progression of keratoconus [5]. An increasing number of published manuscripts is now also available assessing CXL in pediatric patients demonstrating also favorable outcomes.

Failure of different protocols of CXL to arrest progression of keratoconus is attributed to different factors; the presence of negative influences such as atopy and allergy, continuous eye rubbing, poorly fitted contact lenses, genetic factors and the stage of keratoconus at the time of CXL procedure. Thereby allergy should be controlled before and after CXL to maintain its effect and decrease the risk of its failure [6].

13.2 Epidemiology of Keratoconus in Pediatric Patients

Keratoconus is usually diagnosed in the second decade of life, and continues to develop until the third and fourth decade. However, earlier onset has been documented in the literature as early as four years old in patients with predisposing factors such as Down syndrome and eye rubbing [7]. In the current literature, the average age of initial diagnosis of keratoconus is approximately 25 years. The prevalence, incidence and onset varies according to different geographical areas; it tends to be more prevalent with earlier presentation in hot and dry areas such as India and middle east compared to other cold areas like the United Kingdom and The Netherlands [8–10]. Saini et al. showed in his study that patients with severe keratoconus presented at a younger average age (18.8 ± 5.35 year) than moderate keratoconus (23.69 ± 8.08 year) [11]. Furthermore, Reeves et al. reported that keratoconus progression was more frequent and more rapid in patients under the age of eighteen, which demonstrate a seven fold higher risk of requiring corneal transplantation in the future [6].

13.3 Indications for Corneal Collagen Crosslinking in Pediatric Keratoconus

Documented progression of keratoconus in the only indication for CXL treatment. Progression is expressed as the increase in the cone apex keratometry of 0.75 diopters (D) or alteration of 0.75 D in the spherical equivalent refraction within a 6 month time interval. Initially, the same indication was also implemented in the pediatric patients as well; nevertheless, due to the aggressive nature of keratoconus in this age group ophthalmologists today tend to treat (CXL) their pediatric patients immediately after initial diagnosis and do not wait for documentation of progression. Chatzis and Hafezi clearly recommend not to wait for progression and to perform CXL in young patients as 52 of 59 eyes enrolled in their study showed progression of keratoconus [12]. However, other authors follow a more conservative approach; Soeters et al. recommend short and frequent follow up visits every 1–3 months in children and apply CXL when progression is documented [13].

The inclusion criteria for CXL in children do not differ from that of the adults. They include corneal thickness of at least 400 μm in thinnest location after epithelial removal (for epithelium off protocols), no corneal opacities, no history of herpetic keratitis, no severe dry eye, absence of autoimmune diseases and endothelial density of more than 1000 cell/mm^2 [14–16].

13.4 Protocols of Corneal Cross Linking in Pediatric Keratoconus

Cooperation during the surgical procedure is a critical issue when treating younger patients. Most studies reported the use of topical anesthesia except in few studies where general anesthesia was necessary [15]. It is also controversial whether to do both eyes in one session in case of general anesthesia to avoid the risks and stress of repetitive general anesthesia. The decision is best made by the ophthalmologist and the parents after discussion about the risks and benefits of both types of anesthesia and after assessment of the cooperation level of the patient.

The protocols of CXL used in pediatric keratoconus do not defer from those used in adults, nevertheless it is advised to utilize the original Dresden protocol in this sensitive patient group as it demonstrates the highest efficacy (the Dresden protocol induces significantly most stromal corneal stiffness when compared to other accelerated or epithelial on protocols as demonstrated in experimental studies) [17]. Transepithelial CXL (Epi-On technique) approaches and accelerated CXL protocols which use higher irradiances to reduce exposure time and the overall surgical time (i.e., 9 mW/cm^2 for 10 min or 30 mW/cm^2 for 4 min instead of 3 mW/cm^2 for 30 min) have been used; most authors present that both the accelerated and transepithelial protocols are equally effective to the original Dresden protocol, nevertheless there are clinical reports that show superiority of the Dresden protocol [12–26].

13.5 Safety of CXL in Pediatric Patients

Most clinical studies showed that CXL is safe in pediatric patients with no major complications in both standard and non-standard techniques. However, adverse effects and complications reported also in adult CXL such as, significant haze, delayed epithelial healing, transient glare and corneal edema have been reported [12–26].

13.6 Efficacy of Standard CXL Protocol in Pediatric Patients

Studies show that CXL stabilizes keratoconus progression in all age groups and sometimes it causes improvement of most the corneal parameters. One of the largest studies conducted by Caporrosi et al. (the Siena CXL pediatrics) involved 152 patients aged

18 years or younger (10–18 years) with a follow up of 36 months, showed a significant improvement in uncorrected distance visual acuity, corrected distance visual acuity, K-readings, asymmetry index values and coma aberrations [23]. Vinciguerra et al. also found a significant reduction in total corneal high order and astigmatic wave front aberrations [16]. On the other hand, Barbara et al. showed in their retrospective study of 29 eyes of 20 children who underwent CXL using the standard protocol that the change of sphere, keratometry, corneal hysteresis, corneal resistance factor and cornea compensated intraocular pressure were statistically insignificant [24]. Efficacy of CXL in pediatrics was also demonstrated by Bakshi et al. in their study, except that the improvement in uncorrected distance visual acuity (UDVA) and corrected distance visual acuity (CDVA) were statistically insignificant [25, 26].

Chatzis et al. retrospective pediatric CXL study showed similar results. This study also noticed a significant K-max reduction up to 24 months after CXL which lost significance at 36 months. However, in their study one eye showed progression despite CXL. This was attributed to continuous eye rubbing and/or vernal keratoconjunctivitis. CXL was repeated in this specific case and keratoconus stabilization was achieved up to 11 months after the repeat CXL [12].

The continuous physiologic corneal collagen turnover which demonstrates a rate of 6–7 years may exceed the capacity of the natural age related corneal collagen crosslinking in the pediatric patients. The natural age related corneal stromal cross linking is believed to play a role in older adults as keratoconus stabilization is naturally demonstrated after the age of 40 years, or rarely seen in pediatric patients with diabetes mellitus [27, 28]. In other words the achieved corneal stromal stiffening effect after CXL in pediatric patients which halts the progression of keratoconus is transient and may wear off after 6–7 years from CXL treatment. The above suggests that young keratoconic patients even after CXL treatment should be followed closely (at least once or twice a year) and be retreated in case of keratoconus reactivation.

13.7 Efficacy of Non-standard CXL Protocol in Pediatric Age Group

None-standard CXL protocols aim either to decrease the duration of treatment as in accelerated cross linking or to decrease the postoperative pain as in transepithelial CXL. Both may increase the cooperation of patients performed under topical anesthesia.

13.8 Transepithelial CXL

The primary outcomes of transepithelial CXL (TE-CXL) are encouraging. A study conducted by Magli et al. comparing standard CXL (epi-off) and transepithelial CXL (epi-on) protocols in 37 eyes of 29 patients between 12 and 18 years old. A significant improvement present for K-max, K-min, K-mean, surface asymmetry index, inferior – superior symmetry index, index of height asymmetry and anterior elevation at the thinnest location and the apex, which occurred similarly in both groups. However, post operative corneal edema noticed in 18 eyes in epi-off group compared to epi-on where no post operative edema was reported. TE-CXL also has the advantage of significantly less pain when compared to epi-off CXL [22].

Furthermore, an intact epithelium blocks adequate penetration of riboflavin into the corneal stroma and hence reduces the effectiveness of CXL. Confocal microscopy showed insignificant changes after TE- CXL compared to epi-off CXL [29].

13.9 Accelerated CXL

In accelerated CXL a higher irradiance is delivered to reduce exposure time; 9 mW/cm^2 for 10 min or 18 mW/cm^2 for 5 min. Accelerated CXL showed satisfactory results in the pediatric population regarding visual acuity and keratometry [30–32]. However, it seems that the depth of treatment reported is less than that achieved with the standard technique. The demarcation line depth averages between 100 and 240 μm in accelerated CXL compared to 300–350 μm in the standard technique [33, 34]. Furthermore, Morchen in ex-vivo experiments showed that the biomechanical stiffness effect on corneal tissue using energies up to 10 mW/cm^{2}is similar to that of standard protocol [35]. In addition, Cinar et al. found that the change in UDVA and CDVA at 6 month post accelerated CXL was statistically significant but inferior to conventional CXL [36].

13.10 CXL Plus Corneal Rings Implantation in Pediatric Keratoconus

The combination of CXL and intracorneal ring segment implantation for stabilization of keratoconus and visual rehabilitation has been also used in pediatric patients. Although many studies have been published on the management of pediatric keratoconus, studies on CXL plus corneal rings are scarce. In addition, most of them need longer follow-up and/or larger samples to be more conclusive.

Abdelmassih et al. evaluated the safety and visual outcome of intracorneal segment implantation followed by crosslinking in pediatric keratoconusin 12 patients (17 eyes) aged 9–14 years with a follow-up up to 4 years. A significant improvement of UDVA, CDVA, keratometry and spherical equivalent was shown and the finding demonstrated stability during the 4 years follow up [37]. Similar results were also reported by Abozaid who performed the CXL treatment in children with vernal keratoconjunctivitis [38].

13.11 Conclusion

Few studies have been published about the effectiveness of CXL in pediatric patients when compared to the plethora of available literature concerning adult CXL. More studies for different protocols with longer follow up are necessary. Nevertheless, CXL can potentially have a great impact on the treatment of pediatric keratoconus, as it may prevent amblyopia, improve the fitting of contact lenses and delay or prevent the need for keratoplasty, providing this sensitive group of patients with improved and stable visual performance which is important for their social and academic development.

Provided the severe form of keratoconus in pediatric patients, we recommend the use of the original Dresden protocol until we have scientific proof that the accelerated and epithelium on protocols achieve equivalent stromal stiffness. Finally, we also suggest not to wait for documentation of progression in patient under the age of 18 years, and rather perform CXL after the diagnosis has been established.

References

1. Rabinowitz YS. Keratoconus. Surv Ophthalmol. 1998;42(4):297–319.
2. Davis LJ, Schechtman KB, Wilson BS, et al. Longitudinal changes in visual acuity in keratoconus. Invest Ophthalmol Vis Sci. 2006;47(2):489–500.
3. Davidson AE, Hayes S, Hardcastle AJ, et al. The pathogenesis of keratoconus. Eye. 2014;28:189–95.
4. Leoni-Mesplie S, Mortemousque B, Touboul D, et al. Scalability and severity of keratoconus in children. Am J Ophthalmol. 2012;154:56–62.
5. Kymionis GD, Grentzelos MA, Liakopoulos DA, et al. Long-term follow-up of corneal collagen cross-linking for keratoconus—the cretan study. Cornea. 2014;33:1071–9.
6. Reeves SW, Stinnett S, Adelman RA, et al. Risk factors for progression to penetrating keratoplasty in patients with keratoconus. Am J Ophthalmol. 2005;4:607–11.
7. Gunes A, Tok L, Tok Ö, Seyrek L. The youngest patient with bilateral keratoconus secondary to chronic persistent eye rubbing. Semin Ophthalmol. 2015;30(5–6):454–6.
8. Shehadeh MM, Diakonis VF, Jalil SA, et al. Prevalence of keratoconus among a palestinian tertiary student population. Open Ophthalmol J. 2015;9:172–6.
9. Hashemi H, Beiranvand A, Khabazkhoob M, et al. Prevalence of keratoconus in a population-based study in Shahroud. Cornea. 2013;32:1441–5.
10. Godefrooij DA, de Wit GA, Uiterwaal CS, et al. Age-specific incidence and prevalence of keratoconus: a nationwide registration study. Am J Ophthalmol. 2017;175:169–72.
11. Saini JS, SarohaV, Singh P, et al. Keratoconus in Asian eyes at a tertiary eye care facility. Clin Exp Optom. 2004;87:97–101.
12. Chatzis N, Hafezi F. Progression of keratoconus and efficacy of corneal collagen cross-linking in children and adolescents. J Refract Surg. 2012;28:753–8.
13. Soeters N, Van der Valk R, Tahzib NG. Corneal crosslinking for treatment of progressive keratoconus in various age groups. J Refract Surg. 2014;30:454–60.
14. Zotta PG, Moschou KA, Diakonis VF, et al. Cornealcollagen cross-linking for progressive keratoconus in pediatricpatients: a feasibility study. J Refract Surg. 2012;28:793–6.
15. Arora R, Gupta D, Goyal JL, et al. Results ofcorneal collagen cross-linking in pediatric patients. J Refract Surg. 2012;28:759–62.
16. Vinciguerra P, Alb'e E, Frueh BE, et al. Two-year corneal cross-linking results in patients youngerthan 18 yearswith documented progressive keratoconus. Am J Ophthalmol. 2012;154:520–6.

17. Wollensak G, Iomdina E. Biomechanical and histological changes after cornealcrosslinking with and without epithelial debridement. J Cataract Refract Surg. 2009;35(3):540–6.
18. Hanna R, Berkwitz E, Castillo E, et al. Collagen cross-linking for the treatment of keratoconus in pediatric patients. Int J Kerat Ect Cor Dis. 2015;4(3):94–9.
19. Panos GD, Kozeis N, Balidis M, et al. Collagen cross- linkingfor paediatric keratoconus. Open Ophthalmol J. 2017 Jul 31;11:211–6.
20. El Rami H, Chelala E, Dirani A, et al. An Update on the safety and efficacy of corneal collagen cross-linking in pediatric keratoconus. Biomed Res Int. 2015;2015:257927.
21. Kankariya VP, Kymionis GD, Diakonis VF, et al. Management of pediatrickeratoconus - evolving role of corneal collagen cross-linking: an update. Indian J Ophthalmol. 2013 Aug;61(8):435–40.
22. Magli A, Forte R, Tortori A, et al. Epithelium-offcorneal collagen cross-linking versus transepithelial cross-linking for pediatrickeratoconus. Cornea. 2013;32(5):597–601.
23. Caporossi A, Mazzotta C, Baiocchi S, et al. Long term results of riboflavin ultraviolet a corneal collagen crosslinking for keratoconus in Italy: the Siena eye cross study. Am J Ophthalmol. 2010;149:585–93.
24. Barbara R, Pikkel J, Garzozi H, et al. Collagen cross-linking and keratoconus in pediatric patients. Int J Keratoco Ectatic Corneal Dis. 2012;1(1):57–60.
25. Bakshi E, Barkana Y, Goldich Y, et al. Corneal cross-linking for progressive keratoconus in children: our experience. Int J Keratoco Ectatic Corneal Dis. 2012;1(1):53–6.
26. Bakshi E, Barequet IS, Aizenman I, et al. Corneal crosslinking in patients younger than 18 years: Long-term follow up in three Israeli medical centers. Int J Kerat Ect Cor Dis. 2014;3(2):84–7.
27. Malik NS, Moss SJ, Ahmed N, et al. Ageing of the human corneal stroma: structural and biochemical changes. Biochim Biophys Acta. 1992;1138:222–8.
28. Kymionis GD, Tsoulnaras KI, Grentzelos MA, et al. Topography-based keratoconus regression. Cornea. 2013;32(10):1402–6.
29. Touboul D, Efron N, Smadja D, et al. Corneal confocal microscopy following conventional, transepithelial, and accelerated corneal collagen cross-linking procedures for keratoconus. J Refract Surg. 2012;28:769–75.
30. Shetty R, Nagaraja H, Jayadev C et al. Accelerated corneal collagen cross-linking in pediatric patients: two-year follow-up results. Biomed Res Int. 2014;894095.
31. Ozgurhan EB, Kara N, K. Cankaya I, et al. Accelerated corneal cross-linking in pediatric patients with keratoconus: 24-month outcomes. J Refract Surg. 2014;12:843–9.
32. Waszczykowska A, Jurowski P. Two-year accelerated corneal cross-linking outcome in patients with progressive keratoconus. Biomed Res Int. 2015.
33. Touboul D, Efron N, Smadja D, et al. Corneal confocal microscopy following conventional, transepithelial, and accelerated corneal collagen cross-linking procedures for keratoconus. J Refract Surg. 2012;28:769–75.
34. Ozgurhan EB, Akcay BIS, Yildirim Y et al. Evaluation of corneal stromal demarcation line after two different protocols of accelerated corneal collagencross-linking procedures using anterior segment opticalcoherence tomography and confocal microscopy. J Ophthalmol. 2014;2014:5 pages.
35. Mrochen M. Current status of accelerated corneal cross-linking. Indian J Ophthalmol. 2013;61(8):428–9.
36. Cınar Y, Cingü AK, Türkcü FM, et al. Comparison of accelerated and conventional corneal collagen cross-linking for progressive keratoconus. Cutan Ocul Toxicol. 2014;33(3):218–22.
37. Abdelmassih Y, El-Khoury S, Dirani A, et al. Safety and efficacy of sequential intracorneal ring segment implantation and cross-linking in pediatric keratoconus. Am J Ophthalmol. 2017;178:51–7.
38. Abozaid MA. Sequential Keraring implantation and corneal cross-linking for the treatment of keratoconus in children with vernal keratoconjunctivitis. Clin Ophthalmol (Auckland, NZ). 2017;11:1891–5.

Chapter 14
Re-evaluating the Effectiveness of Corneal Collagen Cross-Linking and Its True Biomechanical Effect in Human Eyes

Damien Gatinel, Cheryl MacGregor, and Muhammed Jawad

14.1 Background and Historical Perspective

In 1997, Spoerl et al. showed that the biomechanical behaviour of corneas obtained from enucleated porcine eyes could be altered by riboflavin and UV irradiation [1]. In keratoconus, where the corneal stiffness is reduced, the concept of strengthening corneal stability offered by artificial cross-linking (with radiation or chemical agents) led to the possibility of a conservative treatment option for keratoconus. The induction of cross-links in corneal tissue to possibly increase its stiffness was further explored in animal studies [2]. There was subsequently ample evidence in vitro demonstrating the alteration in biomechanical behaviour of the cornea by combined riboflavin/UVA-induced collagen cross-linking.

By the late 1990s, numerous studies had shown that cross-linking with riboflavin and UV could potentially stabilize the human cornea. The initial results of the first clinical trials suggested that CXL could provide a useful conservative treatment modality to delay or halt the progression of keratoconus and post-LASIK keratoectasia [3, 4]. In contrast to preliminary in vitro studies, the evaluation of biomechanical changes in vivo could not be performed in the first clinical studies, because instruments for measuring the corneal biomechanical properties in vivo did not exist at the time. Therefore, the parameters used to monitor CXL efficacy and safety in early clinical studies were visual acuity testing, corneal topography and measurements of endothelial cell density, instead of the key parameter in determining the efficacy of the strengthening effect of CXL on the cornea, that of biomechanics.

Source of Support I thank Cordelia Chan, MD, for assisting and providing critical revision of the manuscript.

D. Gatinel (✉) · C. MacGregor
Ophthalmology Department, Queen Alexandra Hospital, Portsmouth, UK

M. Jawad
Ophthalmology Department, North Hampshire Hospital, Basingstoke, UK

A. Barbara (ed.), *Controversies in the Management of Keratoconus*,
https://doi.org/10.1007/978-3-319-98032-4_14

14.2 Clinical Evaluation of the Biomechanical Changes Occurring In Vivo After CXL

In vivo evaluation of the biomechanical properties of the cornea was made possible in 2005 with the introduction of the Ocular Response Analyzer instrument (ORA, Reichert, Buffalo, NY, USA) into clinical practice [5]. This instrument uses a rapid air pulse to indent the cornea and an electro-optical system to monitor the bi-directional deformation of the cornea. Two primary indicators of corneal visco-elastic behaviour are extracted from this measurement process, namely Corneal Hysteresis (CH) and Corneal Resistance Factor (CRF). The method of operation of the device and evidence for the clinical utility of these parameters are described extensively in the literature [5]. Keratoconus, Fuchs' dystrophy, Glaucoma, Marfan syndrome and post-LASIK patients have been found to have low CH and CRF [6–13].

The Corneal Visualization Scheimpflug Technology tonometer (Corvis ST tonometry: CST; Oculus, Wetzlar, Germany) was introduced more recently and allows quantitative and visual assessment of the biomechanical properties of the cornea [14]. The Corvis ST is a non-contact tonometer with an integrated ultra-high-speed Scheimpflug camera, enabling the direct visualisation of corneal movement during the application of a rapid air-puff. The instrument's high-speed camera is capable of obtaining two-dimensional images of the cornea in cross section during its deformation. The device measures several parameters such as amplitude of corneal deformation, area of applanation and deformation velocity, which in turn provide information on corneal biomechanical properties.

Both ORA and CST have been used to assess the effects of CXL on keratoconus.

A pilot study was conducted to investigate, using the ORA, corneal biomechanical changes after CXL with UV-A-riboflavin. There were no significant differences in biomechanical properties as measured with the parameters CH and CRF [15]. In another study, Sedaghat et al. compared CH and CRF before and after CXL for keratoconus, and found no significant change in CH or CRF measured by biomechanical waveform analysis [16].

These were similar to the results published by Gkika et al. in which no significant change in CRF parameters were found in keratoconic eyes before and after UV-A-riboflavin corneal CXL [17].

In another paper, no significant changes in CH and CRF were found after a 24-month follow up period of 57 eyes of 55 patients with progressive keratoconus who were treated with CXL. Interestingly, in the subgroup of patients with decreased *K* max readings (measured with the Pentacam corneal topographer) 24 months after treatment, both CH and CRF showed a significant reduction [18]. Spoerl et al. did not detect significant changes in CH and CRF after cross-linking, and concluded that keratoconic corneas display altered biomechanical properties which remain different from those observed in healthy corneas [19]. Analysing the waveform signs of the ORA measurements, they found that the area under peak 2 significantly increased after CXL, suggesting that this parameter is more sensitive than CH or CRF at detecting biomechanical changes after CXL. Kiliç and Roberts reported a significant increase in the height of peak 1 after transepithelial cross-linking, and attributed it to an increase in corneal stiffness [20]. These findings have not been replicated since. The increase in the height of peak 1 or the area under peak 2 area could be the result of a modified corneal surface which provided improved reflectivity due to improved corneal homogeneity and regularity, which has been reported after CXL [21].

A prospective study was conducted to evaluate the relationship between corneal biomechanical and morphological data in healthy eyes, eyes that underwent myopic photorefractive keratectomy (PRK), eyes with keratoconus, and keratoconic eyes that underwent corneal CXL [22]. Tomographic (Pentacam, Oculus, Wetzlar, Germany) and biomechanical (Corvis ST, Oculus, Wetzlar, Germany) evaluations were performed. Corneas that were affected by keratoconus and CXL treated keratoconic eyes appeared to be easier to applanate, compared to healthy and post-PRK eyes, showing a lower resistance to deformation. Surprisingly, the resistance to deformation was lower in eyes that had undergone CXL than in untreated keratoconic corneas. Post-CXL corneas also took longer to return to the applanation position and recover their original shape. Interestingly, post-PRK corneas displayed similar resistance to deformation to normal eyes.

Bak-Nielsen et al. also described corneal deformation characteristics using rapidly applied forces via an air pulse with ultra-high-speed Scheimpflug technology in keratoconic eyes [23].

Significant differences in deformation parameters were found in both untreated and CXL-treated keratoconic eyes compared with normal eyes. Again however, no significant differences were found between patients with untreated keratoconus and CXL-treated keratoconus.

Tomita et al. investigated shorter duration ultraviolet light exposure in corneal CXL based on the notion that higher power delivered over shorter time periods could provide the same corneal strengthening as lower power over longer time periods [24]. Irrespective of the surgical protocol, no statistically significant difference between biomechanical parameters was found before and after CXL by the ORA and Corvis ST. Additionally, no significant difference in the measured parameters between the accelerated and conventional CXL was found.

Despite great effort, no significant and reproducible change in clinical parameters related to corneal biomechanics have been demonstrated in eyes that have undergone CXL for progressive keratoconus.

14.3 How Then Can We Explain the Lack of Clearly Documented Biomechanical Changes After CXL?

We put forward several hypotheses to explain these puzzling results.

Firstly, it has been suggested that biomechanical changes induced by CXL are too subtle to be measured by the ORA and Corvis ST, or have attributes not well classified by these technologies. However, it has been demonstrated that the ORA and Corvis ST have the capacity to record even subtle biomechanical differences in non-treated keratoconic corneas of differing ectatic degree [6–8]. Furthermore, CH and CRF values have been shown to be altered in patients with diabetes (correlated with Hb1AC levels) [25], in smokers [26, 27], Marfan syndrome [12], and in other instances where altered corneal biomechanics consistent with modified collagen properties would be expected [28]. The reduction in CH and CRF values after LASIK and surface ablation procedures have also been demonstrated [29–32]. The same authors who concluded that the Corvis ST may not be reliable to quantify the effect of CXL in keratoconus eyes, have demonstrated that it is possible to evaluate corneal biomechanical properties after LASIK, ReLEx FLEx, and ReLEx SMILE [33].

In contrast to the above scenarios, the changes induced by CXL on parameters such as CH and CRF seem to be too subtle to detect, or perhaps too subtle to be clinically relevant.

Perhaps CH and CRF are inadequate metrics to detect the possible stiffening achieved by CXL on keratoconic corneas. CH and CRF are not only influenced by the viscoelastic properties of corneal tissue, but other parameters such as corneal thickness and intraocular pressure. The cornea is a highly complex anisotropic tissue with a distinctive collagen fibre arrangement interacting with a complex collagen matrix. During ORA and Corvis ST measurements, the force acts perpendicular to the cornea, and the acquired signals are determined by its bending stiffness. The resistance to the bending of the cornea depends on the collagen fibres and the ground substance in which the fibres are embedded, which consists of glycosaminoglycans and proteoglycans. If the viscosity of the cornea is determined mainly by the ground substance, the creation of links between collagen fibrils or fibres may not significantly alter the value of CH and CRF parameters. The lower CH values observed after CXL may therefore, be derived from decreased glycosaminoglycans due to cell death.

The absence of measurable biomechanical changes in living keratoconus corneas after CXL contrasts with the results of ex vivo experiments, which show significant stiffening effects with standard and some modified CXL protocols, including evidence of increased elastic modulus and increased stiffness. It is possible that in vivo human corneas with progressive keratoconus do not respond to CXL in the same manner as animal models. This difference could be due to CXL inducing insignificant mechanical strengthening compared to the marked weakening caused by the pre-existing alteration of the collagen structure in progressive keratoconus. The disorganisation of collagen fibre intertwining and the compromised structural–mechanical homogeneity induced by the disease may be too overwhelming in progressive keratoconic corneas to be improved by CXL in any of its current (i.e. accelerated or conventional) in vivo modalities. In experimental and theoretical models, the biomechanical behaviour of corneal structures is estimated via stretch forces parallel to the corneal surface direction. Due to the lack of a comprehensive and cohesive theoretical model, bending forces are not considered.

Intensive eye rubbing may be the predominant, if not necessary, deformation mechanism responsible for the resultant corneal ectasia in keratoconus [34]. Eye rubbing produces a marked elevation in intraocular pressure, and the cornea is squeezed between compressive forces, resulting in significant corneal tissue trauma. The shearing forces produced by the fingers or knuckles (rotary or grinding movements on the corneal structure) may alter the fibre adherence and reduce the viscosity of the ground substance of the corneal matrix. In the central corneal region, which is directly exposed to the rubbing trauma, the resistance to bending may be reduced focally, causing local arching of the cornea and the characteristic deformation observed in keratoconus corneas (steep paracentral area surrounded by a flatter peripheral zone). CXL may improve the resistance of the cornea to lateral forces, but in contrast has little effect on bending forces. Indirect evidence of the predominant effect of bending compared to lateral shearing forces in keratoconus deformation is provided by a study which showed that the surface area of keratoconus corneas is remarkably insensitive to curvature change near the vertex [35]. Flattening seen in the periphery of corneas with keratoconus suggests that biomechanical coupling compensates for any increase in curvature occurring in the region of the cone itself. This study also suggested that keratoconus is not a true ectasia unlike keratoglobus, but is instead a specialized type of warpage, at least in the mild to moderate forms of the disease.

One promising technique for rapid evaluation of corneal stiffness is shear wave elastography. This method has been used ex vivo to measure the corneal biomechanics of animal corneas, but data regarding in vivo stiffening after CXL on keratoconic corneas is not yet available [36, 37].

14.4 The Need to Re-evaluate the Effectiveness of CXL: An Alternative Hypothesis

Based on current evidence, it may be challenging for clinicians to accept the alleged biomechanical effects induced by CXL. In keratoconus, post-corneal refractive surgery and corneal oedema where corneal stiffness is reduced [6–9, 13, 29–32], CH and CRF are concomitantly reduced. Why then do CH and CRF not increase in CXL-treated corneas if the primary effect of CXL is to stiffen the cornea? It is difficult to accept that the stiffening effect of CXL is too subtle to be detected by the same instruments that are used to detect changes in keratoconus and other corneal conditions with altered biomechanics.

In traditional mechanics, dynamic laws are deterministic and reversible with time. If the reduction in corneal hysteresis that occurs during the evolution of keratoconus or after corneal refractive surgery can be monitored by an instrument, this same instrument should be able to detect the increase in corneal hysteresis following the reduction of keratoconus severity following CXL procedure.

As the intended purpose of CXL is to increase the rigidity of the treated cornea by creating chemical bonds between collagen fibres, the lack of documented biomechanical improvement in CH and CRF parameters could be regarded as lack of effectiveness [38]. Before in vivo evidence of increased corneal visco-elastic properties is found, one cannot exclude the simple yet controversial hypothesis that CXL fails to significantly change the biomechanical properties of keratoconic corneas.

14.5 Caution in Interpreting the Topographic Response to CXL

Parameters such as corneal curvature, visual acuity, and topographic changes after CXL have been shown to be influenced by CXL. These sequelae were not chief objectives of the CXL treatment protocols, which were aimed primarily at increasing corneal stiffness. In many studies, the results of CXL were evaluated solely with non-biomechanical investigations, such as keratometry, topographic astigmatism magnitude, etc. In contrast to the lack of biomechanical alterations, significant topographical changes have been reported after CXL [18, 39–42] in patients with keratoconus and corneal ectasia. There were significant improvements in the index of surface variance, index of vertical asymmetry, keratoconus index, and minimum radius of curvature at 1 year [43]. A reduction in corneal and ocular high order aberrations (HOAs) was also observed after CXL, implying an improvement in corneal shape [44].

The delayed onset and degree of topographical improvements strongly suggests that the improvements in keratometric readings and visual quality reported after CXL may be due to healing mechanisms as detailed below.

The threshold values of keratometric changes used to determine keratoconus progression or post CXL improvement should also be carefully defined. Topographic measurements in keratoconus patients can be highly variable, so caution should be taken during clinical interpretation. We have recently assessed the repeatability of the corneal topography functions of Orbscan IIz (Bausch & Lomb, Rochester, NY), OPD-Scan III (Nidek, Gamagori, Japan), and iTrace (Tracey Technologies, Houston, TX) in keratoconic eyes and in a control group of normal patients [45]. For the maximum keratometry measurement, repeatability limit was 1.73, 1.49, and 1.41 D in the stage I-IV keratoconic eyes group, 1.11, 1.02, and 0.98 D in the stage I-II keratoconic eyes group, and 0.61, 0.37, and 1.02 D in the normal eyes group with Orbscan II, OPD-Scan III, and iTrace, respectively. These results illustrate that topographies performed in keratoconic eyes are less repeatable than those performed in normal eyes. A recent meta-analysis aiming to assess the efficacy and safety of epithelial removal (ER) and transepithelial (TE) corneal CXL for the treatment of keratoconus reported that based on the analysis of 27 studies on ER CXL, the median value of the reduction in maximal keratometry was −1.01D (range −0.14 to −6.16D) [46]. The conclusions in many of these studies aimed at evaluating preoperative progression and post- CXL stability are based on the assumption that instruments used in this assessment were accurate. It is important to consider topographic variation when interpreting results reporting treatment effect especially if the magnitude of the variations of the maximum keratometry in keratoconus eyes failed to exceed the repeatability limits of the devices used.

14.6 Could Epithelial Wound Healing Account for Most of the Changes Observed After CXL?

Cross-linking of collagen refers to the ability of collagen fibrils to form chemical bonds with adjacent fibrils. This requires both UV light and a photosensitizer to strengthen chemical bonds in the cornea; the simultaneous presence of both riboflavin and UVA is required to produce significant cross-linking of the fibrils. Hence, suppression of UV irradiation will result in interruption of the cross-linking reaction. The supposed biomechanical and topographic changes incurred by CXL should therefore happen during the procedure itself, and be measurable within a few days, right after the re-epithelialization period. Surprisingly, initial topographical changes usually show a mild central steepening, whilst mild flattening occurs typically months after the CXL procedure [18, 41, 42]. This late-onset flattening that has been attributed to the primary effect of CXL should therefore be attributed to a healing response, as any chemically induced response from the concomitant UVA irradiation (as in CXL) would have occurred during the procedure itself, or shortly after.

Phototherapeutic keratectomy produces a similar central flattening with significant gain in corrected distance visual acuity, even when shallow ablation with no refractive correction is performed, as for recurrent erosion syndrome [47]. Based on Munnerlyn's simplified equation (Thickness/Ablation depth, (μm) = 1/3 × Intended correction (D) × (OZ diameter (mm))^2), a reduction of two diopters (D) within the central 3-mm zone could result from a variation of less than 10 μm in epithelial thickness within this optical zone diameter. The importance of epithelium regrowth in the changes seen post-CXL is substantiated by the fact that CXL with de-epithelialization (epi off) has been shown to be more effective than transepithelial (epi on) CXL [46, 48–50]). Therefore, it is reasonable to conclude that the variation in keratometric readings and visual quality observed after CXL may be related to epithelial remodelling, rather than biomechanical changes.

We conducted a study to further investigate the role of the corneal epithelium in the topography of the anterior surface of the cornea [51]. In this study, preoperative OPD-Scan topography was performed on each eye 10 min before photorefractive keratectomy (for myopia) and the administration of topical anaesthesia. Removal of the epithelium allowed us to obtain a specular image of the topography of Bowman's membrane in normal, low to moderately myopic eyes. In 90 eyes of 51 patients, the topography of Bowman's layer was shown to be significantly steeper than that at the epithelial surface. The epithelial layer was demonstrated to decrease the degree of astigmatism and prolateness of Bowman's layer. This compensatory effect of the corneal epithelium was found to be more pronounced in eyes with keratoconus [52]. Interestingly, in the diseased corneas, the degree of change in keratometry after de-epithelialisation was higher than that reported after cross-linking. In the diseased eyes, the central epithelium was never totally removed before undergoing CXL, and yet, was able to remodel the anterior corneal surface with an improved contour. This strongly suggests that it is regrowth of corneal epithelium that may account for the slight topographic changes that have been reported in the long postoperative course after CXL.

14.7 What Is the Place of CXL Today and in the Future?

Since its introduction to ophthalmic practice in 2003 [3], a number of reports have concluded that CXL may slow or halt the progression of keratoconus and post-LASIK ectasia. In contrast, the Cochrane Database of Systematic Reviews' conclusion was more conservative and stated that the evidence was limited due the lack of properly conducted randomized controlled trials (RCTs) [53]. However, these considerations may still be insufficient to discourage ophthalmologists performing CXL in patients with progressive keratoconus. A recent Editorial in the Journal of Ophthalmology concluded that the recent United States Food and Drug Administraton (FDA) approval for the technique might have been triggered more by an unmet medical need rather than evidence based medicine [54]. Currently, other than minimising risk factors for progression (such as eye rubbing), there are no other alternative conservative solutions to halt the progression of keratoconus.

A secondary benefit of CXL could be that patients, following the procedure, may be reluctant to touch or rub their eyes, which further helps stabilise or stop disease progression.

14.8 Conclusions

Regardless of the place of CXL in keratoconus management, the inability to document alleged biomechanical improvement after CXL with currently available methods in keratoconus patients should invite scepticism from clinicians and researchers alike. In science, we are advised to take the null hypothesis as the default position. In the context of cross-linking studies, the null hypothesis would state that CXL has no biomechanical effect on the cornea. Analysis of current literature, particularly with regards to in vivo biomechanical studies, does not provide strong evidence to reject the null hypothesis.

The widespread positive perception of CXL among the ophthalmic community may reflect a confirmation bias, which is the tendency to search for or interpret information in a way that confirms one's preconceptions.

With the current protocols, the evidence shows that only corneal curvature, visual acuity, and topography can be influenced by CXL. These parameters, and not biomechanical strengthening, have been used by both surgeons and patients as yardsticks to qualify success of CXL and justify the need to perform the procedure. Ignoring the evidence that CXL is not a biomechanically efficient strengthening technique in vivo may prevent researchers from improving and refining current treatment modalities. Our feeling is that the discrepancy between the in vivo and in vitro biomechanical changes of the cornea after CXL warrants focus and further investigation. The documented effects of epithelial wound healing after CXL should be explored in depth, as it may explain most if not all the topographic changes observed over time. In this field, the newer high-resolution OCT techniques may be of particular interest. More importantly, establishing why the current CXL protocols have failed to reverse the clinically measurable corneal biomechanical impairment in keratoconic eyes, may be a prerequisite to understanding and discovering new, truly efficacious and biomechanically sound CXL techniques for ectatic corneas.

References

1. Spoerl E, Huhle M, Seiler T. Induction of cross-links in corneal tissue. Exp Eye Res. 1998;66(1):97–103.
2. Spoerl E, Seiler T. Techniques for stiffening the cornea. J Refract Surg. 1999;15(6):711–3.
3. Wollensak G, Spoerl E, Seiler T. Riboflavin/ultraviolet-A-induced collagen crosslinking for the treatment of keratoconus. Am J Ophthalmol. 2003;135(5):620–7.
4. Kohlhaas M, Spoerl E, Speck A, Schilde T, Sandner D, Pillunat LE. A new treatment of keratectasia after LASIK by using collagen with riboflavin/UVA light cross-linking. Klin Monatsbl Augenheilkd. 2005;222(5):430–6.
5. Luce D. Determining in vivo biomechanical properties of the cornea with an ocular response analyzer. J Cataract Refract Surg. 2005;31:156–62.
6. Shah S, Laiquzzaman M, Bhojwani R, Mantry S, Cunliffe I. Assessment of the biomechanical properties of the cornea with the ocular response analyzer in normal and keratoconic eyes. Invest Ophthalmol Vis Sci. 2007;48(7):3026–31.
7. Saad A, Lteif Y, Azan E, Gatinel D. Biomechanical properties of keratoconus suspect eyes. Invest Ophthalmol Vis Sci. 2010;51(6):2912–6.
8. Ali NQ, Patel DV, McGhee CN. Biomechanical responses of healthy and keratoconic corneas measured using a non-contact Scheimpflug-based tonometer. Invest Ophthalmol Vis Sci. 2014;55:3651–9.
9. del Buey MA, Cristóbal JA, Ascaso FJ, Lavilla L, Lanchares E. Biomechanical properties of the cornea in Fuchs' corneal dystrophy. Invest Ophthalmol Vis Sci. 2009;50(7):3199–202.
10. Prata TS, Lima VC, De Moraes CG, et al. Factors associated with topographic changes of the optic nerve head induced by acute intraocular pressure reduction in glaucoma patients. Eye (Lond). 2011;25:201–7.
11. Deol M, Taylor DA, Radcliffe NM. Corneal hysteresis and its relevance to glaucoma. Curr Opin Ophthalmol. 2015;26(2):96–102.
12. Beene LC, Traboulsi EI, Seven I, Ford MR, Sinha Roy A, Butler RS, Dupps WJ Jr. Corneal deformation response and ocular geometry: a noninvasive diagnostic strategy in Marfan syndrome. Am J Ophthalmol. 2016;161:56–64.e1.
13. Chen S, Chen D, Wang J, Lu F, Wang Q, Qu J. Changes in ocular response analyzer parameters after LASIK. J Refract Surg. 2010;26(4):279–88.
14. Koprowski R. Automatic method of analysis and measurement of additional parameters of corneal deformation in the Corvis tonometer. Biomed Eng Online. 2014;13:150.
15. Goldich Y, Barkana Y, Morad Y, Hartstein M, Avni I, Zadok D. Can we measure corneal biomechanical changes after collagen cross-linking in eyes with keratoconus?-a pilot study. Cornea. 2009;28(5):498–502.
16. Sedaghat M, Naderi M, Zarei-Ghanavati M. Biomechanical parameters of the cornea after collagen crosslinking measured by waveform analysis. J Cataract Refract Surg. 2010;36(10):1728–31.

17. Gkika MG, Labiris G, Kozobolis VP. Tonometry in keratoconic eyes before and after riboflavin/UVA corneal collagen crosslinking using three different tonometers. Eur J Ophthalmol. 2012;22(2):142–52.
18. De Bernardo M, Capasso L, Lanza M, Tortori A, Iaccarino S, Cennamo M, Borrelli M, Rosa N. Long-term results of corneal collagen crosslinking for progressive keratoconus. J Optom. 2015;8(3):180–6.
19. Spoerl E, Terai N, Scholz F, Raiskup F, Pillunat LE. Detection of biomechanical changes, after corneal cross-linking using ocular response analyzer software. J Refract Surg. 2011;27(6):452–7.
20. Kiliç A, Roberts CJ. Biomechanical and refractive results of transepithelial cross linking treatment in keratoconic eyes. Int J Kerat Ect Cor Dis. 2012;1(2):75–8.
21. Vinciguerra P, Albè E, Trazza S, Rosetta P, Vinciguerra R, Seiler T, Epstein D. Refractive, topographic, tomographic, and aberrometric analysis of keratoconic eyes undergoing corneal crosslinking. Ophthalmology. 2009;116(3):369–78.
22. Lanza M, Cennamo M, Iaccarino S, Irregolare C, Rechichi M, Bifani, Gironi Carnevale AU. Evaluation of corneal deformation analyzed with Scheimpflug based device in healthy eyes and diseased ones. BioMed Res Int. 2014;2014:748671. 9 pages.
23. Bak-Nielsen S, Pedersen IB, Ivarsen A, Hjortdal J. Dynamic Scheimpflug-based assessment of keratoconus and the effects of corneal cross-linking. J Refract Surg. 2014;30(6):408–14.
24. Tomita M, Mita M, Huseynova T. Accelerated versus conventional corneal collagen crosslinking. J Cataract Refract Surg. 2014;40:1013–20.
25. Scheler A, Spoerl E, Boehm AG. Effect of diabetes mellitus on corneal biomechanics and measurement of intraocular pressure. Acta Ophthalmol. 2012;90(6):e447–51.
26. Schweitzer C, Korobelnik JF, Boniol M, Cougnard-Gregoire A, Le Goff M, Malet F, Rougier MB, Delyfer MN, Dartigues JF, Delcourt C. Associations of biomechanical properties of the cornea with environmental and metabolic factors in an elderly population: the ALIENOR Study. Invest Ophthalmol Vis Sci. 2016;57(4):2003–11.
27. Kilavuzoglu AE, Celebi AR, Altiparmak UE, Cosar CB. The effect of smoking on corneal biomechanics. Curr Eye Res. 2017;42(1):16–20.
28. Spörl E, Terai N, Haustein M, Böhm AG, Raiskup-Wolf F, Pillunat LE. Biomechanical condition of the cornea as a new indicator for pathological and structural changes. Ophthalmologe. 2009;106(6):512–20.
29. Qazi MA, Sanderson JP, Mahmoud AM, Yoon EY, Roberts CJ, Pepose JS. Postoperative changes in intraocular pressure and corneal biomechanical metrics Laser in situ keratomileusis versus laser-assisted subepithelial keratectomy. J Cataract Refract Surg. 2009;35(10):1774–88.
30. Kamiya K, Shimizu K, Ohmoto F. Comparison of the changes in corneal biomechanical properties after photorefractive keratectomy and laser in situ keratomileusis. Cornea. 2009;28(7):765–9.
31. Kamiya K, Shimizu K, Ohmoto F. Time course of corneal biomechanical parameters after laser in situ keratomileusis. Ophthalmic Res. 2009;42(3):167–71.
32. Barbara R, Nassar A, Zadok D, Barbara A. Corneal biomechanical properties post-LASEK for the correction of myopia. Int K Kerat Ect Cor Dis. 2014;3(1):23–6.
33. Pedersen IB, Bak-Nielsen S, Vestergaard AH, Ivarsen A, Hjortdal J. Corneal biomechanical properties after LASIK, ReLEx flex, and ReLEx smile by Scheimpflug-based dynamic tonometry. Graefes Arch Clin Exp Ophthalmol. 2014;252(8):1329–35.
34. Gatinel D. Eye rubbing, a sine qua non for keratoconus? Int J Kerat Ect Cor Dis. 2016;5(1):6–12.
35. Smolek MK, Klyce SD. Is keratoconus a true ectasia? An evaluation of corneal surface area. Arch Ophthalmol. 2000;118(9):1179–86.
36. Nguyen TM, Aubry JF, Fink M, Bercoff J, Tanter M. In vivo evidence of porcine cornea anisotropy using supersonic shear wave imaging. Invest Ophthalmol Vis Sci. 2014.28;55(11):7545–52.
37. Touboul D, Gennisson JL, Nguyen TM, Robinet A, Roberts CJ, Tanter M, Grenier N. Supersonic shear wave elastography for the in vivo evaluation of transepithelial corneal collagen cross-linking. Invest Ophthalmol Vis Sci. 2014.28;55(3):1976–84.

38. Gatinel D. Effectiveness of corneal collagen crosslinking in vivo for corneal stiffening. J Cataract Refract Surg. 2014;40(11):1943–4.
39. Goldich Y, Marcovich AL, Barkana Y, et al. Clinical and corneal biomechanical changes after collagen cross-linking with riboflavin and UV irradiation in patients with progressive keratoconus: results after 2 years of follow-up. Cornea. 2012;31:609–14.
40. Raiskup-Wolf F, Hoyer A, Spoerl E, Pillunat LE. Collagen crosslinking with riboflavin and ultraviolet-A light in keratoconus: long-term results. J Cataract Refract Surg. 2008;34:796–801.
41. Vinciguerra P, Albè E, Frueh BE, Trazza S, Epstein D. Two-year corneal cross-linking results in patients younger than 18 years with documented progressive keratoconus. Am J Ophthalmol. 2012;154:520–6.
42. Caporossi A, Mazzotta C, Baiocchi S, Caporossi T. Long-term results of riboflavin ultraviolet a corneal collagen cross-linking for keratoconus in Italy: the Siena eye cross study. Am J Ophthalmol. 2010;149:585–93.
43. Greenstein SA, Fry KL, Hersh PS. Corneal topography indices after corneal collagen crosslinking for keratoconus and corneal ectasia: one-year results. J Cataract Refract Surg. 2011;37(7):1282–90.
44. Greenstein SA, Fry KL, Hersh MJ, Hersh PS. Higher-order aberrations after corneal collagen crosslinking for keratoconus and corneal ectasia. J Cataract Refract Surg. 2012;38(2):292–302.
45. Guilbert E, Saad A, Elluard M, Grise-Dulac A, Rouger H, Gatinel D. Repeatability of keratometry measurements obtained with three topographers in keratoconic and normal corneas. J Refract Surg. 2016;32(3):187–92.
46. Shalchi Z, Wang X, Nanavaty MA. Safety and efficacy of epithelium removal and transepithelial corneal collagen crosslinking for keratoconus. Eye (Lond). 2015;29(1):15–29.
47. Starr M, Donnenfeld E, Newton M, Tostanoski J, Muller J, Odrich M. Excimer laser phototherapeutic keratectomy. Cornea. 1996;15:557–65.
48. Vinciguerra P, Romano V, Rosetta P, Legrottaglie EF, Piscopo R, Fabiani C, Azzolini C, Vinciguerra R. Transepithelial iontophoresis versus standard corneal collagen cross-linking: 1-year results of a prospective clinical study. J Refract Surg. 2016;32(10):672–8.
49. Stojanovic A, Chen X, Jin N, Zhang T, Stojanovic F, Raeder S, et al. Safety and efficacy of epithelium-on corneal collagen cross-linking using a multifactorial approach to achieve proper stromal riboflavin saturation. J Ophthalmol. 2012;2012:498435.
50. Filippello M, Stagni E, O'Brart D. Transepithelial corneal collagen crosslinking: bilateral study. J Cataract Refract Surg. 2012;38(2):283–91.
51. Salah-Mabed I, Saad A, Gatinel D. Topography of the corneal epithelium and Bowman layer in low to moderately myopic eyes. J Cataract Refract Surg. 2016;42(8):1190–7.
52. Touboul D, Trichet E, Binder PS, Praud D, Seguy C, Colin J. Comparison of front-surface corneal topography and Bowman membrane specular topography in keratoconus. J Cataract Refract Surg. 2012;38(6):1043–9.
53. Sykakis E, Karim R, Evans JR, Bunce C, Amissah-Arthur KN, Patwary S, McDonnell PJ, Hamada S. Corneal collagen cross-linking for treating keratoconus. Cochrane Database Syst Rev. 2015;(3):CD010621.
54. Bennie HJ, Marjan F, Patel SV, Schwab IR. Corneal cross-linking for keratoconus: a look at the data, the Food and Drug Administration, and the future. Ophthalmology. 2016;123(11):2270–2.

Chapter 15
Alternative Corneal Cross-Linking Agents

Arie L. Marcovich

Corneal stiffening via cross-linking can be achieved by several agents. Cross-linking can be induced through chromophores that produce reactive oxygen species following illumination by a specific wavelength or by chemical reaction that does not require light. The clinically used RF is activated by UVA light at 365 nm. There are drawbacks to the RF/UVA treatment. UVA was shown experimentally to be toxic to corneal endothelium in rabbits and there were several reports of corneal edema after RF/UVA cross-linking [1–4]. A minimal corneal thickness of 400 μ is required for safety and RF/UVA was not efficient in thin corneas [1, 2, 5]. Epithelial debridement is usually performed to facilitate RF penetration and ensure deep corneal cross-linking. These limitations promoted research of other chromophores that are excited by green light at 532 nm (rose bengal [6–10], eosin [11, 12]) or near infrared (NIR) light at 755 nm (WST-D [13–15]) and chemical cross-linkers like genipin [16–18] and galacorin [19].

15.1 Photoactivated Cross-Linkers

15.1.1 Rose Bengal

RB is a diagnostic dye for corneal and conjunctival surface. It's excitation by green laser light at 532 nm in the presence of oxygen, leads to production of singlet oxygen [10]. Several studies demonstrated its ability to stiffen the cornea in rabbits ex-vivo and in-vivo and increase the resistance of treated corneas to collagenase

A. L. Marcovich (✉)
Department of Ophthalmology, Kaplan Medical Center, Rehovot, Israel

Department of Plant and Environmental Sciences, Weizmann Institute of Science, Rehovot, Israel

A. Barbara (ed.), *Controversies in the Management of Keratoconus*,
https://doi.org/10.1007/978-3-319-98032-4_15

digestion [6–8, 11]. RB 0.1% in phosphate buffered saline is applied to deepithelialized cornea for 2 min followed by illumination of green light (532 nm) at 0.25 W/cm^2 for 3.3–10 min with repeated application of RB every 3.3 min for 30 s. Corneal stiffness increased 3.8-fold ex-vivo and 2.8-fold after 28 days in vivo compared to untreated controls. RB penetration to the corneal stroma is limited to 100 μ. Corneal stiffening increases in this region as demonstrated by Brillouin microscopy [6]. When applied in vivo RB/green light treatment induced reduction of keratocyte counts in the 120 μ anterior stroma that recovered after 28 days [8]. The green light intensity of 0.25 W/cm^2 is relatively high. Histology, transmission electron microscopy and fluorescein angiography didn't detect retinal damage in rabbits after treatment on day 1 or day 28 [8]. The restricted penetration of RB may enable cross-linking of thin corneas without risking the endothelium with minimal toxicity to keratocytes [6, 8].

15.1.2 Eosin Y

Eosin Y (yellowish) is a water-soluble fluorescent xanthene stain that binds to proteins containing arg and lys. It's absorption peak is at 514 nm. When activated with green light (514 nm or 525 nm) it becomes excited producing oxygen radicals [11, 12]. Experiments conducted in rabbits in-vivo demonstrated corneal stiffening similar to RF/UVA treatment. For corneal penetration the epithelium was removed. Full corneal penetration was observed after 10 min [11]. Eosin was applied in gel formulation of 0.04% eosin in 3% carboxymethylcellulose for 5 min followed by illumination with green light (525 nm) at 6 mW/cm^2 for 10 min. Less phototoxicity to keratocytes and endothelium was reported compared to RF/UVA treatment of 30 min impregnation with 0.1% RF and 30 min UVA illumination at 3 mW/cm^2. Corneal epithelialization was observed after 7 days [11]. Eosin is an efficient cross-linker that requires low illumination intensity at a visible green wavelength.

15.1.3 WST-D

WST-D is a watersoluble palladium bacteriochlorin 130-(2-sulfoethyl)amide dipotassium salt (WST11) that generates O_2 – and •OH radicals when illuminated with near infrared (NIR) light at 755 nm [13]. The drug is approved in Europe and Mexico for the photodynamic treatment of prostate cancer when injected intravenously (http://ec.europa.eu/health/documents/community-register/html/h1228.htm). When formulated with dextran T-500 WST-D penetration into the deepithelialized cornea is restricted to 50% of the stroma [13]. Ex vivo and in vivo studies in rabbits demonstrated 4.7-fold increase in corneal stiffening ex vivo and 2.7-fold after 1 month in vivo after impregnation of depithelialized cornea with WST-D 0.25% in 20% dextran T-500 for 20 min and NIR illumination with 10 mW/cm^2 for 30 min [13]. No rise in corneal temperature was detected during the treatment [13]. A long term follow up of 8 months treatment in rabbits in vivo demonstrated a sustained corneal stiffening [15]. Histology detected loss of keratocytes in the anterior 40% of the corneal stroma 1 week after treatment, with full repopulation after 8 months. No endothelial damage was evident [15]. An ex vivo and in vivo study was performed to determine the required duration of NIR illumination at 10 mW/cm^2 after 20 min of 0.25% WST-D impregnation. A comparable and significant stiffening effect of WST-D/NIR was achieved even with a reduced irradiation time of only 1 min ex vivo and 5 min in vivo, without increasing irradiance [14]. NIR light causes no intrinsic damage to cells by itself and is, within ranges, considered safe to patients and environment by the International Commission of Ionizing Radiation Protection (ICNIRP) [20]. NIR can however cause thermal damage to ocular structures, in particular to the retina, at high irradiance and/or exposure time. The ICNIRP considers NIR irradiance at 10 mW/cm^2, as used in this study, to be safe to the cornea and lens for longer than 17 min. For 5 min of illumination this would mean a safety threshold of 25 mW/cm^2 [20]. The ability to limit the corneal penetration of WST-D with dextran and the safe nature of NIR light enable to treat safely thin corneas. Other applications like scleral cross linking for myopia and treatment of corneal infections are possible.

15.2 Chemical Cross-Linkers

15.2.1 Genipin

Genipin is a natural protein crosslinker extracted from the plant gardenia jazminoides. In ex-vivo porcine corneas it induced stiffening and resistance to enzymatic digestion in a concentration dependent ratio [16]. In-vivo, genipin 0.25% was applied for 5 min to deepithelialized corneas in rabbits. It flattened the cornea in treated eyes by 4.4 diopters ±0.5 [SD] compared to control eyes. Pachymetry and IOP were stable. The treatment didn't affect the endothelium. Minimal corneal edema was observed 4 days after treatment. Epithelialization was complete after 5 days, with light blue coloration [17]. Comparing treatment of rabbit corneas with 0.2% genipin showed minimal toxicity toward keratocytes and endothelial cells and appeared safer than RF/UVA crosslinking [18]. Genipin is biocompatible. Implantation of chitosan membranes containing genipin in the anterior chamber of rabbits for 24 weeks didn't induce inflammation [21]. Genipin injected sub tenon didn't show retinal toxicity. In vivo scleral crosslinking in guinea pigs with genipin effectively reduced form deprivation myopic eye growth without histological damage to the retina or choroid [22]. In summary genipin demonstrated in-vivo flattening of the cornea and retardation of induced myopia without evidence of corneal or retinal toxicity.

15.2.2 Galacorin®

Galacorin® (decoron) is a recombinant human decorin. Decorin is a 100 kDa proteoglycan that consists of 40 kDa protein and a glycosaminoglycan chain of chondroitin sulfate/dermatan sulfate disaccharides that resides in the extracellular matrix of collagen fibrils. Collagen fibrils interact with decorin among other extracellular components to organize and stabilize collagen structure [23]. Galacorin® demonstrated increased corneal rigidity ex-vivo in human and porcine corneas [19]. Galacorin®'s molecular weight is 40 kDa and cannot diffuse through intact epithelium. In order to facilitate its passage through the epithelium a penetration enhancer needs to be used. A pretreatment solution (an alkaline 0.2 M disodium phosphate pH 9.0) is applied for 45–60 s followed by an acetylation agent (7.5 mg glutaric anhydride powder dissolved in an alkaline pH of 9.12, 0.3 M disodium phosphate solution) applied for 45–60 s. The cornea is then rinsed with saline drops and Galacorin® is applied for 45–60 s using another clean eye cup. The whole treatment lasts 3–4-min and does not require epithelial debridement. One limitation of the report is that there was no control group receiving the pretreatment alone [19].

15.3 In conclusion

Several promising novel cross-linking agents are available in various pre-clinical stages. They may be added to the currently available riboflavin/UVA cross-linking, or treat patients with thin corneas unsuitable for the existing treatment. Chemical cross-linkers do not require light application, which facilitates their use while photodynamic therapy allows better control of the intensity of the treatment.

Other applications for cross-linking like infections or scleral stiffening to arrest myopia are undergoing research.

References

1. Spoerl E, Mrochen M, Sliney D, Trokel S, Seiler T. Safety of UVA-riboflavin cross-linking of the cornea. Cornea. 2007;26(4):385–9.
2. Wollensak G, Spoerl E, Wilsch M, Seiler T. Endothelial cell damage after riboflavin-ultraviolet-A treatment in the rabbit. J Cataract Refract Surg. 2003;29(9):1786–90.
3. Bagga B, Pahuja S, Murthy S, Sangwan VS. Endothelial failure after collagen cross-linking with riboflavin and UV-A: case report with literature review. Cornea. 2012;31(10):1197–200.
4. Sharma A, Nottage JM, Mirchia K, Sharma R, Mohan K, Nirankari VS. Persistent corneal edema after collagen cross-linking for keratoconus. Am J Ophthalmol. 2012;154:922–6.
5. Hafezi F. Limitation of collagen cross-linking with hypoosmolar riboflavin solution: failure in an extremely thin cornea. Cornea. 2011;30:917–9.
6. Cherfan D, Verter EE, Melki S, Gisel TE, Doyle FJ Jr, Scarcelli G, et al. Collagen cross-linking using rose bengal and green light to increase corneal stiffness. Invest Ophthalmol Vis Sci. 2013;54:3426–33.

7. Bekesi N, Kochevar IE, Marcos S. Corneal biomechanical response following collagen cross-linking with rose bengal-green light and ribo avin-UVA. Invest Ophthalmol Vis Sci. 2016;57:992–1001.
8. Zhu H, Alt C, Webb RH, Melki S, Kochevar IE. Corneal crosslinking with Rose Bengal and green light: efficacy and safety evaluation. Cornea. 2016;35:1234–41.
9. Kochevar IE, Redmond RW. Photosensitized production of singlet oxygen. Methods Enzymol. 2000;319:20–8.
10. Fadlallah A, Zhu H, Arafat S, Kochevar I, Melki S, Ciolino JB. Corneal resistance to keratolysis after collagen crosslinking with rose bengal and green light. Invest Ophthalmol Vis Sci. 2016;57:6610–4.
11. Schwartz DM, Mattson MS, Kornfield JA, Maloney RK, Grubbs RH, inventors. Photochemical therapy to affect mechanical and/or chemical properties of body tissue. US patent 20080114283. May 15, 2008.
12. Huynh J. Factors governing photodynamic cross-linking of ocular coat. Dissertation (Ph.D.), California Institute of Technology; 2011. http://resolver.caltech.edu/CaltechTHESIS:05202011-143758537.
13. Marcovich AL, Brandis A, Daphna O, et al. Stiffening of rabbit corneas by the bacteriochlorophyll derivative WST11 using near infrared light. Invest Ophthalmol Vis Sci. 2012;53:6378–88.
14. Brekelmans J, Goz A, Dickman MM, Brandis A, Sui X, Wagner HD, Nuijts RM, Scherz A, Marcovich AL. Corneal stiffening by a bacteriochlorophyll derivative with dextran and near-infrared light: effect of shortening irradiation time up to 1 minute. Cornea. 2017;36:1395–401.
15. Brekelmans J, Goz A, Dickman MM, Brandis A, Sui X, Wagner HD, Nuijts RM, Scherz A, Marcovich AL. Long-term biomechanical and histological results of WST-D/NIR corneal stiffening in rabbits, up to 8 months follow-up. Invest Ophthalmol Vis Sci. 2017;58:4089–95.
16. Avila MY, Navia JL. Effect of genipin collagen crosslinking on porcine corneas. J Cataract Refract Surg. 2010;36:659–64.
17. Avila MY, Narvaez M, Castañeda JP. Effects of genipin corneal crosslinking in rabbit corneas. J Cataract Refract Surg. 2016;42:1073–7.
18. Song W, Tang Y, Qiao J, Li H, Rong B, Yang S, Wu Y, Yan X. The comparative safety of genipin versus UVA-riboflavin crosslinking of rabbit corneas. Mol Vis. 2017;23:504–13.
19. Metzler KM, Roberts CJ, Mahmoud AM, Agarwal G, Liu J. Ex vivo transepithelial collagen cross-linking in porcine and human corneas using human decorin core protein. J Refract Surg. 2016;32:410–7.
20. ICNIRP (International Commission on Non-ionizing Radiation Protection). Guidelines on limits of exposure to broad-band incoherent optical radiation (0.38 to 3 microM). International Commission on Non-Ionizing Radiation Protection. Health Phys. 1997;73:539–54. http://www.ncbi.nlm.nih.gov/pubmed/9287105
21. Lai J-Y. Biocompatibility of genipin and glutaraldehyde crosslinked chitosan materials in the anterior chamber of the eye. Int J Mol Sci. 2012;13:10970–85.
22. Wang M, Corpuz CCC. Effects of scleral cross-linking using genipin on the process of form-deprivation myopia in the guinea pig: a randomized controlled experimental study. BMC Ophthalmol. 2015;15:89.
23. DeVore DP, DeWoolfson BH, Glady GE, Hoopes PJ, Moodie KL, Roberts CJ. Decorin core protein for organizing and stabilizing stromal collagen structure. Poster presented at: 9th International Congress of Corneal Crosslinking; December 6–7, 2013; Dublin.

Chapter 16
PRK and Corneal Cross-Linking in the Management of Keratoconus

Arthur Cummings

Very few corneal specialists working in the keratoconus area would doubt the benefits that corneal crosslinking (CXL) have provided keratoconus patients [1–7]. Fundamental to most surgical management of keratoconus approaches would be the immediate cessation of eye rubbing followed by CXL. Today when treating keratoconus, the decision needs to be made as to whether the primary reason for treatment is:

1. Stabilisation of the keratoconus
2. Visual rehabilitation, then stabilised with CXL

The patient that has progressive keratoconus but is still seeing well, requires stabilisation only and this is provided by CXL. To the contrary, the patient where CDVA has already been affected or where visual quality is inadequate, may not want that particular state of affairs made permanent by CXL. In these cases, it is appropriate to first regularise the corneal shape either by topography-guided PRK, PTK removal of the epithelium prior to CXL, Intacs or other intrastromal ring segments, thermal procedures such as conductive keratoplasty (CK) and such like procedures, and then once the improved corneal shape has been obtained, then to stabilise this new improved shape with CXL.

This chapter deals with the use of the excimer laser only in conjunction with CXL [8–14]. The other treatment modalities are discussed elsewhere in the book.

When treating with the excimer laser, there are several issues to consider:

1. The timing of the CXL: is it done prior to the PRK, simultaneous with the PRK [10–12] (i.e. immediately afterwards) or after the PRK (weeks to months to years).
2. The mode in which the excimer laser is used: PTK, standard PRK or Topography-guided PRK (TG-PRK).

A. Cummings (✉)
Wellington Eye Clinic and Beacon Hospital, Dublin, Ireland
e-mail: abc@wellingtoneyeclinic.com

A. Barbara (ed.), *Controversies in the Management of Keratoconus*,
https://doi.org/10.1007/978-3-319-98032-4_16

3. Concerning the CXL aspect of the treatment: is it performed epi-ON [15–18] or epi-OFF and when is it standard CXL and when is it accelerated CXL (ACXL)? [7, 15, 19–21]

This chapter is going to address these questions and attempt to provide guidance on possible approaches.

The author's approach to the use of the excimer laser is mostly indicated by the level of vision that the patient presents with: if the CDVA and even more significantly, the UDVA is good, then CXL only is typically applied and the excimer laser is not employed. When the CDVA has been reduced by the corneal irregularity and the visual quality has been negatively affected, then the use of the excimer laser is indicated. The basic concept here is that the excimer laser is used to regularise the cornea and then once this has been achieved, the cornea is stabilised with CXL.

Corneal regularisation can be achieved in many ways using the excimer laser:

1. Using the PTK mode to remove the corneal epithelium prior to epi-OFF CXL
2. Using manual epithelial removal followed by TG-PRK to regularise the cornea
3. Using a combination of the above: PTK plus TG-PRK
4. Using all three options above but with a wavefront-guided (WFG) modality
5. Using the first three options above with a wavefront-optimised (WFO) profile

In addition, when using the excimer laser, there are distinctly different potential aims of treatment:

1. Simply regularise the cornea, thereby improving quality of vision and reducing higher order aberrations. This leads to improved CDVA but not necessarily improved UVDA. In some cases, UDVA may in fact be worse.
2. Regularize the cornea and correct the underlying refractive error: in these cases, both UDVA and CDVA are improved.
3. Correct the refractive error with a WFO profile: here the UDVA is improved but not necessarily the CDVA.

It is imperative to discuss this clearly prior to the procedure and ensure that the patient is fully informed and has realistic expectations.

Some centres are treating the full refractive correction while others are treating no refractive error (only corneal higher order aberrations (HOAs)) or partial refractive error (mostly cylinder). Again, it is imperative to inform the patient of your intentions so that their expectations are aligned.

If the cornea was entirely stable after the excimer laser application, the challenge would not be nearly as great as it is. As we know, the cornea is not stable in keratoconus necessarily and CXL may be indicated. Although very few doubt the value of CXL, most would concede that they cannot predict the effect of CXL. Sometimes it leads to nothing more than stabilising the cornea, sometimes the cornea flattens and on occasion, the cornea flattens very significantly. This all results in refractive unpredictability. Therefore, the manner of CXL applied [15–18] (epi-ON or epi-OFF), the fluence (CXL or ACXL) [7, 15, 19–21] and the timing are all so important. In the author's experience, the strongest CXL effect achieved is the combined, simultaneous procedure of TG-PRK followed immediately by CXL. This leads to a very good Riboflavin soak given that Bowman's membrane has been removed and hence to a very significant CXL effect. This observation has been noted over the decade of employing this treatment (TG-PRK plus CXL) in the author's own experience.

The least predictable CXL application in terms of refractive predictability is epi-OFF CXL, especially when Bowman's membrane has been removed either with PTK or PRK. Corneal flattening can be very modest or very significant. Corneal flattening can occur in the first few months or even years later. One example of this is a patient that was −7.00D at the time of SimLC (simultaneous laser crosslinking – a phrase employed by the author to differentiate this treatment from all other combined treatments and always referring to the treatment of the HOAs only – i.e. no refractive correction) where for the first 4 years after the procedure, the refraction remained around the −7.00D mark. Two years ago, the patient presented with a −2.50D refraction and 1 year ago with −1.00D. At his most recent postoperative visit, he was +1.50D with all the corneal flattening occurring 4 years after the initial treatment. This late flattening has been reported by Theo Seiler and others too. On the other hand, the CXLO approach to epi-ON CXL has led to very predictable corneal changes [13, 18]. Using their protocol, the cornea achieves stability and progressive steepening is halted. When corneal flattening does occur (and this is in over 50% of cases in the author's experience with this protocol over the past 5 years), the flattening is modest and typically less than 1D. This provides more refractive predictability for both the patient and the surgeon.

The timing of the CXL plays a very significant role too in the refractive outcomes, the corneal flattening expected and the visual recovery. There are three options concerning timing:

1. First do CXL, wait for some level of corneal stability to occur and then do PRK.
2. Do PRK or PTK, followed immediately by CXL. The author has named this SimLC when there is no refractive input and many other protocols exist. The best-known protocol is the Athens Protocol [10] where some of the astigmatism is corrected.
3. First do the PRK and then monitor the cornea for stability. If any sequential steepening occurs, then apply CXL. This could be weeks, months or years later and in many cases, especially where the patient has completely ceased with eye rubbing, never. The PRK alone suffices in terms of correcting the HOAs or even the refractive error (if low enough) and it provides corneal and refractive stability. It is imperative, as with all keratoconus patients, that the patient is fully aware of the need for regular follow up examinations. At the first sign of progression, CXL can be applied to halt the progression and stabilise the improved vision.

Timing of the CXL has further implications in terms of the final corneal stability and corneal biomechanical strength. Most would agree that epi-OFF CXL provides the greatest biomechanical strength gains but if laser ablation is applied at some time later, the strongest of these collagen fibres is being ablated. This then weakens the initial CXL effect. If the TG-PRK is done first, many would agree that there is a redistribution of corneal strain in the collagen fibres and a better shape results. If the cornea continues to steepen however, epi-ON CXL can now be applied. The resultant final corneal biomechanical strength in these two examples may ultimately be quite similar [22]. With the first example however, there are two distinct disadvantages: the ablation is done on cornea that has undergone CXL and second, epi-OFF CXL has a less predictable effect. There is much to be said in the author's view for the second approach when it is feasible.

The final piece of the puzzle concerns the CXL itself. The latest nomenclature as suggested by J. Bradley Randleman, MD; Marcony R. Santhiago, MD, PhD; George D. Kymionis, MD, PhD and Farhad Hafezi, MD, PhD in the Journal of Refractive Surgery in November 2017, is the use of the terms CXL for corneal crosslinking and A-CXL for accelerated CXL [23]. Furthermore, it has been suggested to use S-CXL for the standard protocol and A-CXL (9*10) for the accelerated protocol where 9 mW was used for 10 min or A-CXL (15*6) where 15 mW was used for 6 min or A-CXL(30*3) where 30 mW was used for 3 min. The standard or Dresden protocol would be stated as S-CXL(3*30). There is an additional difference in the UV-lamps and that concerns their beam profile. The original IROC UV-X 1000 has most of its fluence centrally while the later UV-X 2000 has most of its fluence in the periphery. The author tends to select the lamp to be used based on where the cornea is thinnest: if it is central, then the UV-X 1000 is used and if it is peripheral, the UV-X 2000 is used.

The factors that impact the final shape of the cornea that originate from the excimer laser can be divided into the following categories:

1. PTK epithelium removal:
   With this approach the epithelium is removed using the excimer laser's PTK mode. If for example the ablation depth is set to 50 μ and the corneal epithelium is only 40 μ thick over the steepest point or cone, then the laser ablation is going to remove these 10 additional stromal microns precisely at the point where the stroma is steepened. The result is significant flattening over the cone and regularisation of the cornea.

Figures 16.1, 16.2, 16.3 and 16.4 illustrate the effect of PTK on the stromal regularity.

2. TG-PRK (or WFG-PRK):
   Here a customised ablation profile is used based either on corneal HOAs (TG-PRK) or on whole eye aberrations (WFG-PRK) and the ablation profile is designed to reduce the measured aberrations. This ablation is applied to the cornea after manual epithelial removal using alcohol or a mechanical method like a brush for example. It is important to note that the TG-PRK data is obtained from the

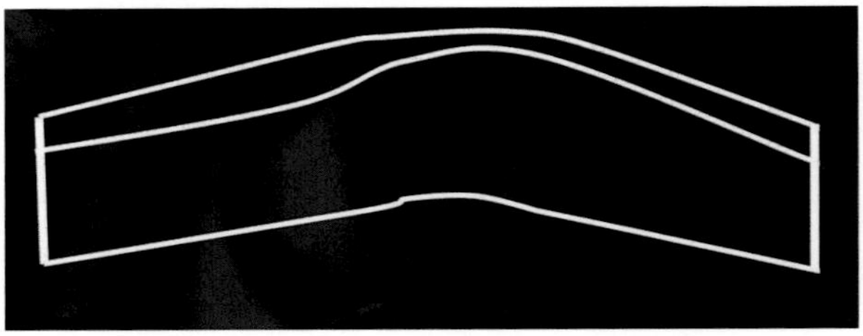

Fig. 16.1 The cornea demonstrating epithelial thinning over the steepest part of the stroma/cone

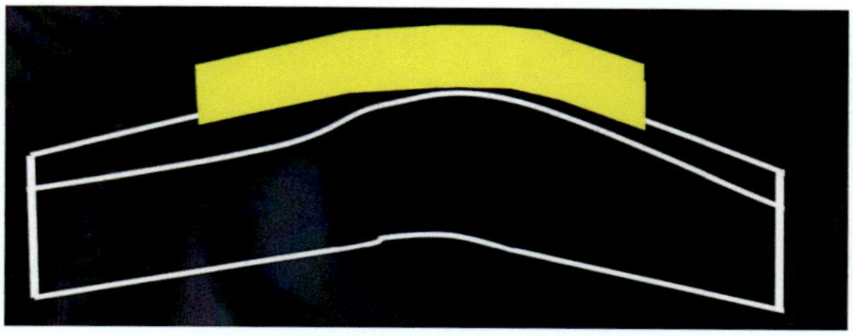

Fig. 16.2 The PTK commences and given that it is a PTK, the overall shape of the ablation is simply equal across the entire optical zone with the intention of removing 50 microns for example of corneal tissue in the pathway of the ablation, whether it be epithelium or stroma

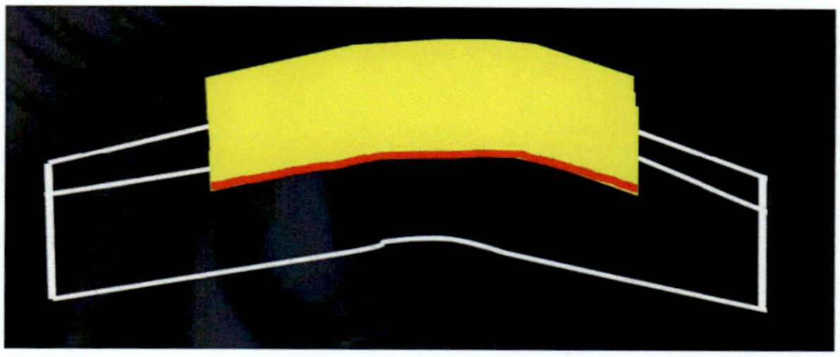

Fig. 16.3 As the PTK progresses into the cornea, there are areas where more stroma has been ablated than other areas

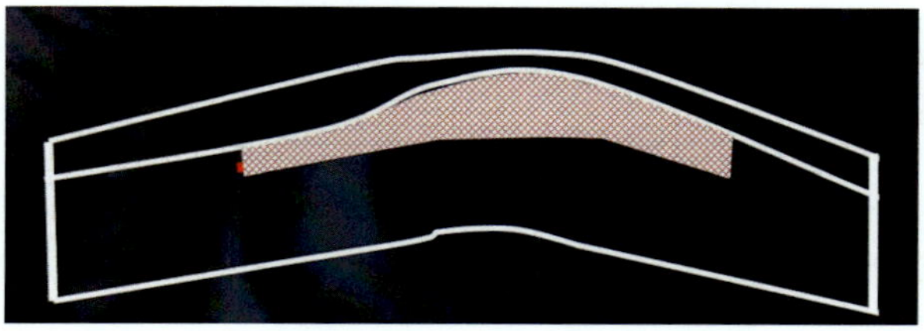

Fig. 16.4 The final stromal ablation has a different shape to the original PTK thanks for the masking of the corneal epithelium. In this instance, a standard PTK has resulted in a topography-guided effect

surface of the corneal epithelium/tear film and hence some of the true stromal topography data is masked by the epithelium's attempt to regularise the cornea.

3. Combined PTK plus TG-PRK/WFG-PRK:
   Here the effects of the PTK and customised PRK are added and this typically leads to greater regularisation of the cornea than either of the two modalities in isolation. This is the approach most commonly adopted by the author. Figure 16.5 below illustrates the typical ablation profile for a keratoconic eye.

The following case illustrates a PTK combined with TG-PRK where CL was applied epi-ON 1 week later. This is not the usual delay that the author uses between PRK and CXL but since the patient was travelling from abroad, the 1-week delay suited best. Figure 16.6 illustrates the preoperative corneal topography centrally, the postoperative image 1 week later prior to CXL on the left and the difference map on the right.

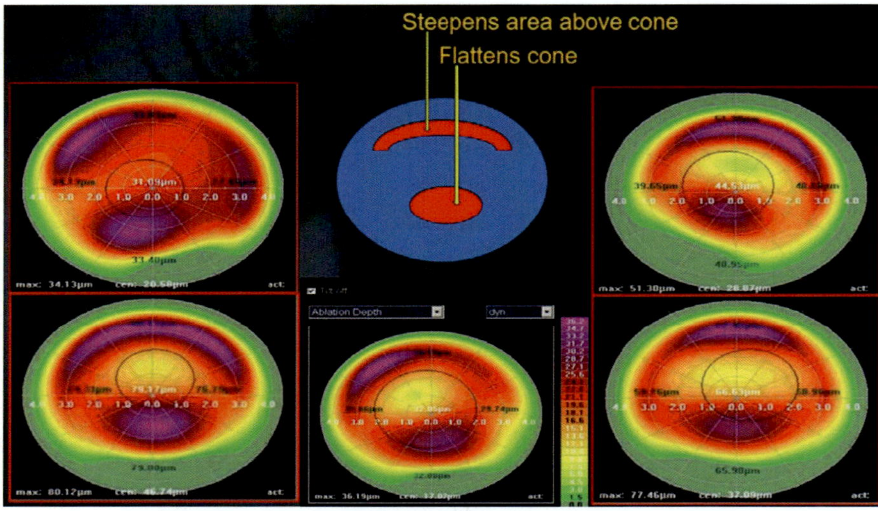

Fig. 16.5 The upper central image is a sketch of the typical ablation profile for keratoconic eyes with flattening of the area over the cone and steepening of the superior central area. This steepening is achieved along similar lines to hyperopic ablation profiles where ablating in the corneal periphery leads to steepening of the cornea that is central to the ablation. The examples on either side of the sketch and below the sketch illustrate just how similar the ablation profiles appear for five different keratoconic eyes

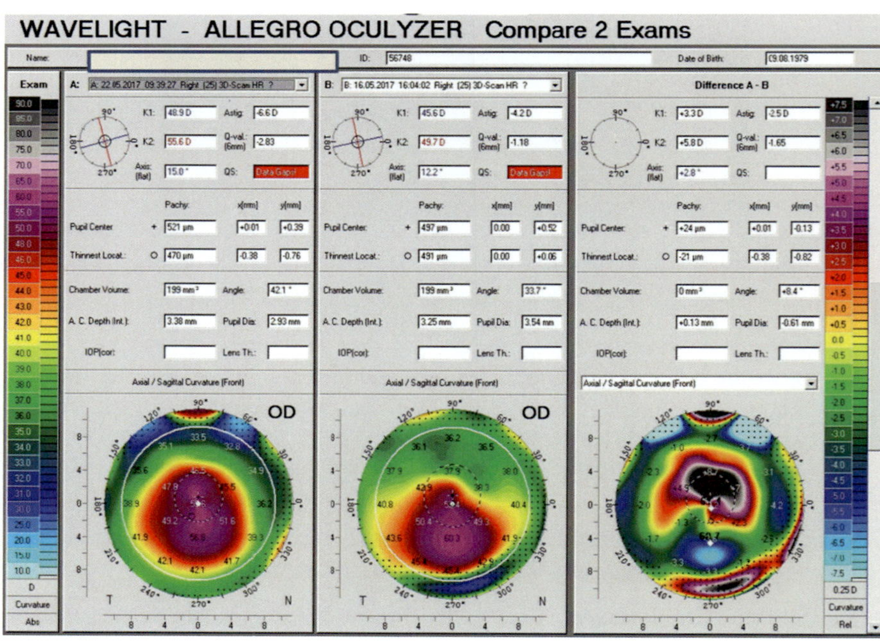

Fig. 16.6 Preoperatively the cone is irregular and displaced inferiorly as is typical for keratoconus (middle). 1 week following the PTK/TG-PRK, the cornea is more regular (left) while the difference map demonstrates 7D of inferior flattening and 7D of superior steepening resulting in 14D of regularisation. The improvement in CDVA was significant and the epi-ON CXL has led to a stable postoperative condition that now allows additional surgery such as a phakic IOL or ICL to be utilised

The UV light source also plays a role in the success of CXL and there is currently a development in this space where more customised light sources are being created that can target the weakened cornea specifically. In the mean time however, the author uses the currently available light sources according to where their energy is most heavily concentrated, either centrally or peripherally. The images below illustrate this point (Figs. 16.7 and 16.8).

This chapter was intended to provide the reader with thoughts to consider when opting to use the excimer laser in conjunction with CXL to manage keratoconus. The literature is saturated with articles and case studies demonstrating different protocols and approaches and some references are included below. This chapter was intended to serve as a review of the different approaches and encourage the use of the most appropriate mode (PTK, TG-PRK, WFG-PRK), the best use of CXL timing, the most appropriate CXL light source and the use of epi-ON versus epi-OFF that suits both the patient and the ophthalmologist delivering the care.

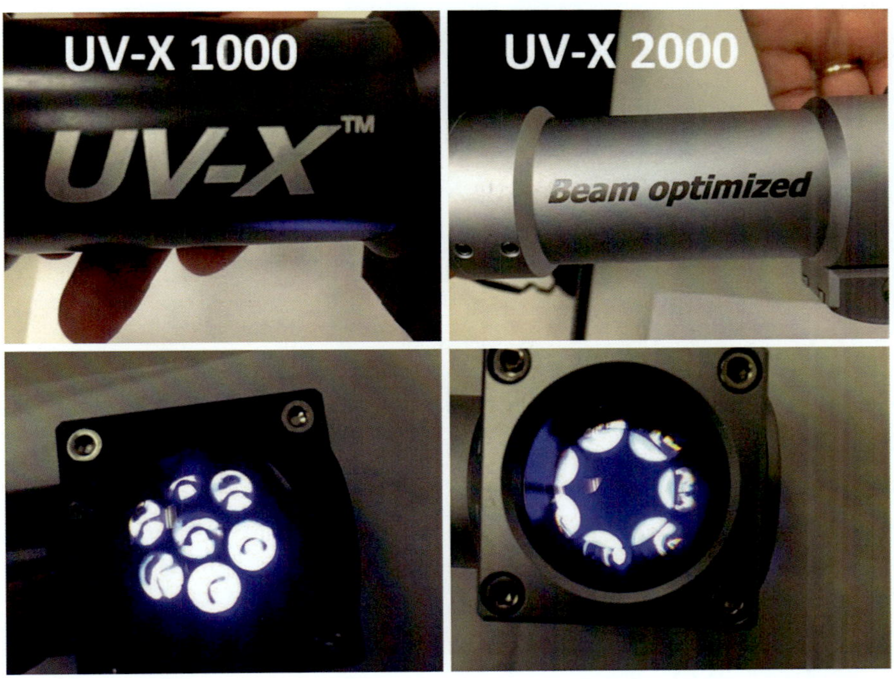

Fig. 16.7 The UV-light sources both comprise 7 Light-emitting diodes (LEDs) but the LEDs are arranged differently. On the left, the UV-X 1000 has 7 LEDs that fill the aperture with 1 LED in the centre and 6 LEDs in the periphery and on the right, the 7 LEDs are arranged with a gap in the centre and 7 LEDs in the periphery

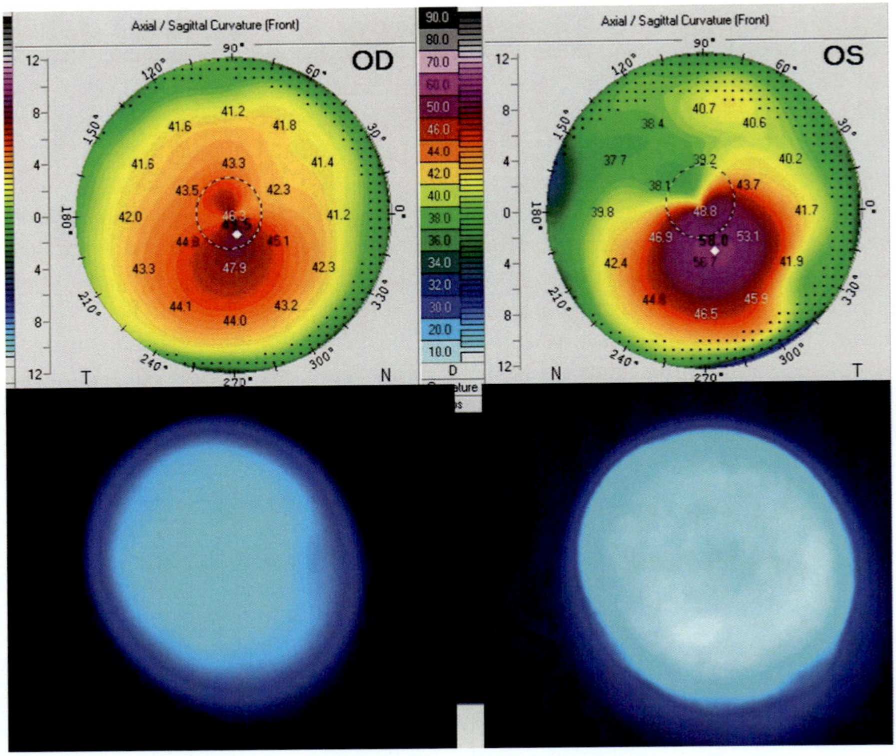

Fig. 16.8 The light energy on the bottom left (UV-X 1000) is concentrated centrally, perhaps better suited to the more central cone (top left) while the light source on the bottom right (UV-X 2000) is concentrated in the periphery, perhaps better suited to the more peripheral cone featured in the top right topography

References

1. Wollensak G, Spoerl E, Seiler T. Riboflavin/ultraviolet-a-induced collagen crosslinking for the treatment of keratoconus. Am J Ophthalmol. 2003;135:620–7.
2. Wollensak G, Spoerl E, Seiler T. Stress–strain measurements of human and porcine corneas after riboflavin-ultraviolet-A-induced cross-linking. J Cataract Refract Surg. 2003;29:1780–5.
3. Hafezi F, Kanellopoulos J, Wiltfang R, Seiler T. Corneal collagen crosslinking with riboflavin and ultraviolet A to treat induced keratectasia after laser in situ keratomileusis. J Cataract Refract Surg. 2007;33:2035.
4. Raiskup-Wolf F, Hoyer A, Spoerl E, et al. Collagen crosslinking with riboflavin and ultraviolet-A light in keratoconus: long-term results. J Cataract Refract Surg. 2008;34:796–801.
5. Zhang Y, Conrad AH, Conrad GW. Effects of ultraviolet-A and riboflavin on the interaction of collagen and proteoglycans during corneal cross-linking. J Biol Chem. 2011;286:13011–22.
6. Randleman JB, Khandelwal SS, Hafezi F. Corneal cross-linking. Surv Ophthalmol. 2015;60:509–23.
7. Kymionis GD, Tsoulnaras KI, Liakopoulos DA, Skatharoudi CA, Grentzelos MA, Tsakalis NG. Corneal stromal demarcation line depth following standard and a modified high intensity corneal cross-linking protocol. J Refract Surg. 2016;32:218–22.

8. Mortensen J, Carlsson K, Ohrstršm A. Excimer laser surgery for keratoconus. J Cataract Refract Surg. 1998;24:893–8.
9. Koller T, Iseli HP, Donitzky C, Ing D, Papadopoulos N, Seiler T. Topography- guided surface ablation for forme fruste keratoconus. Ophthalmology. 2006;113:2198–202.
10. Kanellopoulos AJ, Binder PS. Collagen cross-linking (CCL) with sequential topography-guided PRK: a temporizing alternative for keratoconus to penetrating keratoplasty. Cornea. 2007;26:891–5.
11. Alpins N, Stamatelatos G. Customized photoastigmatic refractive keratectomy using combined topographic and refractive data for myopia and astigmatism in eyes with forme fruste and mild keratoconus. J Cataract Refract Surg. 2007;33:591–602.
12. Cennamo G, Intravaja A, Boccuzzi D, Marotta G, Cennamo G. Treatment of keratoconus by topography-guided customized photorefractive keratectomy: two-year follow-up study. J Refract Surg. 2008;24:145–9.
13. McQuaid R, Cummings AB, Mrochen M. The theory and art of corneal cross-linking. Indian J Ophthalmol. 2013;61:416–9.
14. Kymionis GD, Grentzelos MA, Portaliou DM, Kankariya VP, Randleman JB. Corneal collagen cross-linking (CXL) combined with refractive procedures: CXL plus. J Refract Surg. 2014;30:566–76.
15. Cummings AB, McQuaid R, Mrochen M. Newer protocols and future in collagen cross-linking. Indian J Ophthalmol. 2013;61:425–7.
16. Vinciguerra P, Romano V, Rosetta P, et al. Transepithelial iontophoresis versus standard corneal collagen cross-linking: 1-year results of a prospective clinical study. J Refract Surg. 2016;32:672–8.
17. Cruzat A, Shukla A, Arafat S, et al. Ex vivo study of transepithelial corneal cross-linking. J Refract Surg. 2017;33:171–7.
18. Cummings AB, Shaw P, Kelly G. 3 year outcomes of epi-on CXL for progressive keratoconus using the CXLO protocol. FP 42560 Epi-ON CXL – Poster Village – ESCRS Lisbon; 2017.
19. Hashemian H, Jabbarvand M, Khodaparast M, Ameli K. Evaluation of corneal changes after conventional versus accelerated corneal cross-linking: a randomized controlled trial. J Refract Surg. 2014;30:837–42.
20. Hammer A, Richoz O, Mosquera S, Tabibian D, Hoogewoud F, Hafezi F. Corneal biomechanical properties at different corneal collagen cross-linking (CXL) irradiances. Invest Ophthalmol Vis Sci. 2014;55:2881–4.
21. Cummings AB, McQuaid R, Naughton S, Brennan EE, Mrochen M. Optimizing corneal cross-linking in the treatment of keratoconus: a comparison of outcomes after standard- and high-intensity protocols. Cornea. 2016;35(6):814–22.
22. Richoz O, Hammer A, Tabibian D, Gatzioufas Z, Hafezi F. The biomechanical effect of corneal collagen cross-linking (CXL) with riboflavin and UV-A is oxygen dependent. Transl Vis Sci Technol. 2013;2:6.
23. Randleman JB, Santhiago MR, Kymionis GD, Hafezi F. Corneal Cross-Linking (CXL): standardizing terminology and protocol nomenclature. J Refract Surg. 2017;33(11):727–9.

Chapter 17
The Athens Protocol: Perform a Partial Topography-Guided Normalization Treatment Separate or Together with Corneal Cross-Linking? Cross-Linking and PRK: Sequential Versus Combined Strategy

A. John Kanellopoulos

Corneal cross-linking (CXL) has established a new paradigm for the treatment of progressive ectasia and keratoconus [1–3]. The visual rehabilitation of patients who achieve stability after CXL can be challenging if they were intolerant of rigid gas permeable contact lenses or if they had poor vision with glasses and/or soft contact lenses prior to treatment. The problem led my colleagues and me to introduce the topography-guided normalization of corneas that remain highly irregular despite some flattening effect from CXL [4, 5].

17.1 Early Efforts

At the outset, we waited at least 6 months after CXL to perform topography-guided partial PRK. Because these were "uncharted waters," we set an arbitrary 50-μm limit to the ablation over the cone. Admittedly, such conservative treatment did little to correct refractive error.

We decided that, if the corneal parameters permitted, we would treat up to 70% of the sphere and cylinder but always maintain that 50-μm maximum ablation over the thinnest part of the cone. The refractive effects of this treatment strategy were impressive: the great majority of patients obtained a BCVA of 20/40. Few complications occurred aside from some PRK-related haze and occasionally delayed epithelial healing [6]. We therefore began to discuss our findings with prospective CXL patients and to offer them the option of CXL and partial topography-guided PRK as a combined, same-day procedure.

A. J. Kanellopoulos (✉)
LaserVision.gr Eye Institute, Athens, Greece

New York University School of Medicine, New York, NY, USA

A. Barbara (ed.), *Controversies in the Management of Keratoconus*,
https://doi.org/10.1007/978-3-319-98032-4_17

17.2 Advantages

Our early experience identified three advantages of our combined approach. First, there is no need to remove cross-linked cornea (the CXL effect is greater closer to the surface). With a sequential approach, surface ablation removes some of the most biomechanically stable corneal tissue produced by CXL [7].

Second, we observed less corneal haze and scarring in these eyes [8]. A third and surprising finding was that performing CXL and topography-guided PRK at the same time had a synergistic effect: we achieved greater corneal flattening and a more dramatic refractive effect [9, 10] (see Box 17.1).

Box 17.1. A Clinical Example

A 23-year-old man had progressive keratoconus in his right eye. In 2008, his refraction was −5.00 −3.00 × 130, and his BSCVA measured 20/60. The patient underwent treatment using the Athens protocol in 2009: topography-guided PRK −2.00 −1.50 × 121 (the topography axis) combined with same-day corneal collagen cross-linking.

Eight years later, his keratoconus is stable, and the patient has a distance UCVA of 20/25. His refraction is currently +0.50 −100 × 050 = 20/20 (Fig. 17.1).

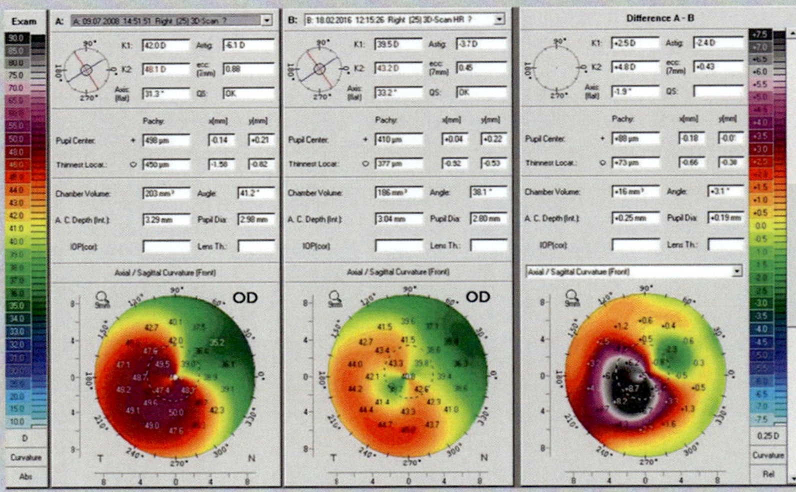

Fig. 17.1 Preoperative measurements (left). Eight years postoperatively (middle). The difference between the pre- and postoperative measurements (right) demonstrates the high degree of treatment accuracy and remarkable flattening of almost 9.00 D at the peak of the cone

17.3 Results and Refinement

We carefully studied our results in approximately 200 procedures of CXL first and topography-guided partial PRK performed 6 months later at the earliest, and we compared them to the results of more than 200 cases in which CXL and PRK were performed simultaneously [6]. We named the combined same-day procedure the "Athens Protocol" and have since reported on over 1000 cases, both primary keratoconus and post-LASIK ectasia, and their long-term follow-up [7].

We have since enhanced the Athens protocol. Because the epithelium of these eyes is invariably highly irregular, we remove the tissue via phototherapeutic keratectomy using a 7-mm optical zone and a depth of 50 μm. We use the epithelium as a "masking agent" for the topography-guided PRK procedure.

Another change we have made is a transition to higher-fluence ultraviolet light for CXL: 6 mW/cm^2 applied for 15 min for the same total energy of 5.4 J [11]. Moreover, like most investigators globally, we use riboflavin solution based in saline rather than dextran for better absorption and less dehydration of the stroma [12].

17.4 Combined Versus Sequential Treatment

The argument against the combined procedure is as follows: one cannot predict the long-term refractive effects of CXL [13], so it is not possible to predict what the refractive error produced by the combination technique will be. We have indeed observed a few cases of a slight refractive overcorrection after more than 10 years of follow-up, when the postoperative refraction was initially on target for the first couple of years **Another significant concern regarding the Athens protocol is the combined UV assault on the epithelium from PRK and CXL, with delayed epithelial healing and stromal loss as potential sequelae** [14]**.**

Sequential treatment is certainly a valid option. After performing CXL, the ophthalmologist monitors the patient's visual rehabilitation and considers the possibility of contact lenses or a phakic IOL [15] if anisometropia or residual refractive error persists. If needed, the surgeon performs a partial topography-guided PRK 6 months or longer after CXL, when most of the healing has taken place. Again, the disadvantage is that PRK will remove some of the most biomechanically stable tissue produced by the CXL procedure.

The combined approach reduces patient morbidity. In our experience, it is also far more attractive to patients. Proper informed consent is needed so they understand that the Athens protocol cannot be a fully predictable refractive procedure—not comparable to today's routine PRK and LASIK [16, 17]. Further visual rehabilitation with soft contact lenses, glasses, or potentially a future refractive procedure on the cornea or with a phakic IOL may be required if emmetropia or a result approaching it is desired.

Our preference is to inform patients about both options, share with them our experience and clinical outcomes, and let them decide. To promote a well-educated and thoroughly discussed decision, we ask the family to be present, because most of our candidates are teenaged boys or young adult men (early 1920s). We have uploaded on YouTube some of these discussions with the patients that I think you may find helpful.

https://www.youtube.com/watch?v=qfCmjTtcRTs

17.5 Conclusion

The big lesson we have drawn from our extensive study of corneal diagnostics is that not everything that looks like ectasia or keratoconus progression on topography or tomography is what it seems. A multifactorial assessment of the cornea is necessary to remove bias for potential epithelial remodeling, the use of contact lenses, etc.

As far as combining CXL with partial PRK or performing the procedures sequentially, once surgeons acquire experience with both approaches, they will determine what best meets their patients' needs.

Financial Disclosure Consultant for Alcon, Avedro, Allergan, i-Optics, Keramed, Zeiss, ISP Surgical.

At a Glance

To promote visual rehabilitation, the author and his colleagues introduced the topography-guided normalization of corneas that remain highly irregular despite some flattening effect from corneal collagen cross-linking (CXL).

Sequential treatment involves performing CXL first and topography-guided partial PRK at least 6 months later. In the combined approach, also termed the "Athens protocol," the two procedures are performed on the same day.

References

1. Kanellopoulos AJ. Post-LASIK ectasia. Ophthalmology. 2007;114(6):1230.
2. Hafezi F, Kanellopoulos AJ, Wiltfang R, Seiler T. Corneal collagen crosslinking with riboflavin and ultraviolet A to treat induced keratectasia after laser in situ keratomileusis. J Cataract Refract Surg. 2007;33:2035–40.
3. Krueger RP, Kanellopoulos AJ. Stability of simultaneous topography-guided photorefractive keratectomy and riboflavin/UVA cross-linking for progressive keratoconus: case reports. J Refract Surg. 2010;26(10):S827–32.

4. Kanellopoulos AJ, Asimellis G. OCT corneal epithelial topographic asymmetry as a sensitive diagnostic tool for early and advancing keratoconus. Clin Ophthalmol. 2014;8:2277–87.
5. Kanellopoulos AJ, Asimellis G. OCT- derived comparison of corneal thickness distribution and asymmetry differences between normal and keratoconic eyes. Cornea. 2014;33(12):1274–81.
6. Kanellopoulos AJ. Comparison of sequential vs same-day simultaneous collagen cross-linking and topography-guided PRK for treatment of keratoconus. J Refract Surg. 2009;25(9):S812–8.
7. Kanellopoulos AJ, Asimellis G. Keratoconus management: long-term stability of topography-guided normalization combined with high-fluence CXL stabilization (the Athens Protocol). J Refract Surg. 2014;30(2):88–92.
8. Kanellopoulos AJ. Sequential versus simultaneous CXL and topography-guided PRK. Cover story – cataract & refractive surgery today Europe. 2009.
9. Kanellopoulos AJ, Asimellis G. Comparison of Placido disc and Scheimpflug image derived topography-guided excimer laser surface normalization combined with higher fluence CXL: the Athens Protocol, in progressive keratoconus. Clin Ophthalmol. 2013;7:1385–96.
10. Kanellopoulos AJ, Asimellis G. Epithelial remodelling after partial topography-guided normalization and high-fluence short-duration crosslinking (Athens Protocol); results up to 1 year. J Cataract Refract Surg. 2014;40:1597–602.
11. Kanellopoulos AJ. Long-term results of a prospective randomized bilateral eye comparison trial of higher fluence, shorter duration ultraviolet A radiation, and riboflavin collagen cross linking for progressive keratoconus. Clin Ophthalmol. 2012;6:97–101.
12. Kanellopoulos AJ, Pamel GJ. Review of current indications for combined very high fluence collagen cross-linking and laser in situ keratomileusis surgery. Indian J Ophthalmol. 2013;61(8):430–2.
13. Kanellopoulos AJ, Moustou V, Asimellis G. Evaluation of visual acuity, pachymetry and anterior-surface irregularity in keratoconus and crosslinking intervention follow-up in 737 cases. J Kerat Ect Cor Dis. 2013;2(3):95–103.
14. Kanellopoulos AJ, Loukas YL, Asimellis G. Cross-linking biomechanical effect in human corneas by same energy, different UV-A fluence: an enzymatic digestion comparative evaluation. Cornea. 2016;35(4) 557–61.
15. Kanellopoulos AJ, Skouteris V. Secondary ectasia due to forceps injury at childbirth: management with combined topography-guided partial PRK and collagen cross-linking (Athens Protocol) and subsequent phakic IOL implantation. J Refract Surg. 2011;27(9):635–6.
16. Kanellopoulos AJ, Perry S. Binder: management of corneal ectasia after LASIK with combined, same –day, topography-guided partial transepithelial PRK and collagen cross-linking: the Athens Protocol. J Refract Surg. 2011;27(5):323–31.
17. Kanellopoulos AJ, Khan J. Topography-guided hyperopic LASIK with and without high irradiance collagen cross-linking: initial comparative clinical findings in a contralateral eye study of 34 consecutive patients. J Refract Surg. 2012;28(11 Suppl):S837–40.

Chapter 18
Combined Corneal Cross-Linking and Photoablation for KC-Risks of

Joseph Frucht-Pery and Denise Wajnsztajn

18.1 CXL 2018

Traditionally, keratoconus (KC) with a pre-existing structural weakness is a contraindication for photoablative procedures. At the present time, corneal collagen cross-linking (CXL) is an accepted treatment to stop progression of KC. It is well documented that CXL significantly increases the rigidity of the KC cornea [1]. The idea of combined CXL and photoablation is based on the ability of CXL to increase the corneal rigidity, while photoablation of limited amount of tissue in KC cornea can safely improve the visual function and comfort. This assumption is correct if a standardized CXL procedure can produce predictable corneal biomechanical changes with constant and permanent biomechanical stability of the KC eye.

However, can we consider KC cornea after CXL a long-lasting, predictable, biomechanically stable structure? Is it comparable to a normal cornea?

18.2 What Do We Know About CXL Procedure in 2018?

A comprehensive review (for ASCRS Cornea Clinical Committee) summarized the outcomes of 3 randomized controlled trials and 24 prospective and retrospective longitudinal studies of CXL for KC with only 3 studies following their patient cohort for more than 3 years [2]. This report summarizes groups of patients between mean ages of 16–35 years with a follow-up duration up to 6 years. In 62–100% of the treated patients the progression of the KC stopped. There was reduction of keratometric

J. Frucht-Pery (✉) · D. Wajnsztajn
Ophthalmology Department, Cornea and Refractive Surgery Service, Hadassah Medical Center, Hebrew University Hospital, Jerusalem, Israel
e-mail: josefr@hadassah.org.il

A. Barbara (ed.), *Controversies in the Management of Keratoconus*,
https://doi.org/10.1007/978-3-319-98032-4_18

measurements (K's) in all the studies, but only half of the reviewed studies presented a significant reduction of K's. The flattening of the cornea measurements varied between mean of 0.01–2.0 and 3.0 D in 24% of the studies. The corrected distance visual acuity (CDVA) improved in all the studies between 0.01 and 0.55 logMAR. There was also improvement of UDVA. The improvement of vision was related to a decrease in corneal curvature and astigmatism, and topographic homogenization of corneal surface. Decrease of high-order aberrations (HOA) and coma also contributed to visual function improvement. The mean spherical equivalent (SE) decreased over 2.0 D in some studies and remained unchanged in others; the maximum keratometry (Kmax) and mean keratometry (Kmean) responded likewise [2]. In the most recent report by Hersh et al. on US multicenter trial of corneal CXL, after 1 year, the Kmax value decreased by 2.0 D or more in 31.4% and the Kmax value increased by 2.0 D or more in 5.6% [3]. Interestingly, improvement of corneal topographic indices does not necessarily correlate with visual acuity [4]. In another major review of corneal CXL, Randleman et al. concluded that prediction of CXL outcome is impossible [5]. In that review, some studies show better functional and morphological improvement between the ages of 18–39 years and others show better outcome over the age 30 compared with a younger group. Some claimed that steeper corneas have greater flattening, not correlated to age. Some steepening patterns may lead to better outcome and some suggest that peripheral topographic cones are less successful [5].

The outcome of CXL at young age is even more controversial and has shorter clinical experience compared to CXL in adults. The stability of the initial CXL effect is in question. Some studies showed a rapid improvement in the first year after the treatment, and recurrence of KC progression in most of the eyes during a longer term [6], which suggests a more aggressive disease and lesser predictability of the outcome in the younger age.

Demarcation line, which supposedly shows the depth of CXL effect in treated corneas, varies among the treated subjects; in some it is less uniform or dense which may suggest non-homogeneous CXL effects in some areas of the treated corneas as compared to others. According to some studies [5], accelerated CXL protocols shows less constant and less homogeneous demarcation lines compared to standard protocol.

Failure of KC stabilization 1 year post-CXL occurs in 7.6–9.8% of patients [7–9]. Topographic flattening can continue up to 6 years after the treatment [10]. In our 10-years-long CXL experience we observed several patients who had clinically significant flattening or steepening of the cornea along the years including cases with initial flattening during the first year followed by steepening in the following years. One of our patients, after standard CXL, had in one eye continuous flattening of 8 D with continuous improvement of CDVA during 5 years of follow-up and in the other eye flattening of only 1.5 D, confirming the unpredictability of CXL outcome even in the eyes of the same person (Fig. 18.1). In another 16-year-old patient a significant flattening stopped after 1 year and recovery of steepening began (Fig. 18.2). Two cases of significant corneal flattening of 7.0 D and 14.0 D 1 year after a standard CXL protocol were reported by Santhiago [11]. Corneal thinning and flattening of greater than 5 D, slowly progressing along the years, in one of the two

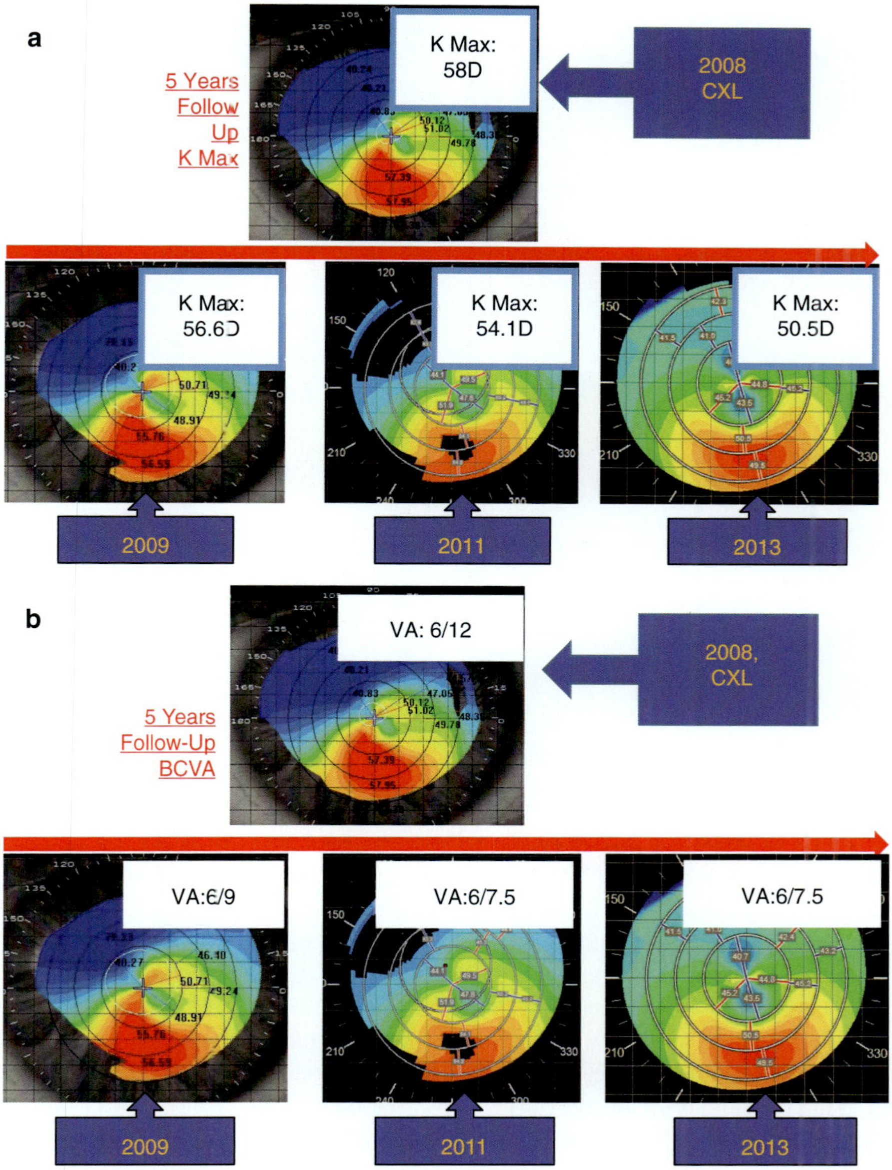

Fig. 18.1 17 year-old male after standard CXL: 5 years follow-up. (**a**) Along the next 5 years the Kmax decreased from 58 to 50.5 D. (**b**) Along the next 5 years; the CDVA improved from 6/12 to 6/7.5

crosslinked eyes was reported by Kymionis [12] and others [13]. The flattening shows a potent ongoing remodeling effect after the surgery and the gradual adjustments caused by a selective stiffening of the cornea. The cases of intense flattening highlight the possible unpredictable response of the cornea after CXL [5].

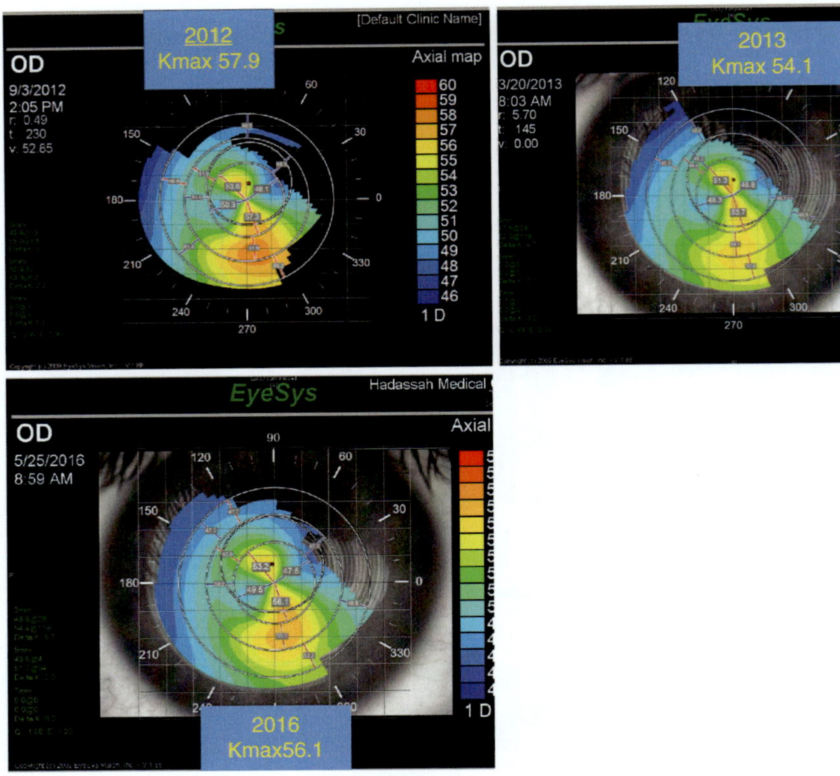

Fig. 18.2 2012: 16 year-old male with progressing KC and Kmax of 57.9D underwent OD Standard CXL. 2013: after 1 year, Kmax decreased to 54.1D. 2016: after 4 years the Kmax increased to 56.1 D

The complication rate after CXL is low but may be severe. The more severe complications such as permanent corneal haze may occur in 8.6% of treated eyes after standard CXL treatment [14]. Loss of 2 lines or more of CDVA is reported in 2.9% by Koller [7] and in 6% in the recently reported study by Hersh [3] who found no potentially contributing cause for loss of CDVA in one of the eyes. Furthermore, KC patients with pre-treatment CDVA of 6/7.5 or better have greater risk for visual loss after CXL [7].

Other reports of severe complications include a variety of infections, corneal melting, persistent corneal edema and endothelial damage [2]. Our over 10-year-long experience include several cases of corneal infections, corneal scarring, loss of CDVA and cases of delayed epithelial healing for more than 14 days.

The current CXL literature has limited evidence-based data, it is mostly short-term and it shows that CXL can stop the progression of the KC with some flattening effect in the majority of the treated cases. However, in an individual case of KC there are no well-established indicators for expectations of visual outcome and long-term stability.

It is therefore clear that CXL has unpredicted outcome and its long-term efficacy and duration of the stiffening effect is yet unknown. However, there is a worldwide consensus that one should do CXL in a progressing KC and that the benefits outweigh the risks of the procedure.

18.3 Combined Photorefractive Keratectomy and Crosslinking

The idea of stabilizing the KC by CXL and remodeling of the corneal shape by topography-guided PRK (tPRK) is very attractive to a refractive surgeon. However, will a significant crosslinked-increase in structural rigidity of the KC cornea [1] withstand tissue loss? Will the loss of the Bowman's membrane, the most rigid part of the cornea, change the remodeling process and the biomechanical response? How will the additional photoablation affect the already unpredictable remodeling response of CXL in the KC eye? Finally, will the benefits of additional photoablation overcome the risks of the procedure in crosslinked eyes?

Initially, the stated purpose of combined procedure was to improve the CDVA in progressing KC eye by a minimal ablation to treat some of the irregular astigmatism. Both sequential and simultaneous CXL and tPRK were evaluated. Kanellopoulos and Binder reported 6/6 UDVA in KC case where a tPRK was done a year after CXL [15].

Kymionis et al. reported favorable outcome following same day CXL and tPRK in a series of patients [16]. Kanellopoulos showed superiority of simultaneous treatment over sequential one in regards to visual outcome and severity of postoperative haze formation [17]. Simultaneous treatment caused stromal haze that improved, but did not resolve at 1 year. The tPRK combined with CXL improves visual acuity, visual function and quality of life indices [18]. Kontadakis et al. compared simultaneous tPRK + CXL with CXL alone in KC eye [19]. After 39 months of follow-up, both groups had the same stability but in the simultaneous tPRK + CXL group the refractive and visual outcomes (UDVA and CDVA) were better. The maximal tissue ablation was 50 μm with a minimal residual corneal thickness of 400 μm. In the combined treatment group, pre-operatively planned under-correction of sphere, cylinder and customization ended with overcorrection, indicating unpredicted flattening effect. In both studied groups, there was no loss of more than two Snellen lines of CDVA while topographic stability was similar [19]. After 6 months, 6.7% in each group showed steepening of keratometry of more than 0.75 D [19]. The remodeling process after PRK + CXL procedure showed different pattern from CXL alone. After combined procedure, there were greater delay of keratocytes repopulation, slower sub-basal nerve plexus recovery and more prominent anterior stromal non-homogeneous reflectance [19]. Alessio et al. in a prospective non-randomized study supported these results [20].

Kymionis addressed his concept of PRK + CXL procedure; primarily the purpose of the procedure is stabilization of progressing KC with additional minor photoablative treatment to improve corneal surface regularization. He suggested not ablating a stable KC with acceptable CDVA. In progressing KC with acceptable CDVA, CXL should be the only required procedure. Only in KC with unacceptable CDVA, is CXL with minimal photoablative intervention suggested [21]. According to this concept one should not offer a combined procedure in a stable KC or topographically defined forme fruste keratoconus (FFKC) with spectacle corrected good CDVA. However, if the vision in progressing KC is unacceptable, the combined PRK + CXL procedure may prevent the need for keratoplasty. This is the most conservative approach in the literature of combined CXL and photoablative procedures. Nevertheless, peer-review literature indicates that in most cross-linked KC eyes the CDVA will improve without photoablation, allowing reasonable and compatible vision with spectacles or contact lenses in most of eyes.

However, even the most conservative approach of Kymionis carries new and unpredictable risks. Any tissue loss in an already biomechanically unstable KC eye will probably increase the risk for the cornea instability in the future. The remodeling processes and corneal biomechanical changes after CXL are unclear. Previous studies have shown that while biomechanical properties after ex-vivo CXL are indicative of corneal stiffening, they may not provide entirely accurate information about the responses to CXL in vivo [22]. It is more complicated and unpredictable after photoablation of Bowman's membrane, the stiffest part of the cornea. Loss of Bowman's membrane may be of significant importance for the future stiffness and stability of the cornea. Bowman's membrane absorbs a considerable part of incident UVA irradiation during the CXL process and most probably provides the majority of the corneal stiffness and resistance to further progression of KC [23, 24]. CXL of KC tissue without Bowman's membrane alters the remodeling process in the cornea, which we do not yet understand after CXL in KC eye without additional ablation. As mentioned above, Kontadakis reported that compared to CXL alone, combined PRK+CXL shows different patterns of haze, cellular repopulation, nerve plexus recovery with unpredicted flattening effect [19]. What will be the value of refractive-PRK-effect if the flattening will progress along time or steepening will recur, as happens in CXL alone? The different scarring effect is also of great concern as already indicated by some reported [25, 26] and unreported data presented in this chapter (cases 1, 2–5). Of even greater concern is our currently limited understanding of keratocytes and collagen turnover in normal cornea and particularly in KC cornea. Most probably, the renewed collagen will not maintain the increased tensile strength properties of the crosslinked-collagen in KC eye. Long-term well-designed randomized control trials (RCT) will clarify the uncertainty that surrounds the long-term effects of photopolymerization, and the post-CXL-ectatic-eye response to decrease of tensile strength at the elder age, particularly in crosslinked eyes of teenagers. Furthermore, one can only speculate on the future of KC eye after combined procedure followed by CXL treatment failures: technically failed procedure or in extremely progressive KC disease as occurs in some of the younger patients with KC. Should one expect unpredictable ectatic changes, loss of initially gained lines of UDVA or CDVA and what will be the remodeling pattern after CXL retreatment? Probably some will require keratoplasty.

Some ophthalmologists use combined CXL+PRK procedures in KC as a refractive tool. They ignore the potential risks of the even conservative concept of Kymionis [21] and aim to correct refractive errors in the KC eye, almost like in a normal eye. The goal of these ophthalmologists is to achieve the maximal correction of vision in KC eye. There is not an accepted consensus for the minimal age of treatment, stability of KC, selection criteria, limits of tissue ablation or a residual stromal thickness (Table 18.1). In general, the concept of these authors is "let's assume that CXL provides a sufficient stiffness and corneal stability to KC eye" and "let's correct some of the cylinder and high-order aberrations and spheres", "let's ablate to a limit of residual bed thickness, that each one decides, in purpose to get the best

Table 18.1 Pre-operative inclusion criteria of combined PRK and CXL studies

Author/Ref.	CCT (μm)	Age range (years)	Kmax/ Steep K range (D)	CDVA (range)	KC status
Kanellopoulos/ [15]	440	26	48.5	0.39^{L}	Progressing
Krueger/[27]	421 and 496	21 and 24	59.7 and 53.1	20/50 and 20/30	Progressing
Kymionis/[28]	>400	19–49	42.7–67.7	0.81 ± 0.65 $(2–0.1)^{L}$	Progressing
Tuwairqi/[29]	>440	19–40	NA	$\geq 0.8^{D}$ 0.025 ± 0.077 $(NA)^{L}$	Progressing
Alessio/[20]	≥450	21–46	NA	0.06 ± 0.08 $(0.3–0.01^{L}$	Progressing
Sakla/[30]	≥400	21–42	41–52.5	0.28 ± 0.20 $(NA)^{L}$ $0.9–0.5^{D}$:60%	NA
Kanellopoulos/ [31]	≥300	17–57	NA	$0.62 \pm 0.23(NA)^{D}$	Progressing
Fadlallah/[32]	≥450	16–54	NA	≥20/30 0.035 ± 0.062 $(NA)^{L}$	Stable or progressing
Shetty/[33]	≥450	23–47	NA	0.28 ± 0.05 $(NA)^{L}$; 0.19 ± 0.06 $(NA)^{L}$	Progressing
Kanellopoulos/ [34]	≥ 300	18–44	NA	0.62 ± 0.24 $(0.10–1.00)^{D}$; 0.63 ± 0.33 $(0.10–1.00)^{D}$	NA
Shaheen/[35]	≥400	21–38	42.0–59.6	0.28 ± 0.24 (0.00–$1.00)^{L}$; ≥20/40: 73.5%	Stable
Sakla/[36]	≥400	15–41	NA	0.41 ± 0.27 $(NA)^{L}$ ≥20/25:11.8 % ≥20/40: 36.5%	NA
Chen/[37]	>400	13–50	41.0–58.25	0.16 ± 0.18 $(-0.08–1.00)^{L}$	Progressing
Kontadakis/[19]	>440	17–39	NA	0.25 ± 0.17 $(NA)^{L}$	Progressing
Grentzelos/[38]	≥400	18–39	NA	0.20 ± 0.23 $(NA)^{L}$	Progressing

Legend: *Ref* reference, *CCT* central corneal thickness, *Kmax* maximum keratometry, *Steep K* steep keratometry, *CDVA* corrected distance visual acuity, *KC* Keratoconus, *L* LogMAR, *D* decimal, *NA* not applicable vision possible". This concept reflects a group of published articles with favorable short-term UDVA and CDVA outcomes, achieved by using varying protocols (Table 18.1). Some authors suggest maximal ablation of 50 μm and no use of mitomycin C (MMC) [16]. Others maintain a minimal residual corneal thickness of 350 μm and use MMC [17]. Others keep a minimal residual corneal thickness of 300 μm and maximal ablation depth of 80 μm [5]. A more conservative approach is to maintain a minimal residual corneal thickness of 400 μm and maximal ablation depth of 50–60 μm [16, 39]. Sakla et al. [30] reported one of the extreme approaches where 70% of cylinder and some of the sphere were ablated to a minimal residual stromal bed of 350 μm, Afterwards, hypotonic riboflavin was used to inflate the cornea before the CXL procedure. Children and adults underwent combined procedures. Chen [37] included patients from the age of 13 years, Sakla et al. [30] from the age of 15 years, Kontadakis et al. [19] from the age of 17 and Fadlallah et al. [32] over the age of 50 years.

Fadlallah et al. [32] treated a group of 79 patients with mild to moderate KC who had initial CDVA of 20/30 or better (mean decimal CDVA 0.93, UDVA 0.45) with or without history of stable KC. Inclusion criteria for treatment included discomfort with spectacles or rigid contact lenses. After 2 years, 71.4% had UDVA of 20/25 or better. Haze and myopic shift caused loss of two lines of UDVA in four eyes and loss of one line in seven eyes. Kontadakis et al. [19] treated patients with progressing KC only. Sakla et al. [30] treated topographically diagnosed KC not related to stability or progression of KC. About 10% had pre-treatment CDVA of 0.9 and more than 60% had CDVA of 0.5. Post-treatment only one eye (3.2%) lost one line of UCVA. Grentzelos treated 55 eyes with progressing KC and mean CDVA of 0.20 ± 0.23 (LogMAR) [38]. At 3 months four eyes had significant haze but at 12 months only one eye (2%) had lost two lines of CDVA [38]. Alessio treated 17 KC eyes with combined PRK and CXL [20]. The mean CDVA was 0.06 ± 0.08 (LogMAR) ranging from 0.3 to 0.00 (LogMAR). There was no loss of CDVA after 2 years of follow-up [20]. Others also included patients with functional CDVA before treatment (Table 18.1).

Most studies in literature report flattening effect after combined CXL and photoablation. Fadlallah et al. [32] after 2 years had a decrease of mean Kmax by 1.3 D (from 47.8 to 46.5 D). Kontadakis et al. [19] had a decrease of mean Kflat by 2.16 D (from 44.85 to 42.69 D). Sakla et al. [30] treated KC patients with steep K between 41.0 and 52.5 D. After 1 year the mean steep K decreased by 2.55 D (from 46.52 to 43.97 D) and the mean flat K decreased by 1.17 D (from 43.69 to 42.52 D).

As compared to CXL for KC, the peer-review literature of combined CXL+ photoablative procedures hardly report any complications. Most of the reports (Table 18.1) deny complications while others have no statements regarding complications.

Occasional studies reported loss of CDVA or UDVA. Out of all the publications in Table 18.1, only one study report loss of two lines of CDVA in one eye [38] and in another report four eyes lost two lines of UDVA [32]. Mild to moderate haze are reported in the early stages after the treatment. Usually the haze decreases or disappears with time (Tables 18.2 and 18.3).

Guell et al. reported a case of persistent deep stromal scarring after PRK and CXL in a patient with forme fruste KC (FFKC) [25]. A 22-year-old man had FFKC with UDVA of 20/30 in OD and 20/40 in OS. CDVA in both eyes was 20/20. Simultaneous PRK and CXL were done. After a month, UDVA was 20/20 in each eye. After 6 weeks, the corneas were clear and topical fluorometholone was discontinued. After 5 months, the UCVA in the OD decreased to 20/25 and deep stromal haze was

Table 18.2 Intra-operative methods of combined PRK and CXL studies

Author/Ref.	Target of treatment	CXL time	Surgical procedure	MMC	Minimal stromal bed	Maximum tissue removed range
Kanellopoulos/[15]	Improve VA	30 min	Sequential/Tg	Yes	NA	50 μm
Krueger/[27]	Normalize cornea, decrease refractive error	30 min	Simultaneous/Tg	Yes	NA	56 and 48 μm
Kymionis/[28]	Decrease cylinder and sphere	30 min	Simultaneous/Tg	No	400 μm	Up to 50 μm
Tuwairqi/[29]	Improve VA	30 min	Simultaneous/Tg	Yes	400 μm	NA
Alessio/[20]	Normalize cornea	30 min	Simultaneous/Tg	No	NA	18–49 μm
Sakla/[30]	Decrease cylinder and sphere	30 min	Simultaneous/Tg	Yes	>350 μm	Up to 50 μm
Kanellopoulos/[31]	NA	10 min	Simultaneous/Tg	No	NA	NA
Fadlallah/[32]	Improve VA	30 min	Simultaneous/Con	No	450 μm	Up to 50 μm
Shetty/[33]	Normalize cornea	4 min	Simultaneous/Tg	No	400 μm	Up to 50 μm
Kanellopoulos/[34]	NA	15 min	Simultaneous/Tg	No	NA	Up to 50 μm
Shaheen/[35]	NA	30 min	Sequential/WFG	Yes	NA	NA
Sakla/[36]	Decrease cylinder	5 min	Simultaneous/Tg	Yes	>350 μm	Up to 50 μm
Chen/[37]	Improve VA	5 or 7.5 min	Simultaneous/Tg	No	400 μm	25–113 μm
Kontadakis/[19]	Decrease cylinder and sphere	30 min	Simultaneous/Tg	No	400 μm	Up to 50 μm
Grentzelos/[38]	NA	30 min	Simultaneous/Con	No	>350 μm	6–50 μm

Legend: *Ref* reference, *VA* visual acuity, *Sequential* PRK done 1 year after CXL, *Simultaneous* PRK followed by same day CXL, *Tg* topoguided, *Con* conventional, *WFG* wave front-guided, *MMC* mitomycin C, *NA* not applicable

Table 18.3 Post-operative results of combined PRK and CXL studies

Author/Ref.	FU (months)	Refraction (SE)	Loss of VA > 2 lines	Stability effect	Complications
Kanellopoulos/[15]	18	−0.25	None	Yes	None
Krueger/[27]	>30	−2.25/−0.50 × 05 and −0.75/−0.75 × 125	None	No	None
Kymionis/[28]	12 to 25	−1.08 ± 2.41	None	Yes	50% – linear haze at 1 year that improved
Tuwairqi/[29]	12	0.05 ± 0.73	NA	NA	NA
Alessio/[20]	24	−0.19 ± 0.65	None	Yes	50% – subepithelial haze at 1 year that disappeared with steroids tapered within 1 month
Sakla/[30]	12	−1.10 ± 1.94	None	Yes	None
Kanellopoulos/[31]	36	NA	NA	Yes	NA
Fadlallah/[32]	24	−0.42 ± 0.60	4 eyes lost 2 lines of UDVA	Yes	9 eyes: grade 2 haze at 1 month, 5 eyes: grade 2 at 6 months and 1 eye: grade 2 haze (or higher) at 2 years
Shettv/[33]	12	−2.79 ± 0.64 and −0.85 ± 0.76	None	NA	None
Kanellopoulos/[34]	12–36	NA	NA	NA	NA
Shaheen/[35]	12	−0.68 ± 0.64	None	NA	None
Sakla/[36]	12	−2.80 ± 4.47	None	Yes	None
Chen/[37]	>6	−0.05 ± 2.01	NA	NA	None
Kontadakis/[19]	39 ± 11	−1.54 ± 3.30	None	Yes	None
Grentzelos/[38]	12	−2.24 ± 2.81	1 eye (2%) lost 2 lines of CDVA	Yes	4 eyes had haze grade 2 at 3 months

Legend: *Ref* reference, *FU* follow-up time, *SE* spherical equivalent, *VA* visual acuity, *UDVA* uncorrected distance visual acuity, *CDVA* corrected distance visual acuity, *NA* not applicable

observed. A few months later, the UDVA in OD decreased to 20/80 and the CDVA with a correction of +2.00 D was 20/25. During 2-year follow-up, the opacification was stable. Both excessive flattening and scar formation caused loss of UDVA and CDVA. The authors concluded that FFKC should remain a contraindication for laser refractive surgery even with the use of CXL.

Prakash et al. [26] reported a 44-year-old male with preoperative OD CDVA of 20/30 (−0.50/−3.50 × 10 D) and OS CDVA of 20/20 (−0.25/−3.50 × 10 D) The corneal thickness was over 580 μm in each eye. Combined PRK and CXL was done, as described in the report, due to a "suspicious topography". The vision improved during the first 3 months and decreased thereafter. After 15 months, deep scars in the anterior stroma in both eyes were observed. In the OD the UDVA was 20/60 and CDVA was 20/30 (+1.25/ −1.00×5 D). In the OS the UDVA was 20/40 and CDVA decreased to 20/25 (+1.50/ −1.50×95 D). The authors claim that this case had similar complication with different preoperative profile from the case described by Guell [25].

There are probably many unreported cases of unsuccessful combined treatments in the world. I have heard of some from ophthalmologists in conferences talks. I have examined some in my practice, and received some nonpublished reports from ophthalmologists elsewhere. Part of it will be reported in the peer-review literature.

18.3.1 Case 1 (Figs. 18.3 and 18.4)

A 28-year-old female from Cyprus had diagnosis of KC from the age of 19 years. KC was stable for years. She used spectacles only for night driving. She claimed that the CDVA before the procedure was 6/6 in each eye. She was told that she would not need spectacles at all after combined PRK and CXL. She agreed to do the procedure in one eye at a time. In November 2012, she underwent simultaneous procedure in OD. She was not happy with the visual outcome and underwent additional OD CXL in October 2013. The vision further decreased. I examined her in June 2014. She could not provide detailed preoperative evaluation. In OS, the untreated eye, she had UDVA of 6/7.5 corrected to 6/6 with +0.25/−1.00×105 D. OS cornea was clear with a thickness of 488 μm. In OD, the UDVA was 6/60 corrected to 6/30 with +3.00 D. The cornea had deep stromal scar up to the Descemet (Fig. 18.3) with corneal thickness of 367 μm. OS topography had questionable mild FFKC. In the OD, topography presented an irregular surface with central flattening (Fig. 18.4). The scar, the UDVA and the DCVA did not improve after 3 months of treatment with high doses of topical dexamethasone phosphate 0.1%. In December 2016, she underwent corneal transplantation in her right eye.

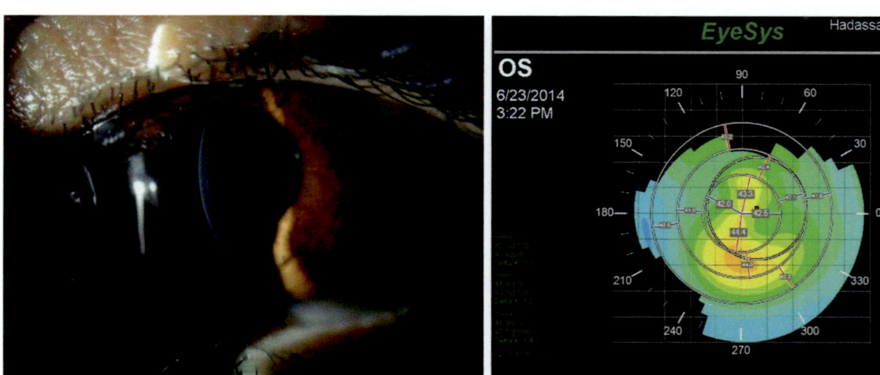

Fig. 18.3 Case 1. OS untreated eye: clear cornea and stable topography compatible with FFKC

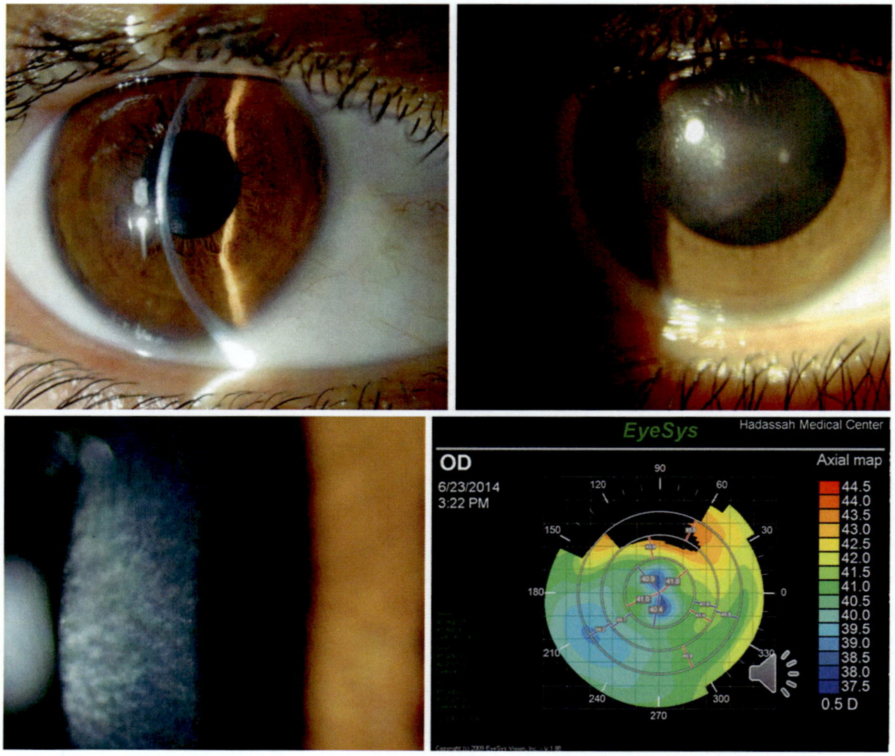

Fig. 18.4 Case 1. OD 2 years after simultaneous standard CXL + PRK and CXL enhancement a year latter. Central dense corneal scar. Topography presents central flattening and irregularity. Upper left, upper right and lower left: Presence of deep stromal scar. Lower right: Irregular post-treatment topography with remarkable flattening

18.3.2 Case 2 (Fig. 18.5)

A 23-year-old male presented with KC diagnosis from the age of 22 years and CDVA 6/6 in each eye. During the next 2 years in the OD there was a myopic increase of 0.5 D and with a correction of $-2.25/-1.00 \times 135$ D, the CDVA was 6/6. In the OS the refraction increased by 2.00 D of cylinder and the CDVA decreased to 0.8 with a refractive correction of Plano/-3.00×105 D. The corneas were clear. He used soft contact lenses and except for some glare and halos at night time driving, did not have any complaints. In January 2015 he was told that combined CXL and photoablation would improve his night function. He hoped that he would be free of lenses or spectacles. In January 2015, he underwent simultaneous PRK and CXL in both eyes. Initially, his vision improved. His CDVA was 6/6 in both eyes. A year later he bitterly complained that his reading ability and distance vision decreased, the night glare increased during driving and he couldn't use soft contact lenses anymore. He refused the enhancement offered by the surgeon.

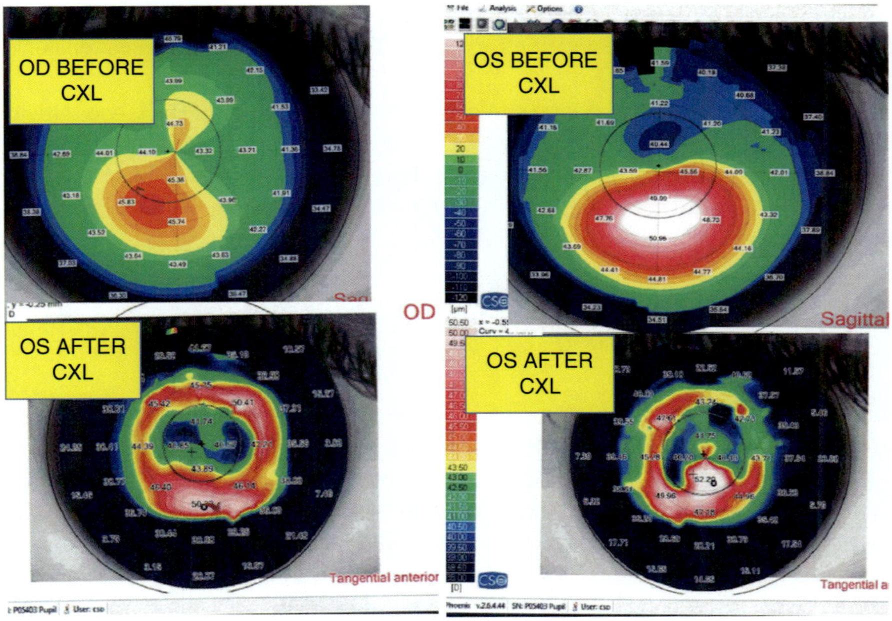

Fig. 18.5 Case2. 23-year-old-male after CXL and PRK. Upper left: Pre-treatment OD FFKC. Upper right: Pretreatment OS KC. Lower right and left: Post-CXL and PRK tangential topographies. Lower right: OS irregular ocular surface. Lower left: OD irregular ocular surface. Topographic changes 2 years after combined CXL+PRK

In January 2017, ophthalmic evaluation in our clinic revealed CDVA of 6/9- in OD with a correction of +0.50/−1.00×97 and CDVA of 6/12 in OS with a correction of +0.50/−2.50×97. He had mild haze in the OD cornea and greater degree of opacity in the OS. The computerized topography showed significant irregularity in both eyes (Fig. 18.5), which explain the decrease of vision and patient's complaint. Currently, he is not able to use spectacles for his daily activity and he uses scleral contact lenses.

18.3.3 Case 3

A 30-year-old male underwent combined CXL and PRK in Cyprus in the year 2007 to be free of the daily-use spectacles. Patient had only partial documentation of eye examinations prior to procedure. He had stable refraction during several years. In 2007 the CDVA in OD was 6/9 with a refractive correction of −1.00/ −3.00×100 D. In OS with a refraction of −0.75/−3.00×85 D his CDVA was 6/6. The corneas were clear. The OD corneal thickness was 559 μm and in OS, 560 μm. The axial topography presented some irregularity (within a normal range) in the OD and normal topography with regular symmetric astigmatism in OS (at the present time, we do not have access to these topographies). Post-operatively, he had long healing process with failure of epithelialization for weeks. This followed with corneal opacification and loss of CDVA.

I examined the patient in our clinic in January 2017. The UDVA was finger counting and the CDVA with HCL was 6/30 in each eye. Both corneas had dense central corneal scarring (5 mm by 4 mm) and excessive tissue loss in the centers of both corneas. Central corneal thickness in OD was 306 μm and in OS it was 122 μm. Recently, this patient underwent PKP in OS.

18.3.4 Case 4 (*Fig. 18.6*)

A 38-years-old male from Germany had longstanding stable KC. His CDVA was 1.0 in each eye, with refractive correction of +0.50/ −1.50 × 80D in OD and +1.50/ −2.25 × 85 D in OS. In the OD, the topographic evaluation presented mild KC with Kmax of 45.2 D and in OS he had FFKC with Kmax of 43.4 D. In March 2014 in Turkey, he underwent bilateral combined procedure of PRK (ablation of 9 μ of tissue in OD and 28 μ in OS) using wavefront technology, followed by CXL. After the procedure his vision in OS decreased. In June 2017, in OS, the UDVA was 0.4 and the CDVA was 0.5 with refractive correction of +2.00/−2.50 × 65 D. He had deep central corneal scar with topographically significant irregularity and flattening of 7.1 D. In OD his UDVA was 0.5. The CDVA was 1.0 with a refractive correction of +1.00/ −1.00 × 100 D. Topographic presented flattening of 4.8 D. The cornea had mild haze.

18.3.5 Case 5 (*Fig. 18.7*)

A 31-years-old female had bilateral KC. Her pre-operative and post-operative CDVA is not available but she claimed that her vision with spectacles was good and stable for years. Pre-treatment, the refractive correction in OD was +0.50/ −0.75 × 165D and in OS plano/ −2.50 × 150 D in. In Turkey, in September 2013, she underwent in OS a combined procedure of PRK (18 μ) and CXL. In OD she had only CXL in November 2013. In December 2013 the OS refraction was +0.50/−0.75 × 165 D. In June 2016 the OS presented remarkable central corneal scarring, topographically significant flattening and irregularity and refraction of +4.50/−0.75 × 55 D. In OD the refraction was −0.50/−2.00 × 15 D.

18.3.5.1 Is Combined CXL and Photoablation a Refractive Surgery?

At the present time, it is well accepted that stable KC or FFKC with spectacle or lenses corrected functional vision should not be crosslinked and/or photoablated. However, the literature clearly reports KC patients with very good functional CDVA

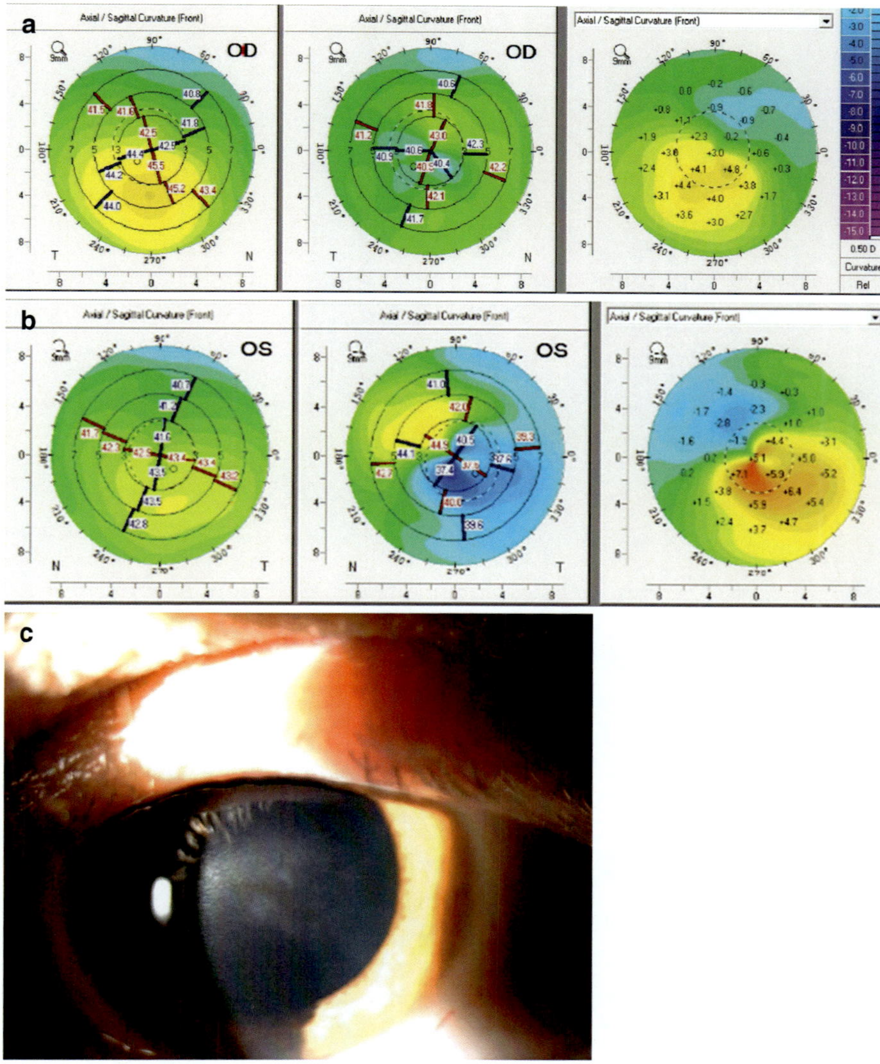

Fig. 18.6 Case 4. (**a**) Topography of OD KC before and after combined CXL+PRK. Left fig: 2014 pre-CXL. Center fig: 2017 post-CXL+PRK. Right fig: difference map presenting 4.8D of flattening. (**b**) Topography of OS KC before and after combined CXL+PRK. Left fig: 2014 pre-CXL. Center fig: 2017 post CXL+PRK. Right fig: difference map presenting 6.4D of irregular flattening. (**c**) OS cornea: 2017. Corneal central scar 3 years after combined CXL+PRK

who underwent CXL + refractive photo-reshaping procedures (Table 18.1). These KC patients have post-refractive surgery expectations, similar to normal-healthy-spectacles-dependent population, after standard refractive procedures in normal eyes. Those patients who undergo CXL for extra stabilization of KC cornea, in order to allow a refractive photoablation, are exposed to all the risks of standard CXL procedure. In addition, some of them, unfortunately those with the better

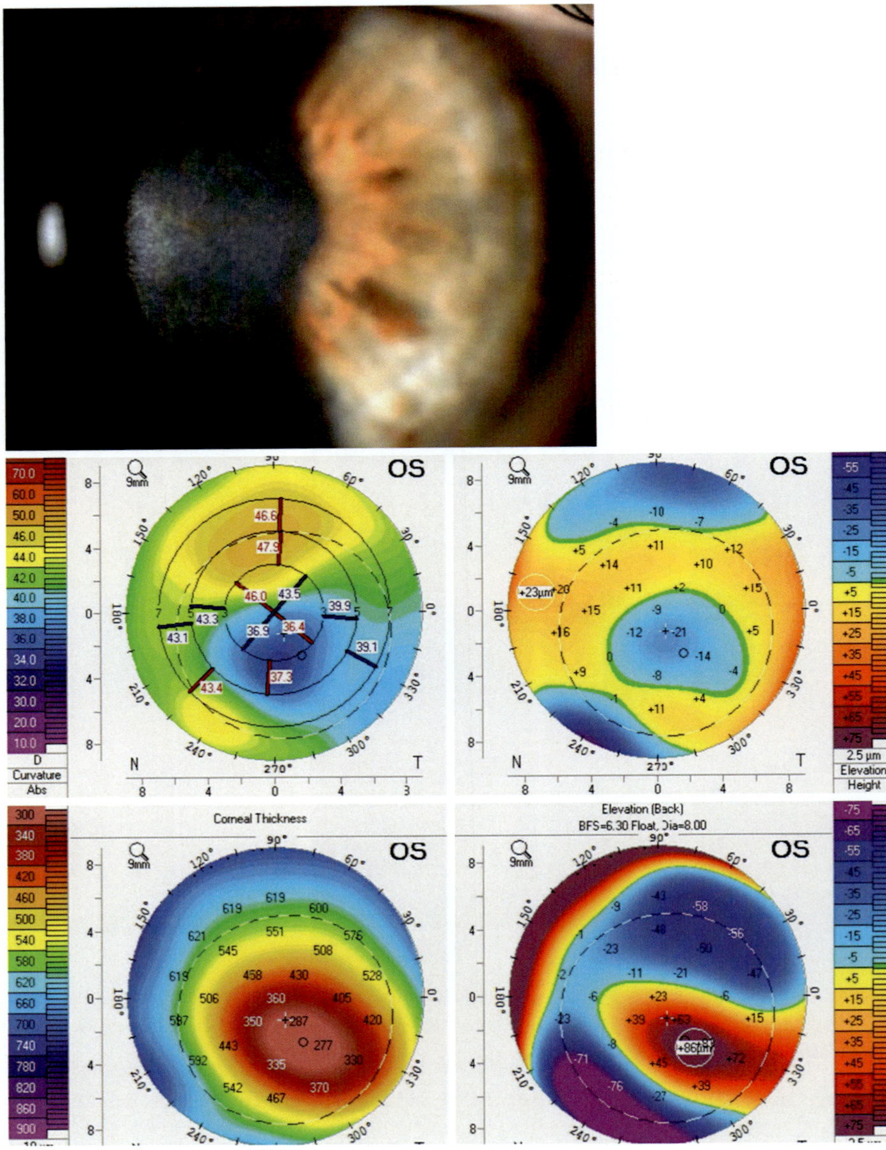

Fig. 18.7 Case 5. OS: 3 years after CXL + PRK of 18 μm. Right fig: OS Central corneal scar. Inferior fig: OS topography presents remarkable irregularity and flattening

pre-treatment CDVA, have greater risk of losing lines of CDVA as reported after CXL in KC eyes with preoperative CDVA of 6/7.5 or better [7]. Furthermore, as in standard CXL the flattening effect may slowly progress over the years with unpredictable and remarkable refractive change and unpredictable final CDVA. Likewise, regressive steepening may as well occur along the time. Therefore, there is no guarantee that the early reports of great success and excellent visual outcome will last in the coming years.

There are several concerning aspects in the CXL combined with photoablation-procedures published literature. There are no RCTs, no long-term studies, the number of treated eyes is small and the data are of very low-quality evidence of the efficacy of combined treatment. Many of the studies (Table 18.1) do not report some of the major selection criteria of the treated candidates such as initial KC severity, KC stability, the minimal age, the limits of tissue ablation. Combined procedures are done in stable KC, in FFKC, in eyes with Kmax 41.0 D, in young adults, at the age of 50 years, and in eyes with functionally good visual acuity. Some authors use standard CXL Dresden protocol. Others use accelerated CXL protocols which reportedly are less effective [40]. Many do not report the rate of complications such as loss of UDVA and CDVA. The goal in some of these studies appears to be primarily refractive surgery with additional CXL, to prevent extra ectasia. Short-term reports suggest good short-term CDVA in KC eyes after PRK +CXL (Table 18.1).

However, the uncertainty of long-term effects of CXL and photo-polymerization will be clarified in the future when well-designed multicenter studies will provide sufficient evidence-based data. Thereafter, only after the disclosure of the risks versus benefits of the combined procedures, will data be available to reevaluate the additive effect of photo-reshaping procedures in post-CXL KC eyes.

At the present time, in well-functioning stable KC, how should one calculate the benefit of initially gaining some vision versus the unknown and unpredictable outcome of vision in the long future? How can one foresee the long lasting remodeling changes of CXL, the flattening effect or failure of CXL treatment due to inefficiently done CXL procedure or continuous progression of KC? What will be the influence of photoablated tissue loss (including Bowman membrane) in these eyes? What should be written in a signed consent of combined CXL and PRK procedures? The cases reported in this chapter comprise a sample of the future to come. Some of the cases have only partial data available, but the outcome is clear. Some of these reported patients had stable FFKC or mild KC with pre-treatment CDVA of 6/6. After simultaneous CXL and PRK patients had corneal scarring, significant flattening, irregular corneas and loss of lines of vision. Two underwent corneal transplants. This small group of patients presents more complications than has been published in the whole peer-review world-literature of combined CXL and PRK procedures. These cases support the report of Guell [25] and his conclusion. There must be many more cases with similar or other complications elsewhere.

Based on such uncertainty, it is unacceptable at the present time to consider crosslinked KC eye as a normal subject for refractive procedure. Why should one offer combined procedures in KC patients at the late 40s or at age of 50 years (Table 18.1)?. Furthermore, it is even less acceptable to PRK children or young adults with KC and follow the rules of the minimal thickness of a residual bed as we use in normal eye refractive PRK procedures. To the best of my knowledge, even in a topographically normal eye many refractive surgeons will hesitate to perform PRK on an eye with pre-operative corneal thickness of 425 μm.

Nevertheless, the published data may mislead an unexperienced ophthalmologist in the field of CXL. They may get an impression of a new concept that allows refractive procedures in KC eyes, and some will be happy to offer great refractive outcomes for a previously laser-contraindicated candidate. Eventually, some will do an unexpected extra step and increase the risks even more.

18.4 In Summary

In the long term, combined procedure of CXL and photoablation of KC eye may carry unknown risks due to a poor understanding of remodeling process in KC cornea. It is not advised to consider these procedures as a new refractive option in a KC eye, where photoablation of KC is still a contraindication among members of ophthalmic community.

One should never offer any procedures in stable KC or combined procedures in progressing KC eyes with satisfactory functional vision. In KC with functionally unacceptable vision, the procedures are per the ophthalmologist's decision. However, signed consent should clearly indicate the unpredictability and the controversy of this subject.

References

1. Wollensak G. Crosslinking treatment of progressive keratoconus: new hope. Curr Opin Ophthalmol. 2006;17:356–60.
2. Ziaei M, et al. Reshaping procedures for the surgical management of corneal ectasia. J Cataract Refract Surg. 2015;41:842–72.
3. Hersh PS, et al. United States multicenter clinical trial of corneal crosslinking for keratoconus treatment. Ophthalmology. 2017;124:1259–70.
4. Greenstein SA, et al. Cornea topography indices after corneal collagen crosslinking for keratoconus and corneal ectasia: one year results. J Cataract Refract Surg. 2011;37:1282–90.
5. Randleman JB, et al. Corneal crosslinking. Surv Ophthalmol. 2015;60:509–23.
6. Chatzis N, Hafezi F. Progression of keratoconus and efficacy of pediatric[corrected] corneal collagen crosslinking in children and adolescents. J Refract Surg. 2011;28:753–8.
7. Koller T, et al. Complication and failure rates after corneal crosslinking. J Cataract Refract Surg. 2009;35:1358–62.
8. Hersh PS, et al. Corneal collagen crosslinking for keratoconus and corneal ectasia: one year results. J Cataract Refract Surg. 2011;37:149–60.
9. Sloot F, et al. Effective corneal collagen crosslinking in advanced cases of progressive keratoconus. J Cataract Refract Surg. 2013;39:1141–5.
10. Raiskup-Wolf F, et al. Collagen crosslinking with riboflavin and ultraviolet-a light in keratoconus: long tem result. J Cataract Refract Surg. 2008;34:796–801.
11. Santhiago MR, Giacomin NT, Medeiros CS, et al. Intense early flattening after corneal collagen cross-linking. J Refract Surg. 2015;31:419–22.
12. Kymionis GD, et al. Excessive corneal flattening and thinning after corneal crosslinking: single case report with 5-year follow-up. Cornea. 2015;34:704–6.

13. Hafezi F, et al. Marked remodeling of the anterior corneal surface following cross-linking with riboflavin and UVA. Br J Ophthalmol. 2011;95:1171–2.
14. Raiskup F, et al. Permanent corneal haze after riboflavin-UVA-induced crosslinking in keratoconus. J Refract Surg. 2009;25:S824–8.
15. Kanellopoulos AJ, et al. Corneal collagen crosslinking [CXL] with sequential topography-guided PRK: a temporizing alternative for keratoconus to penetrating keratoplasty. Cornea. 2007;26:891–5.
16. Kymionis GD, et al. Simultaneous topography guided PRK followed by corneal collagen crosslinking for keratoconus. JRS. 2009;25:S807–11.
17. Kanellopoulos AJ. Comparison of sequential vs same-day simultaneous collagen crosslinking and topography guided PRK for treatment of keratoconus. JRS. 2009;25:S812–8.
18. Labiris G, et al. Impact of keratoconus cross-linking and cross-linking combined with photorefractive keratectomy on self reported quality of life. Cornea. 2012;31:734–9.
19. Kontadakis GA, et al. Long term comparison of simultaneous topography guided collagen photorefractive keratectomy followed by corneal cross-linking versus corneal cross-linking alone. Ophthalmology. 2016;123:974–83.
20. Alessio G, et al. Photorefractive keratectomy followed by crosslinking versus cross-linking alone for management of progressive keratoconus: two-year follow-up. Am J Ophthalmol. 2013;155:54–65.
21. Kymionis GD, et al. Corneal collagen crosslinking [CXL] combined with refractive procedures for the treatment of corneal ectatic disorders: CXL plus. J Refract Surg. 2014;30:566–76.
22. Bekesi N, Gallego-Muñoz P, Ibarés-Frías L, et al. Biomechanical changes after in vivo collagen cross-linking with rose bengal-green light and riboflavin-UVA. Invest Ophthalmol Vis Sci. 2017;58:1612–20.
23. Kymionis GD, et al. Corneal collagen crosslinking mushroom shape demarcation line profile after limited Bowman membrane removal by photorefractive keratectomy. Open Ophthalmol J. 2015;9:17–9.
24. Kolozsva'ri L, et al. UV absorbance of the human cornea in the 240 to 400-nm range. Invest Ophthalmol Vis Sci. 2002;43:2165–8.
25. Guell JL, et al. Late onset of a persistent deep stromal scarring after PRK and corneal cross-linking in a patient with forme fruste keratoconus. J Refract Surg. 2014;30:286–8.
26. Prakash G, et al. Persistent stromal scar after PRK and CXL: different preoperative findings, similar complication. J Refract Surg. 2015;31:211.
27. Krueger RR, Kanellopoulos AJ. Stability of simultaneous topography-guided photorefractive keratectomy and riboflavin/UVA cross-linking for progressive keratoconus: case reports. J Refract Surg. 2010;26:S827–32.
28. Kymionis GD, et al. Simultaneous topography-guided photorefractive keratectomy followed by corneal collagen cross-linking for keratoconus. Am J Ophthalmol. 2011;152:748–55.
29. Tuwairqi WS, Sinjab MM. Safety and efficacy of simultaneous corneal collagen cross-linking with topography-guided PRKin managing low-grade keratoconus: 1-year follow-up. J Refract Surg. 2012;28:341–5.
30. Sakla H, et al. Simultaneous topography guided partial photorefractive keratectomy and corneal collagen crosslinking for keratoconus. J Cataract Refract Surg. 2014;40:1430–8.
31. Kanellopoulos AJ, Asimellis G. Keratoconus management: long-term stability of topography-guided normalization combined with high-fluence CXL stabilization (the Athens protocol). J Refract Surg. 2014;30:88–93.
32. Fadlallah A, et al. Non-topography guided PRK combined with CXL for correction of refractive errors in patients with early stage keratoconus. J Refract Surg. 2014;30:688–93.
33. Shetty R, et al. Cone location-dependent outcomes after combined topography-guided photorefractive keratectomy and collagen cross-linking. Am J Ophthalmol. 2015;159:419–25.
34. Kanellopoulos AJ, Asimellis G. Novel placido-derived topography-guided excimer corneal normalization with cyclorotation adjustment: enhanced Athens protocol for keratoconus. J Refract Surg. 2015;31:768–73.

35. Shaheen MS, et al. Wave front-guided photorefractive keratectomy using a high-resolution aberrometer after corneal collagen cross-linking in keratoconus. Cornea. 2016;35:946–53.
36. Sakla H, et al. Simultaneous topography-guided photorefractive keratectomy and accelerated corneal collagen cross-linking for keratoconus. Cornea. 2016;35:941–5.
37. Chen X, et al. Epithelial thickness profile change after combined topography guided transepithelial PRK and corneal cross-linking in treatment 634 of keratoconus. J Refract Surg. 2016;32:626.
38. Grentzelos MA, et al. Combined transepithelial phototherapeutic keratectomy and conventional photorefractivekeratectomy followed simultaneously by corneal crosslinking for keratoconus: Cretan protocolplus. J Cataract Refract Surg. 2017;43:1257–62.
39. Stojanovic A, et al. Topography-guided transepithelial surface ablation followed by corneal collagen crosslinking performed in a single combined procedure for the treatment of keratoconus and pellucid marginal degeneration. J Refract Surg. 2010;26:145–52.
40. Wernli J, et al. The efficacy of corneal cross-linking shows a sudden decrease with very high intensity UV light and short treatment time. Invest Ophthalmol Vis Sci. 2013;54:1176–80.

Chapter 19
Intracorneal Ring Segments and Keratoconus

Alfredo Vega-Estrada, Jorge Alio del Barrio, and Jorge L. Alio

19.1 Introduction

Intracorneal ring segments (ICRS) are small devices made of synthetic material which are implanted within the corneal stroma in order to induce a change in the geometry and the refractive power of the tissue (Fig. 19.1). Blevatskaya in 1966, was whom first introduced the idea of implanting a corneal ring in order to change the refractive power of the eye [1]. Such a ring was composed of a 360° device which led to a several complications mainly due to the metabolic alterations in the corneal stroma which

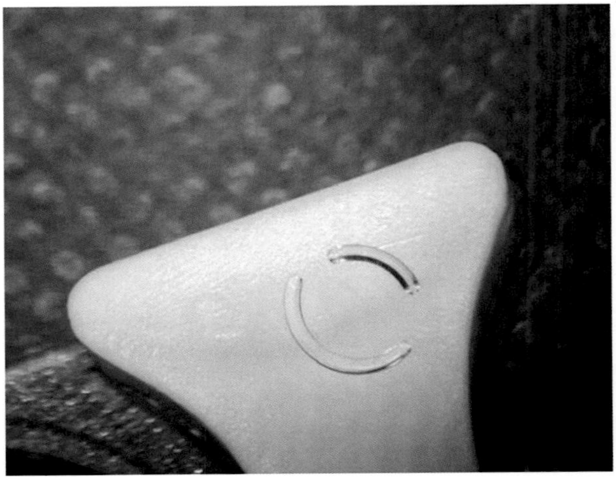

Fig. 19.1 Intracorneal ring segments

A. Vega-Estrada · J. Alio del Barrio · J. L. Alio (✉)
Keratoconus Unit, Vissum/Instituto Oftalmológico de Alicante, Alicante, Spain

Division of Ophthalmology, Universidad Miguel Hernández, Alicante, Spain
e-mail: jlalio@vissum.com

A. Barbara (ed.), *Controversies in the Management of Keratoconus*,
https://doi.org/10.1007/978-3-319-98032-4_19

was the reason to abandoned the 360° ring designs; afterwards, a new approach with the segments types that we know nowadays begins to be studied. During the decades of the 1970 and 1980, ring segments designs were widely investigated in order to provide the efficacy necessary to treat refractive errors. In the decade of the 1990, specifically in 1996, Intacs Technology, received the CE certificated and later in 1999, the FDA approval for the use of intracorneal ring segment (ICRS) implantation in the correction of myopic refractive errors [2]. Although several theoretical models as well as clinical research demonstrate the efficacy and predictability of this novel technology in the correction of low to moderate myopia, ICRS was rise above by the upcoming corneal excimer laser surgery due to the excellent refractive results of the latest technology [2]. In despite of the aforementioned, in the year 2000, Prof. Joseph Colin proposed to take advantage of the corneal modelling abilities of ICRS and use it for the treatment of keratoconus [3]. Afterwards, several investigators have reported good results when treating keratoconus patients using intracorneal ring segments, as well as delaying and also avoiding more complex surgeries as keratoplasty procedures.

Corneal ectatic disorders are a group of diseases characterize for progressive alterations in the morphology of the corneal tissue that negatively impact in the visual function and the optical quality of the patients [4]. Keratoconus is by far the more frequent pathology among this group of entities; its main features are corneal thinning, gradual corneal protrusion, and progressive irregular astigmatism [5]. The incidence in the general population is relatively low and variable, between 4/1000 and 6/1000 nine with other authors reporting that the current incidence is 1/2000 per year [6]. In addition, the incidence may vary according to the geographic region; though there are also studies supporting the fact that the prevalence is higher in zones with higher UV exposure or with a combination of genetic and environmental factors [7]. Regarding the therapeutic approaches, several treatment has been proposed in order to treat this disease, such as, contact lens wearing, thermokeratoplasty procedures, corneal collagen cross linking, intracorneal ring segment (ICRS) implantation and lamellar and penetrating keratoplasty [8–11].

The purpose of the present chapter is to update the main features of intracorneal ring segment implantation in the treatment of patients suffering from keratoconus.

19.2 Intracorneal Ring Segments Designs

Currently we have several models of ICRS that are commercially available; the ones that are widely spread used in the clinical practice are the hexagonal cross section segments represented by the Intacs (Addition technologies) (Fig. 19.2) and the triangular cross section represented by the Kerarings (Mediphacos) (Fig. 19.3). The main characteristics of these two types of ring segments are summarize in Table 19.1. Moreover, there is a variation of the Intacs, known as the Intacs SK, that because of the smaller diameter and different design have a more flattening capabilities and are reserved for those keratoconic cases that present high myopic refractive errors. The only true ring with a total 360° diameter that is currently available on the market is

Fig. 19.2 Intacs ICRS

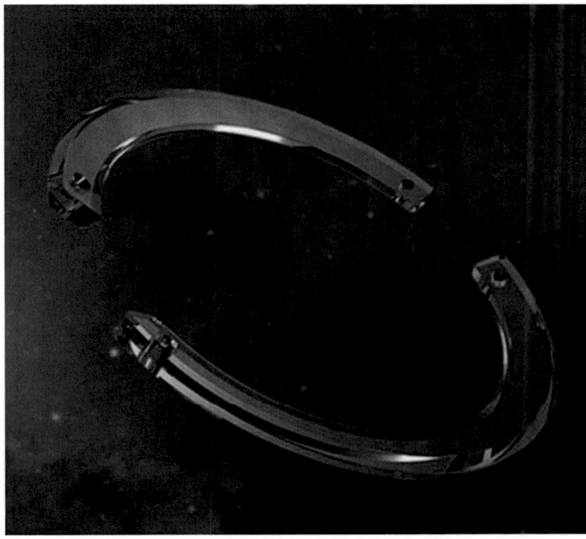

Fig. 19.3 Keraring ICRS

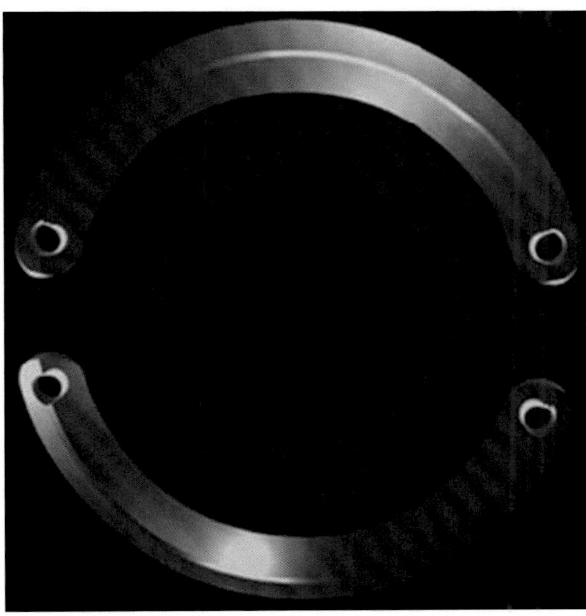

the Myoring from Dioptex (Fig. 19.4). Due to the full ring design, this model of ICRS is special used in those keratoconus that showed a topographic pattern with a center steepening, high keratometries and a high myopic refractive error.

In recent years, Mediphacos developed an interrupted ring of 355°, which is available in a diameter of 5.7 mm and a thickness ranging from 200 to 300 µm. Although there are just few studies published in the literature reporting results with

Table 19.1 Intracorneal ring segment main characteristics

Model	Intacs	Kerarings
Arc length (degrees)	150°	90–210°
Cross section	Hexagonal	Triangular
Thickness (mm)	0.25–0.35	0.15–0.35
Inner diameter (mm)	6.77	6.00
Outer diameter (mm)	8.10	7.00

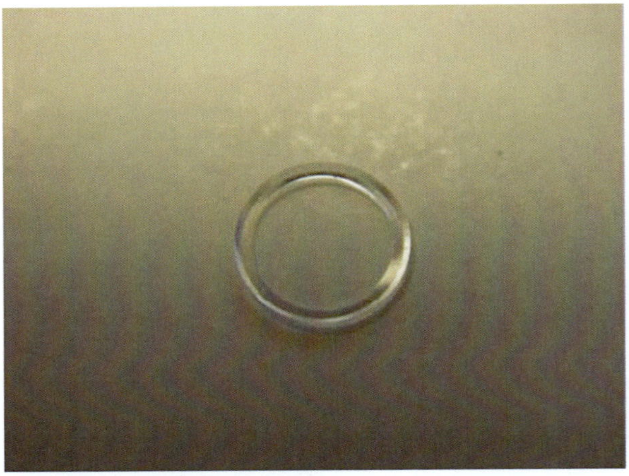

Fig. 19.4 Myoring ICRS

this type of ring, they show an improvement in the visual and refractive status of patients with central keratoconus. On another hand, our investigation team recently developed a new type of ICRS, the V-R technology, which is not yet commercially available and combines an asymmetric design in an almost completely full ring of 350° of arc length (Fig. 19.5). The potential advantages of the latest design is that will achieved both, the reduction of the asymmetry of the cornea that is observed when the segments are implanted and the significant flattening induced when using the full ring devices. Additionally because it is an incomplete ring can be implanted through a single incision in the cornea.

19.3 Mechanism of Action of the ICRS

Intracorneal ring segments acts as spacer elements between the collagen fibres of the corneal tissue [12]. Thus, ICRS induce an arc shortening effect of the geometry that in consequence flattens the central area of the cornea. Some theoretical models based on finite element analysis have proven that the flattening observed after ICRS implantation is directly proportional to the thickness of the segment and inversely proportional to the corneal diameter where is implanted. This means that the thicker and the smallest the diameter, the higher the flattening effect that will be induced by the segment [13]. Nevertheless, these theoretical models apply just to normal

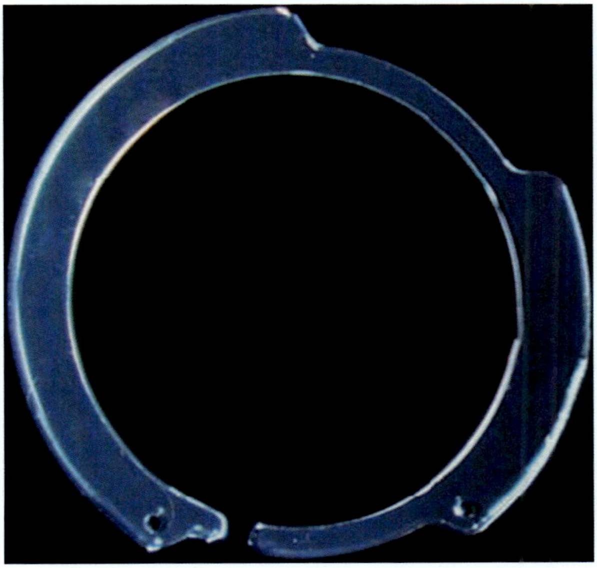

Fig. 19.5 V-R technology ICRS

corneas where there is an orthogonal arrangement of the collagen fibers. As have been demonstrate, in patients with keratoconus this special arrangement of the collagen fibers is lost, which leads to a more unpredictable result when evaluating the effect of corneal implants in this type of patients [14]. Another theory that may explain the mechanism of action of the ICRS is the "Thickness law" proposed by Barraquer which quote that when tissue is added to the periphery of the cornea or tissue is removed from the center a flattening of the cornea will be achieved and vice versa [15]. However, there is not enough scientific data published in the literature that supports the latest theory to explain the flattening effect of ICRS.

19.4 Surgical Techniques

In order to implant the intracorneal ring segments into the deep of the stroma we need to performed channels in the corneal tissue where the rings will be inserted. These channels or tunnels can be created manually or assisted by the femtosecond laser. In the following lines we will explain both procedures.

In the mechanical or manual technique, the surgeon must mark the center of the pupil in order to use it as a reference point during the procedure. Then a calibrated diamond knife is used to create an incision at a depth of 70% of the corneal pachymetry. A suction ring is placed around the corneal limbus in order to fixate the eye during the dissection of the corneal stroma. Then, two semicircular dissectors are placed through the incision and advance in the deep stroma in a clockwise and counter clockwise movement aiming to perform a tunnel within the corneal lamellas (Fig. 19.6). Once the channel is created, the ICRS is inserted.

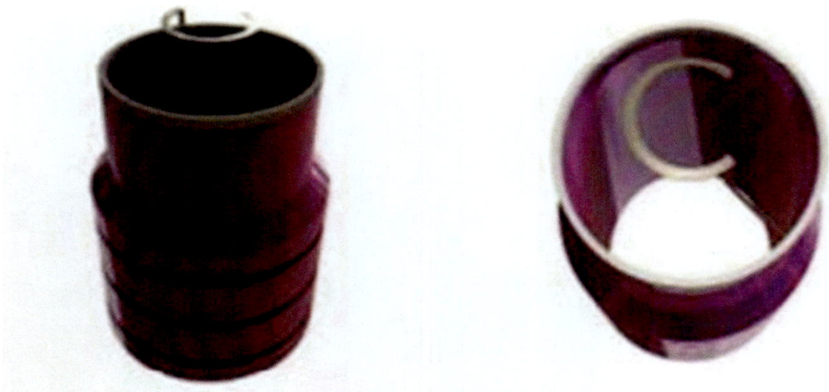

Dissectors (Clock Wise) Dissectors (Counter Clock Wise)

Fig. 19.6 Manual stromal dissectors for ICRS implantation

The other technique to create the tunnels is using the femtosecond laser assisted technique. In this case, a disposable suction ring of the femtosecond laser system is placed and centred. Afterwards, the cornea is flattened with a disposable aplannation cone which allows a precise focus of the laser beam thus creating a dissection on the desire depth. Then the tunnel is created at approximately 70% or 80% of the corneal pachymetry without direct manipulation of the eye. Finally, ICRS are inserted in the created tunnels.

Independently of the procedure used in order to perform the stromal tunnels in some exceptional cases and just if the surgeons considered that is necessary a 10-0 nylon suture can be placed to close the incision site.

Finally, in order to insert the full ring design ICRS, the Myoring, into the deep of the stroma a pocket must be created within the corneal lamellas. This pocket can be performed using a system device design for this purpose by the manufacturer known as the PocketMaker microkeratome [16]. The other approach to create this space in the middle in the corneal stroma is by using the femtosecond laser assisted technique with an entrance to the pocket of aprox. 5 mm [17].

19.5 Nomograms for Implantation

In order to choose the arc length, number, thickness and position of the segments in the cornea, we need to use the implantation nomograms. Even when several authors have reported good results when implanting ICRS in keratoconic eyes, the main limitations that nomograms have is that most of them are based in anecdotic clinical data or variables that are very subjective in patients with keratoconus, such as, spherocilyndrical refraction and topographic pattern of the cone. For instance, in an investigation conducted by our research group it was found that based on the topographic pattern of the keratoconus the best choice was to implant one segment in those cases of inferior steepening and two segments in central cones [18].

Other works published in the literature support that the best location to implant the segments is by placing the corneal incision in the temporal site of the cornea [19–23].

There are other works that have reported good results when implanting the ICRS guided by the comatic axis [24]. Recently, our research team published a scientific work in which we concluded that the best outcomes for implanting ICRS were observed in those cases where the refractive and topographic cylinder did not differ in more than 15° [25].

As we can see, there are different approaches regarding the guidelines to be used when implanting ICRS. Nevertheless, today the most widespread nomograms that are used in the clinical practice are those developed by the main manufacturers of ICRS.

Our research team is currently working with artificial intelligence (AI) software approach in order to optimize and refined the results of ICRS implantation [26]. Specifically, together with the CSO manufacturer an informatic software was developed based on a neural network which analyzed clinical data in order to provide a simulation of the best combination of ICRS that will induce the best optical function to a specific cornea. The main advantage of this approach is that a system based on AI is able to train itself by the inclusion of continuous input (cases implanted) that is upload on its system. This way, in the mean that we simulate more cases, the better the optical quality that can be predicted by the system thus providing better results after ICRS implantation. Figure 19.7 shows a screen display of a simulation provided by the neural network.

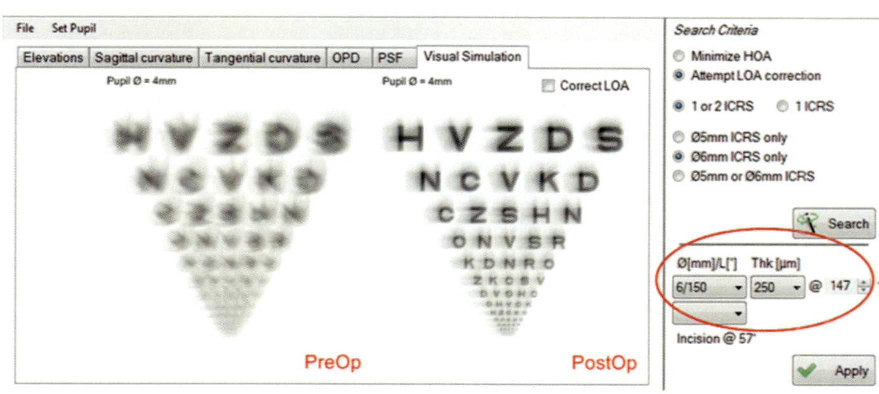

Fig. 19.7 Screen display of the neural network used for ICRS implantation guidance showing a preoperative (preop) and postoperative (postop) visual simulation of a patient. Red circle: segment type and location where the incision should be placed

19.6 ICRS Clinical Outcomes

Since the first report in the year 2000 when Colin and col. published their results after ICRS implantation for the treatment of keratoconus [3] several authors have demonstrate the efficacy of this surgical technique in reducing the spherical equivalent and keratometric readings as well as improving the visual function in patients with keratoconus [27–31]. The majority of those studies report an improvement in the uncorrected and corrected visual acuity, as well in the spherical equivalent and a reduction in the corneal astigmatism. Most of the authors observed a central flattening of the cornea that is consistent with a mean reduction of the keratometric readings that goes between 3 and 5 diopters [27–31]. Additionally, investigations that have assessed the optical quality by analysing the changes in anterior corneal higher order aberrations have found a reduction in these variables after ICRS implantation, specifically an improvement of the asymmetric aberrations (coma and coma-like) which are the ones that more limitations induces in keratoconic patients. These changes observed in the aberrometric coefficient are expected to occur due to the capability of the implants in regularizing the geometry of the corneal tissue [31–33].

As we can see most of the authors who have analysed the results of implanting ICRS in patients suffering of keratoconus agreed in the good outcomes regarding the visual function, refraction and anterior corneal higher order aberration; nevertheless, in a recent multicentric study performed by our research team it was found that the efficacy of ICRS implantation was related to the visual limitation of the patients at the moment of the surgery [31]. In that study we aimed to assess the outcomes of the surgical procedure based on a grading system that takes into account the visual acuity of the patients diagnose of keratoconus [34]. We observed that those patients with good spectacle corrected visual acuity at the moment of the surgery were more prone to lose lines of corrected vision after ICRS implantation; on the other hand, those cases with a severe limitation of the visual function before the procedure were the ones that benefit the most from the surgical procedure [31] (Table 19.2). These findings lead us to the consideration that ICRS implantation in cases with keratoconus and good vision should be undertaken with extreme caution because of the risk of loosing vision in this group of patients.

In relation to long-term results of ICRS implantation for the treatment of keratoconus there have been some controversies regarding the stability of the procedure after long period of time. While some studies reported the long term stability of this technique [22, 33, 35]. There is a clear limitation in most of these investigations as they do not state whether or not the patients that they are evaluating within their

Table 19.2 Percentage of corrected visual acuity after ICRS implantation according to the vision of keratoconic patients

Visual acuity	Gain ≥1 line CDVA	Lost ≥1 line CDVA	Lost ≥2 lines CDVA
CDVA ≥ 0.6 Grade I + II	37%	36%	25%
CDVA ≤ 0.4 grade IV + plus	82%	10%	4%

cohort belong to cases with the progressive or stable form of the disease, or they just analyze patients with stable form of keratoconus. In a recent study carried out by our research group was observed that long term stability of ICRS implantation depends on the progression pattern of keratoconus at the moment of the surgical technique. Thus, in those cases with the stable form of the disease, ICRS implantation remains without significant changes after long period of follow up. Nevertheless, in those cases that shows clinical signs of progression, the benefit achieved immediately after the procedure is expected to be lost after long period of time. From that work, we conclude that stability of the keratoconus should be established before considering ICRS in patients with keratoconus [36].

In relation to long arc length types of ICRS or completely full ring devices, most of the published data agree that these designs induce a more pronounced corneal flattening than those achieved by the conventional segments. Alio and co workers published in 2011 a pilot study analysing the clinical results of Myoring implantation where it was found that a mean reduction of around 8 diopters in the mean keratometric reading 6 months after Myoring implantation can be achieved [17]. In the same way, Jadidi et al. conducted a study where the authors analysed the 355° arc length ICRS manufactured by Mediphacos and they found that the mean keratometry was reduced in more than 5 diopters 6 month after ICRS impantation [37]. In a recent study conducted by a our research team where results of a 350° asymmetric intracornealring, V-R technology, were analysed, it was found that 1 year after the surgical procedure a mean reduction of more than 7 diopters can be observed in the spherical equivalent of patients with keratoconus [38].

19.7 Complications

Implanting ICRS in keratoconic patients is considered to be a safe surgical procedure mainly due to the advent of the femtosecond technology that provides more precise and predictable size and depth of the stromal tunnels. Even when rare, most of intraoperative complications have been describe when performing the channels with the manual technique.

Complications after ICRS implantation can be divided in: surgical related complications, postoperative complications and optical related complications.

Among the surgical procedure related complications after ICRS implantation, as previously commented, they are often seen when using the manual technique and very rarely with the femtosecond assisted procedure. These complications are usually related to an inadequate depth of the stromal channels, segment decentration or asymmetric position of the segment within the tunnels [39]. The most severe surgical related complication is corneal perforation which usually occurs during the rotational movement with the manual dissector. Complications related to femtosecond laser assisted technique usually are mild, like suction ring lost, subconjuntival hemorrhage and just in less than 0.6% of the cases a corneal perforation may be observed [40].

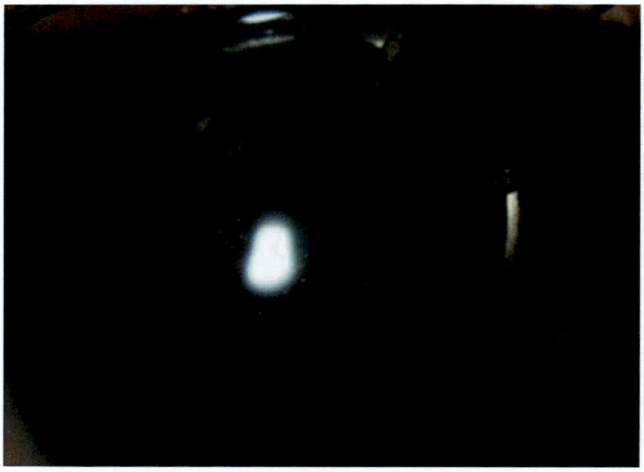

Fig. 19.8 Segment migration. In the lower part of the image contact between the two segments can be seen

Postoperative complications are not often present and when they are most of it usually does not represent a major risk for the eye of the patient. In any case, one of the most fear complications after this surgical technique is infectious keratitis; although, is have been reported to be less than 0.1% of the cases when dissecting the tunnels using the femtosecond laser assisted technique [41].

Extrusion and migration (Fig. 19.8) of the segment are among other of the complications that might be seen after ICRS implantation. Once again most of the published data agree that this complication is more often observed when using the mechanical technique [39, 41]. When present, extrusion or migration of the segments does not represent a clinically relevant event and may induce just a mild refractive change in the cornea thus the case might be followed just by observation. However, in some cases, severe photic phenomena, recurrent epithelial defect and stromal inflammation that could even lead to more severe complications like infectious keratitis and corneal melting may appear and in these cases segment explantation should be perform [42].

Corneal neovascularisation (Fig. 19.9) is other of the postoperative complications that may appear usually at late stages after ICRS implantation. Although rare when appear is mainly due to dissection of the tunnel to close to the corneal limbus.

A postoperative event that is often observed after ICRS complications are white deposits within the stromal tunnel (Fig. 19.10). Even when its incidence have been reported by some authors to be as high as in 60% of the cases [42]. These channel deposits does not induce any optical or structural alteration and are considered to be completely benign thus any specific treatment should be performed when they are observed [43].

Another complication that can be present after ICRS implantation and that is very severe is corneal melting. Even when the incidence is very low, around 0.2% according some authors [39], when present explantation of the ICRS should be perform.

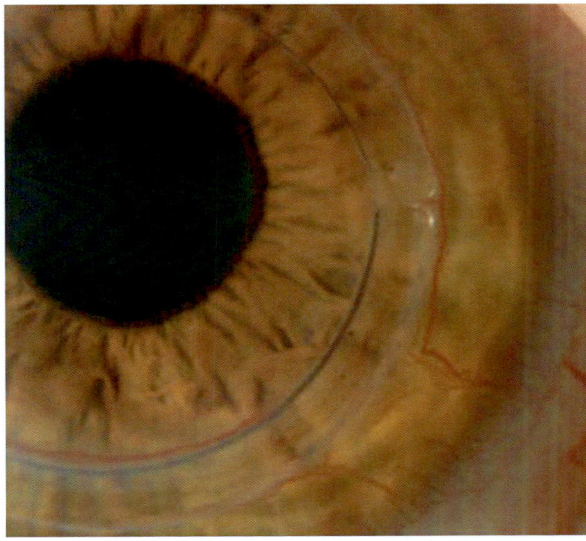

Fig. 19.9 Corneal neovascularization through the stromal channel

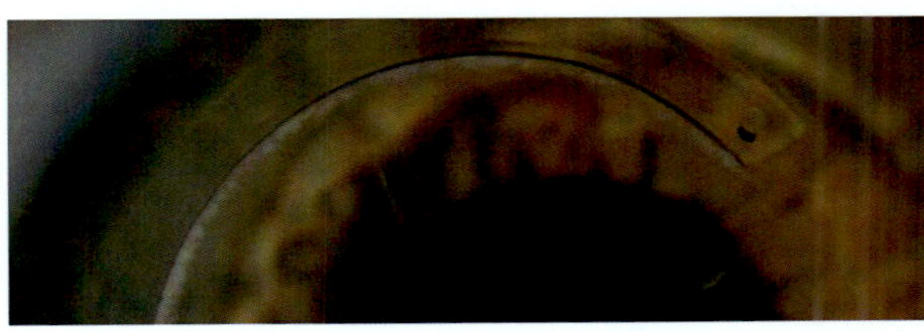

Fig. 19.10 Corneal deposit within the segment tunnel

In relation to optical complications after the procedure, photic phenomena as halos and glare might be present usually when the dissection of the tunnel has been decenter or when severe migration of the segment occurs during the postoperative period. Losing corrected visual acuity can be other complication observed in patients with keratoconus and good visual function. Our research team conducted a clinical investigation were it was demonstrate that those patients with more than 0.9 of corrected visual acuity in the decimal scale have around 50% of risk of losing lines of vision after ICRS implantation [31].

Finally, with the advent of new long arc length design an increasing number of complications related to corneal melting and extrusion of the segment have been reported which makes necessary to conduct long term studies analysing a higher number of patients implanted with segments of more than 340° of arc length [37].

In this point it is worth to mention that one of the main advantages that ICRS implantation has is it reversibility. Even when some of the above mentioned complications might appear, some studies have shown that segment explantation can be safely performed with visual, refractive and topographic variables coming to preoperative levels [44].

19.8 Futures Perspective

Nowadays, there is enough scientific based evidence demonstrating the efficacy of ICRS for the treatment of keratoconus. We can have access today to technology and materials that allow us to develop new designs that combines the main features and advantages of different type of rings, as is the case of the currently available long arch length ring type designs, in order to provide a better results to our keratoconic patients. Additionally, there is every time more publications that show the benefit effect of combining different treatment approaches as ICRS together with corneal collagen cross-linking. Moreover, with the advent of artificial intelligence systems and neural network software as well as technology of enormous amount of data analysis we will be able to refine our nomograms of implantation and the predictability of the outcomes based on the analysis of the clinical results from previous success cases implanted with ICRS.

19.9 Summary

In conclusion we can say that ICRS is an effective procedure in the treatment of keratoconus patients. This surgical procedure induces a change in the morphology of the corneal stroma leading to an improvement in the visual function and the quality of life leading in many times to avoid more complex procedures as keratoplasty in patients with keratoconus. Currently, there are many research teams working in improvement of the implantation nomograms; new approaches as using artificial intelligence or big data analysis to increase the predictability of the outcomes after ICRS implantation is nowadays in practice. Although there are some reports analysing the long term stability of the procedure most of the published data agree that ICRS is a stable technique after long period of follow up specifically in those patients with stable keratoconus. ICRS implantation are considered to be a safe and reversible technique and the few complications that are reported is usually when using the manual technique in order to performed the stromal channels. Finally our increased in knowledge and understanding of ICRS together with new designs and better nomograms of implantation will certainly improve the outcomes of implanting ICRS in patients with keratoconus.

References

1. Blevatskaya ED. Intralamellar homoplasty for the purpose of relaxation of refraction of the eye. Arch Soc Am Ophthalmol Optom. 1968;6:311–25. (translated from Oftalmol Zh 1966;7:530–537).
2. Vega-Estrada A, Alió JL. The use of intracorneal ring segments in keratoconus: a review. Eye Vis (Lond). 2016;3(8):2326–0254.
3. Colin J, Cochener B, Savary G, Malet F. Correcting keratoconus with intracorneal rings. J Cataract Refract Surg. 2000;26:1117–22.

4. Tan DT, Por YM. Current treatment options for corneal ectasia. Curr Opin Ophthalmol. 2007;18:284–9.
5. Rabinowitz YS. Keratoconus. Survey Ophtalmol. 1998;42:297–319.
6. Kennedy RH, Bourne WM, Dyer JA. A 48-year clinical and epidemiologic study of keratoconus. Am J Ophthalmol. 1986;101:267–73.
7. Malecaze F, Ancele E, Butterworth J. Chap. 1: Epidemiology of Keratoconus. In: Barbara A, Rabinowitz YS, editors. Textbook on Keratoconus: new insights. New Delhi: Jaypee Brothers Medical Publishers; 2012.
8. Barnett M, Mannis MJ. Contact lenses in the management of keratoconus. Cornea. 2011;30:1510–6.
9. Vega-Estrada A, Alió JL, Plaza Puche AB, Marshall J. Outcomes of a new microwave procedure followed by accelerated cross-linking for the treatment of keratoconus: a pilot study. J Refract Surg. 2012;28:787–93.
10. Snibson GR. Collagen cross-linking: a new treatment paradigm in corneal disease – a review. Clin Exp Ophthalmol. 2010;38:141–53.
11. Busin M, Scorcia V, Zambianchi L, Ponzin D. Outcomes from a modified microkeratome-assisted lamellar keratoplasty for keratoconus. Arch Ophthalmol. 2012;130:776–82.
12. Silvestrini T, Mathis M, Loomas B, Burris T. A geometric model to predict the change in corneal curvature from the intrastromal corneal ring (ICR). Invest Ophthalmol Vis Sci. 1994;35:2023.
13. Burris TE, Baker PC, Ayer CT, Loomas BE, Mathis ML, Silvestrini TA. Flattening of central corneal curvature with intrastromal corneal rings of increasing thickness: an eye-bank eye study. J Cataract Refract Surg. 1993;19(l):182–7.
14. Daxer A, Fratzl P. Collagen orientation in the human corneal stroma and its implication in keratoconus. Invest Ophthalmol Vis Sci. 1997;38:121–9.
15. Albertazzi R. Tratamiento del queratocono con segmentos intracorneales. In: Albertazzi R, editor. Queratocono: pautas para su diagnóstico y tratamiento. Buenos Aires: Ediciones cientificas argentina para la keratoconus society; 2010. p. 205–68.
16. Daxer A, Mahmoud H, Venkateswaran RS. Intracorneal continuous ring implantation for keratoconus: one-year follow-up. J Cataract Refract Surg. 2010;36(8):1296–302.
17. Alio JL, Piñero DP, Daxer A. clinical outcomes after complete ring implantation in corneal ectásica using the femtosecond technology: a pilot study. Ophthalmology. 2011; 118(7):1282–90.
18. Alió JL, Artola A, Hassanein A, Haroun H, Galal A. One or 2 Intacs segments for the correction of keratoconus. J Cataract Refract Surg. 2005;31:943–53.
19. Colin J, Cochener B, Savary G, Malet F, Holmes-Higgin D. Intacs inserts for treating keratoconus. One year results. Ophthalmology. 2001;108:1409–14.
20. Hellstedt T, Mäkelä J, Uusitalo R, Emre S, Uusitalo R. Treating keratoconus with Intacs corneal ring segments. J Refract Surg. 2005;21:236–46.
21. Kanellopoulos AJ, Pe LH, Perry HD, Donnenfeld ED. Modified intracorneal ring segment implantations (Intacs) for the management of moderate to advanced keratoconus. Efficacy and complications. Cornea. 2006;25:29–33.16.
22. Alió JL, Shabayek MH, Artola A. Intracorneal ring segments for keratoconus correction: long-term follow-up. J Cataract Refract Surg. 2006;32:978–85.
23. Shetty R, Kurian M, Anand D, Mhaske P, Narayana KM, Shetty BK. Intacs in advanced keratoconus. Cornea. 2008;27:1022–9.
24. Alfonso JF, Lisa C, Merayo-Lloves J, Fernández-Vega Cueto L, Montés-Micó R. Intrastromal corneal ring segment implantation in paracentral keratoconus with coincident topographic and coma axis. J Cataract Refract Surg. 2012;38(9):1576–82.
25. Peña-García P, Alió JL, Vega-Estrada A, Barraquer RI. Internal, corneal, and refractive astigmatism as prognostic factors for intrastromal corneal ring segment implantation in mild to moderate keratoconus. J Cataract Refract Surg. 2014;40(10):1633–44.
26. Sanz P, Vega-Estrada A, Alio JL, Versaci F, Faini S. Neural network to guide keratoconus treatment with ICRS. Copenhagen: European Society of Cornea and Ocular Surface Disease Specialists (EUCORNEA); 2016.

27. Piñero DP, Alio JL. Intracorneal ring segments in ectatic corneal disease – a review. Clin Exp Ophthalmol. 2010;38(2):154–67.
28. Siganos D, Ferrara P, Chatzinikolas K, Bessis N, Papastergiou G. Ferrara intrastromal corneal rings for the correction of keratoconus. J Cataract Refract Surg. 2002;28:1947–51.
29. Coskunseven E, Kymionis GD, Tsiklis NS, et al. One year results of intrastromal corneal ring segment implantation (KeraRing) using femtosecond laser in patients with keratoconus. Am J Ophthalmol. 2008;145:775–9.
30. Alió JL, Shabayek MH, Belda JI, Correas P, Feijoo ED. Analysis of results related to good and bad outcomes of Intacs implantation for keratoconus correction. J Cataract Refract Surg. 2006;32(5):756–61.25.
31. Vega-Estrada A, Alio JL, Brenner LF, Javaloy J, Plaza Puche AB, Barraquer RI, Teus MA, Murta J, Henriques J, Uceda-Montanes A. Outcome analysis of intracorneal ring segments for the treatment of keratoconus based on visual, refractive, and aberrometric impairment. Am J Ophthalmol. 2013;155(3):575–84.
32. Shabayek MH, Alió JL. Intrastromal corneal ring segment implantation by femtosecond laser for keratoconus correction. Ophthalmology. 2007;114:1643–52. 27
33. Vega Estrada AL, Alió JL, Brenner LF, Burguera N. Outcomes of intrastromal corneal ring segments for treatment of keratoconus: five-year follow-up analysis. J Cataract Refract Surg. 2013;39:1234–40.
34. Alió JL, Piñero DP, Alesón A, Teus MA, Barraquer RI, Murta J, Maldonado MJ, Castro de Luna G, Gutiérrez R, Villa C, Uceda-Montanes A. Keratoconus-integrated characterization considering anterior corneal aberrations, internal astigmatism, and corneal biomechanics. J Cataract Refract Surg. 2011;37:552–68.
35. Torquetti L, Berbel RF, Ferrara P. Long-term follow-up of intrastromal corneal ring segments in keratoconus. J Cataract Refract Surg. 2009;35(10):1768–19. 73
36. Vega-Estrada A, Alió JL, Plaza-Puche A. Keratoconus progression following intrastromal corneal ring segments in young patients: five-year follow-up. J Cataract Refract Surg. 2015;41(6):1145–52.
37. Jadidi K, Mosavi S, Nejat F, et al. Intrastromal corneal ring segment implantation (keraring 355°) in patients with central keratoconus: 6-month follow-up. J Ophthalmol. 2015;2015:916385.
38. Alió JL, Vega-Estrada A, Chorro E, et al. Visual, refractive and aberrometric outcomes of a new asymmetric intracorneal ring segment. Presented as poster in the: American Academy of Ophthalmology. 2017.
39. Miranda D, Sartori M, Francesconi C, Allemann N, Ferrara P, Campos M. Ferrara intrastromal corneal ring segments for severe keratoconus. J Refract Surg. 2003;19:645–53.
40. Coskunseven E, Kymionis GD, Tsiklis NS, Atun S, Arslan E, Siganos CS, Jankov M, Pallikaris IG. Complications of intrastromal corneal ring segment implantation using a femtosecond laser for channel creation: a survey of 850 eyes with keratoconus. Acta Ophthalmol. 2011;89(1):54–7.
41. Kwitko S, Severo NS. Ferrara intracorneal ring segments for keratoconus. J Cataract Refract Surg. 2004;30:812–20.
42. Ferrer C, Alió JL, Uceda-Montañes A, et al. Causes of intraestromal corneal ring segment explantation: clinicopathologic correlation analysis. J Cataract Refract Surg. 2010;36(6):970–7.
43. Ruckhofer J, Twa MD, Schanzlin DJ. Clinical characteristics of lamellar channel deposits after implantation of Intacs. J Cataract Refract Surg. 2000;26:1473–9.
44. Alió JL, Artola A, Ruiz-Moreno JM, et al. Changes in keratoconic corneas after intracorneal ring segment explantation and reimplantation. Ophthalmology. 2004;111:747–51.

Chapter 20
Can Intrastromal Corneal Ring Segments Halt Keratoconus Evolution?

Leonardo Torquetti, Guilherme Ferrara, and Paulo Ferrara

The implantation of intrastromal corneal ring segments (ICRS) is a minimally invasive surgical option for reshaping the cornea in keratoconus and other secondary ectasias. Intrastromal corneal ring segments have been used to correct ectatic corneal diseases, reduce the corneal steepening, reduce irregular astigmatism and improve the visual acuity [1–4]. Besides, the ICRS is a surgical alternative to at least delay, if not eliminates, the need of lamellar or penetrating keratoplasty.

The stability of keratoconus after intrastromal corneal ring segments implantation (ICRS) remains a debate among keratoconus specialists. Some of them agree that ICRS stabilizes the disease; some agree that it reduces the speed of progression and some believe that it has just an ortophedic effect, correcting the deformity without direct influence in the evolution of the disease.

There are few studies carried out to assess the long-term results of ICRS implantation, and they give different findings concerning stability [5–9]. Most of them conclude that the procedure is stable. However, one study found that the procedure was not stable when keratoconus was in progression at the time of surgery [8].

The two primary surgical options for the actual treatment of keratoconus are crosslinking (CXL) [10, 11] and ICRS implantation. The corneal transplantation, despite significant advances in the last years in lamellar techniques, still is a more invasive and risky procedure, which are usually reserved for more advanced cases [12].

CXL is successful in halting the progression of the disease [13]. The work of the Dresden group revolutionized the field by showing that CXL could not only do this

L. Torquetti (✉)
Centro de Excelência em Oftalmologia, Pará de Minas, MG, Brazil

Paulo Ferrara Eye Clinic, Belo Horizonte, Brazil
e-mail: leonardo@ceoclinica.med.br

G. Ferrara · P. Ferrara
Paulo Ferrara Eye Clinic, Belo Horizonte, Brazil

A. Barbara (ed.), *Controversies in the Management of Keratoconus*,
https://doi.org/10.1007/978-3-319-98032-4_20

but in some cases also leads to an improvement in many anatomical and refractive indices in keratoconus [14, 15]. However, despite the value of CXL in halting the progression of keratoconus, several investigators have raised concerns about its significant vision-threatening complications [16, 17]. These include corneal infiltrates [18], melting [19], infections [20], and scar formation [21], all of which may lead to a reduction in CDVA.

In a long-term follow-up study in CXL [15], it was demonstrated the ability of CXL to slow down KC progression in pediatric patients, improving functional performance. Long-term stability was correlated with a CXL-induced delay in corneal collagen turnover and with spontaneous age-related KC stabilization. A 24% regression rate could be contemplated in the patients who were aged 15 years and younger at the time of inclusion in the treatment protocol.

Considering CXL and ICRS the two major treatments before corneal transplantation in keratoconus patients, the long-term efficacy of both procedures should be evaluated to define the adequate treatment for each patient.

20.1 Long-Term Follow-up After ICRS Implantation in Keratoconus

We retrospectively reviewed patient records of 94 eyes of 76 patients, which were consecutively operated (Ferrara ICRS implantation) [5]. There were 33 female and 61 male. The average age of the patients was 28.1 years. All procedures were performed by the same surgeon (PF), between June of 1996 and September of 2007. Patients included in the study presented clear cornea and a minimal corneal thickness of 300 μm at the ICRS track. Patients were intolerant to contact lens and/or showed a progression of the ectasia.

Fifty-eight subjects underwent to a single eye treatment, whereas 18 subjects had both eyes treated. Seventy-three eyes had a 2 years follow-up, 66 eyes had a 3 years follow-up, 48 eyes had a 4 years follow-up, and 34 eyes had a 5 years follow-up. All patients completed at least a 2 years follow-up. No intraoperative complications occurred. All patients returned for ocular examination on day 1, 1 week and a month after the surgery and then 3, 6 and 12 months. After that, the following eye examinations occurred yearly.

Preoperative and postoperative UDVA, CDVA, and keratometry data were collected from all patients. The mean UDVA (decimal) at the preoperative period was 0.12, and the mean CDVA (decimal) was 0.41. At the 1st month, the mean UDVA improved to 0.25, and the mean CDVA improved to 0.56. At the 2nd year follow-up, the mean UDVA improved from 0.12 preoperatively to 0.29. At the 3rd year follow-up, the mean UDVA improved to 0.34, at the 4th year follow-up, the mean UDVA improved to 0.42, and at the 5th year follow-up, the mean UDVA decreased to 0.31 postoperatively. The mean CDVA, at the 1st month, improved to 0.56. At the 2nd year follow-up, the mean CDVA improved from 0.41 preoperatively to 0.68. At the 3rd year follow-up, the mean CDVA decreased to 0.63, at the 4th year follow-up, the mean CDVA improved to 0.65, and at the 5th year follow-up, the mean CDVA decreased to 0.59 postoperatively.

The mean keratometry decreased significantly from the preoperative to the last postoperative follow-up. Preoperative mean keratometry was 50.36, which reduce to 47.29 at 1st month postoperative follow-up. The mean keratometry follow-up along the 2nd to 5th years was 45.96; 45.83; 46.44 and 46.24, respectively.

A study published by Pesando et al. [22] found similar results, in a 5-year follow-up. A total of 93.84% (122 patients) of the eyes gained lines of UDVA, and only 1.53% (2 eyes) lost them. A total of 97.69% (127 patients) of the treated eyes gained lines of CDVA, and no eyes lost them. The value of K1 and K2 were considerably reduced over 5 years. The preoperative value of K average of 49.27 D became 4.68 D postoperatively. Both the UDVA and the CDVA showed an increase. The UDVA changed from 0.14 lines preoperatively to 0.32 postoperatively while the BCVA improved from 0.40 to 0.59. The spherical equivalent changed from −8.34 D before the operation to −2.83 D after the surgery.

In 2014 we published a paper [23] with the longest follow-up ever described, after ICRS implantation. The mean UDVA (logMAR) improved from 1.01 ± 0.28 to 0.71 ± 0.38 at 5 years (P = .000) and 0.67 ± 0.25 at 10 years (P = .735). The mean CDVA (logMAR) improved from 0.45 ± 0.45 to 0.24 ± 0.19 at 5 years (P = .004) and 0.29 ± 0.09 at 10 years (P = .292). The mean maximum K value decreased from 54.99 ± 6.33 to 50.58 ± 5.11 D at 5 years (P = .000) and 50.65 ± 5.17 D at 10 years (P = .854). The mean minimum K value decreased from 48.85 ± 5.70 to 46.90 ± 5.08 D at 5 years (P = .000) and 47.12 ± 4.22 D at 10 years (P = .945). The central corneal thickness decreased from 457.42 ± 58.21 to 421.34 ± 74.12 μm at 5 years (P = .039) and 434.32 ± 77.65 μm at 10 years (P = .427).

There is some criticism of this paper. First, the mean age of patients at the time of surgery was 28.6 years. We agree that keratoconus tends to be stable approximately after 30 years of age [24]. Therefore, the results regarding stability could be influenced by the mean age of the studied patients. However, we could include in this paper only patients with came back for revision at 5 and 10 years after the surgery. As we are a reference center for ICRS implantation in Brazil and receive patients from all over the country, several patients are missed to follow-up. This could be considered a bias of selection; however, only the patients that came back for follow-up could be included in this study.

20.2 ICRS Implantation in Pediatric Keratoconus Patients

One recently published study evaluated the long-term efficacy of ICRS implantation in pediatric patients [9]. A small sample of patients (14 eyes) was evaluated; the follow-up was 5 years.

Baseline average UCVA and BCVA were 0.07 ± 0.09 and 0.34 ± 0.21, respectively, and they improved to 0.25 ± 0.15 and 0.54 ± 0.17 after ICRS implantation ($p < 0.01$ and $p = 0.011$, respectively). During follow-up, both UCVA and BCVA remained almost constant, reaching, at the end of follow-up, 0.3 ± 0.21 and 0.55 ± 0.13 without statistically significant differences from those observed at 6–12 months postoperatively. Until the end of follow-up, no patient needed additional procedures, besides the use of optical correction with glasses or contact lenses.

In this study, there were no statistically significant differences in keratometric readings over time. Regarding visual acuity, it was observed maintenance of the visual gains achieved with ICRS implantation. Despite these findings, the authors of this study conclude that ICRS implantation does not halt the progression of keratoconus over time and it is essential to consider the use of alternative treatments or combination of different treatment modalities in the management of pediatric keratoconus.

Vega-Estrada et al. [8] and Alió et al. [7] observed that the long-term stability of ICRS implantation depends on the progression pattern of keratoconus at the time of surgery, suggesting that in cases of stable keratoconus the results remained stable, in opposition to progressive disease where the short-term outcomes could change after an extended period.

Ferrara et al. [25] published a paper in which they evaluated 58 eyes of 37 children with keratoconus. Thirteen eyes remained untreated, and three eyes underwent lamellar keratoplasty due to advanced keratoconus. The mean age of patients was 13 ± 2.1 years old (range 8–16 years). All patients completed at least 6 months of follow-up (average 20 months, range 6–81). No perioperative or postoperative complications occurred.

In this study, the minimum and maximum keratometry decreased from the presurgical evaluation to the 1st month, while the values of asphericity and pachymetry increased during this same period. Between the 1st month of follow-up to the 2nd year, we observed that minimum keratometry did not change over time, and maximum keratometry had a slight increase over time. The value of asphericity does not change over time; the pachymetry did not change over time. Although there was a slight increase in maximum keratometry over time (0.7 diopters per year, on average), this increase was not clinically significant. In this study, two patients (5.4%) underwent keratoplasty, and one patient (2.7%) underwent corneal crosslinking due to keratoconus progression.

20.3 Conclusion

Based on our personal (unpublished) data, about 5% of patients go to penetrating or lamellar keratoplasty due to progressive corneal scarring, despite proper ICRS implantation. It is important to emphasize that these patients usually had ring implantation in very advanced phases of the disease and did not mean necessarily keratoconus evolution but rather an unsatisfactory visual outcome.

ICRS implantation could be a valuable tool to provide a topographic and visual improvement in children and adults with keratoconus. The younger the patient at the moment of implantation (considering more aggressive kertoconus in very young patients) and the more advanced the case at the time of implantation, the more chance of additional procedures (as keratoplasty) after ICRS implantation. Corneal re-steepening can occur after ICRS implantation. It plays an important role in delaying the progression of keratoconus and postpones a corneal grafting surgery.

Financial Disclosure Dr. Paulo Ferrara and Guilherme Ferrara have a proprietary interest in the Ferrara ICRS. Dr. Leonardo Torquetti does not have a financial interest in any device cited in this review.

References

1. Piñero DP, Alio JL, Uceda-Montanes A, El Kady B, Pascual I. Intracorneal ring segment implantation in corneas with post-laser in situ keratomileusis keratectasia. Ophthalmology. 2009;116(9):1665–74. https://doi.org/10.1016/j.ophtha.2009.05.030.
2. Torquetti L, Ferrara G, Ferrara P. Predictors of clinical outcomes after intrastromal corneal ring segments implantation. Int J Keratoconus Ectatic Corneal Dis. 2012;1:26–30.
3. Torquetti L, Ferrara G, Almeida F, Cunha L, Ferrara P, Merayo-Lloves J. Clinical outcomes after intrastromal corneal ring segments reoperation in keratoconus patients. Int J Ophthalmol. 2013;6(6):796–800. http://www.pubmedcentral.nih.gov/articlerender.fcgi?artid=3874518&tool=pmcentrez&rendertype=abstract
4. Ferrara G, Torquetti L. Intrastromal corneal ring segments: visual outcomes from a large case series. Clin Exp Ophthalmol. 2012;40(5):433–9. http://onlinelibrary.wiley.com/doi/10.1111/j.1442-9071.2011.02698.x/full
5. Torquetti L, Berbel RF, Ferrara P. Long-term follow-up of intrastromal corneal ring segments in keratoconus. J Cataract Refract Surg. 2009;35(10):1768–73.
6. Colin J, Cochener B, Savary G, Malet F, Holmes-Higgin D. INTACS inserts for treating keratoconus: one-year results. Ophthalmology. 2001;108(8):1409–14. https://doi.org/10.1016/S0161-6420(01)00646-7.
7. Alió JL, Shabayek MH, Artola A. Intracorneal ring segments for keratoconus correction: long-term follow-up. J Cataract Refract Surg. 2006;32(6):978–85. https://doi.org/10.1016/j.jcrs.2006.02.044.
8. Vega-Estrada A, Alió JL, Brenner LF, Burguera N. Outcomes of intrastromal corneal ring segments for treatment of keratoconus: five-year follow-up analysis. J Cataract Refract Surg. 2013;39(8):1234–40. https://doi.org/10.1016/j.jcrs.2013.03.019.
9. Abreu AC, Malheiro L, Coelho J, Neves MM, Gomes M, Oliveira L, Menéres P. Implantation of intracorneal ring segments in pediatric patients: long-term follow-up. Int Med Case Rep J. 2018;7(11):23–7.
10. Spoerl E, Mrochen M, Sliney D, Trokel S, Seiler T. Safety of UVA-riboflavin cross-linking of the cornea. Cornea. 2007;26(4):385–9. https://doi.org/10.1097/ICO.0b013e3180334f78.
11. Sorkin N, Varssano D. Corneal collagen crosslinking: a systematic review. Ophthalmologica. 2014;232(1):10–27. https://doi.org/10.1159/000357979.
12. Krumeich JH, Knulle A, Krumeich BM. Deep anterior lamellar (DALK) vs. penetrating keratoplasty (PKP): a clinical and statistical analysis. Klin Monatsbl Augenheilkd. 2008;225(7):637–48. https://doi.org/10.1055/s-2008-1027485.
13. Gatinel D. Effectiveness of corneal collagen crosslinking in vivo for corneal stiffening. J Cataract Refract Surg. 2014;40(11):1943–4. https://doi.org/10.1016/j.jcrs.2014.09.026.
14. Wollensak G. Corneal collagen crosslinking: new horizons. Expert Rev Ophthalmol. 2010;5(2):201–15. https://doi.org/10.1586/eop.10.7.

15. Mazzotta C, Rechichi M, Traversi C, Baiocchi S, Polito MS, Caragiuli S. Slowing the progression of keratoconus – turning to corneal crosslinking. Expert Rev Ophthalmol. 2016;11(1):41–8. https://doi.org/10.1586/17469899.2016.1136788.
16. Koller T, Mrochen M, Seiler T. Complication and failure rates after corneal crosslinking. J Cataract Refract Surg. 2009;35(8):1358–62. https://doi.org/10.1016/j.jcrs.2009.03.035.
17. Dhawan S, Rao K, Natrajan S. Complications of corneal collagen cross-linking. J Ophthalmol. 2011;2011:1–5. https://doi.org/10.1155/2011/869015.
18. Arora R, Jain P, Gupta D, Goyal JL. Sterile keratitis after corneal collagen crosslinking in a child. Contact Lens Anterior Eye. 2012;35(5):233–5. https://doi.org/10.1016/j.clae.2012.06.002.
19. Gokhale NS, Vemuganti GK. Diclofenac-induced acute corneal melt after collagen crosslinking for keratoconus. Cornea. 2010;29(1):117–9. https://doi.org/10.1097/ICO.0b013e3181a06c31.
20. Abbouda A, Abicca I, Alió JL. Infectious keratitis following corneal crosslinking: a systematic review of reported cases:management, visual outcome, and treatment proposed. Semin Ophthalmol. 2016;31(5):485–91. https://doi.org/10.3109/08820538.2014.962176.
21. Kymionis GD, Portaliou DM, Pallikaris IG. Additional complications of corneal crosslinking. J Cataract Refract Surg. 2010;36(1):185. https://doi.org/10.1016/j.jcrs.2009.07.028.
22. Pesando PM, Ghiringhello MP, Di Meglio G, Romeo S. Treatment of keratoconus with Ferrara ICRS and consideration of the efficacy of the Ferrara nomogram in a 5-year follow-up. Eur J Ophthalmol. 2010;20(5):865–73. http://www.ncbi.nlm.nih.gov/pubmed/20491049. Accessed 10 Feb 2016.
23. Torquetti L, Ferrara G, Almeida F, et al. Intrastromal corneal ring segments implantation in patients with keratoconus: 10-year follow-up. J Refract Surg. 2014;30(1):22–6.
24. Rabinowitz YS. Keratoconus. Surv Ophthalmol. 1998;42(4):297–319. doi:S0039625797001197 [pii].
25. Ferrara G, Ferrara PTL. Intrastromal corneal ring segments in children with keratoconus. Int J Keratoconus Ectatic Corneal Dis. 2017;6(2):1–4.

Chapter 21
Can We Improve Visual Acuity After Intrastromal Corneal Ring Segments Implantation for Keratoconus and Post LASIK Ectasia

Adel Barbara, Sajjad Abbas, and Ramez Barbara

21.1 Introduction

Keratoconus (KC) is an ectatic corneal disease which causes irregular astigmatism that cannot be corrected by spectacles. The irregular astigmatism leads to loss of uncorrected and corrected visual acuity (VA) and leads to a deterioration in the quality of the vision. Contact lenses (CL) improves the VA but cannot be tolerated in many cases due to a variety of reasons including loss of motivation and atopic/allergic conjunctivitis which is frequently seen in patients with KC.

Intrastromal corneal ring segments (ICRS) are crescent shape PMMA segments, produced in different geometric shapes, thicknesses and lengths. They are inserted in the periphery of the cornea at a depth of 70–80% of the corneal thickness as measured by pachymetry at the incision site. The incision and the tunnels through which the ICRS are inserted may be created either mechanically or by femtosecond laser. The whole procedure is performed under topical anesthesia and is reversible are currently three groups of commercially available ICRS:

1 **Intacs:** These have a hexagonal shape, are 150 degrees (°) of arc long, have a 7 mm optical zone with variable thicknesses (250–450 um in a 50 μm steps), **Intacs SK** (SK 'severe keratoconus') have an oval shape, possess a 6 mm optical, variable length of arc: 90°, 130° and 150° zone and are 400–450 μm thick. Both are produced by AJL Ophthalmic, Spain.

Similar review was published in 2014 by A. Barbara et al in "The International Journal of Keratoconus & Ectatic Corneal Diseases", www.ijkecd.com.

A. Barbara (✉)
Medical Director of IVISION, Refractive Surgery and Keratoconus Treatment Center, Haifa, Israel

S. Abbas
Bournemuoth Eye Unit, Royal Bournemouth Hospital, Bournemouth, UK

R. Barbara
Southampton Eye Unit, Southampton General Hospital, Southampton, UK

A. Barbara (ed.), *Controversies in the Management of Keratoconus*,
https://doi.org/10.1007/978-3-319-98032-4_21

2 **Ferrara Rings**: These have a pyramidal shape, a fixed flat base of 600 μm, have a 5 mm optical zone (also available with a 6 mm optical zone) with a variable thickness (150–350 μm) in 50 μm increments and a length of 90°, 120°, 160°, 210° and 340° of arc. Ferrara rings are yellow in order to reduce haloes and glares and are produced by AJL Ophthalmic, Spain. **Kerarings** are similar to Ferrara Rings and are produced by Mediphacos, Brazil.
3 **MyoRing**: This is a round ring (360°) which is inserted into a pocket created by a special keratome or by femtosecond laser at a depth of 300 μm. These rings vary in thickness between 200 and 320 μm, they were developed by Alber Daxer and are marketed by Dioptix, Austria.

ICRS implanted in keratoconic eyes improve uncorrected visual acuity (UCVA) and best spectacle corrected visual acuity (BSCVA).They also reduce myopia, regular and irregular astigmatism, high order aberrations (HOA) and regularizes the cornea. Similar results are achieved in the treatment of post LASIK and post PRK ectasia. These results have also been realized in long-term follow up [1–11]. The more advanced the KC is the greater the magnitude of effect of the ICRS is but with a lower resulting functional VA being finally achieved, whilst the reverse is true for less advanced KC. Thicker rings are more effective with smaller optical zones achieving a greater effect.

The aim of ICRS implantation in KC is not to be free of glasses or CL but to enable the patient to see better with glasses or to allow them to tolerate CL in order to prevent or delay the need for penetrating keratoplasty (PKP) or deep anterior lamellar keratoplasty (DALK).

In many cases we can achieve a functional and satisfactory UCVA with no need for glasses in patients with non-advanced KC. In many other cases the UCVA and BSCVA, though improved post ICRS implantation are unsatisfactory and further means are needed to improve them.

21.2 How to Improve VA After ICRS?

There are **non surgical and surgical** options to improve VA after ICRS.

21.2.1 Non Surgical Options

1 Glasses: All the studies mentioned above report improvement in BSCVA, unlike patients undergoing refractive surgery, glasses are welcomed by patients suffering from KC.
2 Contact lenses (CL): ICRS flatten the cornea, making it more regular hence facilitating CL tolerance in patients suffering from KC.

A study of 12 contact lens intolerant keratoconic eyes that underwent Intacs implantation with no intra- or postoperative complications found improved measures in UCVA, best corrected visual acuity (BCVA) and K readings. Eight eyes were then able to wear contact lenses [12]. Sixty percent of patients suffering from KC tolerated CL after Intacs implantation [13]. Guel et al. reported on one patient who was successfully fitted with a soft CL (SCL) after Intacs implantation for KC [14]. Most of the studies mentioned in this chapter report better tolerance of CL after ICRS. A central thickness of the SCL equal or superior to 0.4 mm seems to decrease the ocular high order aberration (HOA) and to improve the visual function in KC patients implanted with ICRS [15].

I have fitted patients following Intacs implantation with SCL, soft KC (Soft K) CL, and rigid gas-permeable (RGP) CL with no special requirements from the manufacturers of the lenses. Some patients who had been intolerant to RGPCL with unsatisfactory VA with soft CLs, achieved satisfactory VA with soft CLs. In a retrospective study of 19 patients who were intolerant to CL prior to ICRS implantation, 2 patients (10.5%) did not achieved good comfort with CL and underwent PKP, the remaining 17 patients showed good or moderate comfort after the implantation of ICRS. Four were fitted with RGP CL, one with a piggyback CL (soft CL and RGP CL over it), three with toric SCL, two with soft K CLs and seven with disposable soft lenses [16]. Piggyback CL was fitted for KC in a patient who was CL intolerant prior to ICRS implantation. The authors of this article concluded that the changes in the corneal anatomy created by the ICRS may make CL fitting more challenging due to corneal irregularity [17]. Another patient was successfully fitted with a soft CL for visual rehabilitation 5 months after Intacs placement [18].

In addition, successful fitting of a newly designed full scleral contact lens in advanced KC with previous implantation of ICRS was reported by Pinero et al. [19] and in patients who were still intolerant to corneal RGP or SCL after ICRS [20]. A Mini scleral rigid contact lens was fitted successfully in a case of advanced keratoconus after implantation of Intacs [21]. Lovisolo et al. reported on several patients who had been "absolutely contact lens intolerant" and subsequently were comfortable wearing RGP contacts on a daily basis after Intacs implantation followed by collagen corneal crosslinking (CXL). This can be explained by the regularization of the anterior corneal surface after the combined treatment [22]. Successful fitting of custom-made hydrogel silicone CL in keratoconus with ICRS has also been reported [23].

In summary ICRS implantation in KC patients promotes improved CL tolerance and thus, by extension, visual improvement.

21.2.2 Surgical Options

21.2.2.1 Re-implantation and Reposition

Under or over correction may occur following ICRS implantation. Pokroy et al. reported on Intacs surgery that required either removal, exchange, addition, or shifting of an Intacs segment in 58 keratoconic eyes. Seven eyes (over 10%) underwent surgical adjustment of intacts. The indications for Intacs adjustment were increased astigmatism in four eyes, induced hyperopia (over correction) in three eyes, and under correction in one eye. Induced astigmatism and hyperopia were usually managed by removing the superior segment whilst the under corrected eye, having initially received a single inferior segment, was treated by implanting a superior segment. This adjustment yielded good results [24].

Alio et al. reported on the visual, refractive, and corneal aberrometric outcomes in eyes with KC that had implantation of new ICRS after previous segment explantation for an unsuccessful outcome due to segment extrusion or poor visual outcomes, 21 eyes from 21 patients were evaluated. There was a significant improvement in UCVA, manifest refraction, keratometry (K) readings and corneal aberrometry analysis 6 months following the second surgery. There were no statistically significant differences in any visual, refractive, keratometric, or aberrometric parameters between eyes that had ICRS explantation for segment extrusion and eyes that had explantation for poor visual outcomes [25]. Subsequent topographic guided repositioning and/or replacement of corneal ring segments resulted in improved topographic, optical, and visual outcomes in three patients in whom the initial result of ICRS implantation was unsatisfactory [26].

21.2.2.2 Kerarings After Intacs

Coskunseven reported on three eyes (two keratoconic patients) with previous Intacs implantation that underwent adjuvant single Keraring ICRS implantation. Improvements in UCVA and BCVA with significant reductions in K readings were reported [27]. Lovisolo et al. reported on a patient who underwent LASIK in a keratoconic eye that was later implanted with four ring segments: a pair of 450 μm Intacs 2 years after excimer surgery, and a pair of 250 μm Ferrara Rings 3 years postoperatively. Eight years after the original surgery, the same eye was treated with CXL. Two years after cross-linking and 10 years after the original surgery, the eye showed topographic and refractive stability and BSCVA of 20/30. For night driving, this patient was fitted with a custom-made RGP CL resulting in 20/20 vision [22].

21.2.2.3 MyoRing After Intacs

A MyoRing was implanted in a keratoconic patient who had a residual refractive error 4 years after initial Intacs implantation. There were no intraoperative or postoperative complications. After 1 year; mean keratometric power decreased from 50.3 to 43.6 diopters (D), UCVA improved from 20/400 to 20/50, and BCVA improved from 20/200 to 20/30 [28].

21.2.2.4 Collagen Corneal Cross-Linking

The aim of CXL is to arrest the progression of KC. Since the introduction of this technique by the Dresden group hundreds of papers were published on the efficacy of this procedure in stabilizing the ectatic process both in KC and in post LASIK ectasia. Moreover, improvement of UCVA, BSCVA, reduction of astigmatism and K readings were reported in the majority of the treated eyes [29–34]. Additive effect of CXL and ISCR has been reported [35]. Better results were achieved if the ICRS were implanted first followed by CXL as opposed to the reverse sequence [36]. Ertan al evaluated the efficacy of transepithelial CXL in keratoconic eyes after Intacs implantation in 25 eyes of 17 patients with bilateral KC. Further improvement was reported in UCVA, BCVA, decrease in spherical refraction, astigmatism and K values [37]. Kamburoglu et al. similarly demonstrated the additive effect of CXL after Intacs SK in a case of post LASIK ectasia [38]. Similar results were reported by El Awady H et al. on 21 eyes of 13 patients with mild to moderate degree of KC. All eyes had implantation of Keraring followed by CXL [39].

21.2.2.5 Photorefractive Keratectomy (PRK)

PRK has been safely used to reduce astigmatism in KC and was first reported by Jes Mortensen [40, 41]. Safety and efficacy of PRK in forme fruste KC has also been reported [42, 43]. ICRS positively changes the biomechanical properties of the cornea by inducing central flattening and peripheral steepening over the rings with subsequent stress redistribution [44, 45]. CXL as a stabilizing procedure gives PRK in KC an additional protective value. Several reports demonstrate predictability, efficacy, stability and safety of PRK combined with CXL, especially if no more than 50 microns (um) are ablated [46–48]. Tan BU et al. report on PRK for the correction of residual refractive error with Intacs in place who developed myopia progression in eight eyes of five patients. At the last follow-up examination (up to 2 years), all eyes were near plano and had a final VA of 20/10–20/25. Furthermore, no delay in epithelial healing was noted. One patient had subepithelial haze in both eyes which resolved following epithelial scraping and mitomycin-C (MMC) application and PTK enhancement [49]. PRK with and without CXL is reported after ICRS in a number of different sequences, Kremer et al. reported simultaneous PRK and CXL in KC after previous femtosecond -assisted Intacs implantation. Six months later wave front-guided PRK and CXL were performed simultaneously. A significant improvement of the UCVA, BCVA, and reduction central K value was achieved [50]. ICRS implantation and CXL were performed sequentially with a 4-week interval in 17 eyes of keratoconic patients. Six months after CXL non-topography-guided PRK was performed. UCVA improved to 0.18 ± 0.06 logMAR and BCVA to 0.15 ± 0.05 logMAR. The mean spherical error and mean cylinder decreased significantly [51]. Al-Tuwairqi W et al. reported on ICRS implantation followed after 6 months (on average) by same-day topographic-guided PRK and CXL in low to moderate KC. Significant improvements were noted in UCVA (0.7 ± 0.32 logMAR vs 0.08 ± 0.08 logMAR), BCVA (0.16 ± 0.19 logMAR vs 0.02 ± 0.04 log-MAR), sphere (-3.65 ± 3.08 D vs 0.06 ± 1.6 D), astigmatism (-3.31 ± 1.5 D vs -0.98 ± 0.75 D), average K (47.28 ± 1.99 D vs 41.42 ± 3.22 D), and coma (2.36 ± 1.23 µm vs 1.47 ± 0.68 µm) ($P < 0.05$). Approximately 63% of eyes gained ≥2 lines of BCVA, whereas no change in BCVA was reported in 27% of eyes. No eyes lost lines of BCVA [52]. Coskunseven E et al. report on Topography-guided transepithelial PRK after ICRS and CXL in a three-step procedure for KC in 10 patients (16 eyes) with progressive KC. All patients underwent topography-guided transepithelial PRK after they initially had Keraring implantation and subsequent CXL. The time interval between both ICRS implantation and CXL and between CXL and topography-guided transepithelial PRK was 6 months. After the three step procedure LogMAR mean UCVA and BCVA improved from 1.14 ± 0.36 to 0.75 ± 0.24 preoperatively to 0.25 ± 0.13 and 0.13 ± 0.06 respectively. Mean spherical equivalent refraction was significantly reduced from -5.66 ± 5.63 D preoperatively to -0.98 ± 2.21 D. Mean steep and flat K values were significantly reduced from 54.65 ± 5.80 D to 47.80 ± 3.97 D preoperatively to 45.99 ± 3.12 D and 44.69 ± 3.19 D respectively [53]. Lovieno A reported on ICRS implantation followed by same-day PRK and CXL in KC in four patients (five eyes). Femtosecond laser-assisted Intacs implantation was performed, 6 months later same-day PRK and CXL were subsequently performed in all patients. Six months after Intacs plus PRK and CXL, significant improvements were noted for UCVA, BCVA, spherical equivalent refraction, K readings, and total aberrations. No patient lost any lines of BCVA or developed haze [54]. Yeung et al. reported on phototherapeutic keratectomy (PTK) combined with implantation of a single ICRS and CXL performed sequentially on the same day in the management of KC with A significant improvement in UCVA, BCVA, and the mean and steep K values. No patient lost BCVA lines [55]. Similar results and sequence of the treatments was reported on 41 eyes with a follow up of 1 year, the PRK in this group was a topography guided PRK (TG-PRK) and on combined corneal wave front-guided transepithelial PRK and high-fluence accelerated CXL after ICRS implantation [56, 57]. In addition, a separate group, demonstrated the effectiveness, safety and stabilization of KC in 11 eyes of 7 patients with progressive KC who were treated with a four-stage procedure with a minimum of 6 months between each procedure: Keraring ICRS implantation followed by CXL, phakic IOL implantation, and TG-PRK, follow-up was 12 months after TG-PRK [58].

In summary PRK combined with CXL is safe and effectively improves UCVA and BCVA. It reduces residual myopia and astigmatism following ICRS.

See Figs. 21.1a–e and 21.2a–g which summarize a combination of ICRS, PRK and CXL in three eyes of two KC patients.

21.2.3 Intraocular Lenses (IOL)

ICRS reduces astigmatism and myopia and improves corneal irregularity. However, high ametropia not correctable by glasses remains in some cases. In patients suffering from residual high ametropia and who are CL intolerant, phakic intraocular lenses (pIOLs) can be considered to correct the refractive error.

The ICRS are usually inserted 3 months before the intraocular lens [59]. Good outcomes have been reported when used in combination with both the Visian ICL and the Verisyse pIOL [60–63]. This is a reversible procedure that is less invasive than PK or DALK. Kamburoglu et al. reported on Artisan toric phakic IOL implan-

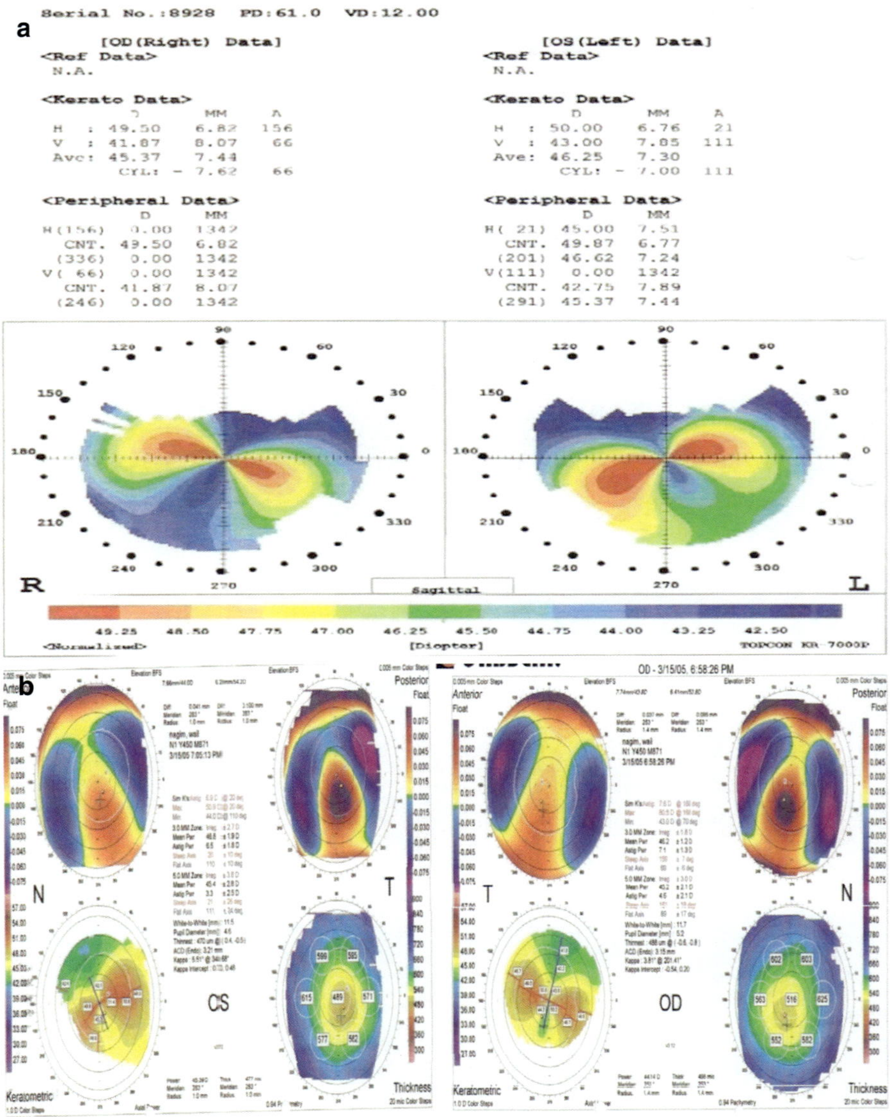

Fig. 21.1 (**a–f**) Topographies of a 26 years old male suffering from KC with astigmatism of 8.5 D in both eyes (BE) treated by single Intacs segment in BE, followed 4.5 years post operatively in right eye (RE) and 8 years in the left eye (LE) by simultaneous PRK and CXL for the correction of residual astigmatism of 5.0 D in BE, the eyes were operated in different dates, with satisfactory refractive results and no post operative complications. (**a**) Pre-operative topography showing KC in BE (Topcon KR-700, Japan). (**b**) Pre-operative Orbscan II (Bausch&Lomb USA). (**c**) Corneal topography after ICRS LE and pre-operative RE (Topcon KR-700, Japan). (**d**) Post PRK & CXL topography (Topcon, KR-700, Japan). (**e**) Topography difference map before and after PRK &CXL RE showing flattening of the cornea (TMS4, Tomey, Japan). (**f**) Topography difference map before and after PRK &CXL LE showing flattening of the cornea (TMS4, Tomey, Japan)

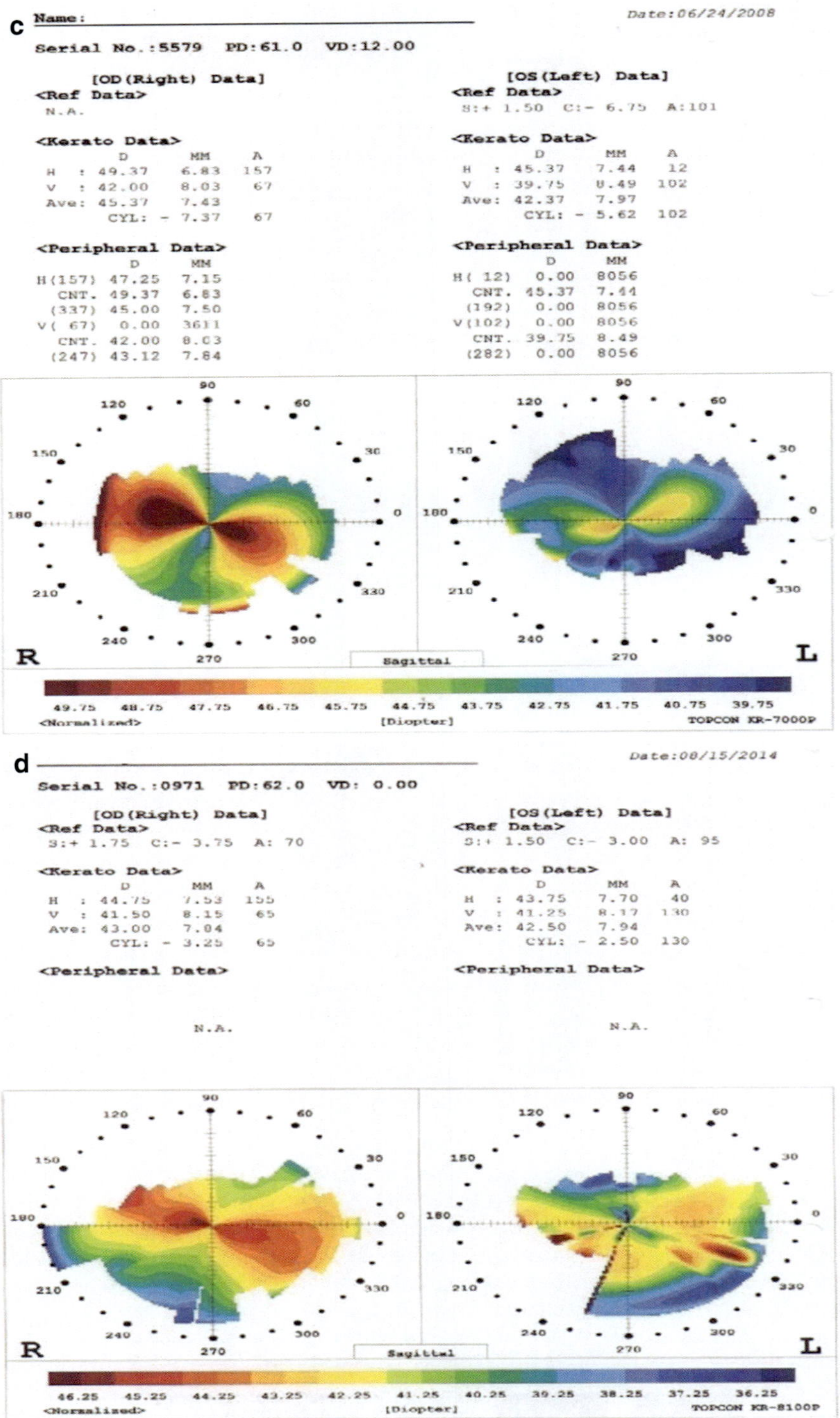

Fig. 21.1 (continued)

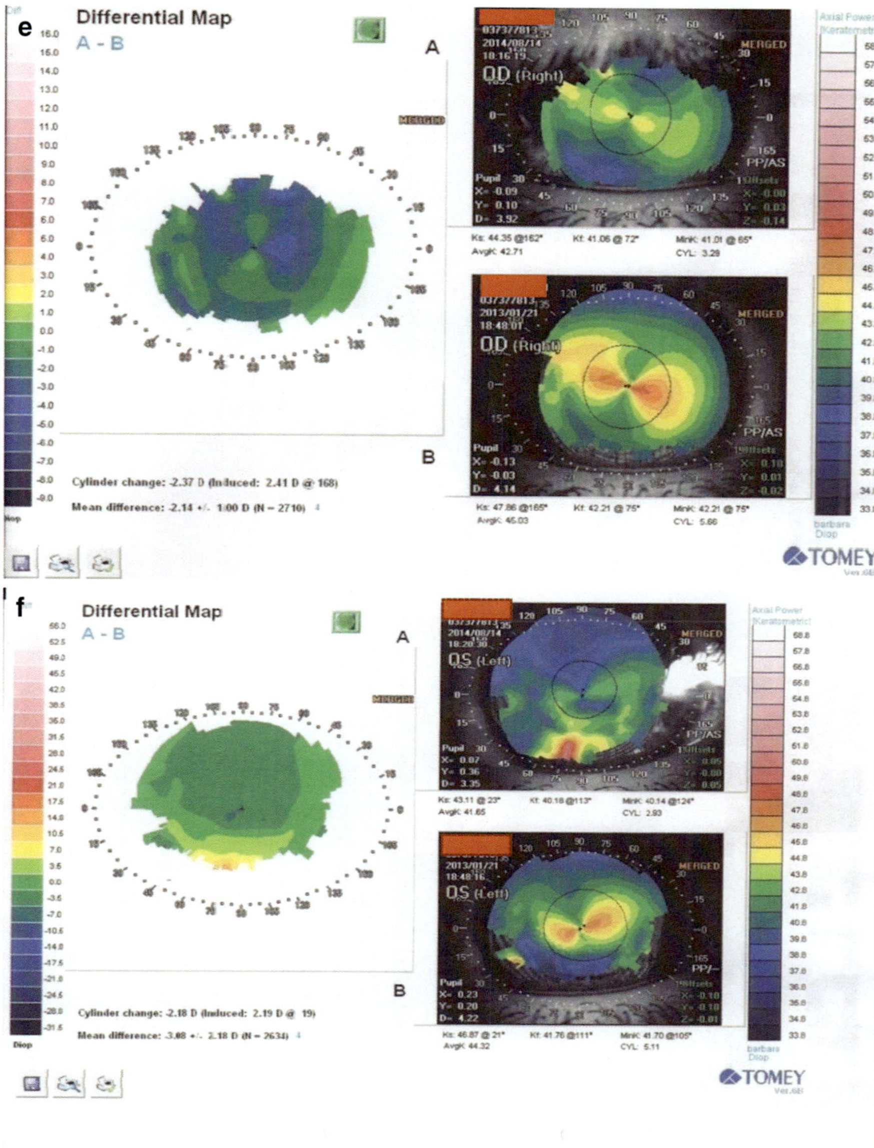

Fig. 21.1 (continued)

tation after Intacs, to correct residual myopia and astigmatism. Five months postoperatively, the UCVA was 0.6 and the BCVA was 0.7 [64]. Budo et al. implanted Artisan pIOLs in both eyes of three patients with KC. Postoperatively, four of the six eyes were within 1.00 D of emmetropia [63]. Colin and Velou implanted an anterior chamber pIOL after Intacs implantation in a patient with KC. The refractive results were satisfactory with minimal residual myopia [62].

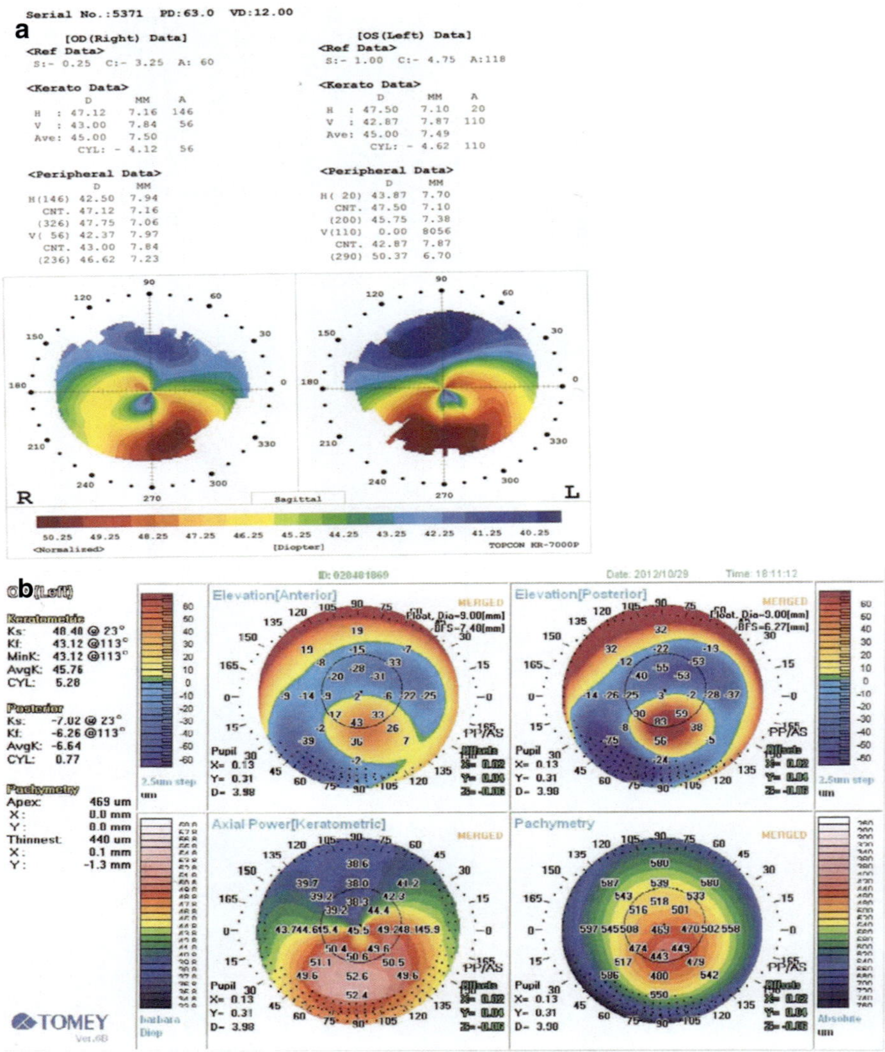

Fig. 21.2 (**a–g**) Describe the LE of a 41 years old female suffering from high astigmatism of 7.0 D because of KC, one Intacs segment was inserted, the astigmatism decreased significantly but a year later returned almost to the preoperative values, PRK and CXL were performed simultaneously the astigmatism decreased to 0.75 D and remained stable till now (February 2018) more than four years post operatively. (**a**) Pre-operative topography showing KC in BE (Topcon, KR-700, Japan). (**b**) Pre- operative topography LE (TMS 5, Tomey, Japan). (**c**) Post Intacs segment topography LE (Topcon, KR-700, Japan). (**d**) Post Intac segment topography LE (TMS5, Tomey, Japan) shows difference map on the right. (**e**) Post PRK & CXL topography LE appears also the RE which was not operated (Topcon, KR -700 Japan). (**f**) Post PRK and CXL topography and difference map LE (TMS 5, Tomey, Japan). (**g**) Colored photo of the Intacs Segment in the cornea LE

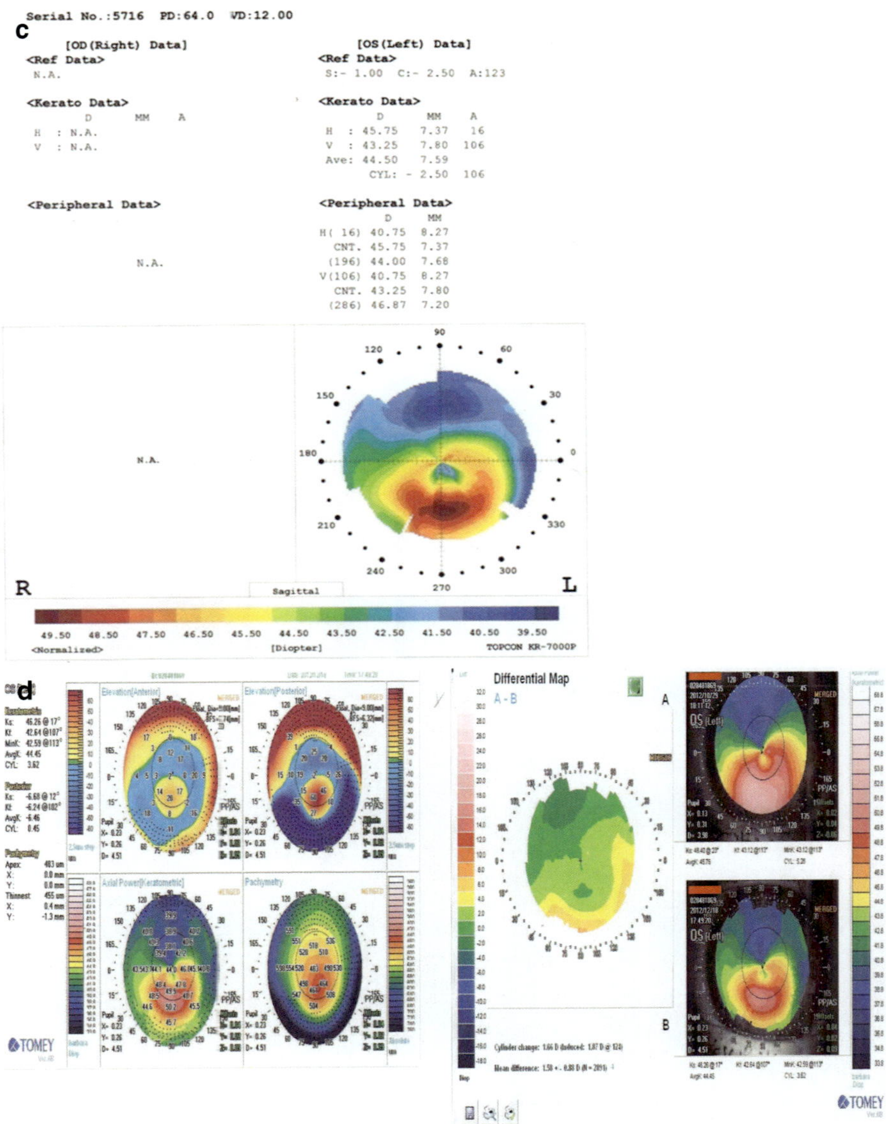

Fig. 21.2 (continued)

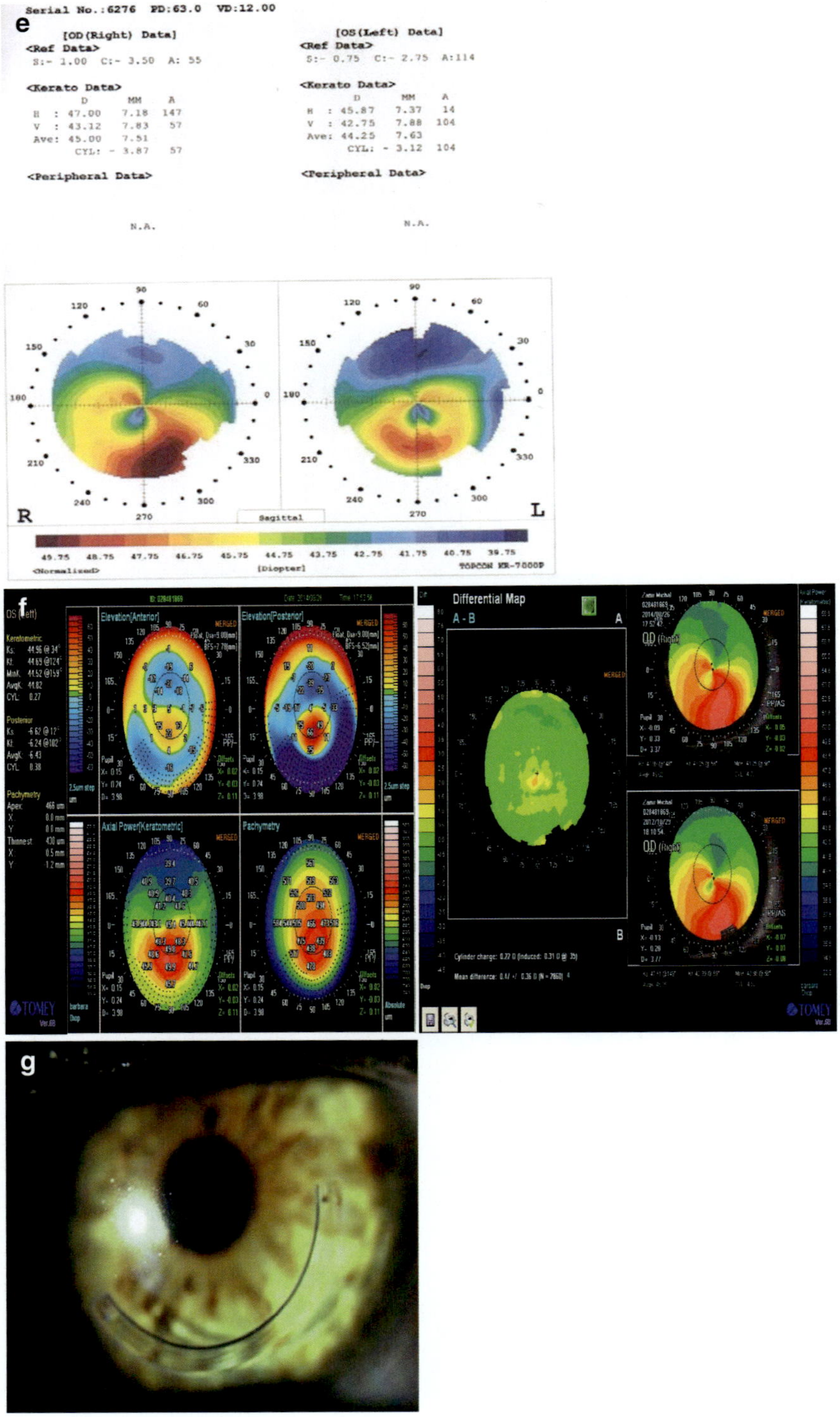

Fig. 21.2 (continued)

El-Raggal et al. conducted a 24 month follow up of eight KC eyes of six patients who had maximum K values of 60 D and underwent sequential Intacs and a Verisyse pIOL implantation for refractive improvement. All eyes achieved UCVA of 20/40 or better. The final spherical error ranged from −1.00 to +1.75 D and the cylindrical error ranged from 1.25 to 2.50 D. No eye lost lines of preoperative BCVA. These results were relatively stable throughout the follow-up period [61]. Guell et al. implanted toric phakic iris-claw Artisan IOL after Intacs implantation with positive results [65]. Moshirfar et al. conducted simultaneous or sequential implantation of Intacs and Verisyse pIOL in 5 eyes with post LASIK ectasia and 14 eyes with KC. Intacs segments were implanted followed by the insertion of a phakic Verisyse lens at the same session (12 eyes) in the "simultaneous group," or several months later (7 eyes) in the "sequential group." At the last follow-up (19 ± 6 months), there was no significant difference in mean UCVA or BSCVA between the two groups preoperatively or postoperatively. No eye lost lines of preoperative BSCVA [66].

Coşkunseven E reported on a case series of ICRS implantation followed by CXL and then toric implantable collagen copolymer pIOL implantation in 14 eyes of 9 patients. After the combined treatments, the mean UCVA and BCVA were significantly improved from 0.01 and 0.14 preoperatively to 0.44 and 0.57, respectively. The mean manifest refraction spherical equivalent decreased from −16.40 D ± 3.56 (SD) to −0.80 ± 1.02 D. The mean refractive astigmatism decreased from −4.73 ± 1.32 D to −0.96 ± 0.35 D. The mean steep and mean flat K values reduced from 60.57 D and 56.16 D to 54.48 D and 53.57 D respectively [67].

Jarade et al. describes sequential implantation of Keraring Implantable Collamer Lens, pIOL implantation and corneal relaxing incisions for refractive correction of KC [68] ICRS implantation (combined with CXL in one study) followed by posterior chamber pIOL, Visian toric ICL and toric Artisan and Artiflex IOLs, yielded improvements in UCVA and BCVA [69–72]. Impressive results with ICRS and cataract surgery has also been shown in advanced keratoconic eyes with improvement in both the UCVA and the BSCVA by eight lines [73].

The drawback of pIOLs in KC like most available treatments for KC is the lack of controlled randomized studies with long term follow-up. There is no consensus on which pIOL to implant and there is a worry about induced corneal endothelial damage through this procedure.

21.3 Summary

ICRS positively alters the corneal shape in keratoconic and post LASIK corneal ectasia eyes and reduces the irregular astigmatism, K readings, myopia, astigmatism and high order aberrations and improves UCVA and BSCVA. ICRS also modifies the biomechanical properties of the cornea and, furthermore, is amenable to visual improvement through spectacles, CLs or via surgical means including CXL, PRK and pIOLs. All these surgical techniques may be combined in a variety of sequences with good reported results. The overall aim to reach satisfactory UCVA and BCVA in order to improve the function and the quality of life of keratoconic patients and avoid keratoplasty.

References

1. Colin J. European clinical evaluation: use of Intacs prescription inserts for the treatment of keratoconus. J Cataract Refract Surg. 2006;32:747–55.
2. Kymionis GD, Bouzoukis DI, Portaliou DM, Pallikaris IG. New INTACS SK implantation in patients with post-laser in situ keratomileusis corneal ectasia. Cornea. 2010;29(2):214.
3. Kymionis GD, Siganos CS, Tsiklis NS, et al. Long-term follow-up of Intacs in keratoconus. Am J Ophthalmol. 2007;143:236–44.
4. Kymionis GD, Tsiklis NS, Pallikaris AI, Kounis G, Diakonis VF, Astyrakakis N, et al. Long-term follow-up of Intacs for post-LASIK corneal ectasia. Ophthalmology. 2006;113(11):1909.
5. Kymionis GD, Grentzelos MA, Diakonis VF, Pallikaris AI, Pallikaris I. Nine-year follow-up of Intacs implantation for keratoconus. Open Ophthalmol J. 2009;8(3):77–81.
6. Barbara R, Zadok D, Pikkel J, Marcovich A, Garzozi H, Nasser O, Lamis Abdelaziz AB. Collagen corneal cross-linking followed by Intac implantation in a case of post-PRK ectasia. Int J Keratoconus Ectatic Corneal Dis. 2012;1:68–72.
7. Salgado-Borges JM, Costa-Ferreira C, Monteiro M, Guilherme-Monteiro J, Torquetti L. Refractive, tomographic and biomechanical outcomes after implantation of Ferrara ICRS in Keratoconus patients. 2012;1(1):16–21.
8. Kwitko S, Severo NS. Ferrara intracorneal ring segments for keratoconus. J Cataract Refract Surg. 2004;30(4):812–20.
9. Salgado-Borges JM, Costa-Ferreira C, Monteiro M, Guilherme-Monteiro J, Torquetti L, Ferrara P, Ambrósio R Jr. Refractive and tomographic and biomechanical outcomes after implantation of Ferrara ICRS in Keratoconus patients. Int J Keratoconus Ectatic Corneal Dis. 2012;1(1):16–21.
10. Pesando PM, Ghiringhello MP, Di Meglio G, Romeo S. Treatment of keratoconus with Ferrara ICRS and consideration of the efficacy of the Ferrara nomogram in a 5-year follow-up. Eur J Ophthalmol. 2010;20(5):865.
11. Barbara A, Barbara R. Long-term follow-up of Ferrara rings segments for the treatment of Keratoconus. 2013;2(1):34–9.
12. Shetty R, Narayana KM, Mathew K, Anand D, Mhaske P, Shetty B. Safety and efficacy of Intacs in Indian eyes with keratoconus: an initial report. Indian J Ophthalmol. 2009;57(2):115–9.
13. Shetty R, Kurian M, Anand D, Mhaske P, Narayana KM, Shetty B. Intacs in advanced keratoconus. Cornea. 2008;27:1022–9.
14. Güell JL, Morral M, Salinas C, Elies D, Gris O, Manero F. Four-year follow-up of intrastraomal corneal ring segments in patients with keratoconus. J Emmetropia. 2010;1:9–15.
15. Carracedo G, Canales J, Gonzalez P, Recchioni A, Carpena-Torres C, Carballo-Álvarez J. The effect of soft contact lens thickness in visual function after intracorneal ring segments surgery. Contact Lens Anterior Eye [Internet]. 2017. [Cited 2018 Feb 11]. Available from: http://www.ncbi.nlm.nih.gov/pubmed/28993070.
16. Moreira LB, Bardal RAC, Crisigiovanni LR. Contact lenses fitting after intracorneal ring segments implantation in keratoconus. Arq Bras Oftalmol. 2013;76(4):215–7.
17. Hladun L, Harris M. Contact lens fitting over intrastromal corneal rings in a keratoconic patient. Optometry. 2004;75(1):48–54.
18. Uçakhan OO, Kanpolat A, Ozdemir O. Contact lens fitting for keratoconus after Intacs placement. Eye Contact Lens 2. 2006;32(2):75–7.
19. Piñero Llorens DP. Fitting of a new design of full scleral contact lens in advanced keratoconus with previous implantation of intracorneal ring segments. Int J Kerat Ect Cor Dis. 2015;4(2):56–9.
20. Rathi VM, Mandathara PS, Dumpati S, Sangwan VS. Scleral lens after intracorneal ring segments in patients with keratoconus. Contact Lens Anterior Eye [Internet]. 2017. [Cited 2018 Feb 11]. Available from: http://www.ncbi.nlm.nih.gov/pubmed/29074305.
21. Dalton K, Sorbara L. Fitting an MSD (mini scleral design) rigid contact lens in advanced keratoconus with INTACS. Contact Lens Anterior Eye. 2011;34(6):274–81.

22. Lovisolo CF, Mularoni A, Mazzolani F. Combining INTACS implantation with other refractive and non-refractive procedures. J Emmetropia. 2010;1(3):148–63.
23. Fernández-Velázquez FJ, Fernández-Fidalgo MJ. Feasibility of custom-made hydrogel contact lenses in keratoconus with previous implantation of intracorneal ring segments. Contact Lens Anterior Eye [Internet]. 2015 [cited 2018 Feb 11];38(5):351–6. Available from: http://www.ncbi.nlm.nih.gov/pubmed/26055226.
24. Pokroy R, Levinger S. Intacs adjustment surgery for keratoconus. J Cataract Refract Surg. 2006;32:986–92.
25. Alió JL, Piñero DP, Söğütlü E, Kubaloglu A. Implantation of new intracorneal ring segments after segment explantation for unsuccessful outcomes in eyes with keratoconus. J Cataract Refract Surg. 2010;36:1303–10.
26. Chan K, Hersh PS. Removal and repositioning of intracorneal ring segments. Cornea [Internet]. 2017 [cited 2018 Feb 11];36(2):244–8. Available from: http://content.wkhealth.com/linkback/openurl?sid=WKPTLP:landingpage&an=00003226-201702000-00019.
27. Coskunseven E, Kymionis GD, Grentzelos MA, Karavitaki AE, Portaliou DM, Jankov MR 2nd, et al. INTACS followed by KeraRing intrastromal corneal ring segment implantation for keratoconus. J Refract Surg (Thorofare, NJ 1995). 2010;26(5):371–4.
28. Behrouz MJ, Hashemian H, Khodaparast M, Rad ASS. Intacs followed by MyoRing implantation in severe keratoconus. J Cataract Refract Surg. 2013;29(5):364–6.
29. Samaras KE, Lake DB. Corneal collagen cross linking (CXL): a review. Int Ophthalmol Clin. 2010;50(3):89–100.
30. Zhang Z-Y, Zhang X-R. Efficacy and safety of transepithelial corneal collagen crosslinking. J Cataract Refract Surg [Internet]. 2012 [cited 2012 Oct 12];38(7):1304; author reply 1304–5. Available from: http://www.ncbi.nlm.nih.gov/pubmed/22727312.
31. Boxer Wachler BS, Pinelli R, Ertan A, Chan CCK, Baiocchi S, Mazzotta C, et al. Safety and efficacy of transepithelial crosslinking (C3-R/CXL). J Cataract Refract Surg. 2010;36(1):186–9.
32. Spoerl E, Mrochen M, Sliney D, Trokel S, Seiler T. Safety of UVA-riboflavin cross-linking of the cornea. Cornea. 2007;26(4):385–9.
33. Wollensak G, Spoerl E, Seiler T. Riboflavin/ultraviolet-A – induced collagen crosslinking for the treatment of keratoconus. Am J Ophthalmol. 2003;135(5):620–7.
34. Hafezi F, Kanellopoulos J, Wiltfang R, Seiler T. Corneal collagen crosslinking with riboflavin and ultraviolet A to treat induced keratectasia after laser in situ keratomileusis. J Cataract Refract Surg. 2007;33(12):2035–40.
35. Vicente LL, Boxer Wachler B. Factors that correlate with improvement in vision after combined Intacs and trans-epithelial corneal crosslinking. Br J Ophthalmol. 2010;94(12):1597–601.
36. Coskunseven E, Jankov MR, Hafezi F, Atun S, Arslan E, Kymionis GD. Effect of treatment sequence in combined intrastromal corneal rings and corneal collagen crosslinking for keratoconus. J Cataract Refract Surg. 2009;35(12):2084–91.
37. Ertan A, Karacal H, Kamburoglu G. Refractive and topographic results of transepithelial cross-linking treatment in eyes with intacs. Cornea. 2009;28(7):719–23.
38. Kamburoglu G, Ertan A. Intacs implantation with sequential collagen cross-linking treatment in postoperative LASIK ectasia. J Refract Surg. 2008;24(7):726.
39. El Awady H, Shawky M, Ghanem AA. Evaluation of collagen crosslinking in keratoconus eyes with Kera intracorneal ring implantation. Eur J Ophthalmol. 2012;22(Suppl 7):S62–8.
40. Mortensen J, Ohrström A. Excimer laser photorefractive keratectomy for treatment of keratoconus. J Refract Surg. 1994;10:368–74.
41. Mortensen J, Carlsson K, Öhrstrom A. Excimer laser surgery for keratoconus. J Cataract Refract Surg. 1998;24(7):893–8.
42. Koller T, Iseli HP, Donitzky C, Papadopoulos N, Seiler T, et al. Topography-guided surface ablation for forme fruste keratoconus. Ophthalmology. 2006;113(12):2198–202.
43. Alpins N, Stamatelatos G. Customized photoastigmatic refractive keratectomy using combined topographic and refractive data for myopia and astigmatism in eyes with forme fruste and mild keratoconus. J Cataract Refract Surg. 2007;33(4):591–602.

44. Dauwe C, Touboul D, Roberts CJ, Mahmoud AM, Kérautret J, Fournier P, et al. Biomechanical and morphological corneal response to placement of intrastromal corneal ring segments for keratoconus. J Cataract Refract Surg. 2009;35(10):1761–7.
45. Barbara A, editor. Textbook of Keratoconus, new insights. 1st ed. New Delhi: Jaypee Brothers Medical Pub; 2011. 30 p
46. Kymionis GD, Kontadakis GA, Kounis GA, Portaliou DM, Karavitaki AE, Magarakis M, et al. Simultaneous topography-guided PRK followed by corneal collagen cross-linking for keratoconus. J Refract Surg. 2009;25(9):807.
47. Kanellopoulos AJ. Short and long term complications of combined topography guided PRK and CXL (the Athens Protocol) in 412 keratoconus eyes (2–7 years follow-up). Invest Ophthalmol Vis Sci. 2101;52(14).
48. Kankariya V, Kymionis G, Kontadakis G, Yoo S. Update on simultaneous topo-guided photorefractive keratectomy immediately followed by corneal collagen cross-linking for treatment of progressive Keratoconus. 2102;1(3):185–9.
49. Tan BU, Purcell TL, Nalgirkar A, Ehrenhaus MP, Torres LF, Schanzlin DJ. Photorefractive keratectomy for the correction of residual refractive error with Intacs intrastromal corneal ring segments in place. J Cataract Refract Surg. 2008;34(6):909–15.
50. Kremer I, Aizenman I, Lichter H, Shayer S, Levinger S. Simultaneous wavefront-guided photorefractive keratectomy and corneal collagen crosslinking after intrastromal corneal ring segment implantation for keratoconus. J Cataract Refract Surg. 2012;38(10):1802–7.
51. Khoueir Z, Chertan G, Jarade E. Non-topographyguided photorefractive keratectomy for the correction of residual mild refractive errors after IGRS implantation and CXL in keratoconus. J Refract Surg. 2014;30(4):266–71.
52. Al-Tuwairqi W, Sinjab MM. Intracorneal ring segments implantation followed by same-day topography-guided PRK and corneal collagen CXL in low to moderate keratoconus. J Refract Surg. 2013;29(1):59–63.
53. Coskunseven E, Jankov MR, Grentzelos MA, Plaka AD, Limnopoulou AN, Kymionis GD. Topography-guided transepithelial PRK after intracorneal ring segments implantation and corneal collagen CXL in a three-step procedure for keratoconus. J Refract Surg. 2013;29(1):54–8.
54. Iovieno A, Legare ME, Rootman DB, Yeung SN, Kim P, Rootman DS. Intracorneal ring segments implantation followed by same-day photorefractive keratectomy and corneal collagen cross-linking in keratoconus. J Refract Surg (Thorofare, NJ 1995). 2011;27(12):915–8.
55. Yeung SN, Low SAW, Ku JYF, Lichtinger A, Kim P, Teichman J, et al. Transepithelial phototherapeutic keratectomy combined with implantation of a single inferior intrastromal corneal ring segment and collagen crosslinking in keratoconus. J Cataract Refract Surg. 2013;39(8):1152–6.
56. Al-Tuwairqi WS, Osuagwu UL, Razzouk H, Ogbuehi KC. One-year clinical outcomes of a two-step surgical management for keratoconus—topography-guided photorefractive keratectomy/cross-linking after intrastromal corneal ring implantation. Eye Contact Lens Sci Clin Pract [Internet]. 2015 [cited 2018 Feb 11];41(6):359–66. Available from: http://www.ncbi.nlm.nih.gov/pubmed/25839343.
57. Lee H, Kang DSY, Ha BJ, Choi JY, Kim EK, Seo KY, et al. Visual rehabilitation in moderate keratoconus: combined corneal wavefront-guided transepithelial photorefractive keratectomy and high-fluence accelerated corneal collagen cross-linking after intracorneal ring segment implantation. BMC Ophthalmol [Internet]. 2017 [cited 2018 Feb 11];17(1):270. Available from: http://www.ncbi.nlm.nih.gov/pubmed/29284455.
58. Coskunseven E, Sharma DP, Grentzelos MA, Sahin O, Kymionis GD, Pallikaris I. Four-stage procedure for keratoconus: ICRS implantation, corneal cross-linking, toric phakic intraocular lens implantation, and topography-guided photorefractive keratectomy. J Refract Surg [Internet]. 2017 [cited 2018 Feb 11];33(10):683–9. Available from: http://www.ncbi.nlm.nih.gov/pubmed/28991336.
59. Rabinowitz YS. Intacs for keratoconus. Int Ophthalmol Clin. 2010;50(3):63–7.

60. Piñero DP, Alió JL, El Kady B, et al. Corneal aberrometric and refractive performance of 2 intrastromal corneal ring segment models in early and moderate ectatic disease. J Cataract Refract Surg. 2010;36:102–9.
61. El-Raggal TM, Abdel Fattah A. Sequential intacs and verisyse phakic intraocular lens for refractive improvement in keratoconic eyes. J Cataract Refract Surg. 2007;33:966–70.
62. Colin J, Velou S. Implantation of Intacs and a refractive intraocular lens to correct keratoconus. J Cataract Refract Surg. 2003;29:832–4.
63. Budo C, Bartels MC, van Rij G. Implantation of Artisan toric phakic intraocular lenses for the correction of astigmatism and spherical errors in patients with keratoconus. J Refract Surg. 2005;21:218–22.
64. Kamburoglu G, Ertan A, Bahadir M. Implantation of Artisan toric phakic intraocular lens following intacs in a patient with keratoconus. J Cataract Refract Surg. 2007;33:528–30.
65. Güell JL, Morral M, Salinas C, Elies D, Gris O, Manero F. Four-year follow-up of intrastromal corneal ring segments in patients with keratoconus. J Emmetropia. 2010;1:9–15.
66. Moshirfar MF, Carlton R, Meyer JJ, Neuffer MC, Espandar L, Mifflin M. Simultaneous and sequential implantation of intacs and verisyse phakic intraocular lens for refractive improvement in keratectasia Cornea. 2011;30(2):158–63.
67. Coşkunseven E, Sharma DP, Jankov MR 2nd, Kymionis GD, Richoz O, Hafezi F. Collagen copolymer toric phakic intraocular lens for residual myopic astigmatism after intrastromal corneal ring segment implantation and corneal collagen crosslinking in a 3-stage procedure for keratoconus. J Cataract Refract Surg. 2013;39(5):722–9.
68. Jarade E, Dirani A, Fadlallah A, Khoueir Z, Antoun JC. Sequential implantation of Keraring intrastromal corneal ring segments (ICRS) and an Implantable Collamer Lens phakic with corneal relaxing incisions for refractive correction of keratoconus. J Cataract Refract Surg. 2013;29(7):444.
69. Alfonso JF, Lisa C, Fernández-Vega L, Madrid-Costa D, Poo-López A, Montés-Micó R. Intrastromal corneal ring segments and posterior chamber phakic intraocular lens implantation for keratoconus correction. J Cataract Refract Surg. 2011;37(4):706–13.
70. Abdelmassih Y, el-Khoury S, Chelala E, Slim E, Cherfan CG, Jarade E. Toric ICL implantation after sequential intracorneal ring segments implantation and corneal cross-linking in keratoconus: 2-year follow-up. J Refract Surg [Internet]. 2017 [cited 2018 Feb 12];33(9):610–6. Available from: http://www.ncbi.nlm.nih.gov/pubmed/28880336.
71. Dirani A, Fadlallah A, Khoueir Z, Antoun J, Cherfan G, Jarade E. Visian toric ICL implantation after intracorneal ring segments implantation and corneal collagen crosslinking in keratoconus. Eur J Ophthalmol [Internet]. 2014 [cited 2018 Feb 11];24(3):338–44. Available from: http://www.ncbi.nlm.nih.gov/pubmed/24242218.
72. Ferreira TB, Güell JL, Manero F. Combined intracorneal ring segments and iris-fixated phakic intraocular lens for keratoconus refractive and visual improvement. J Refract Surg [Internet]. 2014 [cited 2018 Feb 11];30(5):336–41. Available from: http://www.ncbi.nlm.nih.gov/pubmed/24654875.
73. Lee SJ, Kwon HS, Koh I. Sequential intrastromal corneal ring implantation and cataract surgery in a severe keratoconus patient with cataract. Korean J Ophthalmol. 2012;26(3):226–9.

Chapter 22 Phakic Intraocular Lens Implantation in Keratoconus

Yonit Krakauer and Tova Lifshitz

22.1 Introduction

Surgical correction of refractive errors in patients with keratoconus remains challenging. Spectacles and contact lenses are the usual optical treatment in the early stages of keratoconus. As the disease progresses, it is usually associated with significant astigmatism and often accompanied by myopia. In the more advanced cases with high corneal astigmatism and stromal opacity, patients may not tolerate contact lenses or there may be no improvement in visual acuity with contact lenses, therefore, many patients with keratoconus may seek refractive procedures.

In patients with still transparent corneas but significant ametropia, less invasive surgical options to delay the need for penetrating keratoplasty (PK) or deep anterior lamellar keratoplasty (DALK) might be considered. Photorefractive keratectomy and laser-assisted in situ keratomileusis were usually considered contraindicated as they may worsen the disease by further thinning the cornea. Topo-guided photorefractive keratectomy (PRK) and Intrastromal corneal rings can reshape the cornea but correct only a small amount of myopia. Despite the encouraging results after intrastromal corneal rings implantation in keratoconic patients, the predictability of such an approach is still low [1]. Collagen crosslinking using riboflavin and ultraviolet light is performed to stabilize or slow the progression of keratoconus. However, regardless of initial promising results, long-term results and safety should be further evaluated [2, 3].

The use of special intraocular lens (IOL) in patients with non progressive keratoconus is a relatively recent development in refractive surgery, with still only a few published articles till date. Long-term outcomes are unknown and data are still

The authors have no proprietary interest in any of the materials or techniques used in this study.

Y. Krakauer (✉) · T. Lifshitz
Department of Ophthalmology, Soroka University Medical Center, Ben-Gurion University of the Negev, Beer-Sheva, Israel

A. Barbara (ed.), *Controversies in the Management of Keratoconus*,
https://doi.org/10.1007/978-3-319-98032-4_22

limited. However, compared to PK or DALK for keratoconus, IOLs are less invasive and less technically demanding, and can result in faster recovery of vision, optimal centration within the eye, and maximization of visual quality and exempts of the risk of complications associated with PK or DALK.

This book chapter aims to review the reports on phakic IOLs (pIOL) in patients with keratoconus: pIOLs (angle-supported phakic IOLs, iris-fixated phakic IOLs, and posterior chamber phakic IOLs), refractive lens exchange (with or without toric IOLs) and sequential surgery (intrastromal corneal ring/PRK and phakic IOLs).

A search of the PubMed database 1966–December 2017 was conducted using various combinations of the key words keratoconus, keratoconic, intraocular lens, phakic intraocular lens, phakic, toric, refractive lens exchange, treatment, management, refractive. Articles in all languages were considered, provided that the non-English articles included English abstracts. Relevant articles that were cited in the reference lists of the retrieved articles were also included.

22.2 Angle-Supported Anterior Chamber Phakic IOL

Angle-supported phakic IOLs have been used around three decades for the correction of high myopia [4, 5]. The first report on the use of angle-supported phakic IOL in patients with keratoconus and myopia was published by Leccisotti in 2003 [6]. Leccisotti & Fields described their experience with the ZSAL-4 (Morcher GmbH) IOL, which is angle-supported, plano-concave, polymethyl methacrylate (PMMA), and single piece IOL with two Z-shaped haptics. Twelve consecutive eyes of eight patients with stage I to II keratoconus, myopia from −6.50 to −14.00 diopters (D), and astigmatism from −1.00 to −5.00 D were included. The minimum follow-up was 12 months. Only the manifest spherical component was considered for IOL power calculation, targeting myopic rather than mixed astigmatism. The IOL power was calculated by the van der Heijde formula [7]. The overall IOL diameter was calculated by adding 1.0 mm to the horizontal (white-to-white) corneal diameter, which was determined by videokeratography. The spherical error in all cases was corrected within ±1.00 D. Astigmatism magnitude did not significantly improve. The uncorrected visual acuity (UCVA) was 20/40 or better in all cases. The best spectacle-corrected visual acuity (BSCVA) was equal or improved in all cases. The safety index (postoperative BSCVA/preoperative BSCVA) was 1.18; the efficacy index (postoperative UCVA/preoperative BSCVA) was 0.77. Three eyes had significant halos that improved considerably over 3 months. Spectacles were permanently used by one patient (two eyes in the study) and only for driving by five patients. Complications were limited to three cases of mild pupil ovalization and one case of IOL rotation. Endothelial loss at 12 months was 7.2%.

On 2015, Assaf and Kotb [8] published their experience with Simultaneous corneal crosslinking and surface ablation combined with phakic intraocular lens implantation for managing keratoconus. This was a prospective non-randomized study on 22 keratoconic eyes with stage I to III keratoconus and a clear central cornea. Follow-up interval was at least 6 months.

The procedure included simultaneous topography-guided photorefractive keratectomy (PRK) and crosslinking (Athens protocol) followed by (2–4 months later) phakic IOL implantation. Eight eyes were implanted with the angle-supported "Cachet" phakic IOL and the rest of the eyes were implanted with an iris claw IOL (VeriFlexTM).

The mean preoperative K (45.57 ± 1.51 D) was significantly reduced at 3 months (44.07 ± 1.88 D) and at 6 months after the procedure (43.82 ± 1.98 D, P\0.001). The mean UDVA (logMAR) improved from 1.03 ± 0.24 preoperatively to 0.37 ± 0.08 postoperatively (P = 0.001). The mean CDVA (logMAR) improved from 0.69 ± 0.3 preoperatively to 0.35 ± 0.01 postoperatively (P = 0.001). The mean SE was significantly reduced from −9.08 ± 2.5 to −0.69 ± 0.67 D, P = 0.001. No complications occurred according to their report. Central corneal haze was noted in some eyes after the procedure, but this gradually faded over 3 months. No significant decrease in the central endothelial cell count was reported throughout the follow-up period ($P > 0.05$).

Risks specific to angle-supported PIOL implantation are corneal endothelial cell loss, chronically elevated intraocular pressure, and subclinical intraocular inflammation. The longest follow-up study on angle-supported phakic IOL in non-keratoconic eyes to date, published in 2007, was performed over 12 years after implantation of the ZB5M lens in 225 eyes [9]. Regarding on endothelial cell density, there was an initial 10.6% reduction noted in the first year, followed by a mean annual rate of decrease of 1.78%. Other complications included pupil ovalization in 78 eyes (34.7%), and bilateral hypertensive uveitis (1.33%).

With the advent of foldable models such as the Kelman Duet phakic IOL (Tekia, Inc.) and the AcrySof Cachet phakic IOL (Alcon, Inc.), PMMA angle-supported pIOLs have been almost abandoned. To the best of our knowledge there are still no reports on foldable phakic angle-supported IOLs in keratoconus.

The results of a 5 year follow up after the implantation of the Acrysof Cachet pIOL in 515 non keratoconic eyes with moderate to high myopia prospective, multicenter European clinical study, were published on 2016 [10]. Mean UDVA in all eyes was 20/20, with 94.7% of eyes having a UDVA of 20/40 or less or better. All incidences of CDVA loss of more than two lines after 3 months were considered to be unrelated to the pIOL and were attributed to nuclear cataract (n = 2), irregular astigmatism (n = 1), patient fatigue (n = 1), and branch vein occlusion (n = 1).

The pIOL achieved good predictability and stability of manifest refraction spherical equivalent (MRSE) through postoperative year 5. Five years after surgery, mean MRSE ± SD was −0.34 ± 0.57 D (range −2.50 to 1.63 D). Most eyes (89.8%) had an MRSE within ±1.00 D of their target refractive error at year 5. No eyes had a surgically induced astigmatism of more than 2.00 D at year 5. Through year 5, the most frequently reported serious adverse events included adhesions between the cornea and the iris (synechiae; 4.9%), secondary surgical intervention (4.1%), cataract formation (3.1%), and elevated intraocular pressure (IOP) that required treatment (2.5%). Between the 6-month and 5-year visits, the mean annualized percentage change in central ECD was −1.3%.

22.3 Iris-Fixated Anterior Chamber Phakic IOL

The iris-supported phakic IOL, Artisan, was developed by Ophtec BV in 1991 and brought to the United States as the Verisyse pIOL by Advanced Medical Optics, Inc. (Santa Ana, CA, USA). The Artisan toric phakic IOL is available in powers ranging from +12.0 to −23.5 D in 0.5 D increments, with additional cylinder from +1.0 to +7.0 D in 0.5 D increments. The Artisan toric phakic IOL is made or Perspex CQ-UV PMMA with ultraviolet filtration. Its overall diameter is 8.5 mm and the optical zone diameter is 5.0 mm. Two models are available: in model A the axis runs through the claws (0°), and in model B the axis is perpendicular to the line that runs through the claws (90°). Complications of Artisan pIOL implantation include the potential for endothelial cell damage, cataract formation, glare, disengagement of the haptics, pigmentary dispersion, and a large corneal incision [11].

The evolution in Refractive Surgery with the wish of using smaller incisions have led to the development of a foldable iris-fixated pIOL type in 2005 which is the Artiflex. It has the advantage over the Artisan pIOL of fitting through a smaller incision size (3.2 mm), thus leading to a decrease in surgically induced astigmatism. Combining the toric technology with this foldable Artiflex pIOL resulted in the creation of the Artiflex Toric. It is a three-piece lens that consists of a flexible, cylindrical 6-mm optic made of ultraviolet-absorbing silicone and two rigid haptics made of PMMA. It is available in spherical powers of −1.0 to −13.5 diopters (D) (in increments of 0.50 D) and cylindrical powers of −1.0 to −5.0 D (in increments of 0.50 D) [12].

Budo et al. [13] reported in 2015 the use of the Artisan lens in three contact lens intolerant patients (six eyes) with keratoconus and clear central corneas. Follow-up ranged from 6 months to 1 year. Postoperative BSCVA was stable from 6 weeks onward and improved in five eyes and remained unchanged in one eye. The safety index was 1.49 and the efficacy index as 1.24. Mean preoperative spherical equivalent (SE) refraction was −13.88 D (range −4.00 to −29.00 D). Mean SE refraction postoperatively was −0.29 D (range +1.00 to −2.00 D). Postoperatively, four of the six eyes were within ±1.00 D of emmetropia. The average magnitude of refractive astigmatism was −3.75 D preoperatively and −1.33 D postoperatively. The reduction in the spherical component of refraction was higher (87.4%) than the reduction in astigmatic error (64.5%), suggesting higher predictability for spherical errors than for astigmatic errors. The average incision-induced cylinder was 1.14 D (range 0.28–3.00 D), and it contributed to the poor predictability of the final outcomes. Endothelial cell count was available at only 6 weeks postoperatively; no endothelial cell loss was observed.

Moshirfar et al. [14] reported the use of the Verisyse non toric phakic IOL (model 204, with an optical zone of 6 mm) in two patients (two eyes) with stable keratoconus and high myopia (−15.25 + 2.50 × 80° and −11.75 + 5.00 × 160°). Both patients had a postoperative UCVA of 20/40. Implanting the Verisyse pIOL was effective in correcting the SE to +0.75 D and +2.13 D. The authors used the van der Heijde formula to select the proper IOL power in these keratoconic patients. Based on their findings, they suggested that IOL selection for emmetropia in keratoconic eyes with high levels of astigmatism may lead to hyperopia. Endothelial cell density showed at most a 4% decrease, and no evidence of keratoconus progression was witnessed.

Venter [15] reported in 2009 a case series on Artisan phakic IOL (toric or myopic) in 18 keratoconic eyes (11 patients). Follow-up period was of 1 year. Preoperative manifest refractive sphere was −4.64 ± 2.74 D (range: −9.75 to 0.00 D) and cylinder was −3.07 ± 2.04 D (range: −7.75 to −0.50 D). The mean manifest refraction spherical equivalent (MRSE) was −0.46 ± 0.60 D (range: −1.88 to 0.13 D). Twenty-two percent (4/18) of eyes had UCVA of 1.0 or better and 94% (17/18) of eyes had a UCVA of 0.63 or better. Sixty-one percent (11/18) of eyes had an MRSE within ±0.50 D of the intended correction, and 72% (13/18) of eyes gained one or more lines of BSCVA and no eyes lost lines of BSCVA. The authors suggested that the increase in BSCVA reported in their study is likely due to the optical effect of implanting the Artisan phakic IOL within the optical system of the eye rather than correction at the spectacle plane. Implantation of an IOL causes magnification on the retina and a decrease in spot size, which can increase BSCVA. Mean endothelial cell counts decreased by 23 cells/mm^2 at 6 months postoperatively.

In 2011 Izquierdo et al. [16] published an article which described the use of Artiflex IOL implantation after Corneal Collagen Cross-linking in keratoconic eyes. This prospective, comparative study, included 11 eyes with stage I–II keratoconus, with no corneal opacities, anterior chamber depth >3.2 mm, spherical equivalent refraction >4.50 diopters (D) (with a cylinder component <2.00 D), and no other treatment for keratoconus other than contact lens. Each patient underwent CXL in the keratoconic eye followed by implantation of an Artiflex IOL 6 months thereafter. Mean preoperative UDVA was 1.40 ± 0.40 logMAR. Postoperative UDVA 6 months after CXL was 1.16 ± 0.46 logMAR and 0.16 ± 0.06 logMAR 6 months after Artiflex pIOL implantation, which shows a statistically significant reduction between the pre- and postoperative follow-up periods (P = .04 and P < .001, respectively). Compared with preoperative UDVA, a postoperative (6 months after Artiflex implantation) UDVA gain of five or more lines was found in 11 (100%) eyes. All eyes achieved 20/40 or better 6 months after last treatment. Mean preoperative CDVA was 0.14 ± 0.06 logMAR and CDVA at 6 months after Artiflex implantation was 0.04 ± 0.05 logMAR, which was statistically significant compared with the preoperative value (P < .001). Compared with preoperative levels, the mean spherical value decreased 0.45 D and 5.43 D 6 months after CXL and Artiflex implantation, respectively, which was statistically significant (P = .03 and P < .001, respectively). In terms of the cylinder value, a statistically significant reduction of 0.55 D 6 months after Artiflex implantation was observed (P = .04). Mean preoperative central endothelial cell count was 2759.64 ± 159.84 cells/mm^2. Postoperative central endothelial cell count 6 months after CXL was 2739.09 ± 156.99 cells/mm^2, which was not statistically significant (*P* = .46), and 6 months after Artiflex pIOL implantation was 2668.82 ± 133.17 cells/mm^2, which was statistically significant (P = .03). There were no intraoperative or serious postoperative complications in this series of patients. The auteurs concluded that Combining CXL with Artiflex pIOL implantation appears safe and efficacious for the treatment of select cases of progressive keratoconus.

Another article regarding the use of the Artisan pIOL was published on 2011 by Sedaghat, and review their experience with 16 keratoconic eyes. This was a prospective, nonrandomized case series in which 14 Artisan pIOLs and 2 toric Artisan PIOLs were implanted in 13 patients (16 eyes) with stable keratoconus who had contact lens intolerance. Mean follow-up was 14.2 ± 7.8 months. Mean final UDVA was 20/28 and CDVA 20/26. The improvements in UDVA and CDVA were statistically significant (P < .0001 and P < .002, respectively). All patients achieved a final UDVA of 20/40 or better, and 84.6% had a final CDVA of 20/32 or better. No postoperative complications occurred except for two cases of sterile uveitis [17].

Alió et al. [18] studied and compare the use of iris-claw (Artiflex) and collagen copolymer posterior chamber pIOL (ICL) in eyes with stable keratoconus. Twenty eyes received an iris-claw pIOL and 28 eyes, a ICL (the use of ICL will be discussed further on page 13). Postoperatively, there was a statistically significant improvement in UDVA (P < .001). The UDVA was 20/50 or better in 94.23%, 20/30) or better in 35 eyes 67.31% and 20/20 or better in 42.31%. The mean efficacy index (postoperative UDVA/preoperative CDVA) was 0.90 ± 0.26. The improvement in the SE after surgery was statistically significant (P < 001). Most patients were near emmetropia; 82.69% were within ± 1.00 D and 71.15% were within ± 0.50 D. There was a statistically significant improvement in cylinder and sphere postoperatively (both P < 0.001). The mean efficacy index was 0.88 ± 0.28 in the ICL group and 0.96 ± 0.22 in the iris-claw pIOL group; there was no significant difference between the groups. Most patients in the iris-claw group were close to ametropia in most cases; however, there was a tendency toward undercorrection in the ICL group. The mean ECD changed from 2995.75 ± 401.75 cells/mm^2 (range 2513–3436 cells/mm^2) preoperatively to 2732.50 ± 262.66 cells/mm^2 (range 2353–2950 cells/mm^2) 12 months postoperatively.

As mentioned in more details before, on 2015, Assaf and Kotb [8] published their experience with Simultaneous corneal crosslinking and surface ablation combined with phakic intraocular lens implantation of iris claw lenses and angle supported lenses for managing keratoconus. (On page 4–5).

In recent years a few reports have been published regarding the complications after Artisan phakic IOL's.

In 2016, Bouheraoua at el. [19] published a 5 year follow up results of Artisan phakic intraocular lens (pIOL) to correct myopia. This was a Retrospective, interventional case series in 68 non keratogenic myopic eyes. Preoperatively, 83.8% eyes had a CDVA of 20/40 or better, and 38.2% eyes had a CDVA of 20/20 or better. A CDVA of 20/40 or better was found in 94.1%, 91.1%, and 92.6% of eyes after 1, 3, and 5 years, respectively. A CDVA of 20/20 or better was found in 47%, 48.5%, and 50% of eyes after 1, 3, and 5 years, respectively. The safety index (ratio of the mean postoperative CDVA to the mean preoperative CDVA) was 1.09, 1.02, and 1.10 after 1, 3, and 5 years, respectively. The efficacy index (mean postoperative UDVA to mean preoperative CDVA) was 0.96, 0.98, and 1.02 after 1, 3, and 5 years, respectively. The annual endothelial cell loss of 6.27%, 4.99%, 0.7%, 2.62%, and 0.57% at 1, 2, 3, 4 and 5 years of follow-up, respectively.

Risks after Artisan/Verisyse phakic IOL implantation were addressed by the U.S. Verisyse Study Group, which describes the 3-year results of the US FDA Clinical Trial [20]. Six hundred sixty-two adults (1140 eyes) were enrolled in the primary analysis group, with axial myopia from – 4.5 to – 22 D. At 3 years, UCVA was 20/40 or better in 84.0% and 20/25 or better in 51.9% of eyes. BSCVA was 20/40 or better for 99–100% of eyes from 1 month to 3 years. Mean change in endothelial cell count was – 4.8% ± 7.8% over 3 years. Adverse events requiring surgical intervention (3.48%) included inadequate lens fixation resulting in IOL subluxation, and insufficient original IOL fixation. Approximately, half of the adverse events were seen in the first ten cases performed by each surgeon.

Several other studies have focused on endothelial cell densities after Artisan IOL phakic implantation in non keratoconic eyes and their correlation to anterior chamber depth (ACD). Saxena et al. [21] reported a mean endothelial cell loss of 8.3% 5 years after the operation. After 3 years, a significant negative correlation between ACD and endothelial cell loss was revealed. The authors recommended that eyes just meeting the minimum endothelial cell density requirement (2000 cells/mm^2) should have greater ACDs to compensate for greater endothelial cell loss, and that patients with shallow anterior chambers (<2.6 mm) should have higher endothelial cell density.

Doors et al. [22] found a significant endothelial cell density loss of 1.28% ± 8.46% 2 years after Artisan phakic IOL implantation, 3.25% ± 8.24% at 5 years, and 5.02% ± 10.40% at 7 years. They suggested that a shorter distance between the edge of the phakic IOL and the endothelium was significantly associated with higher endothelial cell density loss. The authors also recommended that postoperative examination should include the long-term evaluation of anterior chamber depth.

Recently, Jonker et al. [23] described a 5 and 10 year follow up study regarding this issue. They have follow 507 eyes of 289 patients receiving the Artisan Myopia or Artisan Toric iris-fixated pIOL for the treatment of myopia or astigmatism. They have found an annual ECD decline of 48 cells/mm^2 and 61 cells/mm^2 in the myopic ($P < 0.001$) and toric ($P < 0.001$) groups, respectively, resulting in a total EC loss of 16.6% and 21.5% from 6 months to 10 years postoperatively, respectively. Risk factors for increased EC loss were a shallow ACD ($P < 0.005$) and a smaller distance between the central and peripheral pIOL edge to the endothelium ($P < 0.005$) [23].

22.4 Posterior Chamber Phakic IOL

Currently, two posterior chamber phakic IOLs are available, the Implantable Collamer Lens (ICL) (Staar Surgical Co.) and the Phakic Refractive Lens (PRL) (Carl Zeiss Meditec). The ICL is currently the most widely used posterior chamber phakic IOL (the PRL was actually abended over the last years) [5]. It incorporates material with increased biocompatibility known as Collamer, a hydrophilic porcine collagen/hydroxyethyl methacrylate copolymer, with an ultraviolet-absorbing chromophore. This material attracts deposition of a monolayer of fibronectin on the IOL surface that inhibits aqueous protein binding and makes the IOL invisible to the immune system. The model of Visian ICL V4, is a rectangular single-piece IOL, 7.5–8.0 mm wide. The available power ranges from −3.0 to −23.0 D for myopic IOLs, from +3.0 to +22.0 D for hyperopic ICLs, and with an added positive cylinder of +1.0 to +6.0 D for toric ICLs correcting myopia. This was later evolved to the Visian ICL V4c model and also Recently, STAAR Surgical launched the EVO+ Visian ICL (the V5 model), a pIOL with an expanded optical zone (6.1-mm optic) which was designed for patients with larger pupils (to reduce diffraction effect, such as halos). The lens is also available in a toric model. The available power ranges from −0.50 to −14.00 D, with a cylinder of up to 6.00 D. Both the V4c and V5 models have a central hole with a diameter of 0.36 mm which is aimed to increase aqueous humor perfusion and thus reduce the risk for secondary cataract formation [24].

To the best of our knowledge, only the following reports have been published on the use of the ICL in keratoconic eyes [25–31]. Kamiya et al. [25] were the first in describing their experience with the toric ICL in two patients (two eyes) with keratoconus. Both patients had a history of contact lens intolerance, and refraction and corneal topography were stable for 3–4 years. Phakic toric ICL power calculation was performed using the astigmatism decomposition method. Phakic toric ICLs were manufactured to minimize rotation to within 22.5° from the horizontal meridian. Preoperatively, the manifest refraction was −10.00 −6.00 × 100 in case 1 and −8.00 −2.75 × 100 in case 2. Postoperatively, the manifest refraction was −0.50 −1.00 × 90 in case 1 and −0.25 −1.25 × 100 in case 2. UCVA and BSCVA were markedly improved after implantation in both patients. No progressive sign of keratoconus was seen during 1-year follow-up.

Alfonso et al. [26] evaluated the myopic ICL to correct myopia associated with keratoconus in 25 consecutive keratoconus eyes of 16 patients. Preoperatively, myopia ranged from −3.00 to −18.00 D and astigmatism from −0.50 to −3.00 D. The results were analyzed 12 months after ICL implantation. Myopic ICL implantation was performed through a corneal incision in the steepest meridian. The mean UCVA and BSCVA after ICL implantation were 0.17 ± 0.19 and 0.12 ± 0.12 logMAR respectively. The efficacy index was 0.98. No eyes lost 2 or more lines of visual acuity, 2 eyes lost 1 line, 18 eyes did not change after surgery, and 5 eyes gained 1 or more lines. The safety index was 1.05. BSCVA significantly improved after ICL implantation. Spherical equivalent refraction was within ±1.00 D of the desired refraction in all cases and 84% of cases were within ±0.50 D. Mean postoperative spherical equivalent refraction was −0.32 ± 0.55 D at 12 months.

The method for optimizing the final central vault of the ICL phakic IOL in eyes with keratoconus and myopia has been also studied [27]. The reason for such study is that an oversized phakic IOL (i.e., one that is too long) can push the iris forward, decreasing the size of the angle; on the opposite side, an undersized phakic IOL (i.e., one that is too short) can result in the absence of vault (phakic IOL–crystalline lens touch), increasing the risk for early anterior subcapsular cataract. The length of the phakic IOL to implant was selected based on the white-to-white (WTW) distance or the sulcus-to-sulcus (STS) distance using the phakic IOL manufacturer's protocol. The final central vault distance was compared a minimum of 3 months postoperatively. The WTW and STS methods both provided adequate final central phakic IOL vault in keratoconic eyes with myopia. The STS calculations gave greater final vault and higher vault predictability, although the difference between the two methods was not statistically significant.

Alfonso et al. [28] also assessed the safety, efficacy, stability, and predictability of the ICL phakic toric IOL implantation to correct myopia and astigmatism in 30 eyes (21 patients) with keratoconus. Preoperatively, the mean SE was −5.38 D ± 3.26 D, and the mean cylinder, −3.48 D ± 1.24 D. The postoperative target in all cases was emmetropia. The correct toric phakic IOL size was determined based on the horizontal WTW distance measured by scanning-slit topography. Power calculation for the toric pIOL was performed using software provided by the manufacturer. At 12 months, 86.7% of the eyes were within ±0.50 D of the attempted refraction and all eyes were within ±1.00 D. The mean Snellen UCVA was 0.81 ± 0.20 and the mean BSCVA, 0.83 ± 0.18; CDVA was 20/40 or better in 29 eyes 96.7% of eyes and 20/25 or better in 22 eyes (73.3%). No eyes lost more than 2 lines of CDVA; 29 eyes (96.7%) maintained or gained 1 or more lines. The efficacy index was 1.07 and the safety index, 1.16. There were no complications or adverse events. The authors emphasized that the refractive and visual outcomes in their study were better than in previous reports. For example, they found a larger reduction in astigmatism and most eyes were within ±0.50 D of the SE refraction, showing high predictability, even for the astigmatic component. The authors suggested that toric pIOL implantation should not be performed until refraction and keratometry are stable and cases with BSCVA 20/50 or better, clear central cornea, keratometry less than 52.50 D, and stable refraction for 2 years. If these criteria are not met, PK or DALK would probably provide better visual outcomes. Thus in the authors' opinion, toric pIOL implantation should not be considered a true alternative to PK or DALK but rather an alternative treatment in cases of early keratoconus with relatively low irregular astigmatism.

As mentioned before, Alio et al. [18] studied and compare the use of iris-claw (Artiflex) and collagen copolymer posterior chamber pIOL (ICL pIOL) in eyes with stable keratoconus and found no statistically significant difference.

In 2014, a 3 year follow up report evaluating the use of toric implantable Collamer (TICL) lens after CXL in the treatment of early-Stage keratoconus was published. Sixteen keratogenic eyes who underwent TICL implantation at least 12 months after having their corneal collagen crosslinked and demonstrated stable refraction during this period were followed.

UDVA significantly improved as the mean for preoperative CDVA was 0.63 ± 0.14 and the mean postoperative UDVA was about 0.8 at 1 week and maintained throughout the rest of the follow-up. Considering the sphere, the preoperative mean was about −6.00 ± 4.00 D, which improved to almost undetectable levels postoperatively. Preoperatively, the mean cylinder was about −5 ± 1.50 D, and this improved to 0.0 D postoperatively. The spherical equivalent preoperatively was −8.50 ± 4.00 D, and this improved postoperatively to less than −0.25 D [29].

Hashemian et al. [30] published in 2013 the result of a 6 month follow up study regarding posterior chamber collagen copolymer phakic intraocular lens (pIOL) implantation to correct myopia and myopic astigmatism associated with keratoconus were published in 2013.Twenty two keratogenic eyes were followed. There were no complications during the surgical procedures. Two eyes needed repositioning due to the off-axis alignment. There was no decentration of the collamer lens and no case of pupillary block was detected. There was no significant increase in intraocular pressure. The mean SE preoperatively was −4.98 ± 2.63 D (ranging from −1.75 to −11.00 D). The mean SE after surgery at 1 week and 6 months were −0.42 and −0.33 D, respectively. The mean pre-operative refractive cylinder was −2.77 ± 0.99 DC (ranging from −1.50 to −4.00 DC). The mean refractive cylinders at one week and 6 months after surgery were −1.25 and −1.23 DC, respectively.

Finally, Kamiya et al. [31] reported the outcomes of toric ICL for the correction of high myopic astigmatism with mild keratoconus in 21 eyes of 11 patients with SE of −9.70 ± 2.33 D and astigmatism of −3.21 ± 1.56 D. Toric ICL power calculation was performed by the manufacturer using the astigmatism decomposition method. In all eyes, emmetropia was selected as the target refraction to reduce the preoperative refractive errors as much as possible. The size of the ICL was also chosen by the manufacturer on the basis of the horizontal corneal diameter and anterior chamber depth with scanning slit tomography (Orbscan IIz). LogMAR CDVA was −0.12 ± 0.07, −0.13 ± 0.08, −0.13 ± 0.09, −0.13 ± 0.10, −0.11 ± 0.09 and −0.12 ± 0.09 at 1, 3 and 6 months and 1, 2 and 3 years postoperatively, respectively. The mean percentage of endothelial cell loss was 4.4% at 3 years postoperatively.

No cataract formation, pigment dispersion glaucoma, pupillary block, axis misalignment, axis rotation, or any other vision-threatening complications were seen at any time during the observation period in this series. The authors pointed out that it is difficult to precisely determine the keratometric readings and the manifest cylinder, resulting in less accuracy for toric ICL power calculation.

One of the risks associated with posterior chamber phakic IOLs, but less so with anterior chamber phakic IOLs, is the development of cataracts. Sanders [32] reported the rates of anterior subcapsular opacities and cataracts 5 years after surgery in the visian ICL FDA trial. The study included 526 eyes with myopia between −3 and −20.0 D. At 12 months postop, UCVA was 20/40 or better in 92.5%. The most common adverse event was anterior subcapsular opacities (in 5.9% of eyes at 7 years or later). Cataracts occurred early: 58% in the first year, 68% in the first 2 years, and 74% in the first 3 years. However, only 1.3% progressed to clinically significant cataract, and those were usually in very high myopes and older patients. To the best of our knowledge, no cases of cataracts have been reported after ICL implantation for keratoconus, although long-follow up data are still limited.

22.5 Refractive Lens Exchange

Refractive lens exchange (RLE), also called clear lens extraction, consists of phacoemulsification of the clear crystalline lens or soft cataracts and implantation of an appropriately powered IOL [33]. It is generally used to correct large spherical errors in patients in the presbyopic age range because it causes loss of accommodation. Myopia associated with keratoconus is not considered yet an indication for RLE because of difficult IOL power calculation. There are only three reports on RLE for keratoconus, with or without toric IOLs. A report from Sauder and Jonas [34] on the use of a toric IOL in two keratoconic eyes with cataract and aphakia respectively will not be discussed, as it does not meet the criteria of RLE procedure.

Leccisotti [35] evaluated the visual results and complications of refractive lens exchange to correct myopia associated with stages I to II keratoconus in 34 eyes (20 patients). Preoperative mean spherical equivalent SE was −11.0 ± 4.65 D. Ultrasound biometry was performed using videokeratographic central K-readings and the Holladay 2 formula. An intraoperative handheld autorefractor was used to check the power of implanted intraocular lenses. A single-piece foldable acrylic IOL (Stabibag [Rockmerd BV]) with a 5.5 mm square-edged optic was inserted in the capsular bag. Intraocular lens exchange due to inaccurate power occurred in 11 eyes (32%; 9 eyes intraoperative, 2 eyes postoperative). At 12 months, mean SE was −1.31 ± 1.08 D and mean defocus equivalent was 1.94 ± 1.57 D. Twenty-two eyes (65%) were within ±2 D of defocus equivalent, 16 eyes (47%) were within ±1 D, and 3 eyes (9%) were within ±0.5. Mean surgically induced astigmatism (vector analysis) was 0.54 ± 0.43 D. Preoperative mean BSCVA was 0.55 ± 0.20, and postoperative mean BSCVA was 0.76 ± 0.23. Postoperative mean UCVA was 0.48 ± 0.25. The safety index was 1.38, and the efficacy index was 0.87. Complications were posterior vitreous detachment (9%) and dysphotopsia phenomena (15%). Corneal endothelial cell density at 12 months decreased by 6.3%. The authors recommended the use of intraoperative autorefractometry to improve refractive outcome. They also commented that the main bias of the study was the limited and heterogeneous (in terms of age and SE) sample, which can explain the low incidence of vitreoretinal complications, which are considered the main drawback of RLE and can occur after years, especially in more myopic eyes. In the authors' opinion, phakic IOLs have the advantage of an almost complete reversibility, but their use is not advised in patients of presbyopic age because of progressive convexity of the crystalline lens, which can induce cataract and pigment dispersion, especially with anterior chamber models. Therefore, RLE may be indicated for presbyopic patients with higher spherical errors.

Finally, Jaimes and Navas et al. [36] published their experience with RLE with toric IOL (AcrySof Toric SN60TT IOL) in 19 eyes of 12 patients with nonprogressive keratoconus and one pellucid marginal degeneration patient. The IOL power calculation and toricity were calculated using the manufacturer's website (www.acrysoftoriccalculator.com), and the SRK II formula was used for the IOL power calculation adjusted for emmetropia. Mean follow-up after RLE was 7.89 ± 6.61 months. Mean preoperative sphere was −5.25 ± 6.40 diopters (D), and mean postoperative sphere was 0.22 ± 1.01 D ($P < .001$). Mean preoperative cylinder was 3.95 ± 1.30 D, which decreased to 1.36 ± 1.17 D postoperatively ($P < .001$). Mean pre- and postoperative SE refractions were −7.10 ± 6.41 D and −0.46 ± 1.12 D, respectively ($P < .001$). Preoperative mean UDVA was 20/447 and postoperative mean UDVA was 20/39 ($P < .001$).

22.6 Sequential Surgery (Intacs + Phakic IOL/PRK + CXL + Phakic IOL)

Intrastromal corneal ring segments (Intacs, Addition Technology, Inc., Sunnyvale, CA) have been shown to stabilize or improve both BSCVA and UCVA for up to 5 years in patients with mild to moderate keratoconus or post LASIK corneal ectasia [37, 38]. However Intacs insertion is not expected to correct more than −4.00 D of myopia in the best of circumstances. Furthermore, these ectatic corneas frequently have steep central cones resulting in high myopia in 1 or both eyes, which may lead to profound anisometropia. Many of these patients ultimately become contact lens intolerant and would traditionally be considered for PK or DALK – lamellar transplant surgery. For those eyes, phakic IOL implantation represents a viable treatment option before transplantation [39]. We briefly herein present the reports on sequential Intacs and phakic IOL (anterior chamber, iris fixated, or posterior chamber) for keratoconus.

Colin and Velou [40] were the first to report the sequential use of Intacs and phakic IOL for keratoconus. Before Intacs implantation, manifest refraction was −9.00 −4.50 × 130 with a UCVA of 0.02 and BCVA of 0.7. Two months after Intacs implantation, the UCVA was 0.05 and the BCVA, 0.6, and the manifest refraction was −8.25 −1.75 × 110. An anterior chamber phakic IOL (Nuvita, Bausch&Lomb, which is not in use anymore) with a power of −8.00 D was implanted. The manifest refraction 2 months after IOL implantation was −1.25 −1.75 × 115 with a UCVA of 0.3 and BCVA of 0.8. The specular endothelial microscopy count was 2640 cells/mm^2.

The following represent the reports on the sequential use of Intacs and Artisan/Verisyse IOL for keratoconus. Kamburoğlu et al. [41] reported the case a 24-year-old man with bilateral keratoconus in whom Intacs were implanted in both eyes. The procedure was followed by Artisan toric phakic IOL implantation to correct the residual myopic and astigmatic refractive error (−6.50 −4.50 × 35 in the right eye and −6.50 −5.00 × 150 in the left eye).

El-Raggal and Abdel Fattah [42] reported eight eyes of six keratoconus patients who underwent sequential Intacs and Verisyse phakic non toric IOL implantation. Eyes had contact lens intolerance, clear corneas, a maximum K-value less than 60.0 D, and minimum corneal thickness greater than 400 mm. Refraction 6 months after Intacs insertion showed residual myopia greater than 6.0 D and residual astigmatism not more than 2.0 D. All eyes achieved UCVA of 20/40 or better. The final spherical error ranged from −1.75 to +1.00 D and the cylindrical error, from 1.25 to 2.50 D. No eye lost lines of preoperative BCVA. These results were relatively stable throughout the follow-up period of 2 years.

Moshirfar et al. [39] compared the simultaneous and sequential implantation of Intacs and Verisyse phakic IOL in selected cases of ectatic corneal disease (5 eyes with post–LASIK ectasia and 14 eyes with keratoconus) and did not find significant differences in refractive outcome. Intacs segments were implanted followed by insertion of a phakic Verisyse lens at the same session (12 eyes) in the simultaneous group or several months later (7 eyes) in the sequential group. No intraoperative or postoperative complications were observed. There were no significant differences in mean UCVA or BSCVA between the two groups preoperatively or postoperatively after 1 year. No eye lost lines of preoperative BSCVA. The authors suggested that possible advantages of a simultaneous approach to surgery include reduced cost and recovery time associated with a single surgery and a more rapid improvement in visual acuity. A technical advantage of the simultaneous implantation is that the sequence of creating stromal channels, followed by Verisyse implantation, and then implanting the corneal ring segments offers a less obstructed view of the enclavation process. On the other hand, advantages of the sequential technique is that patients may undergo a trial of contact lenses before proceeding to Verisyse implantation because some patients may regain contact lens tolerance after Intacs insertion, and also the possibility of obtaining K values after Intacs insertion, which theoretically allows for better prediction of the Verisyse lens power before implantation.

Coskunseven et al. [43] reported the use of sequential Intacs and toric ICL in three keratoconic eyes (two patients) with extreme myopia and irregular astigmatism. Time between Intacs and ICL implantation ranged between six and 10 months. No intraoperative or postoperative complications were observed. An improvement in UCVA and BSCVA was found. All eyes were emmetropic within 1 D whereas the mean manifest refractive SE refraction reduced from −18.50 ± 2.61 D (range, −16.75–−21.50 D) to 0.42 D (range, plano to −0.75 D). The mean difference between preoperative and last follow-up UCVA and BSCA was a gain of 6.67 ± 1.15 lines and 4.33 ± 2.52 lines respectively.

Dirani et al. [44] published on 2014 a report on Visian toric ICL implantation after intracorneal ring segments implantation and corneal collagen crosslinking in 11 eyes of seven patients with moderate to severe keratoconus. The two procedures (ICRS-CXL) were performed sequentially at an interval of 4 weeks and TICL implantation was performed at least 6 months after CXL. The two procedures (ICRS-CXL) were performed sequentially at an interval of 4 weeks and TICL implantation was performed at least 6 months after CXL. No intraoperative or postoperative complications occurred.

Finally, Ferreira and Güell [45] evaluated, over a 12 month period, and published their data on 2014, the use of ICRS and Iris Fixated Phakic IOL (Artisan or Artiflex toric lenses were used) in 21 keratogenic eyes. The mean UDVA 12 months after ICRS and pIOL implantation increased from 20/2000 to 20/35 ($P < .001$). The mean CDVA increased from 20/40 to 20/25 ($P = .039$). Mean sphere improved from −9.14 ± 6.87 D (range: −18.00 to −0.75 D) to +0.14 ± 0.45 D (range: −0.50 to +1.00 D) ($P = .012$) and mean cylinder improved from −3.25 ± 1.2 D (range: −5.0 to −2.0 D) to −1.2 ± 1.18 D (range: −3.0 to 0.0 D) ($P = .021$). Predictability of refractive results was good, with spherical equivalent refraction within ±0.50 diopter of the attempted correction in 61.9%of the eyes and within ±1.00 diopter in 90.5%. Both PIOLs used had similar visual and refractive results. Mean central endothelial cell density decreased from 2513 ± 245 cells/mm^2 preoperatively to 2312 ± 263 cells/mm^2 ($P = .402$). The efficacy index was 1.06 and the safety index was 1.40.

The use of term "sequential surgery" has been widened in the last few years and now we can find in the literature reports on the use of PRK, CXL and IOL implantation as was mentioned before in the article published by Assaf and Kotb [8].

Coskunseven et al. [46] reported on 2013 a case series of 14 eyes with progressive keratoconus who had ICRS implantation, then CXL, and then pIOL (Visian Implantable Collamer Lens – ICL) implantation (minimum 6 months between procedures). The mean interval between ICRS and CXL was 7.0 months, and the mean interval between CXL and toric pIOL implantation was 8.4 months. All patients were followed for at least 1 year after pIOL implantation. The manifest refraction spherical equivalent (MRSE) decreased from a mean of −16.40 ± 3.56 D (range −11.50 to −22.50 D) to −9.81 ± 2.71 D 6 months after ICRS implantation ($P < .0001$, Bonferroni test). Six months after CXL treatment, the mean MRSE was −9.67 ± 2.79 D; the difference was not statistically significant. One year after toric pIOL implantation, the MRSE decreased to a mean of −0.80 ± 1.02 D (range −2.00 to +2.00 D) ($P < 0001$). The refractive astigmatism decreased from −4.73 ± 1.32 D (range −3.00 to −7.00 D) to −2.36 ± 0.58 D 6 months after ICRS implantation ($P < .0001$, Bonferroni test). Six months after CXL treatment, it decreased to −2.09 ± 1.31 D; the difference was not statistically significant. One year after toric pIOL implantation, the refractive astigmatism decreased to −0.93 ± 0.31 D (range −0.50 to −1.50 D) ($P < .01$). The mean UDVA increased from 0.01 ± 1.3 lines to 0.03 ± 5 lines 6 months after ICRS implantation and to 0.06 ± 4.3 lines 6 months after CXL treatment; the difference was not statistically significant at either time point. One year after toric pIOL implantation, the mean UDVA increased to 0.45 ± 1.1 lines ($P < .01$). After pIOL implantation, the CDVA was significantly better than after ICRS implantation ($P < .05$) but not statistically significantly better than after CXL.

Just recently, the same author [47] published their work on evaluating a four-stage combined treatment for keratoconus including intrastromal corneal ring segment (ICRS) implantation followed by corneal cross-linking (CXL), toric phakic IOL (toric Visian Implantable Collamer – TICL) implantation, and topography-guided photorefractive keratectomy (TG-PRK) in 11 eyes with progressive keratoconus. There was a minimum of 6 month between each stage. Minimum follow-up was 12 months after TG-PRK. The maximum stromal ablation depth was 50 μm and the attempted correction was approximately 80% of the refraction. The four-stage procedure produced a significant improvement in visual acuity, with all eyes achieving better postoperative UDVA than preoperative (spectacle) CDVA. After the four-stage procedure, mean UDVA improved from 20/1000 preoperatively to 20/29, ($P < .0001$), whereas mean CDVA improved from 20/222 to 20/27, ($P < .0001$). All eyes achieved postoperative UDVA of 20/33 or better. There were no intraoperative or postoperative complications. No eye lost any line of CDVA. All eyes gained at least one line of CDVA after the four-stage procedure. All eyes had high myopic astigmatism with a MRSE between 11.25 D and −22.13 D. The final MRSE for all eyes was within 1.375 D of target, with 4 eyes (27%) having a hyperopic MRSE (maximum +0.875 D). Mean MRSE reduced from 16.78 ± 3.58 D to 0.59 ± 0.89 D after the four-stage procedure ($P < .0001$). In addition, the final result had a significant reduction in refractive astigmatism, from −5.16 ± 1.86 to −0.82 ± 0.28 D ($P < .0001$).

22.7 Conclusion

The use of phakic IOLs is a promising area of refractive surgery which is gaining more and more popularity. The use of IOLs in keratoconus represents just a small part of this area. The majority of reports pointed that a keratoconic eye suitable for IOL implantation should have a central clear cornea, mild astigmatism, stable refraction and good BSCVA. Many of the studies discussed previously suggest good predictability, efficacy, and safety. However there are still many questions to answer. The studies presented consist of relatively small number of cases and lack long-follow-up data. With the available information till date, direct comparison between different IOLs models and designs or surgical techniques (IOL with or without Intacs or PRK and CXL) in keratoconus is not possible, so the best IOL choice for keratoconic eyes is not clear. In addition, when combing procedures, the schedule and timing of the different stages of the procedures is still debated.

While Izquierdo et al. [16] stated that IOL transplantation should be done at least 6 month after the CXL, Assaf and Kotb [8] found according to their experience that a period of 2 month was a sufficient “stabilization period”.

It is also imported to remember that IOL power calculation is not as accurate as in non-keratoconic eyes, and IOL implantation is not exempt of risks. The spectrum of keratoconus management modalities is changing and continues to evolve. Although much research have been done on this subject in the last few years, further studies are required to refine and establish a precise algorithm of indications for the use of IOLs in keratoconic eyes.

References

1. Güell JL. Are intracorneal rings still useful in refractive surgery? Curr Opin Ophthalmol. 2005;16(4):260–5.
2. Jhanji V, Sharma N, Vajpayee RB. Management of keratoconus: current scenario. Br J Ophthalmol. 2011;95(8):1044–50.
3. Samaras KE, Lake DB. Corneal collagen cross linking (CXL): a review. Int Ophthalmol Clin. 2010;50:89–100.
4. Chang GC, Pineda R 2nd. Phakic intraocular lenses. Int Ophthalmol Clin. 2010;50:119–28.
5. Güell JL, Morral M, Kook D, Kohnen T. Phakic intraocular lenses part 1: historical overview, current models, selection criteria, and surgical techniques. J Cataract Refract Surg. 2010;36:1976–93.
6. Leccisotti A, Fields SV. Angle-supported phakic intraocular lenses in eyes with keratoconus and myopia. J Cataract Refract Surg. 2003;29:1530–6.
7. van der Heijde GL. Some optical aspects of implantation of an IOL in a myopic eye. Eur J Implant Refract Surg. 1989;1:245–8.
8. Assaf A, Kotb A. Simultaneous corneal crosslinking and surface ablation combined with phakic intraocular lens implantation for managing keratoconus. Int Ophthalmol. 2015;35:411–9.
9. Javaloy J, Alio JL, Iradier MT, et al. Outcomes of ZB5M angle-supported anterior chamber phakic intraocular lenses at 12 years. J Refract Surg. 2007;23:147–258.
10. Kohnen T, Maxwell WA, Holland S. Correction of moderate to high myopia with a foldable, angle-supported phakic intraocular lens. Results from a 5-year open-label trial. Ophthalmology. 2016;123(5):1027–35.

11. Maloney RK, Nguyern LH, John ME. The Artisan lens study group. Artisan phakic intraocular lens for myopia: short-term results of a prospective, multicenter study. Ophthalmology. 2002;109:1631–41.
12. Doors M, Budo CJ, Christiaans BJ, Luger M, Marinho AAP, Dick HB, Güell JL, Nuijts RMMA. Artiflex toric foldable phakic intraocular lens: short-term results of a prospective European multicenter study. Am J Ophthalmol. 2012;154(4):730–9. e2
13. Budo C, Bartels MC, van Rij G. Implantation of Artisan toric phakic intraocular lenses for the correction of astigmatism and spherical errors in patients with keratoconus. J Refract Surg. 2005;21:218–22.
14. Moshirfar M, Grégoire FJ, Mirzaian G, Whitehead GF, Kang PC. Use of Verisyse iris-supported phakic intraocular lens for myopia in keratoconic patients. J Cataract Refract Surg. 2006;32:1227–32.
15. Venter J. Artisan phakic intraocular lens in patients with keratoconus. J Refract Surg. 2009;25:759–64.
16. Izquierdo L, Henriquez MA, McCarthy M. Artiflex phakic intraocular lens implantation after corneal collagen cross-linking in keratoconic eyes. J Refract Surg. 2011;27:482–7.
17. Sedaghat M, Ansari-Astaneh MR, Zarei-Ghanavati M, Davis SW, Sikder S. Artisan iris-supported phakic IOL implantation in patients with keratoconus: a review of 16 eyes. J Refract Surg. 2011;27(7):489–93.
18. Alio JL, Pena-Garcia P, Abdulla GF, et al. Comparison of iris-claw and posterior chamber collagen copolymer phakic intraocular lenses in keratoconus. J Cataract Refract Surg. 2014;40:383–94.
19. Bouheraoua N, Bonnet C, Labbé A, Sandali O, Lecuen N, Ameline B, Borderie V. Laroche L Iris-fixated phakic intraocular lens implantation to correct myopia and a predictive model of endothelial cell loss. J Cataract Refract Surg. 2015;41(11):2450–7.
20. Stulting RD, John ME, Maloney RK, Assil KK, Arrowsmith PN, Thompson VM, U.S. Verisyse Study Group. Three-year results of artisan/verisyse phakic intraocular lens implantation. Results of the United States food and drug administration clinical trial. Ophthalmology. 2008;115(3):464–72. e1
21. Saxena R, Boekhoorn SS, Mulder PG, Noordzij B, van Rij G, Luyten GP. Long-term follow-up of endothelial cell change after Artisan phakic intraocular lens implantation. Ophthalmology. 2008;115:608–13. e1
22. Doors M, Cals DW, Berendschot TT, de Brabander J, Hendrikse F, Webers CA, Nuijts RM. Influence of anterior chamber morphometrics on endothelial cell changes after phakic intraocular lens implantation. J Cataract Refract Surg. 2008;34:2110–8.
23. Jonker, SMR, Berendschot, TTJM, Ronden, AE, Saelens, IEY, Bauer, NJC, Nuijts, RMMA. Long-term endothelial cell loss in patients with artisan myopia and artisan toric phakic intraocular lenses: 5- and 10-year results. Ophthalmology. 2017. pii: S0161-6420(17)31290-3.
24. Domínguez-Vicent A, Ferrer-Blasco T, Pérez-Vives C, et al. Optical quality comparison between 2 collagen copolymer posterior chamber phakic intraocular lens designs. J Cataract Refract Surg. 2015;41(6):1268–78.
25. Kamiya K, Shimizu K, Ando W, Asato Y, Fujisawa T. Phakic toric implantable collamer lens implantation for the correction of high myopic astigmatism in eyes with keratoconus. J Refract Surg. 2008;24:840–2.
26. Alfonso JF, Palacios A, Montés-Micó R. Myopic phakic STAAR collamer posterior chamber intraocular lenses for keratoconus. J Refract Surg. 2008;24:867–74.
27. Boxer Wachler BS, Vicente LL. Optimizing the vault of collagen copolymer phakic intraocular lenses in eyes with keratoconus and myopia: comparison of 2 methods. J Cataract Refract Surg. 2010;36:1741–4.
28. Alfonso JF, Fernández-Vega L, Lisa C, Fernandes P, González-Méijome JM, Montés-Micó R. Collagen copolymer toric posterior chamber phakic intraocular lens in eyes with keratoconus. J Cataract Refract Surg. 2010;36(6):906–16.

29. Shaheen S, El-Kateb S, El-Samadouny MA. Evaluation of a toric implantable collamer lens after corneal collagen crosslinking in treatment of early-stage keratoconus: 3-year follow-up. Cornea. 2014;33(5):475–80.
30. Hashemian SJ, Soleimani M, Foroutan A, Joshaghani M, Ghaempanah J, Jafari ME. Toric implantable collamer lens for high myopic astigmatism in keratoconic patients after six months. Clin Exp Optom. 2013;96(2):225–32.
31. Kamiya K, Shimizu K, Kobashi H, Komatsu M, Nakamura A, Nakamura T, Ichikawa K. Three-year follow-up of posterior chamber toric phakic intraocular lens implantation for the correction of high myopic astigmatism in eyes with keratoconus. Br J Ophthalmol. 2015;99(2):177–83.
32. Sanders DR. Anterior subcapsular opacities and cataracts 5 years after surgery in the visian implantable collamer lens FDA trial. J Refract Surg. 2008;24:566–70.
33. Packer M, Hoffman RS, Fine IH, Dick HB. Refractive lens exchange. Int Ophthalmol Clin. 2006;46:63–82.
34. Sauder G, Jonas JB. Treatment of keratoconus by toric foldable intraocular lenses. Eur J Ophthalmol. 2003;13:577–9.
35. Leccisotti A. Refractive lens exchange in keratoconus. J Cataract Refract Surg. 2006;32:742–6.
36. Jaimes M, Xacur-Garcia F, Alvarez-Melloni D, et al. Refractive lens exchange with toric intraocular lenses in keratoconus. J Refract Surg. 2011;27:658–64.
37. Colin J, Malet FJ. Intacs for the correction of keratoconus: two-year follow-up. J Cataract Refract Surg. 2007;33:69–74.
38. Kymionis GD, Tsiklis NS, Pallikaris AI, et al. Long-term follow-up of Intacs for post-LASIK corneal ectasia. Ophthalmology. 2006;113:1909–17.
39. Moshirfar M, Fenzl CR, Meyer JJ, Neuffer MC, Espandar L, Mifflin MD. Simultaneous and sequential implantation of intacs and verisyse phakic intraocular lens for refractive improvement in keratectasia. Cornea. 2011;30(2):158–63.
40. Colin J, Velou S. Implantation of Intacs and a refractive intraocular lens to correct keratoconus. J Cataract Refract Surg. 2003;29:832–4.
41. Kamburoğlu G, Ertan A, Bahadir M. Implantation of Artisan toric phakic intraocular lens following Intacs in a patient with keratoconus. J Cataract Refract Surg. 2007;33:528–30.
42. El-Raggal TM, Abdel Fattah AA. Sequential Intacs and Verisyse phakic intraocular lens for refractive improvement in keratoconic eyes. J Cataract Refract Surg. 2007;33:966–70.
43. Coskunseven E, Onder M, Kymionis GD, Diakonis VF, Arslan E, Tsiklis N, Bouzoukis DI, Pallikaris I. Combined Intacs and posterior chamber toric implantable Collamer lens implantation for keratoconic patients with extreme myopia. Am J Ophthalmol. 2007;144:387–9.
44. Dirani A, Fadlallah A, Khoueir Z, Antoun J, Cherfan G, Jarade E. Visian toric ICL implantation after intracorneal ring segments implantation and corneal collagen crosslinking in keratoconus. Eur J Ophthalmol. 2014;24(3):338–44.
45. Ferreira TB, Guell JL, Manero F. Combined intracorneal ring segments and iris-fixated phakic intraocular lens for keratoconus refractive and visual improvement. J Refract Surg. 2014;30:336–41.
46. Coskunseven E, Sharma DP, Jankov MR 2nd, Kymionis GD, Richoz O, Hafezi F. Collagen copolymer toric phakic intraocular lens for residual myopic astigmatism after intrastromal corneal ring segment implantation and corneal collagen crosslinking in a 3-stage procedure for keratoconus. J Cataract Refract Surg. 2013;39:722–9.
47. Coskunseven E, Sharma DP, Grentzelos MA, Sahin O, Kymionis GD, Pallikaris I. Four-stage procedure for keratoconus: ICRS implantation, corneal cross-linking, toric phakic intraocular lens implantation, and topography-guided photorefractive keratectomy. J Refract Surg. 2017;33(10):683–9.

Chapter 23
Phakic Intraocular Lenses in Patients with Keratoconus, the Dilemma

Yishay Weill and David Zadok

Since their introduction over half a century ago, phakic intraocular lenses (pIOLs) have made quite a few transformations [1]. Different types were developed and new surgical techniques were introduced. Following these developments, pIOLs implantation had become safer and higher success rates are being recorded. Currently there are three types of pIOLs; angle supported anterior chamber pIOLs, iris-claw anterior chamber pIOLs and collamer posterior chamber (PC) pIOLs. Each model has its own special surgical technique, success rate and potential complications. Within the United States there are only two FDA approved pIOLs:Verisyse iris-claw pIOL (Abbott Laboratories Inc., Abbott Park, IL, USA) and Visian collamer PC pIOL (Staar Surgical, Monrovia, CA, USA). Both are approved for patients with high myopia and low astigmatism (2.5D>) [1–4]. Toric pIOLsare currently not FDA approved. In Europe, the popular Verisyse lens is branded Artisan (Ophtec BV, The Netherlands) and newer models of different pIOLs are in use under the CE mark approval, including toric pIOLs [1].

When comparing pIOLs to refractive lens exchange (RLE) and corneal refractive surgery, pIOLs offer some key advantages. Compared to RLE, where the innate lens is removed, pIOLs hold the obvious advantage of preserving the natural lens and accommodation [5]. Although corneal refractive surgery attempts to re-shape the abnormal cornea while pIOLs merely correct spherical/astigmatism errors, pIOLs have some advantages when compared to corneal refractive surgery. Phakic IOLs offer treatment to larger range of refractive errors [1–5], they do not depend on corneal thickness and do not carry the known potential complications of corneal ablation therapy. Finally, pIOLs carry the vital advantage of reversibility, since the implanted IOL can be replaced or removed practically at any time [2].

Y. Weill · D. Zadok (✉)
Department of Ophthalmology, Shaare Zedek Medical Center, Hebrew University, Jerusalem, Israel
e-mail: zadokd@szmc.org.il

A. Barbara (ed.), *Controversies in the Management of Keratoconus*,
https://doi.org/10.1007/978-3-319-98032-4_23

However, pIOL implantation is not without risks. Corneal endothelium loss, iritis, pupillary block, pupillary ovalization, pigment dispersion, intraocular pressure rise, induced cataract (mainly anterior subcapsular), lens dislocation, halos and glares are only some of the documented significant complications of pIOLs implantation [2–8]. Additionally, as an intraocular surgery, pIOLs implantation carry all the well-known complications of intraocular procedure. In particular; endophthalmitis, intraocular hemorrhage, retinal detachment and surgically induced astigmatism.

In general, criteria for implanting pIOL with relatively safe and predictable outcomes, includes, inter alia: age >21, no ocular pathology or systemic disease, clear crystalline lens, stable refraction, irido-corneal angle ≥30°, appropriate mesopic pupil size (<5.0–6.0 mm), adequate anterior chamber depth (>2.7–3.0 mm) and sufficient endothelial cell count (ECC) (>2500 cells/mm^2) [2]. This broad list makes selecting a suitable candidate for pIOL implantation a difficult task, but failure to adhere to these criteria could lead to poor outcomes, especially in a patient with keratoconus.

When approaching the controversial topic of pIOL implantation in the setup of keratoconus, we need to address disease and IOL related issues. When one considers implanting any type of pIOL in an eye of a patient with keratoconus, it is important to differentiate four categories of keratoconus- newly diagnosed, progressive, stable and advanced keratoconus. In the case of recently diagnosed disease, pIOL implantation could give unfavorable long-term results since the natural course of keratoconus is to progress during its early stages, thus necessitating future additional interventions, in the form of IOL replacement or corneal intervention. For similar reasons, it is not recommended to implant pIOLsin a case of progressive keratoconus [1, 2, 9, 10]. Implantation of pIOL is also not appropriate in the scenario of advanced keratoconus which is accompanied by significant corneal pathology, irregular astigmatism and high-order aberrations which are not corrected by the pIOLs, spherical or toric [10–12]. Kurian et al. [13], analyzed optical performance described in terms of modulation transfer function (MTF), Strehl ratio and objective scatter index (OSI) in keratoconic eyes implanted with pIOL. While their patient's refractive results were excellent, the mean post-treatment MTF and Strehl ratio were indicative of poor visual quality and the mean OSI was indicative of significant scattering. This leaves only patients with stable keratoconus disease to be potential candidates for pIOL procedure. The period of time to be considered as stable refraction is also unclear and varies in different studies from 6 months to 2 years [10].

As with other IOLs implantation, precise calculations and meticulous measurements are key factors for a successful procedure and patient satisfaction. The commonly used method to calculate pIOL power consider patient's subjective refraction, keratometry and anterior chamber depth. In the setup of keratoconus, IOL measurement is a significant challenge and often yield unpredictable final results due to reduced repeatability of subjective refraction and difficulty in determining axis and power of preoperative astigmatism [10, 11, 14]. Accurate toric alignment is a fundamental demand for precise refractive correction with toric pIOLs. Each degree of misalignment yields astigmatism under-correction of 3.3%, with virtually complete loss of IOL cylinder power whenever the IOL is misaligned by 30° [15].

Once again, these unfavorable outcomes are difficult to manage, and adjustments are sometimes impossible postoperatively since contact lens and corneal refractive procedures are often not feasible [16].

Other concerning issues are IOL related. As mentioned above, there are several potential significant complications in pIOL implantation [2–8]. Endothelial cell (EC) loss remains an important issue in the context of pIOL. The presumed mechanism for the EC loss is either by direct mechanical damage to the EC by the pIOL or indirect injury by interference to the natural aqueous humor flow [6, 8, 17]. Different studies had documented around 5% EC loss 1 year after pIOL implantation of any type, with slower pace of deterioration thereafter. A recent long-term report by Jonker et al. [17] found EC loss of 21.4% 10 years after Artisan toric pIOL implantation. They also identified younger age as a risk factor for EC loss, presumably due to anterior displacement of the crystalline lens during accommodation, which is much more prominent in younger patient. This should be taken into consideration due to the young age of the potential candidates for pIOL implantation.

At last, we need to keep in mind that once a toric pIOL is implanted in a patient's eye, contact lens fitting becomes challenging [16]. Additionally, Once the patient needs gas permeable contact lens after pIOL implantation, the irregular astigmatism is virtually eliminated by the rigid lens, so that the patient ends up with a large degree of residual astigmatism due to the toric pIOL. This is a crucial issue especially since we have established earlier that the candidates for pIOL implantation belong to the moderate and stable keratoconus patients, that potentially can still achieve very good CDVA when wearing contact lens.

In conclusion, in one hand, based on small studies, toric pIOL provides the potential benefit of an increased spectacle independence but in the other hand this potential benefit may induce serious contact lens fitting difficulties, if significant residual astigmatism is present along with poor visual quality and the risk of cataract formation and corneal decompensation along the years.

Conflicts of interest All authors declare they have no conflicts to disclose.

Funding This work received no funding.

References

1. Güell J, Morral M, Kook D, Kohnen T. Phakic intraocular lenses part 1: historical overview, current models, selection criteria, and surgical techniques. J Cataract Refract Surg. 2010;36:1976–93.
2. Pineda R, Chauhan T. Phakic intraocular lenses and their special indications. J Ophthalmic Vis Res. 2016;11:422–8.

3. Lovisolo C, Reinstein D. Phakic intraocular lenses. Surv Ophthalmol. 2005;50:549–87.
4. Barsam A, Allan B. Excimer laser refractive surgery versus phakic intraocular lenses for the correction of moderate to high myopia. Cochrane Database Syst Rev. 2014. https://doi.org/10.1002/14651858.cd007679.pub4.
5. Nanavaty M, Daya S. Refractive lens exchange versus phakic intraocular lenses. Curr Opin Ophthalmol. 2012;23:54–61.
6. Kohnen T, Kook D, Morral M, Güell J. Phakic intraocular lenses part 2: results and complications. J Cataract Refract Surg. 2010;36:2168–94.
7. Chen L, Chang Y, Kuo J, Rajagopal R, Azar D. Metaanalysis of cataract development after phakic intraocular lens surgery. J Cataract Refract Surg. 2008;34:1181–200.
8. Kohnen T, LaFontaine L, Andrew R. Long-term safety follow-up of an anterior chamber angle-supported phakic intraocular lens. J Cataract Refract Surg. 2017;43:1163–70.
9. Alfonso JF, Palacios A, Montes-Mico R. Myopic phakic STAAR collamerposterior chamber intraocular lenses for keratoconus. J Cataract Refract Surg. 2008;24:867–74.
10. Esteve-Taboada J, Domínguez-Vicent A, Ferrer-Blasco T, Alfonso J, Montés-Micó R. Posterior chamber phakic intraocular lenses to improve visual outcomes in keratoconus patients. J Cataract Refract Surg. 2017;43:115–30.
11. Kamiya K, Shimizu K, Ando W, Asato Y, Fujisawa T. Phakic toric Implantable Collamer Lens implantation for the correction of high myopic astigmatism in eyes with keratoconus. J Cataract Refract Surg. 2008;24:840–2.
12. Miháltz K, Kovács I, Kránitz K, Erdei G, Németh J, Nagy Z. Mechanism of aberration balance and the effect on retinal image quality in keratoconus: optical and visual characteristics of keratoconus. J Cataract Refract Surg. 2011;37:914–22.
13. Kurian M, Nagappa S, Bhagali R, Shetty R, Shetty BK. Visual quality after posterior chamber phakic intraocular lens implantation in keratoconus. J Cataract Refract Surg. 2012;38:1050–7.
14. Naderan M, Rajabi M, Zarrinbakhsh P. Distribution of anterior and posterior corneal astigmatism in eyes with keratoconus. Am J Ophthalmol. 2016;167:79–87.
15. Ma J, Tseng S. Simple method for accurate alignment in toric phakic and aphakic intraocular lens implantation. J Cataract Refract Surg. 2008;34:1631–6.
16. Lindsay R, Connell B, Snibson G. Contact lens management of keratoconus in a patient with residual astigmatism resulting from implantation of a toric intraocular lens. Clin Exp Optom. 2013;96:238–41.
17. Jonker S, Berendschot T, Ronden A, Saelens I, Bauer N, Nuijts R. Long-term endothelial cell loss in patients with artisan myopia and artisan toric phakic intraocular lenses. Ophthalmology. 2017. https://doi.org/10.1016/j.ophtha.2017.08.011.

Chapter 24
Toric IOLs in Keratoconus Patients with Cataract

Luba Rodov and Guy Kleinmann

Keratoconus (KC) is a common ectatic disorder involving the central or paracentral cornea, that generates corneal protrusion, irregular astigmatism, and decreased vision [1]. A recent large epidemiologic study from the Netherlands found an annual incidence of 1:7500 in patients aged 10–44 years and estimated prevalence of 1:375 in the general population (265 cases per 100,000). This five- to tenfold increase compared to previous estimations might be due to recent increase in the availability of corneal imaging techniques, resulting in increased accuracy with respect to diagnosing KC [2]. Risk factors for KC development include constant eye rubbing, floppy-eyelid syndrome, allergies, family history of KC, Down syndrome. Nearly all cases are bilateral, though often of asymmetric severity. Sometimes the less affected eye shows only high regular astigmatism. The disease tends to progress during the adolescent years and into the second and third decades. Later on in life progression of KC is rare, and the cornea usually stabilizes. While progression occurs, the apical thinning of the central cornea worsens, and extreme degrees of irregular astigmatism can develop [1].

The diagnosis of KC relies on clinical exam including biomicroscopic examination, combined with corneal imaging such as corneal topography and tomography. In moderate and advanced stages, clinical signs include stromal thinning, Munson sign, Fleischer ring, Vogt striae or hydrops. Subclinical KC, known as form fruste KC, refers to abnormal corneal topography with localized steepening or an asymmetric bowtie but normal appearing cornea on biomicroscopy, plus at least one of the complementary signs (K > 47.0 D, oblique cylinder >1.5 D, central corneal thickness (CCT) <500 μ, clinical KC in the fellow eye). At an early stage of KC, the epithelial thinning over the cone partially compensates for the elevation of the anterior part of the cornea. Systems based on the rotating Scheimpflug camera, such as Pentacam, Galilei, or Sirius systems, offer the possibility of obtaining tomographic

L. Rodov · G. Kleinmann (✉)
Ophthalmology Department, Kaplan Medical Center, Rehovot, Israel

A. Barbara (ed.), *Controversies in the Management of Keratoconus*,
https://doi.org/10.1007/978-3-319-98032-4_24

with additional pachymetric, and aberrometric information. Tomography offers the advantage of direct measurement of the corneal posterior elevation, which is an early sign in KC. Tomographic measurements using optical coherence tomography (OCT) are another option. Specific indices are used for the detection of corneal ectasia, such as the Inferior–Superior index (I-S), surface asymmetry index (SAI), surface regularity index (SRI), corneal irregularity measurement (CIM), and skew of steepest radial axis (SRAX). Algorithms and predictive models that combine data from different systems and analyses can be used for diagnosis in an incipient or subclinical stage [3].

Ambrósio et al. derived a Tomographic and Biomechanical Index (TBI), which combines Scheimpflug based corneal tomography and biomechanics for enhancing ectasia detection. Pentacam HR and Corvis ST (Oculus Optikgeräte GmbH, Wetzlar, Germany) parameters were analyzed and combined using different artificial intelligence methods. The TBI generated by the RF/LOOCV method provided greater accuracy for detecting ectasia and was found to be sensitive for detecting subclinical (form fruste) ectasia among eyes with normal topography in patients with very asymmetric disease severity. The TBI may also confirm unilateral ectasia, potentially characterizing the inherent ectasia susceptibility of the cornea [4].

There are many treatment modalities for the different stages of KC. Spectacles, soft lenses, soft toric, or custom soft toric contact lenses may be used in early KC cases to correct myopia, regular astigmatism, and mildly irregular astigmatism. However, as the disease progresses, it becomes more difficult to achieve satisfactory vision because of high irregular astigmatism and significant anisometropia. Rigid gas-permeable (RGP) lenses or various specialized lenses, such as hybrid lenses, piggyback, or scleral lenses, may be required for advanced KC [5].

Intrastromal corneal ring segments (ICRS) implantation was suggested as a safe and reversible technique that can achieve corneal flattening and improve visual outcomes. Candidates for this procedure are patients with corrected distance visual acuity (CDVA) below 0.9, who are intolerant to contact lens use and have no corneal scarring. Most authors report satisfactory results after ICRS implantation in terms of visual acuity and optical quality. Patients with poor visual acuity at the time of surgery but stable disease are most likely to benefit from the procedure [5].

For advanced cases of KC penetrating keratoplasty (PKP) or Deep Anterior Lamellar Keratoplasty (DALK) are necessary to restore vision [5].

Corneal Cross-Linking uses riboflavin (vitamin B2) in combination with ultraviolet A (UV-A) irradiation to achieve a strengthening effect of corneal tissue and arrest KC progression. This method was proven beneficial using the standard Dresden protocol and accelerated cross linking [5, 6]. Transepithelial techniques are controversial [5].

In keratoconic eyes small changes in lens clarity can significantly impact upon the visual axis and reduce vision. Keratoconic patients also tend to develop lens opacification earlier on in life. As cataract surgery becomes necessary, specific issues regarding IOL selection and surgical technique need to be addressed [7].

Acquiring reliable keratometric values for IOL calculation is challenging in KC patients as corneal topography measurements seem to be more variable for steeper corneal curvatures and in the presence of corneal irregularity and scarring. The reliability of corneal topography and K measurements in KC can be adversely affected by fixation difficulties and a displaced visual axis during measurements [7]. Limited repeatability of keratometric measurements in patients with KC remained a problem using different devices (Pentacam, Eyesys, Orbscan, IOLMaster, Javal manual keratometer), particularly in patients with maximal K reading >55 D [8]. One option to increase reliability in cases with difficult and unreliable corneal measurements is to perform a two-step surgery: first perform cataract extraction and a few weeks later determine aphakic refraction and use the refractive vergence formula developed by W. Hill to choose the appropriate IOL power for secondary implantation [9].

Intraoperative wavefront aberrometry (ORA), is another approach for IOL power calculation. It was tested in eyes with high axial myopia, and found better than all formulas based on preoperative biometry and as effective as the AL-optimized Holladay 1 formula in predicting residual refractive error and reducing hyperopic outcomes [10]. This method was also tested in patients with bilateral cataracts having toric IOL implantation. Compared with standard methods, the use of intraoperative aberrometry system increased the proportion of eyes with postoperative refractive astigmatism of 0.50 D or less and reduced the mean postoperative refractive astigmatism at 1 month [11]. However, its' use was not evaluated in KC patients.

The accuracy of standard IOL calculation formulas is reduced, especially in cases of moderate to advanced KC [7]. For K readings greater than 46.00 D, myopic errors are more likely using the SRK/T and Hill-RBF formulas and hyperopic errors using the Olsen C-constant and Haigis [12].

There are several intraoperative considerations unique to KC patients. The main incision may have an unpredictable impact on the structurally abnormal keratoconic cornea. Aiello et al. [7] recommend to plan its' location during preoperative examination according to the peripheral corneal thickness rather than the astigmatism axis. They suggest that in cases with corneal scarring, the main incision should be placed 90° apart from the scar location. To reduce the risk of post-operative wound leak and induce less change in corneal shape they suggested either creating a two steps sclero-corneal incision or standard temporal corneal incisions, made as close to the limbus as possible. Use of a corneal suture to secure the wound may sometimes be necessary. Capsular staining dye may be considered to enhance capsular visualization during continuous curvilinear capsulorhexis. The authors also suggested to minimize intraocular pressure during surgery to reduce stress on the cornea. Chen et al. showed that the use of hydroxypropyl methylcellulose 2% on the corneal surface provided significantly better optical clarity than BSS during cataract surgery [13]. Aiello et al. [7] suggested it could also improve intraocular visibility and reduce image distortion during cataract surgery in KC patients.

Toric IOLs were designed for patients with regular corneal astigmatism, currently up to 4.00 D in the United States. Outside the US, there is a wider range of toric IOLs, and customized IOLs are also available. Previous studies demonstrated significant reduction in spherical and astigmatic refractive errors using toric IOLs, with good efficacy, safety, and predictability in cataract patients with regular astigmatism [14].

KC is the classical example of irregular astigmatism and therefore KC patients are not obvious candidates for toric IOL implantation. However, for some keratoconic corneas a regular astigmatic component may be isolated in the central area. Such cases may benefit from toric IOL correction. This is particularly important for elderly patients, who often have difficulty using contact lenses. Another consideration is the lenticular component in manifest astigmatism, which in some cases might partially balance the corneal astigmatism. For such patients cataract extraction with non-toric IOL implantation might lead to worsening of astigmatism.

Toric IOL implantation should be avoided in patients who might require future keratoplasty and in patients that are going to return to rigid gas permeable (RGP) contact lens or scleral contact lens after surgery. Effective astigmatism of the cornea is expected to change after penetrating or deep lamellar keratoplasty, leaving an IOL with wrong toric power and axis in the eye, which may be even more difficult to correct. Therefore toric IOLs should only be considered in patients with stable KC, who are not candidates for corneal transplantation. Use of RGP or scleral contact lens eliminates the corneal impact on total astigmatism, so that the toric IOL causes manifest astigmatism [15].

Although to date there are no large prospective clinical trials to provide definite evidence and guidelines, several case studies have been published regarding different aspects of toric IOL implantation in KC patients.

Mol et al. retrospectively studied 17 eyes of 16 patients with three corneal conditions (KC, postkeratoplasty, and post-pterygium surgery) who underwent phacoemulsification with toric IOL implantation for visually significant cataract. The KC group was not evaluated separately from the others. Inclusion criteria were fairly regular corneal astigmatism of 1.25 D or more, a bow tie-like pattern on corneal topography and corneal-based astigmatism correctable with spectacles. They also had to be stable during multiple tomography examinations. Exclusion criteria included endothelial cell count <1500/mm^2, irregular astigmatism unable to be corrected with spectacles and ocular comorbidities that could have an impact on capsular bag stability, affect visual acuity, or the quality of vision. Patients with severe KC (average K readings >55 D) were excluded from this study. At 1 year follow-up, the mean BCVA improved from 0.59 ± 0.44 logMAR, before surgery, to 0.13 ± 0.13 logMAR after surgery. Corrected distance Snellen visual acuity was 20/32 or better in 14 eyes (82%) and 20/25 or better in ten eyes (59%). The mean refractive SE decreased from −3.10 ± 3.95 D preoperatively to 0.22 ± 1.53 D postoperatively. The mean refractive cylinder decreased from 6.3 ± 4.7 D preoperatively to 1.5 ± 1.5 D postoperatively. The authors concluded that phacoemulsification with toric IOL implantation for visually significant cataract was a safe and effective procedure in topographically stable KC, with fairly regular (although sometimes very high) corneal astigmatism. They recommend to remain on the conservative (myopic) side with choice of target SE, as steep keratoconic corneas produce a tendency toward hyperopic outcomes. In eyes with severe KC biometry tends to overestimate the corneal power and underestimate the IOL power, therefore they were not included in this study [16].

Hashemi et al. investigated the results of cataract surgery using AcrySof toric IOL implantation in patients with mild, moderate or severe but stable KC. Twenty three eyes of 17 patients were evaluated. Inclusion criteria were stable KC with a clear cornea in the visual axis and cataract. Exclusion criteria were corneal scaring in the visual axis, endothelial cell count of less than 1500/mm^2, glaucoma, diabetic retinopathy, positive history of ocular inflammation, and macular disorders. IOL power calculation formula was selected according to AL: The Hoffer Q for AL shorter than 22 mm, SRK II for AL of 22–24.5 mm, Holladay I for AL of 24.5–26 mm, and SRK/T formula for AL longer than 26 mm. The placement axis for the IOL was calculated using the AcrySof toric online calculator. Surgically induced astigmatism was estimated as 0.25 D. At 3 months post-surgery, uncorrected distance visual acuity (UCDVA) and best corrected distance visual acuity (BCDVA) improved in all KC severity groups: UCDVA was 0.90 ± 0.64 logMAR, 1.00 ± 0.48 logMAR, and 1.30 ± 0 logMAR before the surgery and 0.27 ± 0.18 logMAR, 0.34 ± 0.19 logMAR, and 0.38 ± 0.29 logMAR after the surgery in the mild, moderate, and severe KC groups, respectively. The refractive cylinder in the three severity groups was 3.00 ± 1.19 D, 3.15 ± 0.82 D and 6.83 ± 3.06 before surgery and 1.83 ± 0.90 D, 1.25 ± 0.96 D and 4.67 ± 2.31 D, 3 month post-surgery. The moderate KC group showed most improvement in BCDVA. Spherical equivalent (SE) also decreased in all KC severity groups. All results were statistically significant for the mild and moderate KC groups but not for the severe group due to its' small size. The preoperative cylinder power of patients in this study was 1.5–10 D, whereas maximum astigmatism correction by the AcrySoftoric IOL is approximately 4 D. Therefore a residual astigmatism was expected for most patients. At 3 months post-surgery this residual astigmatism was measured using manifest refraction and compared to that, anticipated before the surgery. The difference was found to be minimal in patients with mild and moderate KC and more significant in patients with severe KC, indicating the lower reliability of keratomtric readings in this group of patients. The degree of IOL rotation in this study was minimal, similar between the groups, and to that reported for toric IOL implantation in patients without KC. The mean absolute error (MAE) was calculated in a retrograde manner for each formula and each method of keratometry used. The lowest MAE was obtained with corneal topography-derived keratometry, manual keratometry, and the SRK/T formula in patients with mild KC, corneal topography-derived keratometry and the SRK/T formula in patients with moderate KC, and corneal topography-derived keratometry, manual keratometry, and SRK/T and SRK II formulas in patients with severe KC [17].

Kamiya et al. prospectively examined 19 eyes of 19 consecutive patients with stable KC, who underwent phacoemulsification with toric IOL implantation. All were RGP lens intolerant. A toric AcrySof lens was selected using K readings obtained by corneal topography at 3 mm diameter, axial length (AL) measured with an IOL master. IOL power calculations performed by the SRK/T formula and optimal cylinder power and alignment axis determined using the AcrySof toric online calculator. UCDVA significantly improved from 1.14 ± 0.50 logMAR preoperatively to 0.46 ± 0.33 logMAR 3 months postoperatively. BCDVA also significantly improved from 0.27 ± 0.45 logMAR preoperatively to −0.01 ± 0.09 logMAR postoperatively. The refractive astigmatism was significantly decreased from −1.92 ± 1.73 D to −0.70 ± 0.60 D. The corneal astigmatism was not significantly changed postoperatively, nor were the corneal higher-order aberrations (HOAs) for a 4 mm pupil. The authors found no significant correlation between logMAR BCDVA and HOAs preoperatively, but a significant correlation between them 3 months postoperatively. This suggests that corneal HOAs play a role in visual performance in keratoconic patients undergoing toric IOL implantation. They concluded that toric IOL implantation was effective for correction of astigmatic errors in eyes with mild non-progressive KC, without a significant induction of corneal HOAs. The authors suggested that selection criteria for toric IOL implantation for KC will include RGP lens intolerance, stable keratometry and refraction, low grade KC and lower corneal HOAs [18].

Alió et al. investigated the visual and refractive outcomes, safety, efficacy and stability of micro-incision cataract surgery (MICS) followed by implantation of toric IOL in eyes with stable KC. This retrospective study included 17 eyes of 10 patients. The Hoffer Q or the SRK/T formula were applied, according to the AL. MICS technique was chosen in an attempt to reduce astigmatic changes at the corneal level. UCDVA changed significantly from 1.33 ± 0.95 logMAR preoperatively to 0.32 ± 0.38 logMAR postoperatively, with 60% of eyes achieving UCDVA ≥20/30. BCDVA also changed significantly from 0.32 ± 0.45 to 0.20 ± 0.36 logMAR. The astigmatism improved significantly from −2.95 ± 1.71 D preoperative to −1.40 ± 1.13 D postoperative. Keratometry remained stable during the follow up period (9.10 ± 5.54 months). AL showed the strongest correlation with final SE (stronger than the preoperative keratometry). No intraoperative or postoperative complications were detected. They suggested that MICS with toric IOL implantation may be considered as a safe and efficient procedure in non-progressive KC, in initial to moderate grades and with central ectasia. They concluded that refractive accuracy was better in patients with higher axial lengths, higher spherical equivalent and when the SRK/T formula was used [19].

Nanavaty et al. retrospectively studied 12 eyes of nine patients with stable mild to moderate KC and cataract, who underwent phacoemulsification with toric IOL implantation, using the AT TORBI 709 M lens, AcriTec. Mean refractive sphere improved significantly from −4.80 ± 5.60 preoperatively to 0.30 ± 0.50 D postoperatively. Total astigmatism also improved significantly from 3.00 ± 1.00 D to 0.70 ± 0.80 D. No intra- or postoperative complications occurred. No eyes had progression of KC or significant IOL rotation during the follow-up time (9.0 + 8.8 months). Patients showed significant improvement in UCDVA, that was 20/40 or better in 75% of eyes postoperatively and in BCDVA, that was 20/40 or better in 83.3% of eyes [20].

Jaimes et al. reviewed post-operative results of patients with nonprogressive KC, without visually significant cataract, treated with refractive lens exchange (RLE) using in-the-bag AcrySof toric IOL implantation. Medical records of 13 patients (19 eyes) were included, of which 12 patients were diagnosed with KC and 1 with pellucid marginal degeneration. Mean follow-up after the surgery was 7.89 ± 6.61 months. Mean sphere improved significantly from −5.25 ± 6.40 D preoperatively to 0.22 ± 1.01 D postoperatively. Mean total astigmatism also decreased significantly from 3.95 ± 1.30 D to 1.36 ± 1.17 D. The UCDVA improved significantly, from 1.35 ± 0.36 logMAR before surgery to 0.29 ± 0.23 logMAR after the surgery. The authors concluded that RLE with toric IOL implantation may be an effective therapeutic option in the optical rehabilitation of patients with stable and non-progressive KC [21].

Abou Samra et al. prospectively evaluated the visual and topographic outcomes of a two-stage approach treatment for selected cases of progressive KC: corneal collagen cross-linking (CXL) followed by phacoemulsification with toric IOL implantation 6 months later. Inclusion criteria were age 35 years or older, mild to moderate progressive KC according to Pentacam indices, a clear cornea in the visual axis and minimal corneal thickness more than 420 mm. Patients with endothelial cell count less than 1500/mm^2, glaucoma, positive history of ocular surgery or inflammation, fundus disorders, a history of chemical injury, or any other ocular or systemic disease that might affect epithelial healing were excluded. Patients who could not be corrected by their refraction to 0.50 logMAR or better were also excluded from the study. Nine eyes of six patients met those criteria. A standard epi-off CXL protocol (30 min of 3 mW/cm^2 irradiation) was implemented. IOL power was calculated using the SRK-II formula. IOL target power was adjusted for a mild myopic shift because CXL may continue to induce corneal flattening with a resulting myopia reduction. The results demonstrated significant improvements in UCDVA (from 1.42 ± 0.52 to 0.30 ± 0.11 logMAR), BCDVA (from 0.35 ± 0.11 to 0.25 ± 0.11 logMAR), sphere (from −5.82 ± 1.91 to −0.33 ± 0.72 D) and total astigmatism (from −4.51 ± 0.95 to −1.10 ± 0.76 D). Topographical parameters demonstrated stability of Kmax and thinnest pachymetry during 1 year follow-up. Measurements of mesopic vision showed significant increase in contrast sensitivity. However glare also increased significantly after this treatment protocol. Subjective parameters and measures such as clarity of vision, patient satisfaction, visual fluctuation, halos and starburst, activity limitations, far and near spectacle dependence improved significantly after the surgery [22].

Farideh et al. prospectively evaluated the clinical results of toric trifocal diffractive IOL (AT LISA 939MP) in ten eyes of five patients with cataract and mild KC. Exclusion criteria were prior ocular surgery, other ocular disease, amblyopia, diabetes patients, corneal astigmatism lower than 2.00 D, active intraocular inflammation and endothelial cell count less than 1200 cells/mm. At 6 month follow-up, UCDVA (logMAR) improved from 0.88 ± 0.09 to 0.13 ± 0.09, uncorrected intermediate visual acuity (UCIVA) improved from 0.43 ± 0.07 to 0.11 ± 0.07 logMAR, and uncorrected near visual acuity (UCNVA) improved from 0.36 ± 0.06 to 0.1 ± 0.06 logMAR. All were statistically significant. Total astigmatism was reduced from 3.5 ± 1.84 preoperatively to 0.58 ± 0.57 D 6 month postoperatively. Postoperative contrast sensitivity and aberration results were comparable with preoperative values. The authors concluded that implantation of trifocal IOLs can provide good visual outcomes for distance, intermediate and near in patients with mild stable KC [23]. Although they reported promising results caution is recommended since these are far from being the ideal patients for multifocal IOLs.

Phacoemulsification with toric IOL implantation can be considered as a treatment option in selected cases of stable KC with reasonable visual potential and consistent keratomentric measurements. It also requires the identification of an astigmatic axis in the central portion of the cornea. The steep K and posterior astigmatism should be considered. Under-correction of astigmatism is recommended. Realistic patient expectations are of great importance. The patient should be counseled that improvement in visual acuity will be partial due the corneal disease and only a portion of the astigmatism will be corrected (the regular component).

Criteria for toric IOL implantation in KC patients
Stable keratoconus
Reasonable visual potential
Consistent keratometric measurements
Realistic patient expectations
Consider under-correction of astigmatism
Consider the posterior astigmatism and steep k

We present several cases from our practice.

24.1 Case 1

A 79 years old woman diagnosed with stable KC presented with decreased vision in both eyes. On examination her UCDVA was 6/60 OD and 6/120 OS. Refraction was +4.50–6.50×46 OD and +0.25–9.00×89 OS. Her BCDVA was 6/15 OD and 6/30+ OS. On slit lamp examination her corneas were keratoconic with guttata, without edema or scars, there was grade 3 nuclear sclerosis cataract in both eyes and normal fundi. Her endothelial cell count was reduced to 958/905 due to the Fuchs endothelial corneal dystrophy. Her topographic and tomographic measurements are presented in Figs. 24.1 and 24.2.

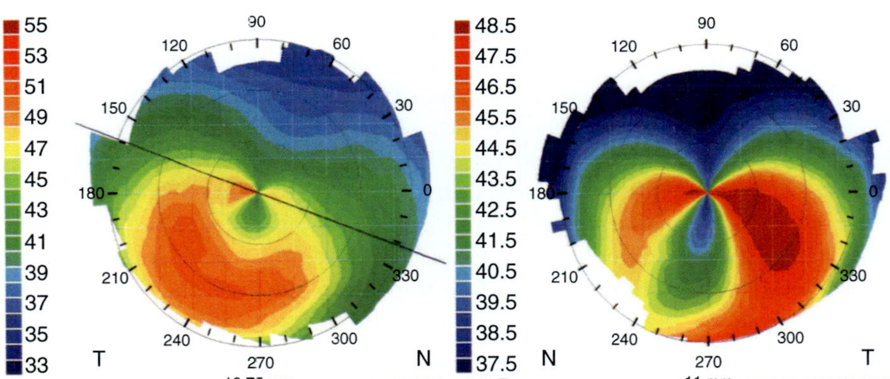

Fig. 24.1 Corneal topography of patient 1 demonstrates keratoconus. An axis of the irregular astigmatism can be defined in both eyes

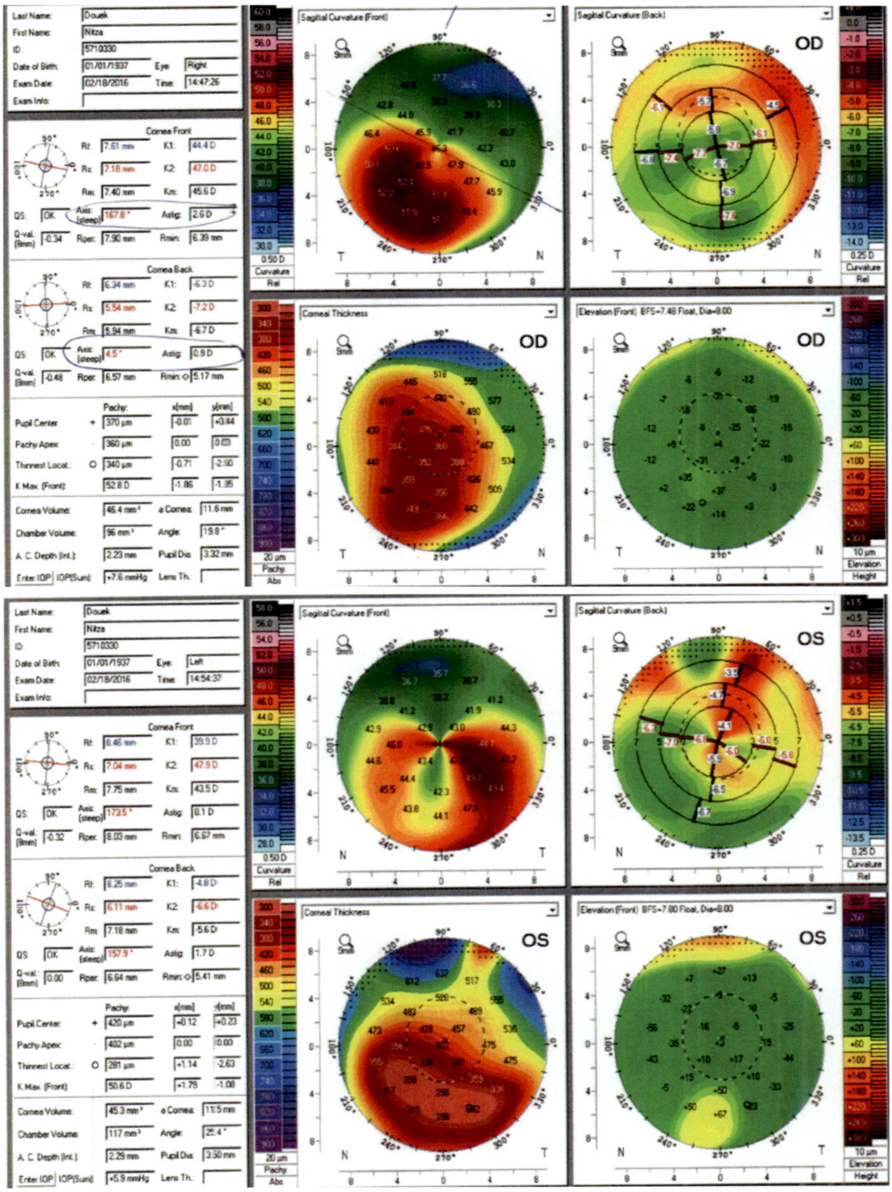

Fig. 24.2 Corneal tomography of patient 1 demonstrates KC. An axis of the irregular astigmatism can be defined in both eyes

Her astigmatism measurements using different devices are presented in Table 24.1.

Since there was a defined central corneal astigmatic axis and good repeatability with different devices, we felt confident to recommend a toric IOL implantation.

Table 24.1 Summary of the corneal astigmatism measurements of patient 1

RE		LE
4.30@157^0	IOL master	9.92@2^0
5.04@162^0	Lenstar	10.17@178^0
3.11@162^0	Atlas	7.82@174^0
4.25X162^0	Refraction	10.50X4^0
2.60@167.8^0	Pentacam Anterior	8.10@174^0
0.90@4.5^0	Pentacam Posterior	1.70@158^0
2.00@161^0	TNP	
4.92@167^0	OA-2000	

We did so despite a low endothelial cell count, as in our practice the majority of such corneas survive surgery without endothelial decompensation. Also, because her corneas were clear, in an event of edema development after cataract surgery, the patient could undergo posterior lamellar transplantation (DSAEK or DMEK) which has little impact on corneal astigmatism. The patient was consulted regarding the risks of surgery, different treatment options and expected outcome, and chose to proceed with cataract surgery with toric IOL implantation. According to this data, the IOLs chosen for implantation were T-FLEX 573T PRM (Rayner, England) SPH 15.50, CYL 6.50@164° in her right eye, and T-FLEX 573T PRM (Rayner, England) SPH 14.50, CYL 11.0@180° in her left eye. At 2 and 3 month follow up her UCDVA were 6/15 in both eyes, refraction was +0.50–1.50×115 in her right eye, and +0.25–2.00×135 in her left eye. The UCDVA for both eyes was 6/12 and the patient was very satisfied with this result.

24.2 Case 2

A 73 years old woman was interested in cataract surgery, specifically with extended depth of focus (EDOF) IOL. Her UCDVA was 6/15 OD and 6/12 OS. Refraction was +2.50–3.00×180 OD and +1.50–0.25×180 OS. BCDVA was 6/9 OD and 6/12 OS. She had clear corneas without signs of KC, significant anterior cortical cataract and normal fundi. Her topographic and tomographic maps showed irregular astigmatism with asymmetric bowties and high Kmax, Figs. 24.3

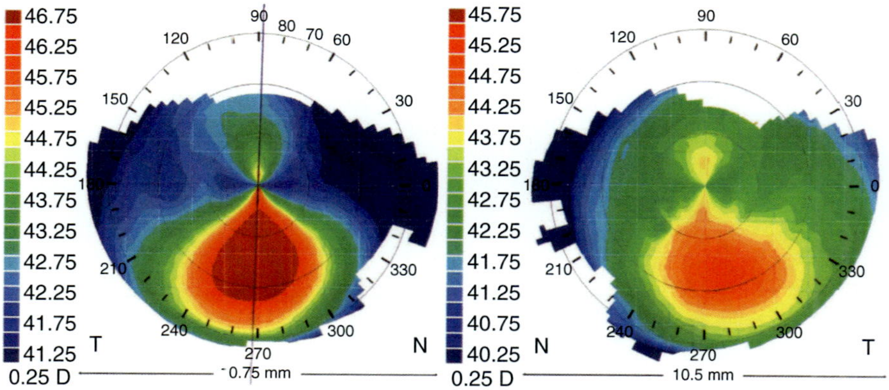

Fig. 24.3 Corneal topography of patient 2 demonstrates an asymmetric bow-tie pattern suggestive of KC. An axis of the irregular astigmatism can be defined in both eyes

and 24.4. She was diagnosed with Form Fruste KC and advised against EDOF IOL implantation. A year later she came back for another consult on cataract surgery. Her UCDVA and BCDVA were the same and the topography and tomography showed no progression.

Astigmatic measurements on both visits using different devices are presented in Table 24.2.

In this patient a defined regular component for central corneal astigmatism was found as well, with similar repeated measurements with different devices and without evidence of progression between the two visits.

The patient had cataract surgery in her right eye, with implantation of Acrysof Toric IQ T5 21.5 D at 89°. Two months post-op her UCDVA was 6/6.6 with −0.5D sphere refraction. BCDVA was 6/6. The patient was extremely pleased with this result.

24.3 Case 3

A 59 years old woman with KC came in for a consult on cataract surgery with toric IOL implantation, because her brother was implanted with toric IOL for high regular astigmatism and was extremely happy with the results. The patient had advanced keratoconus with corneal scars, and she used piggyback contact lenses. She had mild cataracts and her vision was stable with the contact lenses. Her UCDVA was CF 2 m OD and CF 1.5 m OS. Refraction was −18.00/−3.50×30 OD and −21.00/−4.00×168 OS. BCDVA was 6/30 for both eyes. The rest of her ophthalmic exam was within normal limits. Her topographic and tomographic maps are shown in Figs. 24.5 and 24.6. No regular component for the astigmatism was noted.

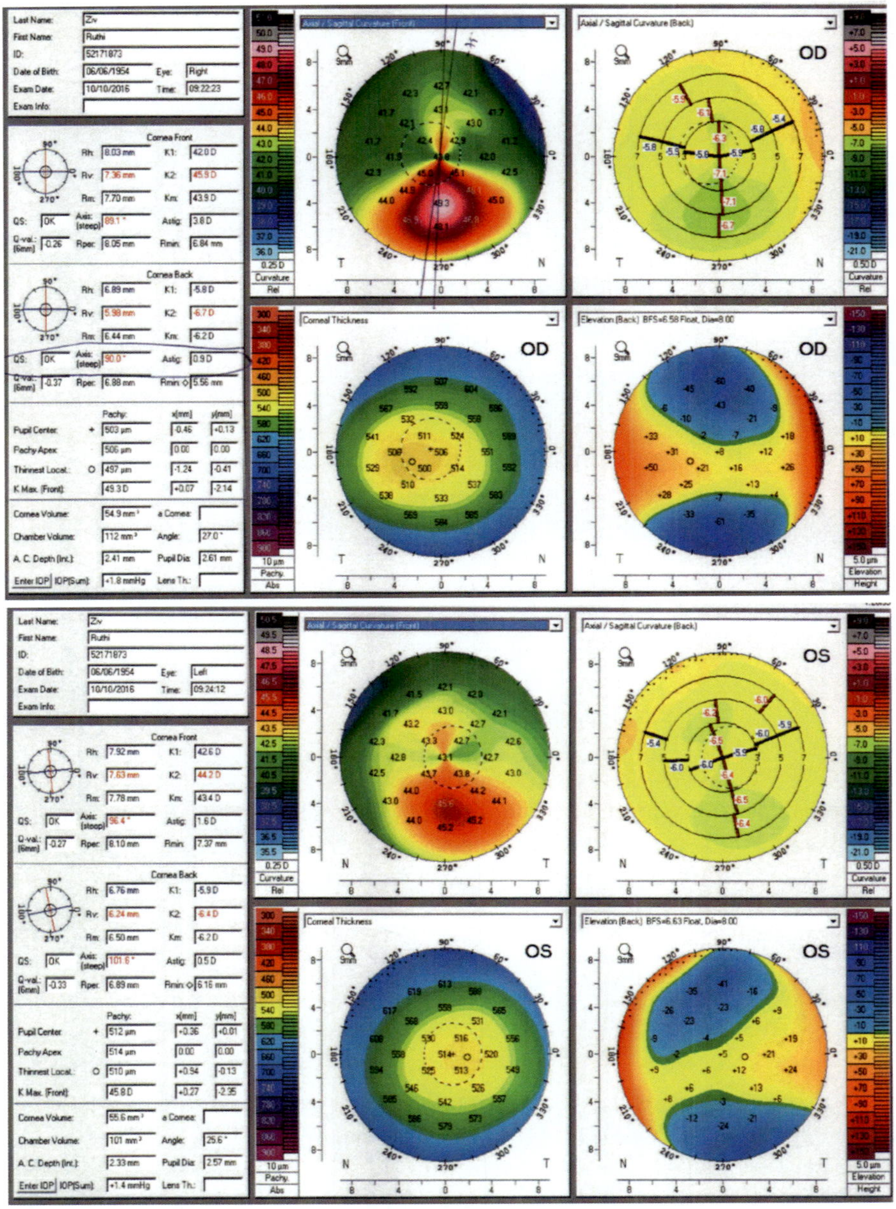

Fig. 24.4 Corneal tomography of patient 2 demonstrates a classic pattern of KC, more prominent in the right eye. An axis of the irregular astigmatism can be defined in both eyes

Table 24.2 Summary of the corneal astigmatism measurements of patient 2, first visit (in blue) and second visit a year later (in black)

RE		LE
3.70@91^{0} *3.93@90^{0}*	IOL master	1.68@97^{0} *1.29@94^{0}*
3.88@87^{0} *3.50@89^{0}*	Lenstar	1.74@99^{0} *1.09@98^{0}*
3.90@94^{0} *3.73@99^{0}*	Atlas	1.52@95^{0} *1.45@96^{0}*
3.0X93^{0} *3.0X90^{0}*	Refraction	1.50@101^{0} *0.25@90^{0}*
3.80@89.10^{0} *3.9@92.2^{0}*	Pentacam Anterior	1.60@96.4^{0} *1.60@95.4^{0}*
0.90@90^{0} *0.9@92.9^{0}*	Pentacam Posterior	0.50@101.6^{0} *0.50@95^{0}*

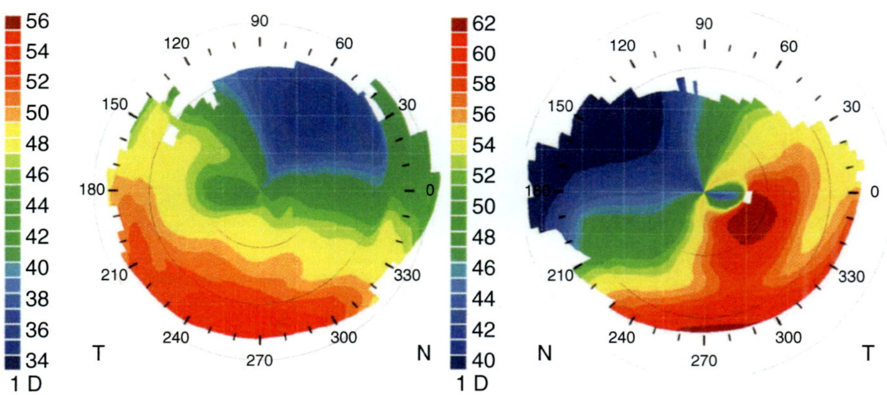

Fig. 24.5 Corneal topography of patient 3 demonstrated a classic pattern of KC. An axis of the irregular astigmatism cannot be defined

Her astigmatism measurements using different devices are presented in Table 24.3, showing poor repeatability.

Due to the severity of KC without a possibility to define a central corneal axis for the astigmatism, poor repeatability of corneal astigmatism measurements by the different devices and the minimal cataract, she was advised against cataract surgery and especially against toric IOL implantation.

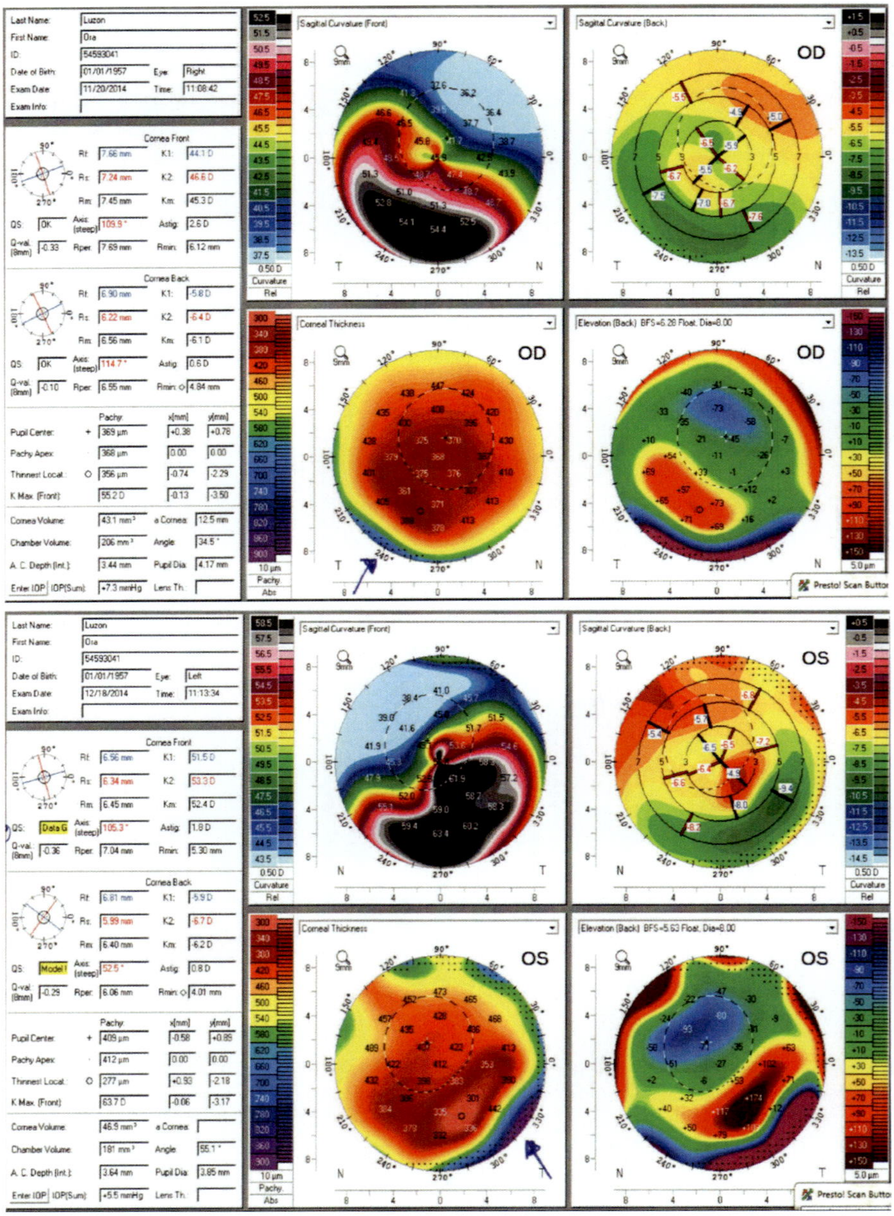

Fig. 24.6 Corneal tomography of patient 3 demonstrated a classic pattern of KC. An axis of the irregular astigmatism cannot be defined

Table 24.3 Summary of the corneal astigmatism measurements of patient 3

RE		LE
4.90 @ 129⁰	IOL master I	8.76 @ 54⁰
	IOL master II	7.07 @ 57⁰
	IOL master III	15.44 @ 49⁰
3.07 @ 122⁰	Lenstar	6.18 @ 71⁰
2.6 @ 109.9⁰	Pentacam	1.8 @ 105.3⁰
5.47 @ 141⁰	Atlas	0.98 @ 35⁰

References

1. Rabinowitz YS. Keratoconus. Surv Ophthalmol. 1998;42:297–319.
2. Godefrooij DA, Ardine de Wit G, Uiterwaal CS, Imhof SM, Wisse RPL. Age-specific incidence and prevalence of keratoconus: a nationwide registration study. Am J Ophthalmol. 2017;175:169–72.
3. Martínez-Abad A, Piñero DP. New perspective on the detection abd progression of keratoconus. J Cataract Refract Surg. 2017;43(9):1213–27.
4. Ambrósio R Jr, Lopes BT, Faria-Correia F, Salomão MQ, Bühren J, Roberts CJ, Elsheikh A, Vinciguerra R, Vinciguerra P. Integration of Scheimpflug-based corneal tomography and biomechanical assessments for enhancing ectasia detection. J Refract Surg. 2017;33(7):434–43.
5. Andreanos KD, Hashemi K, Petrelli M, Droutsas K, Georgalas I, Kymionis GD. Keratoconus treatment algorithm. Ophthalmol Therapy. 2017;6(2):245–62.
6. Wang YM, Chan TC, Yu MCY, Jhanji V. Comparative evaluation of progression rate in keratoconus before and after collagen crosslinking. Br J Ophthalmol. 2017;33(9):632–8.
7. Aiello F, Nasser QJ, Nucci C, Angunawela RI, Gatzioufas Z, Maurino V. Cataract surgery in patients with keratoconus: pearls and pitfalls. Open Ophthalmol J. 2017;11:194–200.
8. Hashemi H, Yekta A, Khabazkhoob M. Effect of keratoconus grades on repeatability of keratometry readings: comparison of 5 devices. J Cataract Refract Surg. 2015;41(5):1065–72.
9. http://www.doctor-hill.com.
10. Hill DC, Sudhakar S, Hill CS, King TS, Scott IU, Ernst BB, Pantanelli SM. Intraoperative aberrometry versus preoperative biometry for intraocular lens power selection in axial myopia. J Cataract Refract Surg. 2017;43(4):505–10.
11. Woodcock MG, Lehmann R, Cionni RJ, Breen M, Scott MC. Intraoperative aberrometry versus standard preoperative biometry and a toric IOL calculator for bilateral toric IOL implantation with a femtosecond laser: one-month results. J Cataract Refract Surg. 2016;42(6):817–25.
12. Reitblat O, Levy A, Kleinmann G, Lerman TT, Assia EI. Intraocular lens power calculation for eyes with high and low average keratometry readings: comparison between various formulas. J Cataract Refract Surg. 2017;43(9):1149–56.

13. Chen YA, Hirnschall N, Findl O. Comparison of corneal wetting properties of viscous eye lubricant and balanced salt solution to maintain optical clarity during cataract surgery. J Cataract Refract Surg. 2011;37(10):1806–8.
14. Miyake T, Kamiya K, Amano R, Iida Y, Tsunehiro S, Shimizu K. Long-term clinical outcomes of toric intraocular lens implantation in cataract cases with preexisting astigmatism. J Cataract Refract Surg. 2014;40(10):1654–60.
15. Moshirfar M, Walker BD, Birdsong OC. Catarct surgery in eyes with keratoconus: a review of current literature. Curr Opin Ophthalmol. 2018;29(1):75–80.
16. Mol IE, Van Dooren BT. Toric intraocular lenses for correction of astigmatism in keratoconus and after corneal surgery. Clin Ophthalmol. 2016;10:1153–9.
17. Hashemi H, Heidarian S, Seyedian MA, Yekta A, Khabazkhoob M. Evaluation of the results of using toric IOL in the cataract surgery of keratoconus patients. Eye Contact Lens. 2015;41(6):354–8.
18. Kamiya K, Shimizu K, Miyake T. Changes in astigmatism and corneal higher-order aberrations after phacoemulsification with toric intraocular lens implantation for mild keratoconus with cataract. Jpn J Ophthalmol. 2016;60(4):302–8.
19. Alió JL, Peña-García P, Abdulla Guliyeva F, Soria FA, Zein G, Abu-Mustafa SK. MICS with toric intraocular lenses in keratoconus: outcomes and predictability analysis of postoperative refraction. Br J Ophthalmol. 2014;98(3):365–70.
20. Nanavaty MA, Lake DB, Daya SM. Outcomes of pseudophakic toric intraocular lens implantation in Keratoconic eyes with cataract. J Refract Surg. 2012;28(12):884–9.
21. Jaimes M, Xacur-García F, Alvarez-Melloni D, Graue-Hernández EO, Ramirez-Luquín T, Navas A. Refractive lens exchange with toric intraocular lenses in keratoconus. J Refract Surg. 2011;27(9):658–64.
22. Abou Samra WA, Awad EA, El Kannishy AH. Objective and subjective outcome of clear lensectomy with toric IOL implantation after corneal collagen cross-linking in selected cases of keratoconus. Eye Contact Lens. 2016.
23. Farideh D, Azad S, Feizollah N, Sana N, Cyrus A, Mohammad G, Alireza BR. Clinical outcomes of new toric trifocal diffractive intraocular lens in patients with cataract and stable keratoconus. Six months follow-up. Medicine (Baltimore). 2017;96(12):e6340.

Chapter 25
Why Perform Deep Anterior Lamelar Keratoplasty and Not Full-Thickness Keratoplasty for the Treatment of Keratoconus

Víctor Sergio Eguiza, Julia Martinez, Merce Morral, Óscar Gris, Daniel Elies, Míriam Barbany, Francisco Bandeira, Spyridoula Souki, Felicidad Manero Vidal, and Jose Luis Güell

25.1 Introduction

Why perform Deep Anterior Lamelar Keratoplasty (DALK) instead of PK (Penetrating Keratoplasty)? In recent years, DALK has experienced improvements in surgical technique that have allowed a much quicker and standardized procedure with similar final visual outcomes but a reduced risk of endothelial rejection compared to PK [1].

Corneal transplantation is one of the most common and successful forms of tissue transplantation in humans. Although PK is a very successful procedure, the overall success rate progressively decreases over time [2–5]. In a recent study, the overall observed 5 and 10-year graft survival after corneal transplantation was 74% and 64% respectively, and the predicted graft survival estimate was 27% after 20 years and 2% after 30 years, because of chronic endothelial failure [2, 4].

Keratoconus (KC) is a corneal ectasia that affects the stroma and the epithelium, which initially manifest as a change in refractive error [3]. In spite of the different treatments we have to improve vision (glasses, contact lenses, intrastromal corneal

V. S. Eguiza · J. Martinez · M. Morral · Ó. Gris · D. Elies · M. Barbany · S. Souki
F. M. Vidal
Cornea and Refractive Surgery Unit at Institut de Microcirurgia Ocular, Barcelona, Spain

F. Bandeira
Federal University of São Paulo, Cornea and External Disease Department, São Paulo, SP, Brazil

J. L. Güell (✉)
Cornea and Refractive Surgery Unit at Institut de Microcirurgia Ocular, Barcelona, Spain

Faculty of the European School for Advanced Studies in Ophthalmology (ESASO), Associate Professor of Ophthalmology at the Universitat Autonoma de Barcelona (UAB), Barcelona, Spain
e-mail: guell@imo.es

A. Barbara (ed.), *Controversies in the Management of Keratoconus*,
https://doi.org/10.1007/978-3-319-98032-4_25

segments [4] and intraocular phakic lenses) [3] and/or to stop their progression (cross-linking) [5], between 10% and 15% —according to the different series, require corneal transplantation [6] as a final treatment. Currently, given that most KC patients have a healthy endothelium the technique of choice is DALK [7].

25.2 History

For almost half a century, PK was the gold standard option for KC [8], but since DALK has been introduced as an alternative, the preference is progressively changing. In the first half of the twentieth century, anterior lamellar keratoplasty (ALK) was associated with poor visual outcomes because of interface scarring and opacification. Then, in the 80s, epikeratoplasty (EKP) was expected to eliminate the risk of interface haze; however, it was abandoned because of inferior visual and refractive results.

During the last decade, the evolution of DALK, particularly when performed in conjunction with the new techniques such as "big bubble" and viscodissection to separate the Descemet's membrane, offered better visual outcomes than traditional ALK and comparable to PK by reducing or eliminating the complications of interface scarring and opacification [9].

The first lamellar keratoplasty was performed by Mühlbauer in 1840 [10]. In 1971, José Barraquer outlined the necessary rules to achieve good visual results with keratoplasty: (1) try to obtain the deepest possible interface to reduce scarring; (2) create a back layer of uniform thickness; (3) make a smooth section of the graft surface as well as of the bed; (4) cut the graft to the appropriate thickness; (5) use the highest quality donor material; (6) ensure good coaptation of the edges and a uniform traction of the sutures, to ensure a perfectly clean interface.

Anwar used air to perform a very deep lamellar dissection to remove as much stromal tissue as possible and baptized the procedure with the name by which we know it today: the "big bubble". The term DALK was originally described by Eduardo Arenas Archila in 1984 [10, 11].

25.3 Advantages

25.3.1 Rejection

Full thickness corneal transplant or PK is the most used keratoplasty in the world, because of its high safety and effectiveness (93–96%) [12]. This is thanks to the avascularity of the cornea and its privileged immune situation [13].

For many years, PK has been the standard treatment for diseases of the corneal stroma with or without an affected endothelium such as KC, infectious keratitis and stromal dystrophies [14], but we must deal with the causes of corneal transplant failures: graft rejection and endothelial decompensation [2]. In DALK, we remove the pathologic stroma while preserving the host's healthy endothelial layer [15], assuming that this eliminates the risk of endothelial graft rejection, (which is 80–90% of all rejection episodes). With little doubt, this is the most important advantage.

On the other hand, we may have, as in any other corneal transplantation, a subepithelial or stromal graft rejection. The best way to prevent these issues is to monitor the wound and the sutures [16].

Several studies have shown a graft failure rate in PK patients of between 10% and 38% after 5 years and between 18% and 37% after 10 years. In DALK patients, the rate was 3% after 5 years. The predicted graft survival was of 41% after 20 years and 3% after 30 years for PK patients, but for DALK patients, this was 63% and 11%, respectively. Therefore, we can conclude that in the long term, as conceptually expected, graft survival is higher in DALK patients compared to PK patients [12]. In another study, a model predicted graft survival of 49 years in the DALK group and of 17.3 years in the PK group [17].

25.3.2 Cell Loss

In average healthy eyes, 0.6% of the endothelial cells (ECD) are lost every year. DALK has been associated with lower levels of endothelial cell loss compared to PK. This may be because of the reduced surgical trauma in DALK [18], because the host's Descemet membrane and endothelium are intact while only the anterior cornea is replaced and this results in less damage to the endothelium with fewer immunologic reactions compared to PK [16], and because of the absence of endothelial cell rejection in patients with DALK. PK induces a decline in the ECD after surgery and a higher annual endothelial cell loss that may persist for many years [18]. After calculating the half-life of the endothelial cell loss, the results were 10.0 years in the PK group and 28.6 years in the DALK group. This means that, in the long term, the ECD decreases by 50% every 10 years after PK and every 29 years after DALK [17]. This has been linked to a higher endothelial residual cell density in the last procedure [16].

25.3.3 Optical and Visual Quality Outcomes

Many studies have compared final visual quality, contrast sensitivity measurement and wavefront aberration measurement as well as the refractive and visual outcome, finding similar results [19–22]. This is especially true since the introduction of advanced techniques to separate the stroma from DM, where clearer interfaces in lamellar keratoplasty are achieved. It is important to differentiate between what we call descemetic DALK (dDALK) and predescemetic DALK (pdDALK): in the first procedure we remove all the stroma, leaving only Descemet's membrane and the recipient endothelium; in the second one we remove almost all the stroma, leaving a thin layer of stroma (Dua's layer and sometimes some posterior layers of the stroma) over Descemet's membrane and recipient endothelium [23, 24].

These procedures imply better postoperative visual results, which are comparable to or better than those achieved with PK. Best corrected visual acuity (BCVA) of 20/40 or greater range between 73% and 91% after PK and between 72% and 92% after dDALK, with no statistically significant differences in terms of uncorrected visual acuity (UCVA) and BCVA between the PK and dDALK [19, 20, 24]. Earlier visual rehabilitation was also observed after DALK surgery compared to PK. Although BCVA, SE, K, and astigmatism values were similar after 1 year, a significantly higher postoperative myopia has been reported in DALK after 12 months [20, 21, 24]. This could be related to the presence of the original Descemet's membrane that may produce a forward pressure after the removal of the sutures. On the other hand, cylinder values remained similar before and after suture removal [21].

No significant differences were found in the topographic astigmatism [7]. The corneal irregularity indices in the 3 and 5 mm zones were similar, which means the procedures are comparable in terms of graft surface irregularity.

One year after the dDALK there was no significant difference in terms of UCVA and BCVA. Comparing contrast sensitivity, no significant difference was found in any spatial frequency, after comparing photopic and scotopic contrast sensitivity functions (CSFs) with dDALK. High order aberrations (HOAs) are irregularities or imperfections of the eye as an optical system, which cannot be corrected by simple spherical or astigmatic corrections. HOAs are usually the responsible for halos, glare, and decreased contrast sensitivity despite normal visual acuity. Total and higher order aberrations were similar, indicating that the graft interface in dDALK does not induce more total HOAs in comparison with PK. The root mean square (RMS) of spherical aberration was significantly higher after DALK, and the RMS of fifth order aberration was higher after PK (Figs. 25.1 and 25.2) [22].

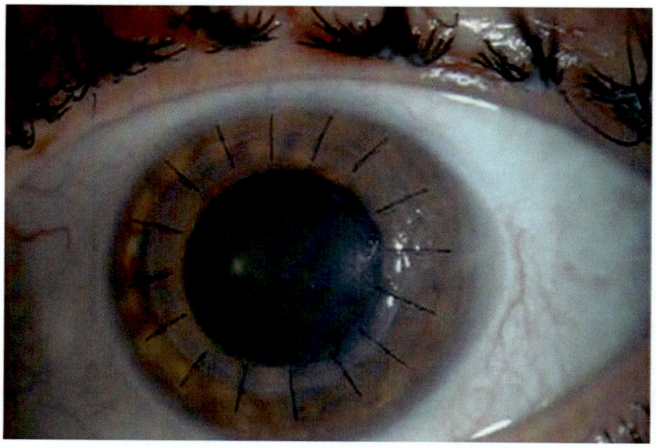

Fig. 25.1 Fourty-eight hours after DALK surgery

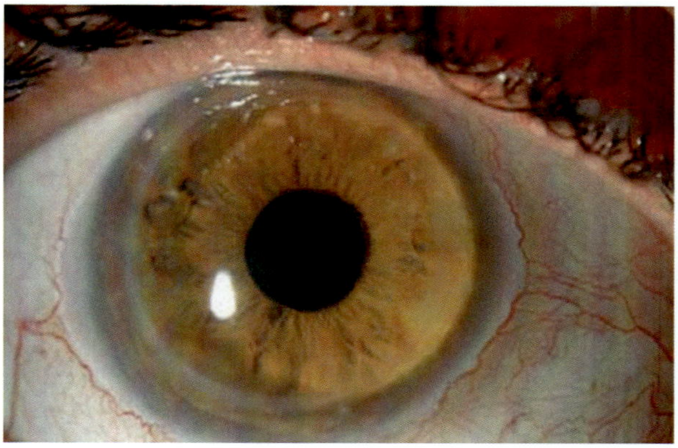

Fig. 25.2 Eighteen months after DALK surgery

25.3.4 *Intra and Postoperative Complications*

25.3.4.1 Intraoperative

DALK avoids most complications encountered during open sky surgery such as development of anterior synechiae, expulsive hemorrhage and endophthalmitis [22]. Descemet's Membrane Ruptures: Descemet membrane (DM) rupture is the most common complication during DALK surgery, even in experienced hands. Different kinds of ruptures can occur. Microperforation is a small DM lesion that usually occurs during the pdDALK approach when the surgeon tries to go *'deeper and deeper'* with the spatula of the scissors. Conversely, macroperforation is a DM rupture that determines an anterior chamber collapse. It generally happens during the removal of residual peripheral stroma using corneal scissors in the dDALK approach but may occur at any time during the full procedure. The ability to repair DM ruptures generally improves when surgeons gradually become more expert [23]. Intraoperative perforation rates vary from 4% to 39% based on five case series, whereas the PK conversion rate has been reported to range from 0% to 14% in four case series. The PK conversion rate gradually decreases as surgeons become more experienced and learn to manage DM ruptures [8]. Excessive trephination is a rare complication that can be avoided by a careful examination of the preoperative pachymetric map and by verifying the trephine calibration [23].

25.3.4.2 Postoperative

Double anterior chambers are usually, though not exclusively, a consequence of DM ruptures (micro or macro). They may also occur because of a retained ophthalmic viscoelastic device, and usually take place when the surgeon does not diligently irrigate the host bed before suturing the donor.

The interface haze seems to be related to several factors, including keratocyte activation, the depth and the smoothness of the recipient bed and the healing process at the interface [23]. It usually resolves spontaneously after 4–8 months post-surgery [23].

Macular edema is a known complication of corneal transplantation surgery; a study revealed no significant difference between both techniques: the PK group showed a 6.5% increase of macular thickness in the first month, a 6.3% increase in the third month and a 4.5% increase in the sixth month while in the DALK group the results were 5.6%, 5.4%, and 2.9%, respectively [25]. Additionally, DALK does not requires such a rigid criteria for donor corneal tissue quality (especially regarding the endothelium), it preserves better the ocular structural integrity against blunt trauma and provides faster visual rehabilitation because of earlier suture removal. We have to take into account the earlier discontinuation of corticosteroids that may also contribute to a stronger wound achieved earlier after DALK [22].

25.4 Disadvantages

25.4.1 Economic

An economic evaluation demonstrated that DALK was more costly than PK. The total costs per patient were €7607 in the DALK group compared to €6552 in the PK group (because of surgery time, and postoperative follow-up). However, the results on the NEI VFQ-25 (National Eye Institute Visual Functioning Questionnaire) was in favor of DALK. It was shown that DALK procedures performed without perforation of the Descemet membrane are more effective. Therefore, the need for retransplantation will be lower in DALK patients compared to PK patients, which will have a positive effect on the long term cost effectiveness of DALK [12]. We must not forget either that we can use the donor cornea for two receptors, where a DALK and a DMEK can be performed, reducing costs, especially in countries that do not have easy access to corneas.

25.4.2 Technique

Perhaps the main disadvantage of DALK is the surgical technique itself. Although DALK has many advantages over PK, it remains a limiting procedure, as mentioned before, due to the risk of perforation of DM, In general, DALK is a complex technique, with longer procedure time and a slower learning curve than the PK [26]. Macroperforation rate in the beginning is 40% and later between 5% and 10% in the last cases. The procedural time was also much higher at the beginning than at the end. Other series demonstrate that in DALK surgeries, intraoperative DM perforation occurred in 15.8% and conversion to PK in 7.9% [22]. On average, DM perforation rate is between 4.0% and 39.2% and DM tears needing conversion to PK is between 2.3% and 27.3% [7].

Some techniques may facilitate surgical intervention and reduce possible complications. The best known techniques are manual dissection layer by layer, hydrodissection, viscodissection (visco-big bubble), and the big bubble with air dissection. For us, the safest technique is the visco bubble dissection. It was described by Shimura and Güell in 2010 and 2014 (Fig 25.3) [27]. We consider it safer since dissection can be performed more slowly and controlled; in addition, visualization of the corneal structures and anterior chamber is much better during dissection and finally, at the moment of opening the bubble with a knife the risk of perforation of the DM is much lower because there is no collapse as it happens with the air bubble [27].

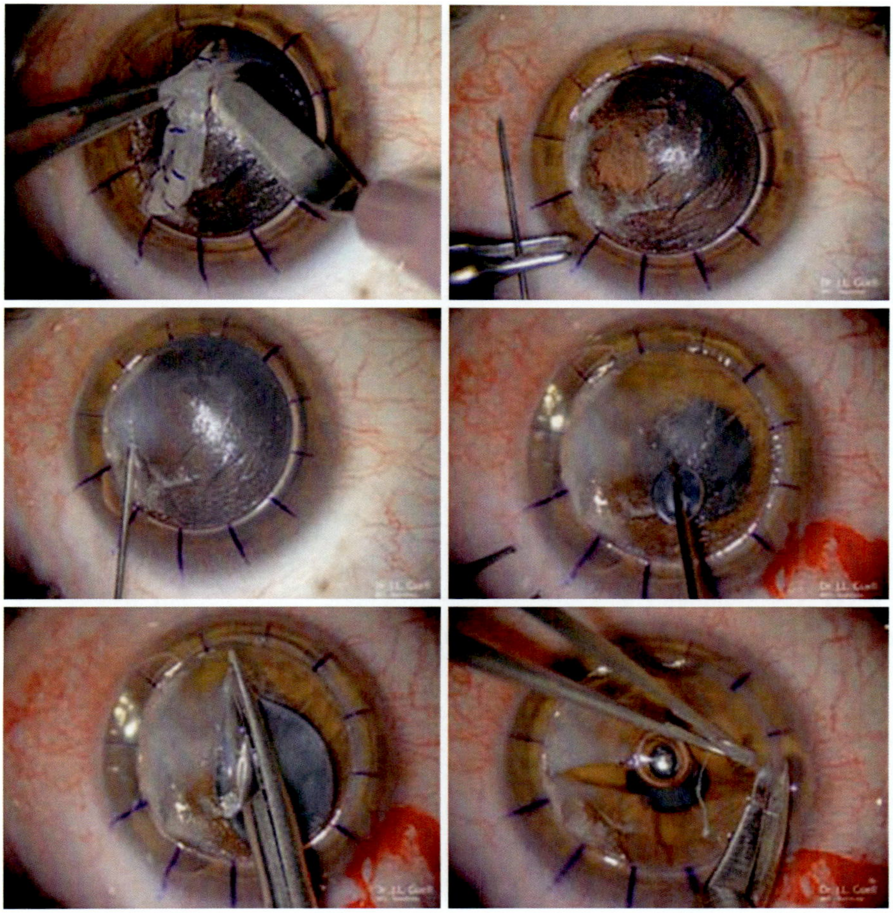

Fig. 25.3 Visco-big bubble technique

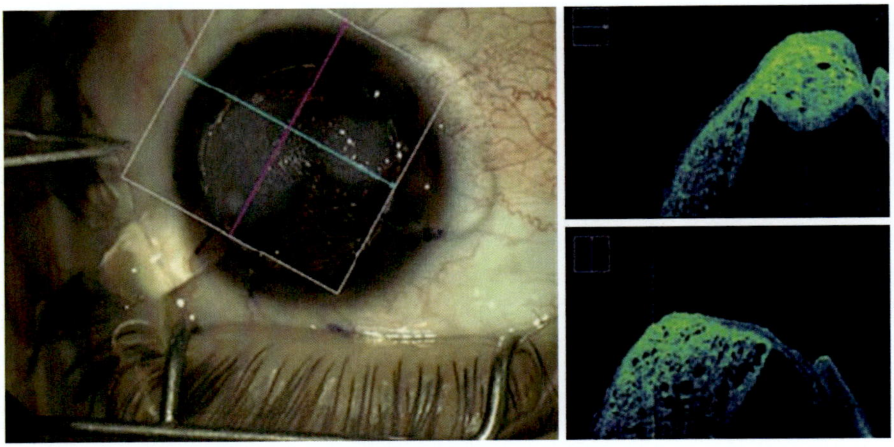

Fig 25.4 Visco- big bubble with OCT during surgery

Nowadays technology may help in improving DALK's safety: For example, with perioperative control by optical coherence tomography (Fig. 25.4), reducing the difficulty and the learning curve.

25.4.3 Recurrence

Rabinowitz suggested that the recurrence may be due either to the existence of the disease in the remaining host tissue or to the presence of subclinical disease in the donor cornea [28]. Maguire believed that most recurrences resulted from incomplete cone excision [29].

Sufficient evidence now confirms that post-transplant recurrence of KC does occur. The possible mechanisms involved may be: (1) the presence of disease in the host cornea (either because it exists in the peripheral cornea or because the cone was incompletely removed during transplant surgery, which may explain why more recurrence is found in DALK: more of the diseased host cornea is left in place, and may be orchestrated by cell migration from host to donor tissue), or (2) presence of disease in the donor cornea [30]. We can also say that recurrent KC in a corneal graft after DALK seems to be much shorter (49 months) than in PK [10]. Eye rubbing and contact lens wear have also been postulated but not associated with a significant number of cases (probably with an "addition effect" [31]. Recently, the early results of PK with crosslinking to prevent KC recurrence are very encouraging (Figs. 25.5 and 25.6).

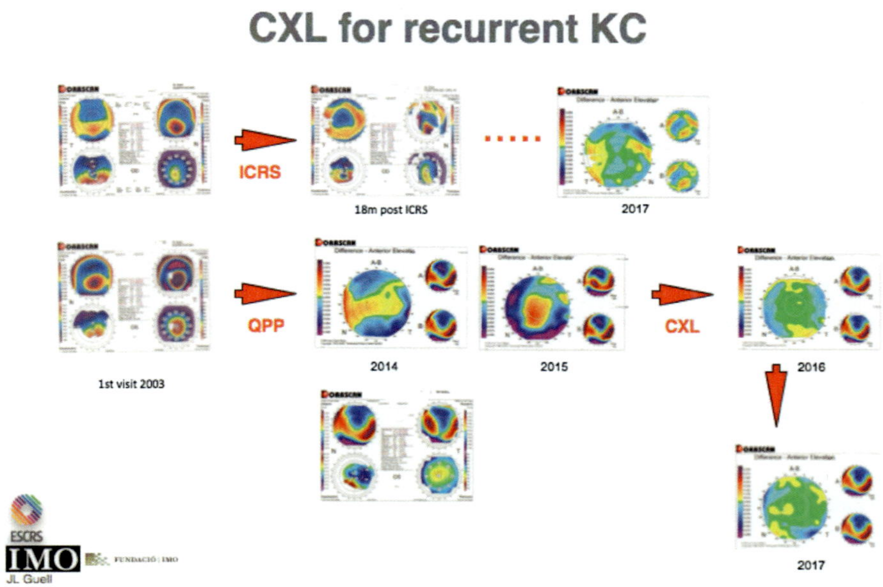

Fig. 25.5 Case with KC, where one eye was treated with ICRS with no recurrence, and the second eye was treated with PKP and after 10 years, we had recurrence of KC. We did crosslinking on the left eye and up until now there is no KC

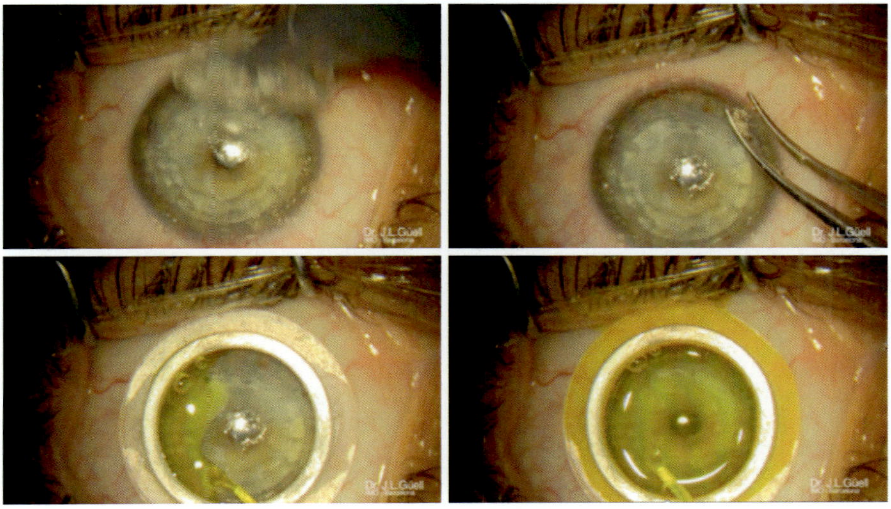

Fig. 25.6 We did peripheral desepithelization with an epiclear corneal scrubber bowman keratectomy of ORCA, leaving a central island of epithelium, and then, we perform a standard 10 min crosslinking

25.5 Conclusion

So returning to the first question, why we should use DALK in KC? Currently, it is clear that DALK is preferred over PK in KC eyes with healthy epithelium because similar or better optical results are obtained while, at the same time, risks during surgery are minimized, and a faster recovery during the postoperative period is seen. Moreover, a lower use of corticosteroids is required and the life of the graft has been shown to be longer and with a better preservation of the globe integrity. DALK can be considered as the first surgical option for patients with KC and possibly other corneal stromal pathologies with normal endothelium, except in three conditions: re-grafting in eyes with PK, prior hydrops with a frank and extensive discontinuity in DM, and deep scars affecting the Descemet's membrane.

References

1. Bahar I, Kaiserman I, Srinivasan S, et al. Comparison of three different techniques of corneal transplantation for keratoconus. Am J Ophthalmol. 2008;146:905–12.
2. Felipe AF, Hammersmith KM, Nottage JM, et al. Indications, visual outcome, and ectasia in clear corneal transplants 20 years old or more. Cornea. 2013;32(5):602–7.
3. Zadok D, Schwarts S, Marcovich A, et al. Penetrating keratoplasty for keratoconus: long term results. Cornea. 2005;24:959–61.
4. Colin J, Velou S. Current surgical options for keratoconus. J Cataract Refract Surg. 2003;29(2):379–86.
5. Espandar L, Meyer J. Keratoconus: overview and update on treatment. Middle East Afr J Ophthalmol. 2010;17(1):15–20.
6. Carlson AN. Keratoconus. Ophthalmology. 2009;116(10):2036–7. author reply 2037–8.
7. Yüksel B, Kandemir B, Uzunel UD, et al. Comparison of visual and topographic outcomes of deep-anterior lamellar keratoplasty and penetrating keratoplasty in keratoconus. Int J Ophthalmol. 2017;10(3):385–90.
8. Tan DT, Dart JK, Holland EJ, et al. Corneal transplantation. Lancet. 2012;379(9827):1749–61.
9. Cohen AW, Goins KM, Sutphin JE, et al. Penetrating keratoplasty versus deep anterior lamellar keratoplasty for the treatment of keratoconus. Int Ophthalmol. 2010;30(6):675–81.
10. Feizi S, Javadi MA, Rezaei KM. Recurrent keratoconus in a corneal graft after deep anterior lamellar keratoplasty. J Ophthalmic Vis Res. 2012;7(4):328–31.
11. Arenas E, Esquenazi S, Anwar M, et al. Lamellar corneal transplantation. Surv Ophthalmol. 2012;57(6):510–29.
12. Rabinowitz YS. Keratoconus. Surv Ophthalmol. 1998;42(4):297–319.
13. Faraj LA, Hashmani K, Khatib T, et al. The changing face of corneal graft rejection. Br J Ophthalmol. 2012;96(8):1049–50.
14. Van den Biggelaar FJ, Cheng YY, Nuijts RM, et al. Economic evaluation of deep anterior lamellar keratoplasty versus penetrating keratoplasty in the Netherlands. Am J Ophthalmol. 2011;151(3):449–59.
15. Sugita J, Kondo J. Deep lamellar keratoplasty with complete removal of pathological stroma for vision improvement. Br J Ophthalmol. 1997;81(3):184–8.
16. Sogutlu Sari E, Kubaloglu A, Unal M, et al. Deep anterior lamellar keratoplasty versus penetrating keratoplasty for macular corneal dystrophy: a randomized trial. Am J Ophthalmol. 2013;156:267–74.

17. Borderie VM, Sandali O, Bullet J, et al. Long-term results of deep anterior lamellar versus penetrating keratoplasty. Ophthalmology. 2012;119(2):249–55.
18. Salouti R, Masoumpour M, Nowroozzadeh MH, et al. Changes in corneal endothelial cell profile measurements after deep anterior lamellar keratoplasty for keratoconus. Cornea. 2013;32(6):751–6.
19. Sogutlu Sari E, Kubaloglu A, Unal M, et al. Penetrating keratoplasty versus deep anterior lamellar keratoplasty: comparison of optical and visual quality outcomes. Br J Ophthalmol. 2012;96(8):1063–7.
20. Chen G, Tzekov R, Li W, et al. Deep anterior lamellar keratoplasty versus penetrating keratoplasty: a meta-analysis of randomized controlled trials. Cornea. 2016;35(2):169–74.
21. Amayem AF, Hamdi IM, Hamdi MM. Refractive and visual outcomes of penetrating keratoplasty versus deep anterior lamellar keratoplasty with hydrodissection for treatment of keratoconus. Cornea. 2013;32(4):e2–5.
22. Javadi MA, Feizi S, Yazdani S, et al. Deep anterior lamellar keratoplasty versus penetrating keratoplasty for keratoconus: a clinical trial. Cornea. 2010;29(4):365–71.
23. Sarnicola E, Sarnicola C, Sarnicola V. Deep anterior lamellar keratoplasty: surgical technique, indications, clinical results and complications. In: Güell JL, editor. Cornea. ESASO course series, vol. 6. Basel: Karger; 2015. p. 81–101.
24. Abdelkader A, Kaufan HE. Descemetic versus pre-descemetic lamellar keratoplasty: clinical and confocal study. Cornea. 2011;30(11):1244–52.
25. Koytak A, Kubaloglu A, Sari ES, et al. Changes in central macular thickness after uncomplicated corneal transplantation for keratoconus: penetrating keratoplasty versus deep anterior lamellar keratoplasty. Cornea. 2011;30(12):1318–21.
26. Shimmura S, Ando M, Ishioka M, et al. Same size donor corneas for myopic keratoconus. Cornea. 2004;23(4):345–9.
27. Güell JL, Aristizábal-Montes D. Viscobubble technique for deep anterior lamellar keratoplasty. J Emmetropia. 2014;5:65–8.
28. Rabinowitz YS. Ectatic disorders of the cornea. In: Foster CF, Azar DT, Dohlman CH, editors. The cornea: scientific foundations and clinical practice. Philadelphia: Lipincott Williams & Wilkins; 2005. p. 839–911.
29. Maguire LJ. Ectatic corneal degenerations. In: Kauffman HE, Barron BA, McDonald MB, editors. The cornea. Boston: Butterworth-Heinemann; 1998. p. 525–37.
30. Bergmanson JP, Goosey JD, Patel CK, et al. Recurrence or re-emergence of keratoconus what is the evidence telling us? Literature review and two case reports. Ocul Surf. 2014;12(4):267–72.
31. Koenig SB. Bilateral recurrent self-induced keratoconus. Eye Contact Lens. 2008;34(6):343–4.

Chapter 26
Why Full-Thickness Penetrating Keratoplasty and Not Deep Anterior Lamelar Keratoplasty for the Treatment of Keratoconus

Hadas Ben-Eli and Abraham Solomon

26.1 Background

Keratoconus (KC) is a corneal ectatic disease of the stromal layer, which initially manifests as a change in refractive error, astigmatism and reduced visual acuity [1]. PKP (Penetrating Keratoplasty) is the ultimate surgical solution in severe KC in patients who cannot achieve reasonable vision or cannot tolerate special contact lenses. For decades PKP was considered as the traditional and only method of corneal transplantation. The most prevalent indication for corneal transplantation in many parts of the world has been KC, with prevalent rates ranging between 14.2% and 45.3% of patients [2–4]. Though in recent years DALK (Deep Anterior Lamelar Keratoplasty) was introduced as an alternative procedure, PKP is still the surgical treatment of choice by most corneal surgeons for KC [4, 5]. The main purpose in DALK is to preserve the host's healthy endothelium and descemet's layer by replacing only the corneal stroma, thus reducing to minimum the likelihood for graft rejections, and minimizing anatomical changes in the anterior chamber as well as some severe intra-ocular complications [6]. However there are still many disadvantages associated with DALK. DALK is a time consuming procedure, technically complicated, and associated with a long and steep learning curve, even for experienced corneal surgeons [6]. At the same time patients after DALK have comparable visual results to those of PKP, as well as comparable results in terms of refractive

H. Ben-Eli
Department of Ophthalmology, Hadassah-Hebrew University Medical Center, Jerusalem, Israel

Department of Optometry and Vision Science, Hadassah Academic College, Jerusalem, Israel

A. Solomon (✉)
Department of Ophthalmology, Hadassah-Hebrew University Medical Center, Jerusalem, Israel

A. Barbara (ed.), *Controversies in the Management of Keratoconus*,
https://doi.org/10.1007/978-3-319-98032-4_26

errors and residual astigmatism [7], and difficulties in accurate measurement of intraocular pressure (IOP) for both DALK and PKP [8].

The aim of this chapter is to summarize the advantages and disadvantages of PKP compared to DALK in the management of KC, and to highlight reasons to prefer PKP rather than DALK as the surgical treatment in KC.

26.2 Advantages of PKP

1. **Transparency of tissue**
   In PKP the likelihood of obtaining a clear corneal stroma is higher compared to DALK. The major drawback in DALK is the reduced stromal transparency which may be caused by the interaction between the host remaining stromal remnants and the donor host. The residual stroma that may remain following incomplete removal may result in interface haze and stromal scarring in DALK [9]. The interface haze is more common in the manual DALK technique (removal of layer by layer) rather than the various 'Big bubble' methods. Patients who underwent the "layer by layer" stromal removal in DALK can produce a large amount of collagen in the host-donor interface, leading to disorganization of the extracellular matrix, which causes haze formation in the posterior stroma and the interface [10]. In a retrospective study, Cohen et al. found that visually significant interface haze occurred in the early postoperative course after DALK [5]. In addition, various types of debris during surgery can accumulate and get trapped between the donor and the host. The presence of this interface debris after DALK [10] can cause inflammatory reaction and scaring of the interface. Thus - stromal remnants and interface debris may lead to significant visual impairment after DALK.

   The stromal tissue in grafts after PKP is usually more transparent compared to grafts after the DALK procedure.
2. ***Visual and refractive outcomes***
   In several studies it was reported that the long-term best-corrected visual acuity (BCVA), mean refractive spherical equivalent, and mean refractive cylinder after DALK were very similar to those after PKP [1, 11, 12]. Amayem et al. demonstrated that in both techniques, the mean BCVA was found to be 0.18 log MAR 12 and 24 months postoperatively. Refractive spherical equivalent means were 24.11 ± 3.4 diopters (D) 2 years after DALK and 21.1 ± 3.6 D after PKP, and mean refractive cylinders were 3.18 ± 1.70 D for the DALK and 3.80 ± 1.80 D for the PKP group. The DALK group was statistically more myopic at 12 and 24 months [1]. This result may indicate the tighter suturing that is required during DALK, as a result of the need to push down the graft against the remaining descemet's membrane, to achieve a smooth surface at the graft-host wound.

   Recently Hamdi reported that after complete removal of all sutures, following stability of refraction, the uncorrected and best spectacle-corrected visual acuity, the mean refractive spherical equivalent and mean refractive cylinder, root mean square of the 3 mm and 5 mm OPD Scan, steep and flat meridians (SimK1 and SimK2, respectively), and the difference between the Sim Ks (the corneal cylinder) were not statistically significantly different between the groups of DALK and PKP [12]. Moreover, in a randomized trial on 81 patients, Javadi et al. reported on the same visual and refractive outcomes, as well as with the contrast sensitivity function, at all tested time points. Yet, comparing the high order aberrations (HOAs), the root mean square (RMS) of the spherical aberrations in the DALK group was significantly higher than that in the PKP group (0.83 ± 0.4 and 0.42 ± 0.3 respectively, p = 0.004), but the RMS of fifth-order aberrations was significantly higher in the PKP than in the DALK group (0.32 ± 0.1 and 0.19 ± 0.2 respectively, p = 0.017). The RMSs of trefoil, coma, third, fourth, total, and higher order aberrations were not statistically different between both techniques [6].

In a prospective, comparative, interventional case series, Kubaloglu et al. have found that though not statistically significant, the mean LogMar BCVA was higher in PKP patients compared to DALK after 3 months period (0.13 ± 0.11 and 0.11 ± 0.09 respectively, P = 0.84), but after 6 month follow up the BCVA was higher in DALK patients compared to PKP (0.13 ± 0.08 and 0.11 ± 0.08 respectively, P = 0.51). The refractive cylinder was lower in the PKP group compared to the DALK group after both follow up periods (after 6 months: −3.31 ± 2.18 and − 3.53 ± 1.62 respectively, P = 0.4), and the keratometric astigmatism was also lower in PKP compared to DALK patients (after 6 months: 3.72 ± 2.18 and 4.17 ± 1.78 respectively, P = 0.37) [13]. This again is probably a result of the tighter suturing that is needed while anchoring the graft in DALK compared to PKP.

Neither DALK or PKP had a significant superiority on the long-term refractive outcomes [11, 14], therefore suggesting, in this respect, that there is no justification in choosing the more complicated procedure of DALK over PKP.

3. ***Endothelial and stromal cell densities***

There are controversial reports on the post-operative endothelial and stromal cell counts and function in PKP vs. DALK.

A long-term follow-up demonstrated lower endothelial cell densities after PKP compared to DALK, suggesting the DALK preserves the endothelial cell counts that are diminished in PKP [14]. However, some studies claim for an increased endothelial cell loss in DALK due to the various manipulations that are performed in close proximity to this layer (including using scissors to cut the stroma, or repeated viscoelastic applications). On confocal microscopy comparison of donor tissues of DALK and PKP it was found that the stroma keratocyte density was significantly reduced and their arrangement was profoundly altered after DALK [10]. The cellular decreased density of keratocytes and endothelial cells after DALK may be a result of the mechanical trauma from the surgical instruments, and from transient dysfunction of the endothelial cells [10].

4. ***Deep pathologies***

A prior requirement to perform DALK is an intact descemet's layer. Corneal disorders involving the deeper layers of the cornea and the descemet's layer, such as hydrops after descemet rapture in KC, penetrating corneal trauma and post herpetic infections, are relative contra-indications for DALK. In these conditions, where the endothelium may be damaged by various diseases, trauma or rupture, PKP may serve as a more reasonable surgical option.

5. ***Complications***
Sight-threatening complications that may occur in both PKP and DALK are post-surgical microbial keratitis and traumatic wound dehiscence [5, 15] In this regard it must be stressed that DALK does not protect from post-surgical wound dehiscence and rupture of the host-graft wound with consequent loss of the lens and vitreous. Complications which associate exclusively with DALK are interface opacification, ocular surface disorders, descemet membrane perforation, as well as stromal rejection [15, 16]. Another rare complication of DALK is retained viscoelastic separating the host descemet membrane from the donor graft, because of incomplete thorough removal of all of the viscoelastic material prior to placing the graft over the descemet. This may lead to a double anterior chamber and to secondary corneal edema (Fig. 26.1). Micro-perforations of the descemet during surgery may also result in a double anterior chamber and corneal edema [5, 15].
6. ***Learning curve***
Röck et al. in 2017 suggested several reasons why the DALK procedure has moderate introduction rates in Cornea practices. These include a long surgical time using the big bubble technique, a higher technical challenge, the introduction of collagen crosslinking in patients with progressive keratoconus, a lower number of patients with the indication for DALK, and a slower and more difficult learning curve for the surgeon [2]. Similarly Rezaei Kanavi claimed that the main reasons for the lack of increase in the trend to perform DALK in comparison with PKP are the longer surgical time and the steep learning curve [4].

The steep learning curve encountered in the "Big bubble" DALK technique is a result of the variation in several critical steps during the procedure. These variations include the level of separation between the stroma and descemet following

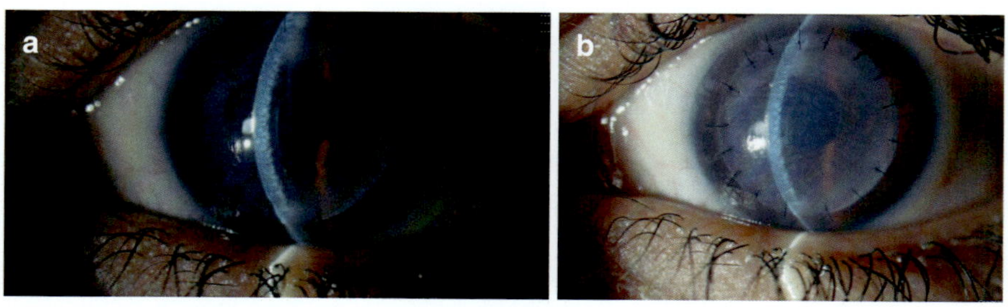

Fig. 26.1 Retained viscoelastic after DALK separating the host descemet's membrane from the donor graft, leading to a double chamber (**a**), and causing corneal edema (**b**). Day 1 post-DALK for keratoconus. (**a**) A separated Descemet's membrane is evident behind the donor graft, leading to a double anterior chamber. (**b**) A secondary corneal edema is demonstrated. (Courtesy: Abraham Solomon, MD)

air injection, the likelihood of a major perforation during entry into the supra-descemetic space with a sharp instrument, and inadvertent perforation which may occur during the excision of the stroma from the descemet. These difficulties are probably a result of the large variation that exists in the composition of the stroma and the descemet between different patients.

7. ***Cost***
   A recent economic evaluation between PKP and DALK procedures by van den Biggelaar et al. demonstrated that the mean total cost per patient was €7607 for DALK compared to €6552 for PKP. These estimates included higher costs of hospitalization, operating room and number of follow-up visits in DALK [17]. However DALK may have a higher cost effective ratio since theoretically one corneal graft can be used for two different patients, one for DALK and the other for DMEK. Practically, this may not be always possible, as the number of cases where descemet's rapture during DALK lead to conversions to full thickness transplantation remains high. The possible conversion from DALK to PKP increases the surgical time, and increases the final costs of DALK over PKP.

26.3 Disadvantages of PKP

1. ***Graft rejection***
   PKP is a procedure identified with higher rates of graft rejection compared to those of DALK. A recent meta-analysis study demonstrated that graft rejection rates were significantly higher in PKP compared to DALK (OR = 0.28; 95% CI 0.15–0.50; $p < 0.001$) [9]. There are consistent reports on higher incidence rates of immunological graft rejection in PKP compared to DALK (11.8% vs. 1.3% respectively, $p = 0.0002$) [15, 18]. Specifically, the graft rejection risk is higher in the pediatric population compared with adults, due to a stronger immunological response in young patients [19]. Overall lamellar keratoplasty procedures are associated with lower graft rejection rates [2]. However, as noted before – other complications such as interface opacification are more common in lamellar transplantations [5].
2. ***Endothelial cell loss***
   The continuous decline of endothelial cell counts at a time point >3 years after PKP, and the greater preservation of the endothelium after DALK, may result in a longer graft survival after DALK compared to PKP [9, 15]. A severe decrease in endothelial cell density may result in corneal edema, and the necessity for a re-transplantation of a full-thickness graft.
3. ***Complications***
   The well known complications of PKP include expulsive hemorrhage, high post-operative intra-ocular pressure, endophthalmitis and architectural disturbances of the anterior chamber (e.g. progressive peripheral anterior synechia and secondary angle-closure glaucoma). Secondary cataract, permanent damage to the

Table 26.1 PKP vs. DALK techniques for keratoconus

	PKP	DALK
Transparency of tissue [5, 10]	No interface debris or haze, transparent tissue	Interface haze
Endothelial and stromal cell densities [9, 10, 14, 15]	Low endothelial cell counts on long-period follow-up, but higher density of stromal keratocytes	Higher endothelial cell counts on short and long-term, but lower density of stromal keratocytes
Graft rejection [9, 15]	Higher rates, more need for re-transplantation	Lower rates, less need for re-transplantation
KC with hydrops, Penetrating trauma or herpes	Suitable for almost any corneal trauma or pathology	Not indicated after healed hydrops, penetrating trauma or herpes
Tight sutures	Easier suturing to maintain a smooth surface at the graft-host junction	Tight sutures to maintain a smooth surface at the graft-host junction resulting in higher astigmatism
Postoperative long-term visual acuity [1, 11, 12]	Comparable or better BCVA	Comparable
Postoperative long-term refraction [1, 11, 12]	Comparable to other technique	Comparable to other technique
Postoperative long-term astigmatism [1, 11, 12]	Comparable to other technique	Comparable to other technique, higher astigmatism in some reports
Descemet rapture [15]	No Descemet rapture during surgery	Descemet rapture during surgery
Steroid use [6]	Increased steroid use, increased risk for cataract and glaucoma	Minimal steroid use, reduction in risk for cataract and glaucoma
Procedure [2, 4]	Easy for the surgeon	Complicated for the surgeon, long and steep learning curve
Surgery time [2, 4]	Short duration	Long duration
Postoperative follow-up [17]	Fewer follow-up visits	More follow-up visits
Cost [17]	Low total cost	High total cost, but one graft can be used for two patients

pupillary sphincter, wound leak, wound dehiscence, and inadvertent iridotomy – are all intra- and post-operative complications which are unique to PKP and do not occur in DALK (Table 26.1).

26.4 Conclusions

Though DALK becomes a more fashionable technique in corneal transplantations, a retrospective data of 47,129 patients revealed that PKP is still the method of choice [4]. The main reason is the long and steep learning curve in DALK, and the longer surgical time required to complete the procedure. On a long-term follow-up PKP is associated with higher rates of graft rejection, while in DALK there is more interface haze and secondary stromal rejection. Whereas DALK is a procedure limited for stromal corneal disorders, PKP can be used for all corneal pathologies that require replacement of the cornea, including descemet abnormalities such as hydrops in severe KC, penetrating trauma and herpetic infections where the endothelium is likely to be involved. On the economic issue, DALK is more expensive as it involves a longer surgical time, longer hospitalization and higher number of postoperative visits. The consistent reports of comparable visual outcomes for both PKP and DALK suggest there is no preference in choosing the more complicated and expensive DALK over PKP. As long as more efficient, reproducible and easy to perform steps in DALK are found, specifically in the big bubble technique, PKP will remain a valid and popular option in corneal transplantation for keratoconus and other anterior stromal disorders.

References

1. Amayem AF, Hamdi IM, Hamdi MM. Refractive and visual outcomes of penetrating keratoplasty versus deep anterior lamellar keratoplasty with hydrodissection for treatment of keratoconus. Cornea. 2013;32(4):30–3.
2. Röck T, Landenberger J, Bramkamp M, Bartz-Schmidt KURD. The evolution of corneal transplantation. Ann Transplant. 2017;22:749–54.
3. Crawford AZ, Mckelvie J, Craig JP, Mcghee CNJ, Patel DV. Corneal transplantation in Auckland, New Zealand, 1999–2009: indications, patient characteristics, ethnicity, social deprivation, and access to services. Cornea. 2017;36(5):546–52.
4. Rezaei Kanavi M, Javadi MA, Motevasseli T, Chamani T, Rezaei Kanavi M, Kheiri BSS. Trends in indications and techniques of corneal transplantation in Iran from 2006 to 2013; an 8-year review. J Ophthalmic Vis Res. 2016;11(2):146–52.
5. Cohen AW, Goins KM, Sutphin JE, Wandling GR, Wagoner MD. Penetrating keratoplasty versus deep anterior lamellar keratoplasty for the treatment of keratoconus. Int Ophthalmol. 2010;30:675–81.
6. Javadi MA, Feizi S, Yazdani S, Mirbabaee F. Deep anterior lamellar keratoplasty versus penetrating. Cornea. 2010;29(4):365–71.
7. Khattak A, Nakhli FR, Abdullah KMA. Comparison of outcomes and complications of deep anterior lamellar keratoplasty and penetrating keratoplasty performed in a large group of patients with keratoconus. Int Ophthalmol. 2017;38:992.
8. Jafarinasab MR, Feizi S, Javadi MA, Hashemloo A. Graft biomechanical properties after penetrating keratoplasty versus deep anterior lamellar keratoplasty. Curr Eye Res. 2011;36:417–21.
9. Liu H, Chen Y, Wang P, et al. Efficacy and safety of deep anterior lamellar keratoplasty vs. penetrating keratoplasty for keratoconus: a meta-analysis. Taylor AW, ed. PLoS One. 2015;10(1):e0113332. https://doi.org/10.1371/journal.pone.0113332.
10. Feizi S, Javadi MA, Kanavi MR. Cellular changes of donor corneal tissue after deep anterior lamellar keratoplasty versus penetrating keratoplasty in eyes with keratoconus : a confocal study. Cornea. 2010;29(8):866–70.
11. Keane M, Coster D, Ziaei M WK. Deep anterior lamellar keratoplasty versus penetrating keratoplasty for treating keratoconus. Cochrane Database Syst Rev. 2014;(7):CD009700.

12. Hamdi IM, Hamdi MM. Quality of vision after deep anterior lamellar keratoplasty (fluid dissection) compared to penetrating keratoplasty for the treatment of keratoconus. J Ophthalmol. 2017;2017:7–9.
13. Kubaloglu A, Coskun E, Sari ES, et al. Comparison of astigmatic keratotomy results in deep anterior lamellar keratoplasty and penetrating keratoplasty in keratoconus. Am J Ophthalmol. 2011;151(4):637–43.
14. Oh BL, Kim MK, Wee WR. Comparison of clinical outcomes of same-size grafting between deep anterior lamellar keratoplasty and penetrating keratoplasty for keratoconus. Korean J Ophthalmol. 2013;27(5):322–30.
15. Shimazaki J, Ishii N, Shinzawa M, Yamaguchi T. How much progress has been made in corneal. Cornea. 2015;34(11):105–11.
16. Kasbekar SA, Jones MNA, Ahmad S, et al. Corneal transplant surgery for keratoconus and the effect of surgeon experience on deep anterior lamellar keratoplasty outcomes. Am J Ophthalmol. 2014;158(6):1239–46.
17. Van Den Biggelaar FJHM, Cheng YYY, Nuijts RMMA, et al. Economic evaluation of deep anterior lamellar keratoplasty versus penetrating keratoplasty in the Netherlands. Am J Ophthalmol. 2011;151(3):449–59.e2.
18. Koytak A, Kubaloglu A, Sari ES, Atakan M, Culfa SOY. Changes in central macular thickness after uncomplicated corneal transplantation for keratoconus: penetrating keratoplasty versus deep anterior lamellar keratoplasty. Cornea. 2011;30(12):2009–12.
19. Gonzalez-salinas R, Hernandez-zimbron LF, Hernandez-quintela E, Sanchez-huerta V. Indications and outcomes of pediatric keratoplasty in a tertiary eye care center. Medicine (Baltimore). 2017;96:1–5.

Chapter 27
Bowman Layer Transplantation for Advanced Keratoconus

Jack S. Parker, Rénuka S. Birbal, Korine van Dijk, Maya Tong, Balamurali Ambati, Lamis Baydoun, Isabel Dapena, and Gerrit R. J. Melles

27.1 Introduction

Bowman layer (BL) transplantation is a relatively new surgical procedure for the treatment of advanced keratoconus (KC). The operation entails the implantation of an isolated, donor BL into a manually-dissected pocket within the mid-stroma of the recipient keratoconic cornea [1]. This results in flattening – by, on average, 8 diopters (D) – and stiffening against further ectasia [2]. Meanwhile, because the operation involves no surface incisions, sutures, or cellular donor tissue, the most

J. S. Parker
Netherlands Institute for Innovative Ocular Surgery (NIIOS), Rotterdam, The Netherlands

Parker Cornea, Birmingham, AL, USA

R. S. Birbal · G. R. J. Melles (✉)
Netherlands Institute for Innovative Ocular Surgery (NIIOS), Rotterdam, The Netherlands

Amnitrans EyeBank Rotterdam, Rotterdam, The Netherlands

Melles Cornea Clinic Rotterdam, Rotterdam, The Netherlands
e-mail: research@niios.com; http://www.niios.com

K. van Dijk · L. Baydoun · I. Dapena
Netherlands Institute for Innovative Ocular Surgery (NIIOS), Rotterdam, The Netherlands

Melles Cornea Clinic Rotterdam, Rotterdam, The Netherlands

M. Tong
Netherlands Institute for Innovative Ocular Surgery (NIIOS), Rotterdam, The Netherlands

Melles Cornea Clinic Rotterdam, Rotterdam, The Netherlands

University of Alberta, Edmonton, Canada

B. Ambati
Pacific Clear Vision Institute, Eugene, OR, USA

A. Barbara (ed.), *Controversies in the Management of Keratoconus*,
https://doi.org/10.1007/978-3-319-98032-4_27

common complications of BL transplantation's predecessor procedures – penetrating and deep anterior lamellar keratoplasty (PK and DALK, respectively) – may be avoided [3].

27.2 Background

It is curious that PK and DALK both enjoy relatively favorable reputations for the treatment of advanced KC considering the wide array of well-known and fairly common post-operative difficulties that appertain to both surgeries. These include: problems with wound healing, suture related complications, tectonic instability, disease progression in the un-operated recipient corneal rim, the persistent risk of allograft reaction and graft rejection, a chronic steroid burden that may predispose to cataract formation and glaucoma, and – often – disappointing visual results [3, 4]. Compared to PK, DALK fares better in most of these categories but nevertheless significant issues remain and are the reason why alternatives to corneal transplantation have been energetically pursued.

In 2003, Wollensak et al. introduced ultra-violet corneal crosslinking (UVCXL) for mild KC, intending to arrest the disease in its early stages and delay or avoid the need for corneal transplantation [5]. Although the results of the procedure have been encouraging – with approximately 90% of treated eyes achieving topographic stability at 1 year postoperatively – certain limitations have applied. For instance, until recently, UVCXL was not FDA approved in the United States and was therefore not widely available. In addition, the procedure may only be indicated in corneas with maximum keratometry (Kmax) values of less than 58 diopters (D) and minimum corneal thicknesses of at least 400 μm; otherwise, the rates of treatment failure vision-threatening complications may significantly increase [6]. Consequently, and especially in the United States, many patients with moderate to advanced keratoconus have found themselves ineligible for UVCXL and, therefore, have had little recourse to arrest the progression of their disease.

Along with UVCXL, intracorneal ring segments (ICRS) have also been applied for the treatment of mild and moderate KC with some success: with the implantation of polymethyl methacrylate (PMMA) segments of various arc lengths, thicknesses, and designs, the keratoconic cornea may be reshaped into a more optically favorable position [7]. In addition, some extra amount of support may be conferred, lessening the chances of progressive ectasia [8]. However, as with UVCXL, similar limitations apply: corneas steeper than 58D are often deemed ineligible for the procedure and a minimum corneal thickness of 400 μm along the intended path of insertion is often regarded as mandatory [9].

As a result, patients with more advanced KC (corneas steeper than 58D or thinner than 400 μm) are often considered poor candidates for both UVCXL and ICRS. This is unfortunate because many of these individuals may retain excellent contact lens (CTL)-corrected vision, but poor CTL tolerance, or acceptable tolerance but are topographically progressing, which imperils that tolerance. What has been badly needed was a new operation to restore or preserve CTL vision in patients with advanced KC, and – thereby – delay or avoid the need for PK or DALK. Hence, BL transplantation was designed.

27.3 Indications

So far, BL transplantation has been successfully performed in patients with advanced KC – too thin and too steep for UVCXL and ICRS – but may also be an option for corneas with pellucid marginal degeneration, post-lasik ectasia, and keratoglobus. Candidate eyes should have "acceptable" CTL-corrected vision but with documented progression or poor CTL tolerance. What constitutes "acceptable" vision is likely to depend on the patient: in our experience, many patients are glad to preserve the vision they have, rather than "gamble" for an upgrade with either a DALK or PK at the cost of incurring significant risks and post-operative obligations.

27.4 Graft Preparation

Isolated BL graft preparation was first described in 2011 in a case report in which an isolated BL graft was harvested, then used as an "onlay" to treat post-refractive laser haze [10]. Now, BL transplantation is used as an "inlay" for the treatment of advanced KC, but the graft preparation technique remains largely unchanged:

From whole globes, corneo-scleral buttons are excised less than 36 h post-mortem, then stored in organ culture until the time of preparation. At which time, they are removed from organ culture, mounted endothelial side up in a custom-made holder with a suction cup, and the Descemet membrane (DM) is carefully stripped free for use in Descemet Membrane Endothelial Keratoplasty (DMEK) in another eye. This step is, of course, optional but is commonly performed at the Amnitrans EyeBank Rotterdam, to enable a single donor cornea to be sectioned for use in multiple patients [11].

Once the DM and endothelium have been removed, the corneo-scleral button is flipped over and mounted epithelial-side up in an artificial anterior chamber, and the epithelium is debrided using a surgical spear. Trypan blue may be dripped over the anterior surface and allowed to stain the (now exposed) BL layer. Then, a 30-gauge needle is used to incise the BL, just inside the limbus, 360° around. After which, McPherson forceps are used to gently and carefully peel the BL free from the underlying stromal attachments. Once the BL has been totally separated, it spontaneously curls into a roll, not unlike a DMEK graft. After which, the donor BL graft is rinsed in 70% alcohol for 30 s, then stored again in organ culture until the time of transplantation (Fig. 27.1).

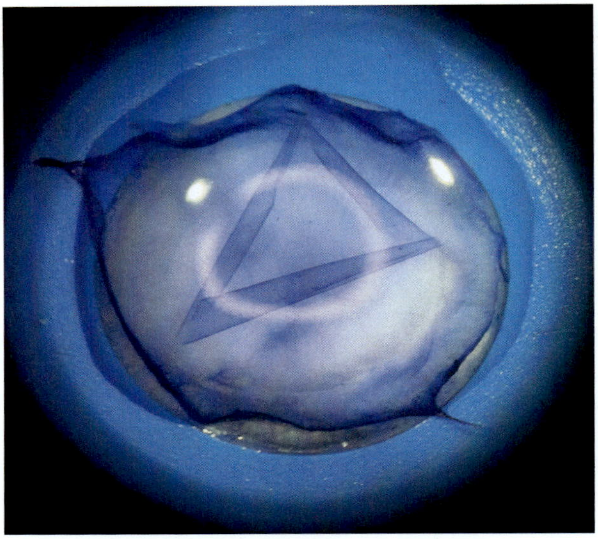

Fig. 27.1 Stained, isolated Bowman layer graft, immediately after stripping

27.5 Surgical Technique

Retrobulbar anesthesia is administered, followed by digital ocular massage and the placement of a Honan balloon for 10 min to obtain a soft eye. After which, a localized, superior conjunctival peritomy is performed and hemostasis may be achieved with cautery. Then, 1–2 mm behind the limbus, a 5-mm partial thickness scleral groove is created, and dissected up into the clear cornea using a crescent knife. A paracentesis is then fashioned, and the anterior chamber is completely filled with air. The intended dissection plane is found using the "air-endothelial reflex", first described for use in Melles manual DALK surgeries. Specifically, when the anterior chamber is filled with air, instruments placed into the peripheral cornea will generate a reflection at their tip, and the distance between the instrument and its reflection in the cornea represents the depth of the ongoing dissection. The closer the two are to meeting, the deeper the dissection, so that – when the two appear to just touch – a 99% dissection depth has been obtained. This is the manner in which a deep controlled dissection for DALK may be achieved [12]. For BL transplantation, a 50% dissection depth is instead preferred (to minimize the risk of inadvertent anterior or posterior perforation), but the air-endothelial reflex is nevertheless valuable for this purpose.

Once the ideal depth has been found, the actual dissection using the Melles manual DALK dissection spatulas may proceed. The objective is to create a mid-stromal pocket, stretching from limbus-to-limbus, 360° around. Once this has been achieved, the air is partially removed from the anterior chamber, and a surgical glide is threaded through the mouth of the corneo-scleral incision and up into the dissected pocket. Then, the donor BL graft is removed from storage, rinsed again with 70% alcohol, then with balanced salt solution (BSS), stained with Trypan blue, and placed atop the glide, where it can be pushed into the eye with the assistance of a cannula (Fig. 27.2). With the graft inside the stromal pocket, the glide is removed and the graft can be unfolded and positioned by the direct action of touches with the cannula, jets of BSS, and strokes on the corneal surface. Once the graft is fully unfolded, the eye is inflated with BSS to a physiologic pressure, the conjunctiva is re-approximated to the superior limbus and the eye is patched shut (Fig. 27.3). Post-operatively, the medication regimen consists of an antibiotic for at least the 1st week and a steroid for the 1st month; thereafter, tapering may proceed according to the surgeon's discretion and, not infrequently, our patients are totally discontinued of all eye drops after the first 6–12 months [1, 2].

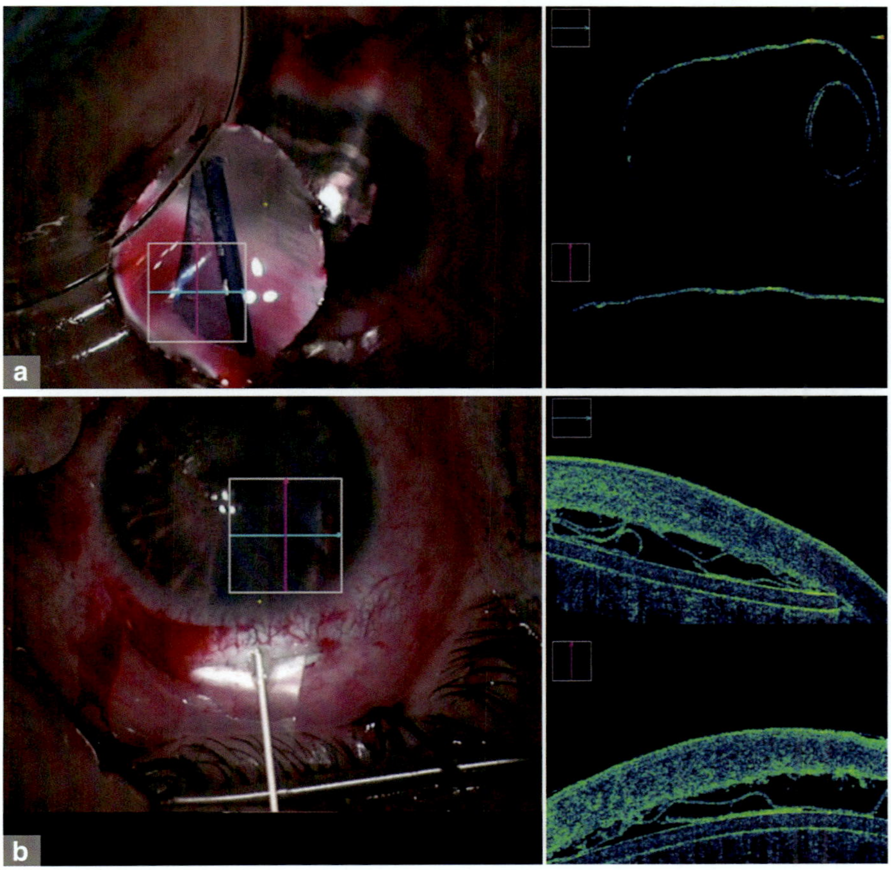

Fig. 27.2 BL graft immediately before insertion (**a**), and after having been pushed into the stromal pocket along the surgical glide, before full unfolding is complete (**b**)

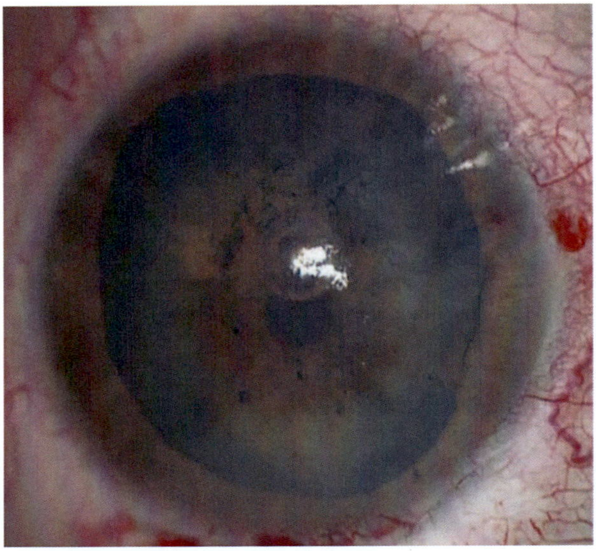

Fig. 27.3 Unfolded BL graft in final position

27.6 Surgical Outcomes

There is good data that describes the postoperative results of BL transplantation through at least the first 5 years after surgery: nearly all eyes experience a significant flattening of their preoperative Kmax values: on average by 8–9 D, which is often achieved by the first post-operative day, and which may be regarded as stable by the 1st month after surgery (Fig. 27.4) [1, 2]. Further, 90% of eyes with "progressive" KC may experience a cessation of ongoing steepening and thinning, which is comparable to the success rate of both UVCXL and ICRS. No significant difference in measured spectacle or contact lens corrected visual acuity is usually attained, although – practically – many patients may enjoy a large improvement in their functional vision, since comfortable contact lens wear may be substantially easier secondary to the large amount of corneal flattening achieved by the procedure. In addition, higher order aberrations, in particular spherical aberration, may be substantially lessened by the operation, perhaps as a result of a "regularizing" of the corneal shape [13]. Meanwhile, clinically, the graft remains only indistinctly visible as a thin white line on slit-lamp examination (Fig. 27.5).

27.7 Complications

The most common complication of BL transplantation may be inadvertent perforation while dissecting the mid-stromal pocket, which was described to occur in 10% of the originally operated cohort of eyes [1, 2]. Perforations may be managed expectantly by aborting the operation, allowing healing to occur, and reattempting BL

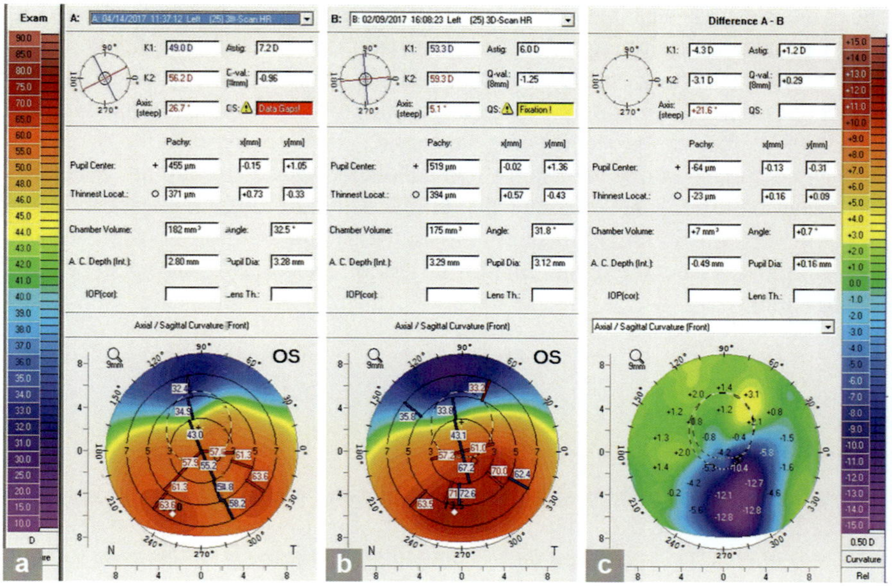

Fig. 27.4 Axial curvature of an eye 10 days after BL transplantation (**a**), compared to before surgery (**b**), which reveals a >10 diopter net flattening effect, concentrated in the infero-temporal cornea (**c**)

Fig. 27.5 Edges of the implanted BL graft only vaguely visible (green arrows)

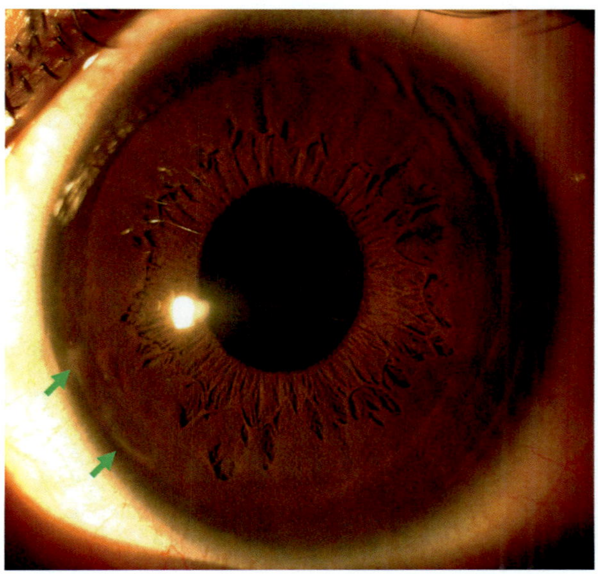

transplantation again at a later date. Alternatively, the surgeon may proceed with PK or DALK, instead, according to his discretion and the wishes of the patient.

No significant postoperative complications stemming from BL transplantation have yet been described. Suture related difficulties are a non-issue (unlike with PK and DALK), since the procedure involves none. Likewise, because the operation involves no corneal-surface incisions, epithelialization problems are not expected. And, because the transplanted tissue is a cellular, allograft reaction may be unlikely (or at the very least, highly amenable to treatment) and therefore topical steroids may be rapidly discontinued, minimizing the risk of glaucoma development or cataract formation.

27.8 Conclusions

In short, BL transplantation seems like a promising way to stabilize eyes with advanced, progressive KC and improve their functional vision by potentially improving their CTL tolerance and by flattening their corneas. In contrast to both PK and DALK, operated eyes are not at significant risk for a wide array of potentially serious postoperative difficulties, and may therefore require less stringent surveillance and less intensive medical therapy.

Financial Disclosure Dr. Melles is consultant for DORC International and SurgiCube International. Drs. Parker, Baydoun, and Dapena are consultants for DORC International. No other author has a financial or proprietary interest in any material or method mentioned.

References

1. van Dijk K, Liarakos VS, Parker J, et al. Bowman layer transplantation to reduce and stabilize progressive, advanced keratoconus. Ophthalmology. 2015;122:909–17.
2. van Dijk K, Parker J, Tong CM, et al. Midstromal isolated Bowman layer graft for reduction of advanced keratoconus: a technique to postpone penetrating or deep anterior lamellar keratoplasty. JAMA Ophthalmol. 2014;132:495–501.
3. Parker JS, van Dijk K, Melles GR. Treatment options for advanced keratoconus: a review. Surv Ophthalmol. 2015;60:459–80.
4. Pramanik S, Musch DC, Sutphin JE, Farjo AA. Extended long-term outcomes of penetrating-keratoplasty for keratoconus. Ophthalmology. 2006;113:1633–8.
5. Wollensak G, Spoerl E, Seiler T. Riboflavin/ultraviolet-a induced collagen crosslinking for the treatment of keratoconus. Am J Ophthalmol. 2003;135:620–7.
6. Wollensak G, Spoerl E, Wilsch M, Seiler T. Endothelial cell damage after riboflavin ultraviolet-A treatment in the rabbit. J Cataract Refract Surg. 2003;29:1786–90.
7. Medical Advisory Secretariat. Intrastromal corneal ring implants for corneal thinning disorders: an evidence-based analysis. Ont Health Technol Assess Ser. 2009;9:1–90.
8. Alió JL, Vega-Estrada A, Esperanza S, et al. Intrastromal corneal ring segments: how successful is the surgical treatment of keratoconus? Middle East Afr J Ophthalmol. 2014;21:3–9.

9. Alió JL, Shabayek MH, Belda JI, et al. Analysis of results related to good and bad outcomes of Intacs implantation for keratoconus correction. J Cataract Refract Surg. 2006;32:756–61.
10. Lie J, Droutsas K, Ham L, et al. Isolated Bowman layer transplantation to manage persistent subepithelial haze after excimer laser surface ablation. J Cataract Refract Surg. 2010;36:1036–41.
11. Groeneveld-van Beek EA, Parker J, Lie JT, et al. Donor tissue preparation for Bowman layer transplantation. Cornea. 2016;35:1499–502.
12. Melles GRJ, Lander F, Rietveld FJR, et al. A new surgical technique for deep, anterior lamellar keratoplasty. Br J Ophthalmol. 1999;83:327–33.
13. Luceri S, Parker J, Dapena I, et al. Corneal densitometry and higher order aberrations after Bowman layer transplantation: 1-year results. Cornea. 2016;35:959–66.

Chapter 28
Management of Keratoconus with Scleral Contact Lenses

David P. Piñero

28.1 Concept of Scleral Contact Lens

Scleral contact lenses have been traditionally defined as those that rests partially or completely in the sclera. Two subgroups were distinguished in scleral lenses depending on the presence of corneal bearing or not: corneo-scleral or semi-scleral, with diameters between 12.5 and 15 mm and which distribute the lens bearing between the cornea and sclera, and lenses that are completely scleral, with diameters between 15 and 18 mm and that only bear on the sclera. Recently, the Scleral Lens Education Society (SLS) has defined a more precise differentiation between different modalities of scleral lenses not only based on the lens diameter, but also on the diameter of visible iris of the eye in which the lens is fitted, as detailed in Table 28.1. Thus, a fully scleral lens of a specific diameter can behave as miniscleral or large-scleral depending on the eye on which it is fitted.

28.2 Indications of Scleral Contact Lenses: Uses in Keratoconus

Scleral contact lenses have always been considered suitable for the correction of irregular astigmatism (post-LASIK, post-keratoplasty), including keratoconus, as they are able to neutralize irregularities with the tear film meniscus that form with the cornea, while maintaining high levels of comfort. However, there are also other

D. P. Piñero Llorens (✉)
Department of Optics, Pharmacology and Anatomy, University of Alicante, Alicante, Spain

Department of Ophthalmology (OFTALMAR), Vithas Medimar International Hospital, Alicante, Spain
e-mail: david.pinyero@gcloud.ua.es

A. Barbara (ed.), *Controversies in the Management of Keratoconus*,
https://doi.org/10.1007/978-3-319-98032-4_28

Table 28.1 Classification of contact lenses according to the Scleral Lens Education Society (SLS)

Type	Subdivision	Bearing
Corneal		All lens bearing on the cornea
Corneo-scleral		Lenses share bearing on the cornea and the sclera
Fully scleral	Mini-scleral Lens is up to 6 mm larger than HVID Large scleral Lens is more than 6 mm larger than HVID	All lens bearing is on the sclera

HVID horizontal visible iris diameter

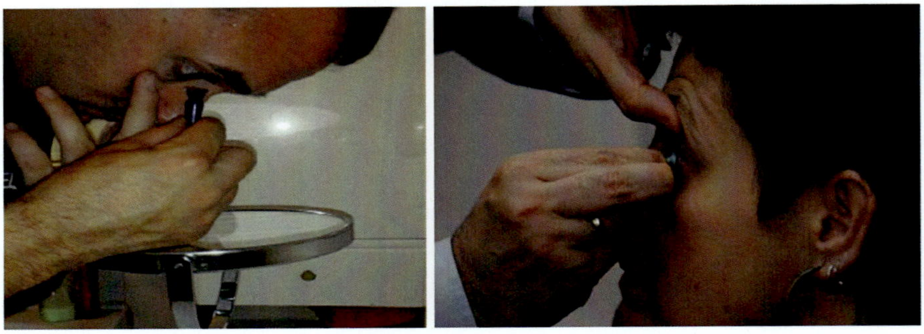

Fig. 28.1 Procedure of insertion (left) and extraction (right) of a fully scleral contact lens

indications feasible for corneo-scleral and fully scleral contact lenses, such as the correction of refractive errors that can not be corrected satisfactorily with rigid gas permeable corneal or soft contact lenses, the introduction of prismatic corrections, for cosmetic purposes and even in healthy corneas due to the advantages of this type of lenses: less palpebral interaction, great comfort as conjuntictival sensitivity is lower than that of the cornea, no possibility of generating corneal distortion if the fitting is adequate and simplified fitting process. In addition, the process of insertion and removal of the lens is simplified by the use of a suction cup, avoiding the contact of the fingers with the eye at all times (Figs. 28.1 and 28.2). Fully scleral contact lenses must be always inserted after being completely filled with saline solution, avoiding the formation of bubbles during the insertion that generates discomfort and poor vision.

According to the peer-reviewed scientific literature, the results of the use of scleral lenses have been described in various types of eyes, including mainly keratoconus, but also in other conditions of the anterior segment, such as post-LASIK ectasia, dry eye or pellucid marginal degeneration. The designs used in all these studies are diverse, but all of them manufactured with materials of high oxygen permeability (Dk between 85 and 189). The diameter used varies greatly from one study to another, not specifying in most cases the specific criteria for the selection

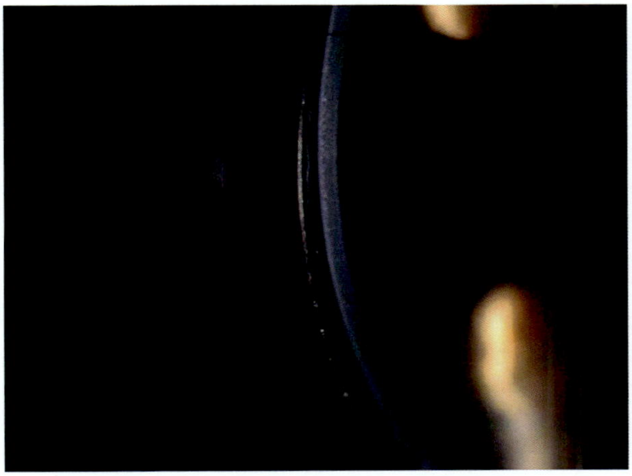

Fig. 28.2 Determination of the apical vault of a fully scleral contact lens ICD fitted in a keratoconus eye by using an optical section with the slit lamp

of one diameter or another. Jiménez and Rodríguez selected the diameter of the scleral lens in their study as a function of the radius of the posterior optical zone, following the trend of a smaller diameter for a smaller radius.

A result that is reported in most of clinical studies on scleral contact lenses conducted to this date is a significant improvement of visual acuity in cases of irregular cornea. This improvement is more limited in advanced keratoconus, as well as in other therapeutic uses, such as post-keratoplasty and irregular astigmatism with secondary nystagmus. The follow-up of all these clinical studies is short in the great majority of cases, being generally of less than 1 year. Therefore, longer-term studies are necessary to know the true behavior of the scleral lens over time and to characterize the possible complications that may appear in the long term. Likewise, in the previous clinical studies, the number of follow-up visits is low, a limitation that should be overcome in future studies considering that these lenses are normally fitted in pathological corneas, such as keratoconus. Another relevant limitation of studies on scleral contact lenses is the sample size, with most of them including a small number of eyes (between 2 and 52 eyes). There is only one study evaluating the results of scleral contact lenses in a large sample including a total of 213 eyes. One of the main reasons for this sampling limitation may be the relatively low prevalence of keratoconus, as well as of other corneal pathological conditions in which scleral lens fitting is performed.

In some studies, there is a significant number of dropouts due mainly to the absence of improvement in visual acuity with scleral lenses. In the study conducted by Schornack et al. a total of 22 eyes of the sample evaluated abandoned the use of scleral lenses. One of the patients who left (2 eyes) was due to the fact that after cataract surgery he noticed a greater improvement in visual acuity with glasses, while in the remaining 20 eyes the reasons for abandonment were very diverse, with some of them reporting the absence of visual acuity improvement with the lenses (8 eyes). The other dropouts reported were due to the following: corrected visual acuity of 20/20 in the eye not wearing the scleral lens in four patients (five eyes), not improvement in visual acuity due to the presence of cataract in two patients (four eyes), no improvement in visual acuity due to corneal wound after transplantation in one patient (one eye), and no coverage of the expenses by the medical insurance in two patients. In a study by Jiménez et al., the number of dropouts was lower (four eyes abandoned), but as in the previous study, 50% of these dropouts were due to an absence of visual acuity improvement with the corneo-scleral lens Rose K2 XL lens (Menicon). Specifically, these patients referred that they had better visión with their previous corneal gas permeable contact lenses. In this same study, the other two dropouts were because the patient preferred the piggyback system in one case and the other one abandoned because the patient needed a lens with peripheral toricity. One of the reasons for the limitation of the visual improvement achieved may be the poor control of the tear film meniscus. It has been shown that thick meniscus (thickness of 300 μm or more) in irregular corneas generate a poorer control of high order aberrations, with even induction of some of them, such as spherical aberration.

Our research group conducted a study to assess the results obtained with the fully scleral contact lens ICD16.5 (Paragon) in corneas with different types of problems. Specifically, this lens has a diameter of 16.5 mm. The study was consecutive and prospective, and was carried out in the Contactology Unit of the Department of Ophthalmology (OFTALMAR) of the Vithas Medimar International Hospital in Alicante. It included a total of 42 eyes of 27 patients, 15 men (55.6%) and 12 women (44.4%). The average age of patients was 39 ± 12 years (range, 14–65 years). Inclusion criteria for the study were: no active ocular disease, no severe dry eye, no previous intolerance to soft or corneal gas permeable contact lenses and signed informed consent. In all cases a very complete pre-fitting examination was carried out that included: filiation data, uncorrected and corrected visual acuity, manifest refraction, biomicroscopy, corneal topography with the Sirius system (CSO), ocular aberration measurements with the iTrace system (Tracey Technologies, Inc.,) and previous anterior segment examination by optical coherence tomography with the 3D OCT-1000 system (Topcon). The patient was evaluated after 1, 3, 6 and 12 months of contact lens wear.

In our study, a total of 25 eyes with keratoconus (59.5%) were fitted, 4 of them with previous implantation of intracorneal ring segments and 10 with previous corneal collagen crosslinking, 6 eyes with irregular cornea after previous LASIK surgery (14.3%), 2 eyes with irregular cornea after radial keratotomy surgery (4.8%), 3 eyes after keratoplasty (7.1%), 1 eye with endothelial corneal decompensation (2.4%)), 2 cases of dry eye (4.8%) and 2 eyes with myopia magna (4.8%). The average spherical refractive error of the sample was −1.81 ± 4.30 D (−11.00 to +8.00 D) and the average manifest cylinder was −3.05 ± 2.34 D (−10.00 to 0.00 D). The mean sagital height required for the fitting was 4294.12 ± 292.56 μm (4000–4900 μm) and the mean optical power was −6.96 ± 6.95 D (−21 to +4 D). After 1 h of wearing, the mean apical vault measured by optical coherence tomography was 299.4 ± 85.56 μm (201–420 μm) (Fig. 28.2). Concerning vision, a significant improvement in decimal visual acuity was achieved with the contact lens after 1 month of wearing compared to that obtained with glasses before fitting ($p < 0.001$),

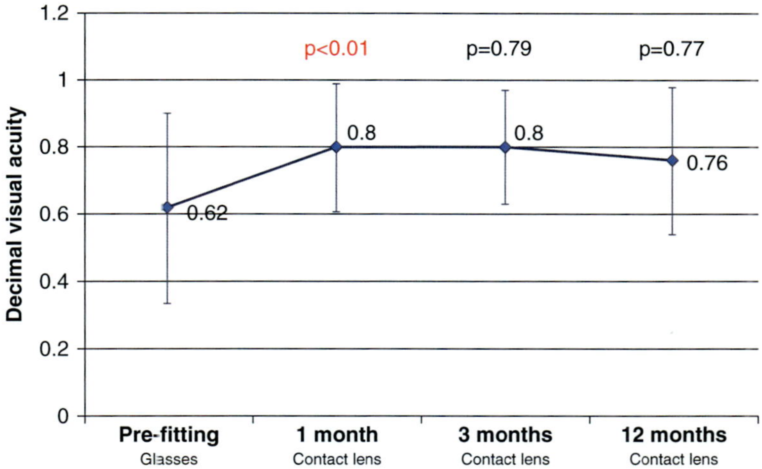

Fig. 28.3 Visual changes with the fully scleral contact lens ICD in a study conducted by our research group

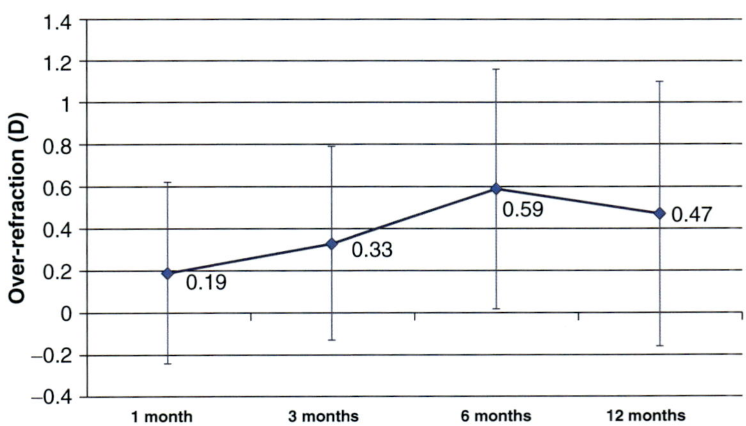

Fig. 28.4 Changes in spherical over-refraction with the fully scleral contact lens ICD in a study conducted by our research group

without significant changes occurring during the rest of the follow-up (Fig. 28.3). There was a tendency to an increasing positive over-refraction during the follow-up, although it did not reach statistical significance ($p = 0.17$) (Fig. 28.4). This change was consistent with a slight anterior ($p = 0.91$) and posterior corneal flattening ($p = 0.37$), which did not reach either statistical significance.

In our study, a small but statistically significant pachymetric increase was also observed at 3 months of wearing (minimum thickness $p = 0.001$, central thickness $p = 0.08$), without significant changes afterwards (minimum thickness $p = 0.86$, central thickness $p = 0.88$). Regarding ocular high-order aberrations, there was a

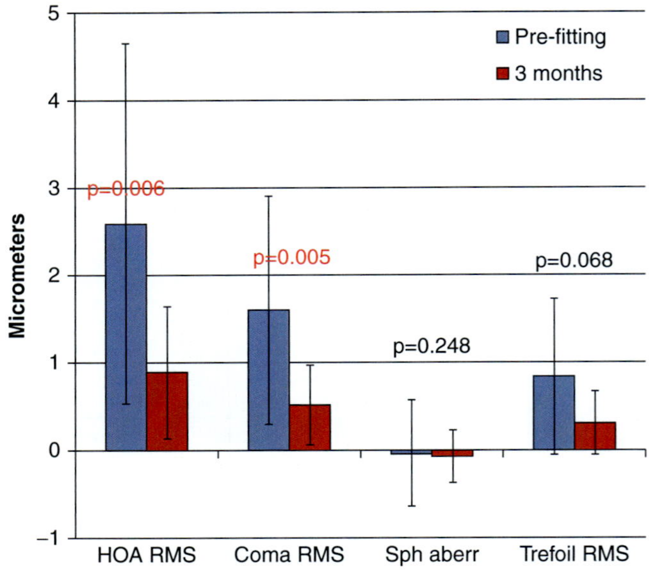

Fig. 28.5 Change in ocular high order aberrations with the wearing of the fully scleral contact lens ICD in a study conducted by our research group. Abbreviations: RMS root mean square, Sph aberr spherical aberration

significant reduction, especially of the primary coma (Fig. 28.5). The tolerance of the contact lens was good in all cases, with the following complications or difficulties reported:

- Abandonment of fitting: three cases (6.8%) due to poor tolerance as a consequence of an excessive lens indentation throughout the day
- Lens power adjustments required during the 1st month (eight cases, 18.2%)
- Adjustments of the scleral landing zone due to lens fogging (five cases, 11.4%) or excessive scleral indentation (two cases, 4.5%)
- Episodes of occasional conjunctival hyperemia (tobradex, thealoz, recugel) (five cases, 11.4%)

One of the indications that has recently been postulated for fully scleral contact lenses is dry eye management. Dr. Carracedo and his team at the Complutense University of Madrid demonstrated in 2016 in a study that included 26 patients with keratoconus fitted with the same model of scleral contact lens (ICD) that 6–9 h of wearing of such lenses generated a significant reduction in the scores obtained with the OSDI questionnaire, osmolarity, and diadenosine tetraphosphate concentration (Ap4A), as well as an increase in MMP-9 concentrations (matrix metalloproteinase 9). Therefore, there was an improvement in the signs and symptoms of dry eye in these keratoconus eyes with the fitting of fully scleral contact lenses.

28.3 Design of Scleral Contact Lenses

Most of designs of scleral contact lenses that are currently available are rotationally symmetrical, with spherical geometry in the optical zone. This zone is the one that provides the desired refractive correction. In fully scleral contact lenses, it should be considered when deciding the power of the optical zone that each 100 μm increase in sagittal height implies an optical power change of 0.12 D. This rule may sometimes fail in keratoconus as well as in other cases of irregular cornea. Likewise, the decentration or displacement of the optical zone of this type of lenses once they are fitted in the eye generates a prismatic effect that may relevant depending on the magnitude of the decentration.

Besides the optical zone, scleral lenses have a transition zone or also called mid-peripheral or limbar zone that is specially relevant when fitting fully scleral lenses, as this zone determines the sagittal height of the lens. Peripherally, the bearing zone or haptic area is the one that directly contacts the conjunctiva, which should be as close as possible to the sclero-conjunctival curvature. Normally this haptic area is characterized geometrically by a fairly flat curve, between 13.5 and 14.5 mm of radius, although there are also tangential designs for this area.

Concerning rotationally asymmetric designs, they are used in more complex fittings requiring peritoric or quadrant designs. These rotationally asymmetric designs are used when a good positioning of the lens with conventional designs is not achieved, as well as when a complete stabilization of the contact lens is needed to introduce toricity in its optical zone. Therefore, rotationally asymmetric designs are aimed at obtaining a more optimized contact lens fit considering the geometric profile of the conjunctival-scleral surface and, therefore, to prevent the scleral lens from being decentered or rotated.

28.4 Scleral Contact Lens Fitting

The fitting criteria are different depending if the contact lens has a sclero-corneal or fully scleral design. In the case of corneo-scleral lenses, the fitting process is commonly guided by keratometry or topography, with very variable criteria for a good fitting among designs. There are designs in which a central alignment is needed with some peripheral tear pooling (Fig. 28.6), while in others the objective is to create a central tear film pooling with contact lens and cornea alignment in the middle periphery (Fig. 28.7). Concerning the evaluation of the alignment of the contact lens at the conjunctival-scleral plane, the "push-in" method is commonly used (Fig. 28.8). This method consists on the induction of a certain level of pressure in the sclera with the help of the eyelid below the edge of the contact lens and on assessing afterwards the level of pressure required to generate bubbles and introduce them in the space between contact lens and eye. If a high level of pressure is necessary, this reveals that an excessive peripheral closure is present, being recommendable to modify the edge lift.

Concerning fully scleral lenses, the fitting is guided by sagital height, not by keratometry as happened with corneo-scleral lenses. The sagital height of the healthy eye is commonly around 4000 μm for a diameter of 15.0 mm. It can vary depending on the diameter considered, radius of curvature, asphericity of the anterior corneal surface, and geometry of the anterior zone of the sclero-conjunctival área. The following steps must be followed for an appropriate fitting of fully scleral lenses:

- Step 1: selection of total diameter
- Step 2: selection of the sagittal height providing a corneal clearance between 200–300 μm

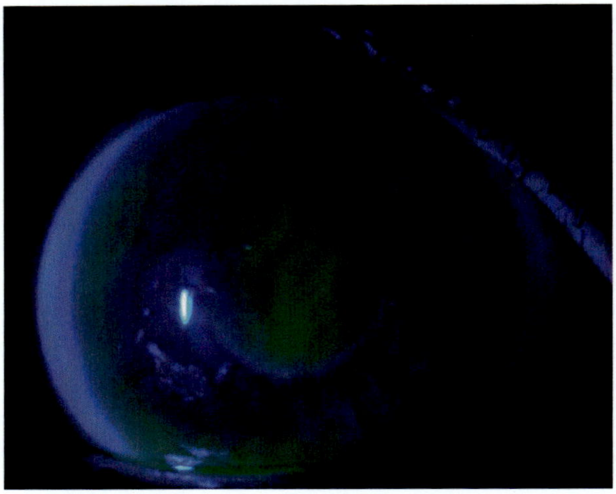

Fig. 28.6 Ideal fluorogram of a corneo-scleral contact lens (Alexa K, Tiedra, Spain) in which a central tear film pooling with contact lens and cornea alignment in the middle periphery is required

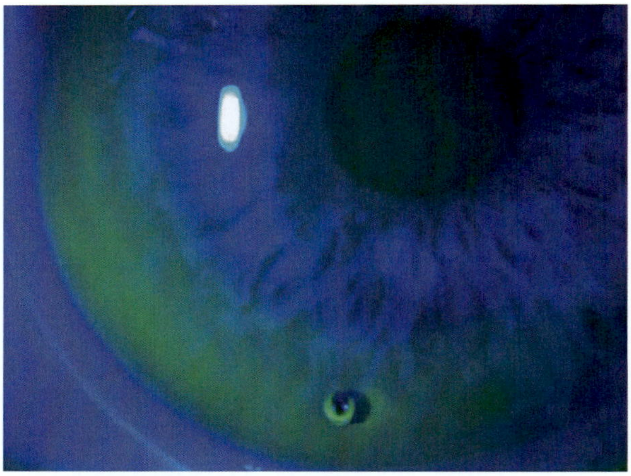

Fig. 28.7 Ideal fluorogram of a corneo-scleral contact lens (SoClear, Tiedra, Spain) in which a central tear film pooling with contact lens and cornea alignment in the middle periphery is required

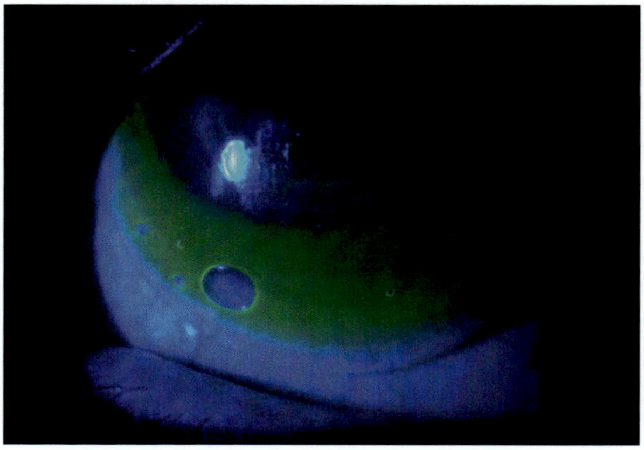

Fig. 28.8 Peripheral bubble generated by conjunctival-scleral pressure induced with the eyelid to assess the closure of the peripheral curve (push-in method)

- Step 3: adjustment of the landing zone of the lens
- Step 4: evaluation of edge lift
- Step 5: selection of a more complex design, such as peritoric or by quadrants if a proper stabilization of the lens is not achieved

The most relevant difficulty in this type of fittings is the selection of the sagital height required for the trial lens. The direct measurement of the sagital height of the eye would be the ideal option by means of optical coherence tomography or devices based on the use of a rotatory Scheimpflug camera. As these options are not available in all clinical settings, empirical nomograms of selection of the sagital height of the lens have been defined for different designs of scleral lenses and the adequacy of this selection is done by comparing in the slit lamp the thickness of the scleral lens, which is commonly around 300–350 μm and the tear film meniscus that must be very similar. Furthermore, recently, new devices have been developed for measuring the corneo-scleral curvature and defining accordingly more accurate estimations of the sagital height required for the trial lens, such as the Eye Surface Profiler (ESP) from Eaglet-Eye (Fig. 28.9). This system allows to measure the sagital height of the eye and to generate a topographic map with XYZ coordinates. This system has the ability of measuring an area of 20 mm of diameter and a total of 250,000 points covering cornea, limbus and sclera. The instillation of fluorescein is necessary to perform the measurement procedure with this device.

28.5 Potential Fitting Problems and Complications

Among the main fitting problems and complications that have been described for scleral contact lenses, the following conditions can be found:

- Presence of bubbles
- Bulbar redness

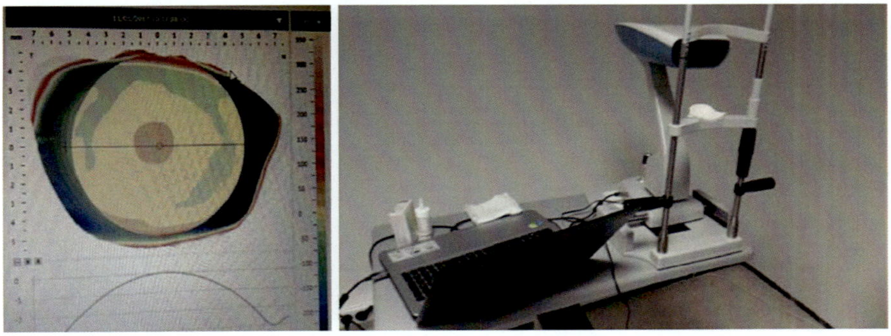

Fig. 28.9 System for the characterization of corneo-scleral geometry ESP (Eye Surface Profiler, Eaglet-Eye). Right, general aspect of the device; left, aspect of the main screen showing the map obtain in a specific case measured with the device

- Conjunctival blanching and staining
- Corneal staining
- Discomfort
- Mucus and debris
- Fogging

The presence of bubbles is associated with discomfort and visual problems, especially when fully scleral lenses are fitted. The main reason for this condition is an inadequate insertion, being recommendable to extract and reinsert the lens again with care (Fig. 28.10). In the case of corneo-scleral lenses, the presence of bubbles, especially in the periphery may be a sign of adjustment problems, being necessary to revise the parameters of the lens.

Several reasons may explain the presence of bulbar redness with scleral lens wear, such as mechanical stress on conjunctiva, corneal hypoxia, toxic reactions, bearing of the lens on cornea or limbus and lens adhesion. For this reason, a careful revision of all fitting parameters will be required as well as to know the real patient's use of the lens. A slight bulbar redness after lens extraction is normal, but it disappears fast.

Conjunctival blanching is a sign of an excessive local pressure of the lens on conjunctiva due to the presence of an irregular geometry of the conjunctival-scleral surface or due to an excess of closure of the edge lift of the lens (Fig. 28.11). This blanching may induce staining as well as local ischemia when the level of indentation is extremely high. This condition can be avoided by modifying the peripheral curvature of the lens as well as the design of the peripheral area of the lens, including toricity or geometric changes by quadrants.

The presence of corneal staining is related to the need for a change in the fitting in terms of lens parameters or patient's use guidelines. If there is a local area of staining, it can be related to an excessive peripheral bearing of a corneo-scleral contact lens or even to the presence of corneal touch with a fully scleral contact lens.

Fig. 28.10 Bubble associated to a wrong insertion of a fully scleral contact lens

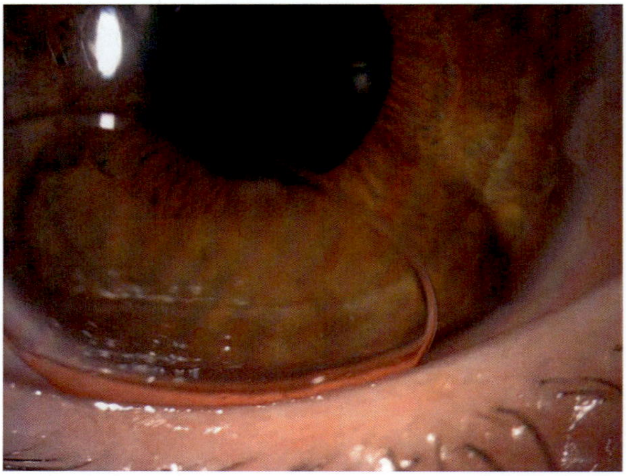

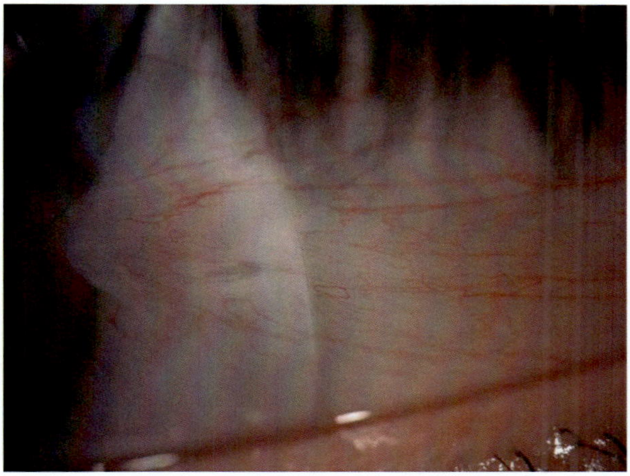

Fig. 28.11 Local área of conjunctival blanching with a fully scleral contact lens due to the presence of pterigium

If the staining is diffuse and general, the possibility of a hypoxic or toxic reaction should be considered.

One of the main characteristics of scleral contact lenses is comfort. If the patient refers discomfort, please consider the presence of corneal or limbus bearing of the lens, a toxic reaction or even a peripheral tight fitting of the lens. Concerning the accumulation of mucus and debris below the lens, it should be consider that may be related to problems of the ocular surface. In this situation, it should be confirmed if blepharitis or Meibomian gland dysfunction are present. If so, an adequate treatment must be prescribed. Before continuing with the fittings, these conditions must be resolved. Likewise, the accumulation of deposits below the lens may be due to an excessive flat periphery of the lens generating an excessive tear film exchange and even to a problem with contact lens solutions.

Finally, the presence of fogging is a complication that the patient describes as very disturbing because it generates loss of visual quality and visual fluctuations. This phenomenon seems to be related to an increase of the tear film temperature below the lens. As possible solutions for this condition, the following options have been described:

- Frequent extraction and re-insertion of the lens
- Change of the edge lift or peripheral curves to facilitate some tear film exchange
- Use of artificial film preserved in the fridge

28.6 Clinical Cases

Case 1: We show a case published previously in Journal of Keratoconus and Corneal Ectatic Diseases, describing the fitting of a scleral lens in a 26-year old man with keratoconus in right eye. Intracorneal ring segment implantation had been performed in this eye 2 years before that generated some corneal remodeling but not eliminating all corneal irregularities (Fig. 28.12). On examination, an uncorrected distance visual acuity of 0.2 was found that improved to 0.3 with the manifest refraction of −3.00 × 55°. Vogat striae were present on slit lamp examination as well as a slight central leukoma (Fig. 28.13). After several trials, a stable and comfortable fit was achieved with a lens of 4600 μm of sagital height and power of −11.25 D (ICD16.5, Paragon Vision Sciences). It provided an apical clearance of 212 μm that decreased to 196 μm after 8–10 h of wearing (Fig. 28.14). With this lens, the patient achieved a decimal visual

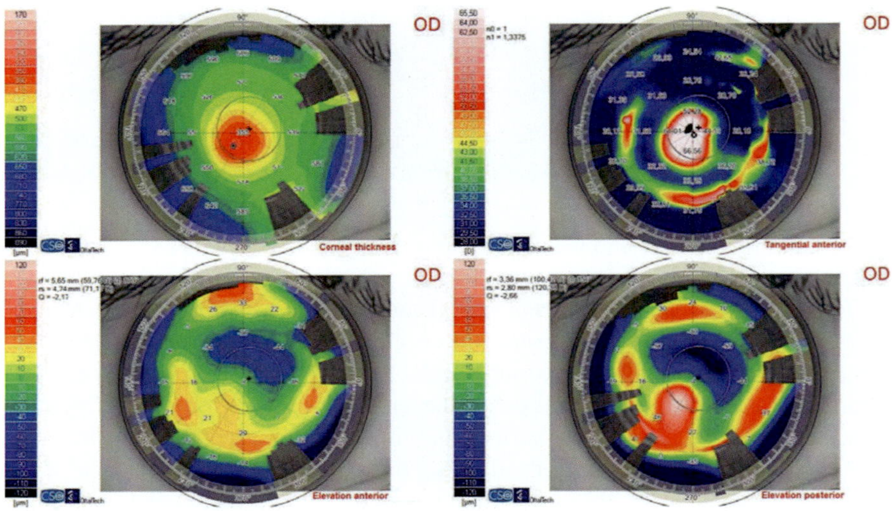

Fig. 28.12 Topographic aspect of the cornea before contact lens fitting in the first clinical case reported

Fig. 28.13 Biomicroscopic aspect of the cornea before contact lens fitting in the first clinical case reported

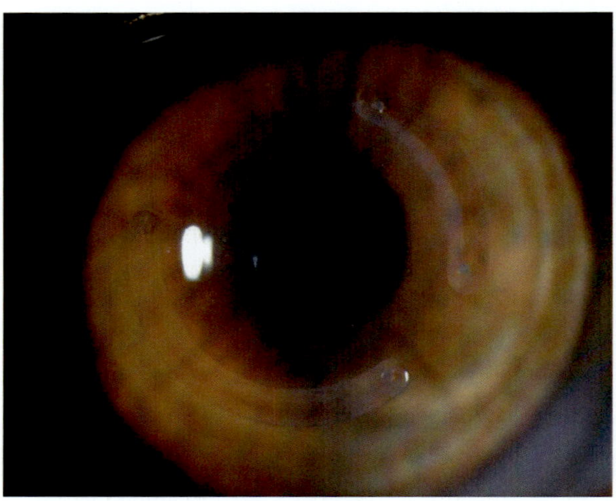

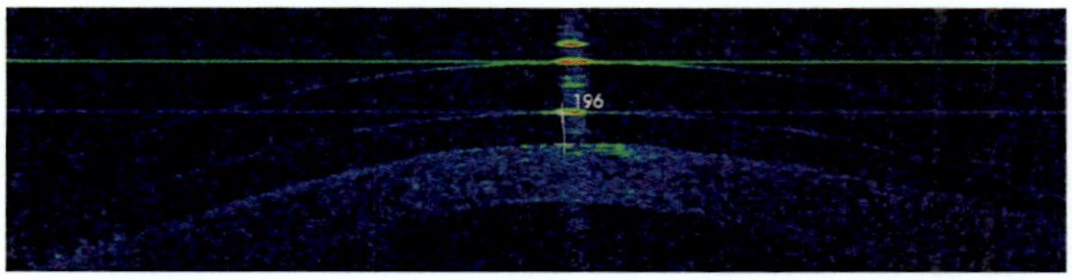

Fig. 28.14 Measurement of the apical clearance achieved with the contact lens fitted in the first clinical case reported

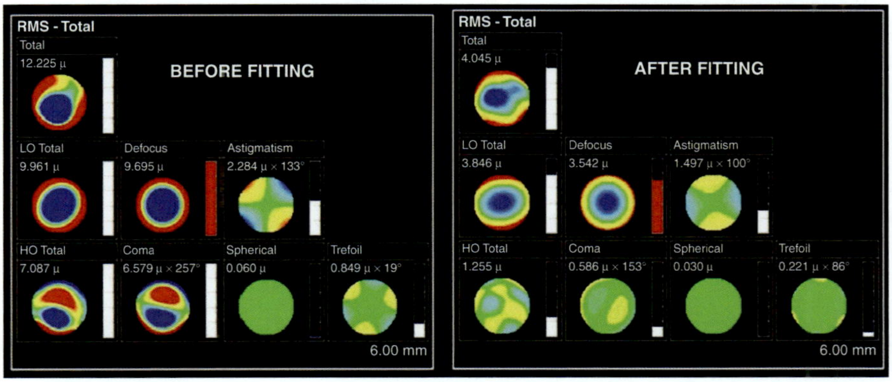

Fig. 28.15 Ocular aberrometric change measured with the i-Trace system induced with the contact lens fitted in the first case reported

acuity of 1.0 and was very satisfied. This high level of satisfaction was also in agreement with the significant reduction of ocular high order aberrations achieved with the lens (Fig. 28.15). This result has been maintained during 3 years after initiating the fitting and wearing of the lens.

Case 2: We report the case of a 35-year-old woman diagnosed with keratoconus since she was 18 years old and wearer of corneal rigid contact lenses. We refitted the case with a fully scleral contact lens (ICD16.5, Paragon Vision Sciences) for obtaining not only a successful visual restoration, but also a comfortable wear. We initiated the fitting with the spherical model of the scleral contact lens, but it failed due to instability of the lens. We confirmed the presence of a clear asymmetry in the anterior scleral geometry in both eyes by using the profilometer eye surface profiler (ESP, Eaglet Eye), with a difference between nasal and temporal sagittal heights of 470 and 170 µm in right and left eyes respectively (Fig. 28.16). Although this profile suggested the need for the fitting of a scleral contact lens with significant peripheral toricity, we followed the manufacturer's guidelines and performed a trial with a lens of moderate peripheral toricity (125 µm of difference between steep and flat meridian). The stability of the contact lens failed again and finally a lens with a peripheral toricity close to that measured with the profilometer was fitted. With this lens, good visual performance, lens stability, and comfort was obtained and maintained during a 1-year follow-up (Fig. 28.17). This case suggests that fully scleral contact lens fitting might be optimized with the use of corneo-scleral profilometers, minimizing potentially the number of trials. This potential benefit should be investigated further in future studies.

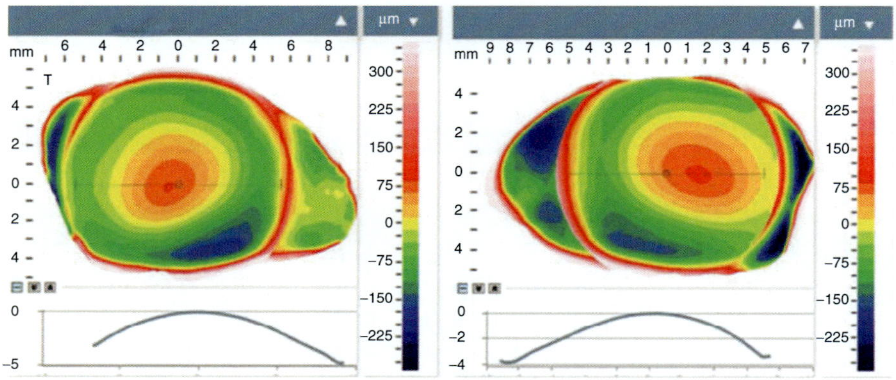

Fig. 28.16 Bisphere elevation map characterizing the corneo-scleral topographic profile obtained with the ESP system (left, right eye; right, left eye) in the second case reported

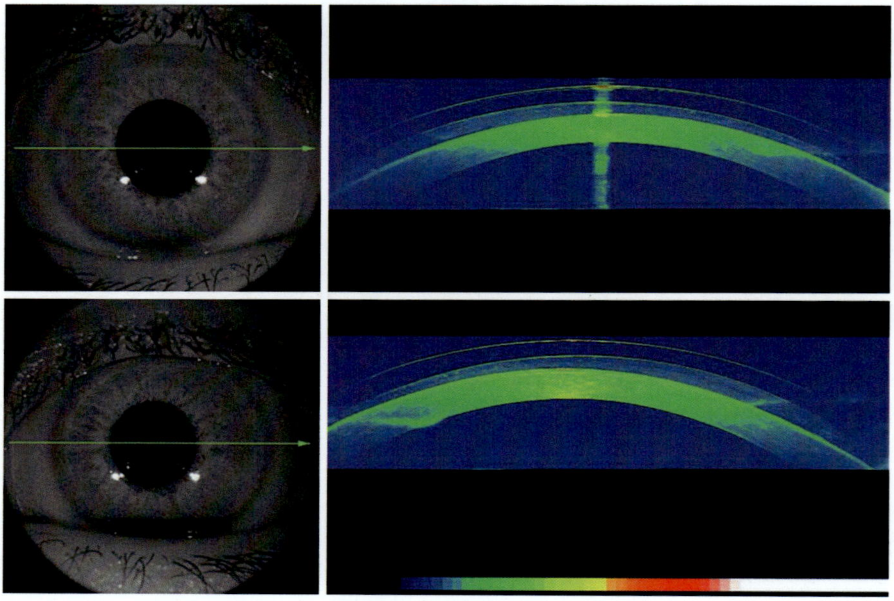

Fig. 28.17 Optical coherence tomography (OCT) analysis of the final scleral lenses fitted in right (up) and left eyes (down) (left: Frontal image of the eye; right: Horizontal OCT scan showing the position of the lens)

Suggested Reading

Alipour F, Rahimi F, Hashemian MN, Ajdarkosh Z, Roohipoor R, Mohebi M. Mini-scleral contact lens for management of poor visual outcomes after intrastromal corneal ring segments implantation in keratoconus. J Ophthalmic Vis Res. 2016;11:252–7.

Asena L, Altınörs DD. Clinical outcomes of scleral Misa lenses for visual rehabilitation in patients with pellucid marginal degeneration. Cont Lens Anterior Eye. 2016;39:420–4.

Barnett M, Lien V, Li JY, Durbin-Johnson B, Mannis MJ. Use of scleral lenses and miniscleral lenses after penetrating keratoplasty. Eye Contact Lens. 2016;42:185–9.

Bleshoy H, Pullum KW. Corneal response to gas permeable impression scleral lenses. J Br Contact Lens Assoc. 1988;11 31–4.

Bray C, Britton S, Yeung D, Haines L, Sorbara L. Change in over-refraction after scleral lens settling on average corneas. Ophthalmic Physiol Opt. 2017;37:467–72.

Bruce AS, Nguyen LM. Acuted red eye (non-ulcerative keratitis) associated with mini-scleral contact lens wear for keratoconus. Clin Exp Optom. 2013;96:245–8.

Carracedo G, Serramito-Blanco M, Martin-Gil A, Wang Z, Rodriguez-Pomar C, Pintor J. Post-lens tear turbidity and visual quality after scleral lens wear. Clin Exp Optom. 2017;100(6):577–82. https://doi.org/10.1111/cxo.12512.

Carracedo G, Wang Z, Serramito-Blanco M, Martin-Gil A, Carballo-Alvarez J, Pintor J. Ocular surface temperature during scleral lens wearing in patients with keratoconus. Eye Contact Lens. 2016;43(6):346–51.

Carracedo G, Blanco MS, Martin-Gil A, Zicheng W, Alvarez JC, Pintor J. Short-term effect of scleral lens on the dry eye biomarkers in keratoconus. Optom Vis Sci. 2016;93:150–7.

Dalton K, Sorbana L. Fitting and MSD (Mini Scleral Design) rigid contact lens in advanced keratoconus with INTACS. Cont Lens Anterior Eye. 2011;34:274–81.

Domínguez-Vicent A, Esteve-Taboada JJ, Recchioni A. Power profiles and in vitro optical quality of scleral contact lenses: effect of the aperture and power. Eye Contact Lens. 2018;44(3):149–58. https://doi.org/10.1097/ICL.0000000000000345.

Esen F, Toker E. Influence of apical clearance on mini-scleral lens settling, clinical performance, and corneal thickness changes. Eye Contact Lens. 2017;43:230–5.

Harthan J, Nau CB, Barr J, Nau A, Shorter E, Chimato NT, Hodge DO, Schornack MM. Scleral lens prescription and management practices: the SCOPE study. Eye Contact Lens. 2017; https://doi.org/10.1097/ICL.0000000000000387. [Epub ahead of print].

Jedlicka J, Johns LK, Byrnes SP. Scleral contact lens fitting guide. Cont Lens Spec. 2010;3:0–36.

Jimenez RM, Rodríguez PF. Utility of a semi-scleral lens design in the management of the irregular cornea. Cont Lens Anterior Eye. 2013;36:146–50.

Kim S, Lee JS, Park YK, Lee SU, Park YM, Lee JH, Lee JE. Fitting miniscleral contact lenses in Korean patients with keratoconus. Clin Exp Optom. 2017;100:375–9.

Navascues-Cornago M, Maldonado-Codina C, Morgan PB. Mechanical sensitivity of the human conjunctiva. Cornea. 2014;33:855–9.

Nixon AD, Barr JT, VanNasdale DA. Corneal epithelial bullae after short-term wear of small diameter scleral lenses. Cont Lens Anterior Eye. 2017;40:116–26.

Otchere H, Jones LW, Sorbara L. Effect of time on scleral lens settling and change in corneal clearance. Optom Vis Sci. 2017;94(9):908–13. https://doi.org/10.1097/OPX.0000000000001111.

Pecego M, Barnett M, Mannis MJ, Durbin-Johnson B. Jupiter scleral lenses: the UC Davis Eye Center experience. Eye Contact Lens. 2012;38:179–82.

Pérez-Cambrodí RJ, Ruiz-Fortes P, Piñero DP. Reverse geometry hybrid contact lens fitting in a case of donor-host misalignment after keratoplasty. Int J Kerat Ect Cor Dis. 2013;2:69–72.

Piñero DP, Soto-Negro R. Anterior eye profilometry-guided scleral contact lens fitting in keratoconus. Int J Kerat Ect Cor Dis. 2017;6:1–4.

Piñero DP. Full scleral lens fitting in an eye with high corneal astigmatism after radial keratotomy and several retreatments. I-Site Newsl. 2017.

Piñero DP. Fitting of a new design of full scleral contact lens in advanced keratoconus with previous implantation of intracorneal ring segments. Int J Kerat Ect Cor Dis. 2015;4:56–9.

Piñero DP, Pérez-Cambrodí RJ, Ruiz-Fortes P, Blanes-Mompó FJ. New-generation hybrid contact lens for the management of extreme irregularity in a thin cornea after unsuccessful excimer laser refractive surgery. Eye Contact Lens. 2014;40:e16–20.

Piñero DP. Um novo conceito de lentes de contacto: a lente de apoio completamente escleral. Look Vision Portugal. 2014;29:44–6.

Porcar E, Montalt JC, España-Gregori E, Peris-Martínez C. Corneo-scleral contact lenses in an uncommon case of keratoconus with high hyperopia and astigmatism. Cont Lens Anterior Eye. 2017. 40(5):351–6. pii: S1367-0484(17)30035-8. https://doi.org/10.1016/j.clae.2017.07.004.

Porcar E, Montalt JC, España-Gregori E, Peris-Martínez C. Corneo-scleral contact lens in a piggyback system for keratoconus: a case report. Cont Lens Anterior Eye. 2017;40:190–4.
Porcar E, España E, Montalt JC, Benlloch-Fornés JI, Peris-Martínez C. Post-LASIK visual quality with a corneoscleral contact lens to treat irregular corneas. Eye Contact Lens. 2017;43:46–50.
Pullum KW, Whiting MA, Buckley RJ. Scleral contact lenses: the expanding role. Cornea. 2005;24:269–77.
Pullum KW, Stapleton FJ. Scleral lens induced corneal swelling: what is the effect of varying Dk and lens thickness? CLAO J. 1997;23:259–63.
Pullum KW, Hobley AJ, Davison C. 100 + Dk: does thickness make much difference? J Br Contact Lens Assoc. 1991;6:158–61.
Rathi VM, Mandathara PS, Dumpati S, Sangwan VS. Change in vault during scleral lens trials assessed with anterior segment optical coherence tomography. Cont Lens Anterior Eye. 2017;40:157–61.
Rathi VM, Mandathara PS, Dumpati S, Vaddavalli PK, Sangwan VS. Boston ocular surface prosthesis: an Indian experience. Indian J Ophthalmol. 2011;59:279–81.
Rocha GA, Miziara PO, Castro AC, Rocha AA. Visual rehabilitation using mini-scleral contact lenses after penetrating keratoplasty. Arq Bras Oftalmol. 2017;80:17–20.
Segal O, Barkana Y, Hourovitz D, Behrman S, Kamun Y, Avni I, Zadok D. Scleral contact lenses may help where other modalities fail. Cornea. 2003;22:308–10.
Severinsky B, Behrman S, Pery JF, Solomon A. Scleral contact lenses for visual rehabilitation after penetrating keratoplasty: long term outcomes. Cont Lens Anterior Eye. 2014;37:196–202.
Schornack MM, Patel SV. Scleral lenses in the management of keratoconus. Eye Contact Lens. 2010;36:39–44.
Suarez C, Madariaga V, Lepage B, Malecaze M, Fournié P, Soler V, Galiacy S, Mély R, Cassagne M, Malecaze F. First experience with the ICD 16.5 mini-scleral lens for optic and therapeutic purposes. Eye Contact Lens. 2016. [Epub ahead of print].
Tomalla M, Cagnolati W. Modern treatment options for the therapy of keratoconus. Cont Lens Anterior Eye. 2007;30:61–6.
Van der Worp E, Bornman D, Ferreira DL, Faria-Ribeiro M, Garcia-Porta N, González-Meijome JM. Modern scleral contact lenses: a review. Cont Lens Anterior Eye. 2014;37:240–50.
Van der Worp E. A guide to scleral lens fitting. Books and monographs. Book. Forest Grove: Pacific University; 2011. (http://commons.pacificu.edu/mono/54).
Vincent SJ, Alonso-Caneiro D, Collins MJ. The temporal dynamics of miniscleral contact lenses: central corneal clearance and centration. Cont Lens Anterior Eye. 2017. pii: S1367-0484(17)30171-6. doi: https://doi.org/10.1016/j.clae.2017.07.002. [Epub ahead of print].
Vincent SJ, Alonso-Caneiro D, Collins MJ, Beanland A, Lam L, Lim CC, Loke A, Nguyen N. Hypoxic corneal changes following eight hours of scleral contact lens wear. Optom Vis Sci. 2016;93:293–9.
Visser ES, Soeters N, Tahzib NG. Scleral lens tolerance after corneal cross-linking for keratoconus. Optom Vis Sci. 2015;92:318–23.
Visser ES, Van der Linden BJJJ, Otten HM, Van der Lelij A, Visser R. Medical applications and outcomes of bitangential scleral lenses. Optom Vis Sci. 2013;90:1078–85.
Visser ES, Visser R, van Lier HJ, Otten HM. Modern scleral lenses part I: clinical features. Eye Contact Lens. 2007;33:13–20.
Walker MK, Bergmanson JP, Miller WL, Marsack JD, Johnson LA. Complications and fitting challenges associated with scleral contact lenses: a review. Cont Lens Anterior Eye. 2016;39:88–96.
Weber SL, de Souza RB, Gomes JÁ, Hofling-Lima AL. The use of the esclera scleral contact lens in the treatment of moderate to severe dry eye disease. Am J Ophthalmol. 2016;163:167–73.e1.
Weber SL, Ambrósio R Jr, Lipener C, Coral-Ghanem C, Hofling-Lima AL. The use of ocular anatomical measurements using a rotating Scheimpflug camera to assist in the Esclera® scleral contact lens fitting process. Cont Lens Anterior Eye. 2016;39:148–53.
Yuksel E, Bilgihan K, Novruzlu Ş, Yuksel N, Koksal M. The management of refractory dry eye with semi-scleral contact lens. Eye Contact Lens. 2016. [Epub ahead of print].

Chapter 29
Navigating the Controversies in the Treatment of Keratoconus

Adel Barbara, Paul R. Meredith, and Ramez Barbara

29.1 What Are the Clinical Challenges in the Management of Keratoconus?

Keratoconus (KC) causes thinning, protrusion and surface irregularity of the cornea. These changes result in progressive deterioration of visual acuity (VA) predominantly due to the induced regular and irregular astigmatism.

In the early stages of disease glasses may help in improving the VA. With progression of the disease and the increase in irregular astigmatism glasses become less beneficial with a loss in best spectacle corrected visual acuity (BSCVA). The more advanced the KC the greater the loss of BSCVA. In the advanced stages of the disease a scar may form in the central area of the cornea which contributes to further reduction in VA.

KC is one of the main indications for keratoplaty, either penetrating keratoplasty (PK) or deep anterior lamellar keratoplasty (DALK).

DALK is becoming the preferred choice over PK in the treatment of KC as it is associated with lower rates of graft rejection. However there is limited evidence of the superiority of DALK over PK in terms of post-surgery astigmatism with better visual outcomes reported with PK [1–3]. A variable rate of conversion from DALK to PK during surgery is reported by cornea surgeons.

Keratoplasty is a major operation with good graft survival rates that decrease overtime [4, 5]. Because of the significant risk of intra-operative, early and late complications after keratoplasty ophthalmologists tend to defer this surgery whenever possible. Even a clear corneal graft may be an optical failure if it is associated with

A. Barbara (✉)
Medical Director of IVISION, Refractive Surgery and Keratoconus Treatment Center, Haifa, Israel

P. R. Meredith · R. Barbara
Southampton Eye Unit, Southampton General Hospital, Southampton, UK

A. Barbara (ed.), *Controversies in the Management of Keratoconus*,
https://doi.org/10.1007/978-3-319-98032-4_29

high astigmatism post-operatively. Astigmatism of five diopters or more has been reported in10–27% [6–8] of cases of keratoplasty and, in our experience the rates of high post-keratoplasty astigmatism are likely under-reported. Progressive astigmatism post-keratoplasty has also been reported. One study that monitored levels of astigmatism in eighty eyes after PKP for KC with a mean follow-up of 20 years (range 15–25) reported stabilization of keratometric astigmatism over the first 7 years (4.39 ± 2.48 D), followed by a progressive increase from 10 years after suture removal until the last follow-up visit (5.48 ± 3.11 D at year 10, 6.43 ± 4.11 D at year 15; 7.28 ± 4.21 D at year 20, and 7.25±4.27 D at year 25) [9]. Recurrence of KC can occur [10, 11] with migration of the disease from host to donor cornea being the most accepted cause. Eye rubbing and contact lens use have also been suggested causative factors [12]. An additional issue with keratoplasty is the shortage of corneas for transplantation particularly in developing countries.

Up until two decades ago there were only two options for managing KC:

1. Contact lenses (CL) – mainly rigid gas permeable (RGP) lenses.
2. Penetrating Keratoplasty.

In the last 20 years huge steps have been made in the diagnosis and management of KC. New topography and tomography devices are available with advanced imaging modalities of the anterior and posterior surface of the cornea. Several new indexes for distinguishing normal from suspect or true KC have been proposed by researchers and manufacturers.

New treatment modalities have emerged such as collagen corneal cross linking (CXL) for arresting the progression of the disease, intra-corneal ring segments (ICRS) for vision improvement, and photorefractive keratectomy (PRK), either alone or combined with CXL, for corneal remolding. Phakic intra-ocular lenses (pIOLs), in particular toric pIOLs, are an additional option for improving VA.

Adding to all this is the development of lamellar keratoplasty, such as DALK, which is replacing PK, in addition to vast improvements in the chemistry and design of CLs such as soft keratoconus lenses, hybrid lenses, scleral and semi-scleral lenses. New horizons of treatment are now available for the keratoconic patient with great potential for improvement in quality of life and increasing levels of patient expectation.

As ophthalmologists we may be confused by the wealth of options and leave our patients equally confused if we do not indicate an appropriate treatment plan, taking into consideration the new treatment modalities at our disposal and adapting them to the clinical situation of the patient and their individual functional, expectations and professional needs.

29.1.1 So How to Approach Patients with Keratoconus?

Several factors influence our approach to patients suffering from KC. The age of the patient. Does the patient suffer from allergic/atopic/vernal keratoconjunctivitis (VKC)? Is the patient an eye rubber? Is the BSCVA satisfactory? Unilateral or bilateral disease? Is the cornea clear? If scarred is the scar deep or superficial?

29.2 The Age of the Patient Is of Great Importance in Choosing the Treatment Modality, Why?

Younger age in the pediatric and adolescent group is a risk factor for progression, with progression possible in as little as a few weeks. An inverse correlation exists between age and severity of KC [13]. In some ethnic groups the disease tends to appear earlier, for example in the UK Asians develop the disease earlier than Caucasians, and it is more severe at the time of diagnosis [14, 15]. Similar patterns of early and advanced KC cases are seen by us in the middle east, with acute corneal hydrops as the presenting symptom of KC reported in five children aged between 5 and 11 years old, four of whom were from the middle east and one from India [16–18]. There is an inverse correlation between age and the severity of acute hydropsas well as the likelihood of developing neovascularisation after its resolution [19]. Patients 30 years or younger have a sevenfold increased risk of transplantation compared with those aged over 40 years [20]. The collaborative longitudinal evaluation of keratoconus (CLEK) study also demonstrated that age is a factor in severity-related outcomes among patient with KC [21].

Chatzis et al. reported on 59 pediatric patients with KC who demonstrated higher rates of progression (in 88% of KC eyes) compared to adult patients with KC [22].

Pediatric KC should be considered as a distinct issue in comparison with adult KC due to:

1. **The accelerated progression of the disease in the pediatric age group**
2. **Coexistence of other ocular morbidities such as VKC**
3. **The negative effect of the visual impairment on their educational, social and psychological development**.

29.3 Arresting Disease Progression Is of Major Importance in the Younger Patient with KC

Since the first publication on CXL for arresting the progression of keratoconus by the Dresden group [23] more than a thousand publications have been published with most reporting the positive effect of CXL in arresting the progression of the disease, improving uncorrected visual acuity (UCVA) and BSCVA, and reducing astigmatism and maximum keratometry (K max.) with benefits persisting even after 10 years [24]. In April 2016CXL was approved for the treatment of keratoconus by the FDA.

Chatzis et al. performed CXL in the previously mentioned pediatric group with reduction of K max and improvement in VA lasting 2 years post-treatment. After 3 years the K values returned to the pre-operative levels. The authors concluded that there is no need to wait for documented progression in order to perform CXL in children and adolescents because of the high rates of disease progression in this group. The treatment should be performed as soon as the diagnosis has been made. Their work however raised doubts about the persistence of the beneficial effects of CXL in this group which might not be as long-lasting as in adults [22].

Other studies have also demonstrated that the efficacy of CXL in pediatric cases is similar to that in adults, with improvements in UCVA and BSCVA, refraction and keratometry indexes showing long-term stability over 1–3 years of follow up [25–30]. Transepithelial CXL (TE-CXL) provided similar outcomes and fewer complications than epithelium-off CXL at 12 and 18 month follow-up [31, 32]. Badawi et al demonstrated that K readings can be reduced safely and remain stable at 1 year follow-up with accelerated CXL (10 mW/cm^2 for 9 min) even in the very young (range: 8–15 years old) [33].

If the surgeon decides to wait for evidence of progression of disease in pediatric KC, patients should be followed very closely (every 3 months rather than 6 months in adults) to identify the earliest signs of progression so that CXL can then be offered. Nevertheless performing CXL without waiting for definite progression is becoming the standard of care.

Keratoconus and Allergy KC is positively associated with allergies and VKC [34, 35]. Multivariate analysis has also shown KC to be associated with eye rubbing, atopy and a positive family history for allergy [36]. The association of KC with higher levels of allergy, itch and eye-rubbing has been reported to hold true across age ranges including teenagers and adults [37]. It has been suggested that eye rubbing may aggravate KC through mechanical and inflammatory mechanisms [38–40]. Eye rubbing in KC causes loss of shear strength and reduction in ground substance viscosity and glue function leading to weakening of the cornea, allowing it to bend and yield in response to intraocular pressure [38, 41]. Some researchers go further and believe that eye-rubbing is not only a risk factor for KC but the direct cause of the disease [39].

Treatment approach Conjunctivitis should be treated aggressively and patients cautioned against eye rubbing.

29.4 How to Relieve Itching, Allergic Irritation and VKC?

1. Try to identify causative allergens and avoid environmental factors that may exacerbate the disease.
2. Education. Verbal counseling to avoid rubbing the eyes may not be successful [42]. Reducing irritation of the eyes and converting eye-rubbing to other remedies may be more helpful.
3. Avoid sun, wind and dust. Use of sun glasses, hat, protective eye-wear and swimming goggles should be recommended,
4. Avoid contact lenses.
5. Cold compresses: flushing the eye with cold water acts as a natural decongestant. Preservative free artificial tears act as an eye wash and dilute the concentration of any allergens or inflammatory mediators.
6. Vasoconstrictors, antihistaminic eye drops, mast cell stabilizers, or ‘dual-acting’ agents (with antihistaminic and mast cell stabilizing properties) may help relieve irritation.

7. In cases of VKC temporary use of steroid eye drops can control symptoms. Fluorometholone, loteprednolorrimexolone should be considered first-line as these induce less of a rise in intraocular pressure. Dosages are chosen based on the inflammatory state of the eye. In severe cases systemic low dose steroids may be required if topical steroids are insufficient. Cyclosporine 1–2% eyedrops are reported to have very good results but usually take 2 weeks before symptoms improve [43, 44]. In the meantime steroid eye drops may be used. Tacrolimus ointment and tacrolimus ophthalmic suspension 0.01%, 0.03% and 0.1% are also used with good effect. Non-steroidal anti-inflammatory agents may be beneficial. Eye drops containing herbal extracts, such as chamomile-containing preparations, should be avoided because they may cross-react with sensitizing allergens [45]. The ophthalmologist should be cautious regarding the side effect of steroids such as cataract and glaucoma. Long-standing VKC may cause limbal stem cell deficiency [46] which may affect future treatment outcomes. Success of PK in VKC patients with KC is less than in patients with KC alone [47].

In summary: KC in the pediatric group is more aggressive and should be managed accordingly. CXL is effective in pediatric KC and should be done at the time of diagnosis otherwise close follow up is mandatory for early detection of progression. Treat any accompanying allergic, atopic or vernal KC and avoid-eye-rubbing.CL should be considered when possible and patients should be encouraged to wear them in order to avoid or delay surgery. In cases of CL failure all other surgical options usually offered to adults may be considered.

29.4.1 KC in the Adult Patient

Is the disease progressing? If the answer is yes then CXL should be offered. The definition of progression therefore determines the timing of treatment as well as evaluation of treatment outcomes, however there is currently no agreed definition of progression.

According to the Global Consensus on Keratoconus and Ectatic Diseases (2015) there is no consistent or clear definition of ectasia progression. The panel defined progression by a consistent change in at least two of the following parameters: steepening of the anterior corneal surface, steepening of the posterior corneal surface, or thinning and/or changes in the pachymetric rate of change. Nevertheless the panel also agreed that specific quantitative data to define progression is lacking. The experts considered that although KC progression frequently leads to a worsening in uncorrected distance VA (UCDVA) and corrected distance VA (CDVA) a change in both UCDVA and CDVA was not required for documenting progression [48].

Here are some of the criteria considered as indicative of progression:

- Increase in Kmax. of 1–1.5 dioptres (D) or more and deterioration in UCVA of more than 0.2 logMAR [49],
- Patient's self-report of deterioration in VA,
- Need for new contact lens fitting more than once in 2 years,

- Increase of ≥1.00 D in manifest refraction astigmatism or ≥0.50 D in manifest refraction spherical equivalent,
- Worsening of UCVA and BSCVA >0.5 Snellen lines,
- Increase in topographic symmetry index SAI/SI >1.00 D,
- ≥10 μm reduction in thinnest point of corneal optical coherence tomography pachymetry or ≥5% decrease in thinnest pachymetry in the preceding 6 months and reduction in corneal thickness (thinnest point) >10 μm lasting more than 6 months [50].

It is worth noting that the different devices for measuring keratometry and corneal thickness cannot be used interchangeably [51–53]. In cases of KC with Kmax readings greater than 55.0 D reduced repeatability is reported even using the same device and measurements should be considered less reliable [54].

If progression is confirmed or the patient decides not to wait for further progression then CXL should be performed. In my opinion the choice of the patient not to wait for further progression of KC is an indication for CXL in itself.

29.4.1.1 Variable Protocols of CXL Are Available

1. **The Dresden protocol** Also known as **standard CXL or conventional CXL (C-CXL)**. The epithelium is removed from the central 8–9 mm of the cornea. Riboflavin 0.1% with dextran 20% is then instilled every 5 min for half an hour until a strong yellow flare is seen in the anterior chamber at the slit lamp. The eye is then irradiated with UVA 365–370 A, 3 mW/cm^{2}from a distance of 5 cm from the eye for half an hour with a total treatment energy of 5.4 J/cm^2. A contact lens is inserted at the end of the treatment. Topical antibiotics are instilled until full epithelization occurs and the contact lens is removed while topical steroids are instilled for 1 month.

The effects of CXL are limited to the anterior 300 μm of corneal stroma. The riboflavin acts as both a photosensitizer and photoprotector. It is highly reactive with oxygen species triggering formation of crosslinks that consist of intra- and inter-fibrillary covalent bonds [55]. A minimum corneal thickness of 400 μm is recommended in order to avoid endothelial cell damage. **So what about the thin cornea?**

Thin Corneas and CXL: in thin corneas (<400 μm thickness) a hypoosmolar riboflavin without Dextran can be used to swell the cornea to beyond 400 μm and the treatment then carried out effectively and safely [56, 57]. Another option is 'epi-on' CXL or partial removal of the epithelium. The epithelium is removed only from the thicker part of the cornea and kept on in the thinner part which is referred to as 'customized pachymetry-guided epithelial debridement' [58].

29.4.1.2 Complications of Conventional CXL

C-CXL is time consuming and carries with it the risk of infection, delayed epithelization and corneal infiltrates. Stromal scars occur in 2.8% of cases [59]. Clinically significant stromal haze was reported in 8.6% of treated eyes. Advanced KC is a risk factor due to the amount of thinning and extreme steepness of the cornea [60]. The presence of an epithelial defect and use of a soft bandage contact lens are risk factors for infective keratitis. Several case reports have been published reporting this complication [61, 62] including one of *Acanthamoeba* keratitis leading to perforation [63]. Corneal perforation after uneventful CXL [64], herpetic keratitis in an individual with no prior history [65] and anterior uveitis [66] have also all been reported. The failure rate of C-CXL or percentage of eyes with continued progression is 7.6% [59].

2. **Cretan Protocol**: This is also an 'epi–off' CXL. Excimer laser is used to remove the anterior 50 μm of "epithelium". The refractive results are superior to C-CXL. The explanation for this beneficial effect of laser ablation of the epithelium is that the epithelium is thinner at the KC apex meaning a few microns of stroma are also removed. This allows more reduction in astigmatism meaning more improvement in VA. It is reported as a PRK combined with CXL [67]. Gaster et al. however reported similar results between laser and manual epithelial removal with no statistically significant difference between the 12- and 24-months postoperatively. At 6-months post-operatively Kmax was flatter in the Cretan protocol group but this effect did not last [68].

In order to avoid the above mentioned complications as well as the pain and irritation experienced after C-CXL alternative treatment protocols have evolved such as the epithelium on protocol (epi-on) named also transepithelial CXL (TE-CXL).

3. **Epi-on CXL:** Riboflavin is instilled without the removal of the epithelium. The results reported in the literature regarding the effectiveness of epi-on CXL are controversial. When the effectiveness is reported the depth of cross linking and the refractive changes (expressed by the reduction of astigmatism and Kmax) are inferior to that achieved in epi–off CXL.

29.4.1.3 Why the Decreased Effect?

1. *Inability of the riboflavin to penetrate the tight junctions of the epithelium.* Although various forms of riboflavin and absorption enhancers have been used the effect in terms of stress and strain measurements after the treatment in porcine eyes was only one-fifth of what is achieved with epi-off treatment. In human cornea a 64% increase in corneal rigidity was reported with epi-on CXL using topical anesthetics and benzalkonium chloride (BK) as enhancers, versus a 320% increase when using epi–off CXL [69–72].
2. *The epithelium is a barrier to UVA.* It absorbs part of the UVA and consumes oxygen which is an essential component in the process of CXL [73]
   Clinically Leccisotti found less pronounced effect than described in the literature after epi–off CXL [74]. On the other hand Stojanovic et al. reported that safe and effective treatment could be achieved using BK to enhance the absorption of a hypotonic riboflavin solution, mechanical disruption of the superficial epithelium and prolongation of the riboflavin-induction time until verification of stromal saturation [75].

Epi-on CXL is useful in cases in which epithelial removal is not desired, such as pediatric cases, uncooperative patients and in thin corneas [76].
Contradictory results are reported even in ex vivo experiments: Epi-on CXL with an extended pretreatment time of 60 min and penetration enhancers (gum cellulose, 0.44% sodium chloride, and 0.01% BK) demonstrated similar results to epi-off CXL [77]. On the other side lower riboflavin concentrations in the anterior corneal stroma when compared to epi–off CXL was reported [78]. In partial epithelial removal the effect of CXL was detected in the stroma under the de-epithelialized corneal areas but only a mild effect was observed under areas of intact epithelium as detected by anterior segment OCT and In vivo confocal microscopy [79]. Similar results demonstrating non –homogeneous uptake in partial grid-pattern epithelial removal have also been reported [80].
To further enhance the absorption of riboflavin through an intact epithelium Iontophoresis CXL (I-CXL) was introduced. In I-CXL an electrical gradient is used to drive negatively charged riboflavin molecules across the intact epithelium. I-CXL has all the advantages of epi–on CXL in terms of post-operative pain reduction, reduced risk of infection and effectively halting the progression of KC, as demonstrated in a 1-year follow up research study [81]. It has the additional benefits of reducing the treatment time and improving riboflavin diffusion [82]. Bibkova et al. reported a decrease in average K and corneal astigmatism, improvement in UCVA and no change in endothelial cell density at 12-months follow-up [83]. Similar out comes to C-CXL were also reported at one- and 3-year follow up but with improved safety and faster recovery of VA [83, 84]. In a study on enzymatic resistance comparing different CXL protocols epi-off CXL was found to be superior to all other protocols while I-CXL was superior to all other epi-on protocols [85]. A similar effect in pediatric KC with over 15-months follow up was reported [86]. Similar stromal riboflavin penetration to epi-off can be achieved if the soaking time is increased, riboflavin concentration increased to 0.25%, BAC 0.01% is added and two cycles of applied current are used instead of one [87]. Similar stiffness of corneas treated by I-CXL or C-CXL in rabbits has been reported [88].

This issue remains controversial some clinicians and researches advocate strongly Epi –on, others are against. Most publications show decreased effect of epi–on CXL versus epi –off CXL.

4. **AcceleratedCXL (A-CXL)**: Several new CXL devices offering higher UVA irradiation intensity with different time settings are available on the market. The aim is to reduce the treatment time by reducing the exposure time of the cornea from 30 to 10 min even to 5 or 3 min while maintaining a total treatment dose of = 5.4 J/cm^2. According to the Bunsen-Roscoe law of reciprocity: 'The effect of a photochemical or photobiological reaction is directly proportional to the total irradiation dose, irrespective of the time span over which the dose is administered'. So if we increase the energy of UVA we can reduce the time of exposure and produce the same effect as long as we keep the total irradiation

dose constant. In CXL the radiant exposure of 5.4 J/cm^2 can be achieved in 30 min at 3 mW/cm^2, 9 min at 10 mW/cm^2, 5 min at 18 mW/cm^2 and 3 min at 30 mW/cm^2.

Does the Bunsen-Roscoe law of reciprocity hold true for the effects of CXL on the cornea? Ex-vivo studies on porcine corneas show this to be only partially true with the law being valid only for illumination intensities up to 40–50 mW/cm^2 and illumination times of greater than 2 min [89]. No significant difference was detected in the median of Young's modulus between the rapid 9 min at 10 mW/cm^{2}and standard 30 min at 3 mW/cm^2 groups [90]. The optimal UV intensity for effective CXL ranges from 3 to 30 mW/cm^2 [91]. Kruger et al. reported on CXL in porcine corneas using variable energies with high versus standard irradiance continuously and fractionated up to15 mW/cm^2 (fractioned with alternate cycles of 30 s "ON" and 30 s "OFF" exposure) and an equivalent radiant exposure of 5.4 mJ/cm^2. The results were comparable in terms of stress strain measurements [92]. On the other hand a decreased stiffening effect with increasing UV-A intensity has also been reported [93].

Clinically Tomita reported on accelerated CXL (3 min at 30 mW/cm^2) compared to conventional CXL and found no statistically significant difference between the two procedures in postoperative change in UCVA, manifest refraction, spherical equivalent or K readings [94]. Similar results were reported for a protocol of 5 min at 18 mW/cm^2 [95–97] while 9 mW/cm^2 accelerated CXL has been shown to stabilize the progression of KC at 12 month follow-up [98].

A-CXL is safe for the endothelium in post-Lasik ectasia and produces a significant reduction in topographic keratometric values and increase in distance BCVA comparable to conventional 3 mW/cm^2 CXL at 2 years follow-up [99].

A-CXL (30 mW/cm^2) was found to be effective in improving UDVA, CDVA, corneal topography readings, total HOA, and coma aberrations during 24-month follow-up [100]. Even accelerated epi-on CXL is reported to be effective in arresting KC progression [101]. Accelerated epi-on for 5 min was compared to C-CXL in progressive KC in patients under the age of 18 years old. Both techniques were effective with progression observed in 5.6% and 12% of eyes in the A-epi-on group and the epi-off group respectively [102]. In another report progression was halted over a 24-month follow-up period with improvement in VA and without relevant side effects in a pediatric KC group [103].

A-epi-on CXL using very high energy intensity up to 45 mW/cm^{2}without removal of epithelium has been reported to be safe and effective with stability and improvement of UCVA and BSCVA reported 12-months after treatment [104]. However Kymionis et al. found the demarcation line (DL) depth to be reduced when using A- CXL of 9 mW/cm^2 (the DL is an optical line that separates treated from untreated stroma and is thought to reflect the depth of treatment) suggesting a reduction in effectivity [105]. A negative effect on topographical outcome after A- CXL of 9 mW/cm^{2}versus C-CXL has also been reported [106]. The DL depth can be significantly increased by prolonging the instillation time of riboflavin from 20 to 30 min when using A-CXL epi-off 18.0 mW/cm^2 for 5 min [107].

Regarding safety of A-CXL to the endothelium: Evidence of a significant reduction in endothelial cell count particularly at 3- and 6-months post A-CXL exists. The coefficient of variance has also been found to be significantly higher at 3- and 6-months postoperatively than the pre CXL value. A slight change in the percentage of hexagonal cells was also noted, however all these changes were transient [108, 109].

In a review of A-CXL Medieros et al. noted that the effect of A-CXL on corneal shape and DL is variable. A-CXL with less riboflavin presoaking time treats largely the superficial cornea which may be of benefit in thin corneas where the distance of A-CXL effect from the endothelium is an advantage [110].

A-CXL has proven to be effective in arresting KC progression but it seems that C-CXL remains the more effective protocol.

Currently we do not know how much CXL is needed in order to arrest the progression of KC. In some eyes epi–on CXL or A– CXL is effective in arresting disease and other eyes not. Even C-CXL has a failure rate of 7.6%.Many KC centers use an energy intensity of 9 mW/cm² for ten minutes as a compromise between high-energy A-CXL and C-CXL.

5. **Acceleated Pulsed CXL(pl-A-CXL):** Oxygen is depleted early in A-CXL because of the higher UVA energies used. Oxygen is necessary for the process of cross-linking [111]. Pulsed protocols with A-CXL delivering ultraviolet light in an on-off pattern may allow better diffusion of oxygen into the corneal stroma producing a deeper response [112]. Advanced oxidation protein product levels indicative of oxygen concentration and reactive oxygen species were found to be higher in accelerated pulsed CXL compared to both C-CXL and A-CXL in rabbit eyes [113]. Lower levels of nitric oxide, a marker of oxidative stress, were measured in the aqueous humor of rabbit eyes treated with pulsed accelerated CXL compared to A-CXL and C-CXL [114]. But do these results in rabbit eyes indicate more efficacy of accelerated pulsed CXL and can we apply this to the human KC cornea?

Similar results were reported in a prospective interventional clinical study 1-year after A-CXL and pl-A-CXL. Stability of KC was achieved in both groups. Functional outcomes were found to be better in epi-off pl-A CXL treatment which produced deeper stromal penetration [115, 116]. Using pulsed rather than continuous light exposure resulted in a significantly deeper DL and deeper apoptotic effect [116, 117]. Using 15 mW/cm² epi-off pl-A-CXL for 6 min (1 s on/1 s off) with UVA exposure of 12 min at a fluence of 5.4 J/cm² resulted in stabilization of KC at 2-year follow-up [118].

Accelerated pulsed CXL seems to yield a deeper effect in the corneal stroma than A-CXL.

6. **Higher Dose A-CXL** Accelerated CXL using a higher UV dose (6.6 J/cm²) and intensity (30 mW/cm²) with reduced irradiation time has been shown to produce a smaller topographic flattening effect than routine C-CXL [119]. Similar findings have been reported when using higher dosage 30 mW accelerated for

4 min continuous or pulsed CXL treatment which, though effective in stabilizing keratoconus progression, was less effective in achieving topographic improvement in comparison with C-CXL or 9 mW/cm ^{2} for 10 min A-CXL [120]. Using higher treatment dosages also does not seem to offer any benefit over standard A-CXL where using a total UV-A radiance of 7.2 J/cm^{2}resulted in similar refractive and topographic outcomes to that for 5.4 J/cm^2 [121]. C-CXL versus 30 mW/cm^2 for 4 min higher dose regime showed similar results and a statistically significant increase in CRF and CH in the second group only [122]. Corneal stromal demarcation line depth also remains similar whether using UV-A 3 mW/cm^2 for 30 min or 9 mW/cm^2 for 14 min [123].

No additional beneficial effect of higher dose CXL was demonstrated versus C-CXL.

7. Low <u>**Dose CXL**</u> has been tested in ex vivo porcine corneas. Similar results were reported comparing a slow low-irradiance CXL setting (1.5 mW/cm^2 for 30 min; fluence 2.7 J/cm^2) with the standard CXL setting (3 mW/cm^2 for 30 min, fluence 5.4 J/cm^2) [124]. **However this protocol has not yet been tested in humans.**
8. <u>**Customized CXL**</u> using up to 10 J/cm^2 centered on the maximum of the posterior float has been reported to produce significantly better results for epithelial healing time, ΔKmax, and regularization index (RI) compared to C-CXL [125]. Mazzotta et al. however found that using three different levels of energy up to 15 J/cm^2 according to the topographic corneal curvature produced similar results to C-CXL although the DL was deeper in areas of cornea irradiated by higher energies [126]. Similar findings were reported at 1-year post-operatively in a prospective non-randomized clinical trial comparing C-CXL to topography guided (TG) CXL involving de-epithelialization focused on the cone, riboflavin application for 10 min and 30 mW/cm^{2}pulsed UV-A irradiance pattern administered according to topography. The demarcation line was found to be of similar depth compared to C-CXL at the top of the cone but it was shallower at the surrounding area in the TG-CXL group [127].

In a prospective randomized study comparing 9 mm 5.4 J/cm^2 pl-CXL with TG –CXL involving an asymmetrical treatment zone centered on the area of maximum corneal steepness and treatment energies ranging from 7.2 to 15.0 J/cm^2, better topographic results were achieved with the TG protocol which was also associated with a greater improvement in VA, though this proved to be non-statistically significant [128].

Though looks very promising, and may be slightly superior to C-CXL, there is no proven conclusion that customized CXL is superior to C-CXL.

Controversy still exists regarding the area of the cornea to be exposed to the higher treatment energies in customized CXL, is it the area of the highest posterior float, the steepest or the thinnest area. The UV-A energies and the doses used in customized CXL remain arbitrary.

29.5 The Significance of the Demarcation Line (DL)

The DL marks the transition zone between cross-linked anterior corneal stroma and untreated posterior corneal stroma. The DL is detectable on slit-lamp biomicroscopy as early as 2 weeks after treatment [129]. The different refractive indices or reflective properties of cross-linked versus untreated corneal stroma creates an area of hyper-reflectivity. This line can be better detected using anterior segment OCT and is considered a measurement of the depth of CXL treatment into the stroma (Figs. 29.1 and 29.2).

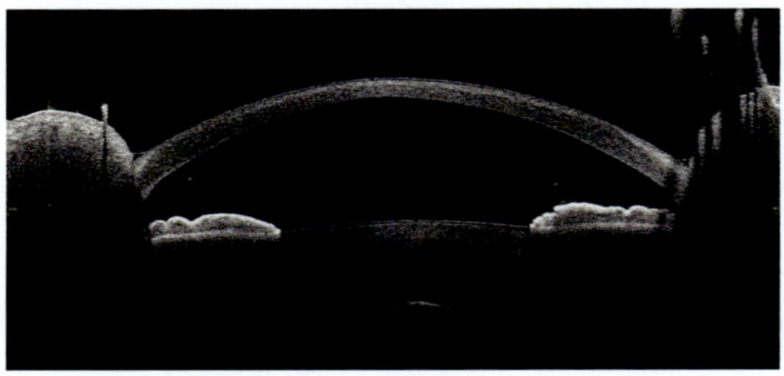

Fig. 29.1 Superficial demarcation line after A-CXL, Casia 2, Tomey, Japan

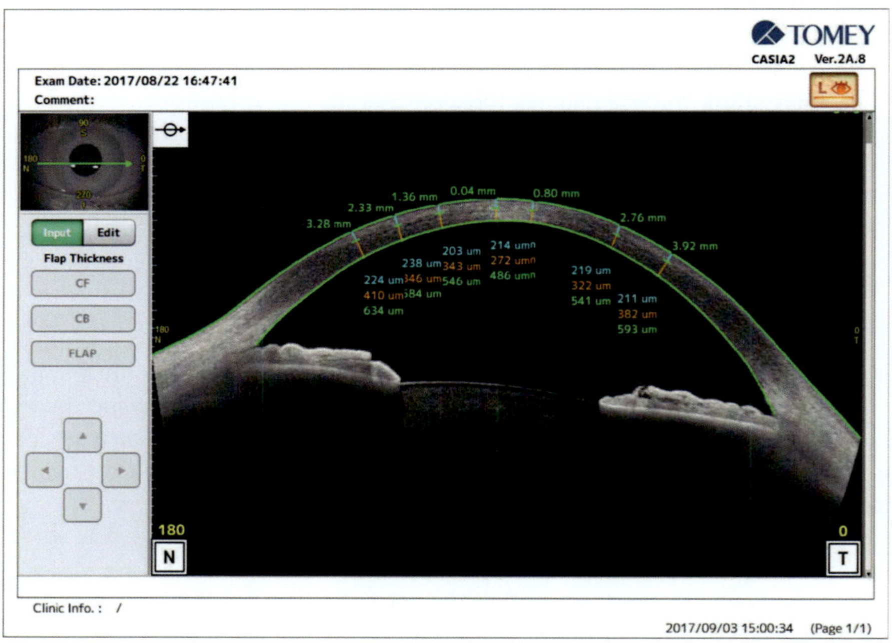

Fig. 29.2 Demarcation Line. Casia 2, Tomey, Japan

In most studies looking at the depth of the DL it is found to increase in the following order: Epi–on CXL proving the most superficial, followed by A-CXL then by the A Pulsed–CXL and the deepest achieved in C-CXL.

A DL which is deeper centrally than peripherally has been observed in some studies. This is probably due to the top-hat beam profile of the UV-A optical system which does not compensate for the natural corneal curvature. The UV-A beam therefore enters the cornea at a non-orthogonal angle in the corneal periphery [130] .

The depth of the demarcation line seems to correlate with the increase in the corneal elastic modulus. It could also be related to the difference in scattering pattern produced by collagen fiber orientation changes induced by the disease [124]. A deeper corneal stromal demarcation line has been correlated to greater corneal flattening [97].

The DL depth could therefore be considered a measure of effectiveness of the CXL i.e. the deeper the better. However some authors believe this approach to be too simplistic for interpreting the clinical importance of the corneal stromal DL [131].

29.6 Why Is There Such Variation in the Results Reported in CXL?

A. KC is not the same in every patient. Even in the same patient there can be asymmetries in shape, anterior and posterior elevation of the cone, the thickness of the cornea, the distribution of this thickness, the degree of corneal irregularity and the rate of progression.
B. The patient may be an eye rubber. Eye rubbing may cause or aggravate KC [40] and will have a profound effect on progression both pre- and post-operatively.
C. A large number of different UVA energies and beam profiles have been used. CXL has been observed to act deeper centrally than peripherally. This is most likely due to the top-hat beam profile mentioned previously [130]. This means that CXL may be more effective in cases of central KC than paracentral KC [132]. There is no evidence to suggest that an enhanced peripheral beam profile provides any superiority over C-CXL. It is worth noting that this change in beam profile was accompanied by an increased beam energy of 9 mW/cm^2, a beam profile introduced by IROC (Zurich, Switzerland).
D. Different riboflavin solutions are used. The riboflavin used may be hypertonic, isotonic or hypotonic, and either with or without dextran. Riboflavin concentrations may vary 0.1–0.25%. A number of different methods of instilling the riboflavin have been employed; with or without lid speculum, the patient adopting a sitting or supine position, varying intervals and duration of instillation and the corneal surface may or may not be rinsed of the riboflavin prior to starting UVA irradiation. Riboflavin may then also be administered during the irradiation process and the quantity may differ in different protocols (Fig. 29.3). In the case of

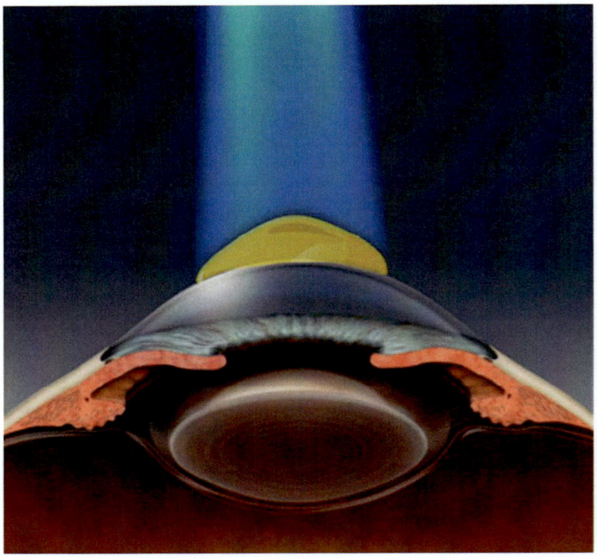

Fig. 29.3 Shows how riboflavin blocks the UVA if applied during irradiation specially if it contains dextran which make the solution more viscous

epi-on CXL what are the enhancers used? Such as BK, Gentamycin, Tetracain. Is alcohol added prior to the riboflavin in order to loosen the tight junctions of the epithelium? Is mechanical disruption of the epithelium performed using a sponge or Daya disrupter (a metallic device for creating multiple small holes in the epithelium)?

E. How much CXL does each KC patient need? We still do not know. In some cases lower doses may be sufficient to halt the progression and this may explain the effectiveness of epi-on CXL reported by some authors.
F. The photochemically induced effect of CXL in the cornea cannot be measured directly by staining methods or microscopy. However changes in the collagen and stroma that occur during treatment can be used as an indirect sign of the cross-linking effect [133].
G. Most studies reporting outcomes of CXL have not been randomized controlled studies (RCS) [49]. Many report only short term outcomes with follow-up periods of only 6 months.
H. Ex vivo experiments provide the opportunity to analyse the effect of all the previously mentioned variables. However we must also consider the age and hydration of the cornea used, the time from death of the specimen, has the whole eye been used or just the cornea? How has the cornea been cut for stress-strain measurements pre- and post-treatment and what device was used to measure the stress and strain? What formulas have been used to compensate for the non-linear distension of the cornea during the stress-strain measurements?
I. For in vivo studies we should consider whether the cornea is from rat, rabbit or pig and can the findings of these animals' studies be transferred to human keratonic eyes?
J. There is no consensus on the definition of KC progression. Therefore the indications for CXL and the evaluation of post-treatment results may vary.

The long list of variables provided above are present in every CXL treatment and will undoubtedly affect individual treatment outcomes. Inconsistency in the parameters used to define progression, and variability in the devices used to measure it, makes the comparison of CXL study results extremely difficult. We still need are liable and accurate technique for measuring corneal biomechanical properties before and after treatment as well as suitably designed prospective randomized controlled trials comparing traditional CXL with each of the alternative procedures. The best treatment protocol that produces the greatest clinical efficacy with the safest outcomes has yet to be defined.

In spite of the controversies CXL should still be offered in cases of progressive KC. Furthermore screening for KC should be performed in schools in order to detect and treat the disease before there is an appreciable deterioration in vision. It is truly frustrating to see young KC patients with advanced stages of the disease who were not diagnosed earlier or even when diagnosed were not offered CXL.

29.7 How to Improve VA in Keratoconic Patients Who Have Unsatisfactory VA with Glasses?

1. Contact Lenses: CL including regular soft CL may correct the refractive error created by KC (myopia and/or astigmatism). However if there is irregular astigmatism then specific CL are required:

(A) Soft KC CL (soft K). These are a special kind of soft CL designed to correct for irregular astigmatism and improve VA. These lenses do not always correct all of the astigmatism but are better tolerated by KC patients.

(B) **RGP CL:** These lenses are descendants of the hard CL composed of PMMA previously used widely for the correction of refractive errors and KC. In the last 30 years new more flexible gas-permeable substances are used. RGP lenses correct for regular and irregular astigmatism and are the most popular lenses for VA improvement in KC patients. In advanced cases these lenses may fall from the eye and are often poorly tolerated.

(C) **Piggyback CL:** These are soft CLs onto which a RGP CL is fitted. Some designs involve a crater on the soft CL in which the RGP CL lies. This provides the comfort of a soft CL with the refractive effect of a RGP CL.

(D) **Hybrid CL:** Hybrid lenses are gas permeable CL surrounded by a skirt of soft CL. These lenses are intended to combine the advantages of a GP CL in terms of astigmatism correction and the advantages of soft CL in terms of better tolerability.

(E) **Scleral and Semi-scleral CL**: These are a special design of GP CL with a larger diameter of 25–30 mm in scleral lenses and 15–19 mm in semi-scleral lenses. The lens lies on the sclera and covers the cornea without "touching" the corneal surface, unlike GP lenses which lie on the corneal surface and are a continuous source of rubbing. These lenses are better tolerated than GP CL and do not irritate the cornea. The semi-scleral lenses are gaining increasing popularity among optometrists, ophthalmologists and KC patient as an effective, tolerable CL even in very advanced cases of KC with irregular corneas.

The wide range and variability of CL design, form, material and producer is enabling more and more KC patients to use CL to improve their vision and quality of life [134]. CL do also have their down sides which should be discussed with patients. The risk of scarring in contact lens wearers is more than twofold that of non-contact lens wearing patients with keratoconus. The findings of the CLEKS suggests a causal effect of CL wear on corneal scarring and optimising CL fit may be important for KC patients [21]. In some cases a proud nodule develops on the surface of the cornea which causes irritation, corneal erosion and makes CL use intolerable. In these cases excimer laser phototherapeutic keratectomy to remove the nodule from the corneal surface can improve CL tolerability [135].

What if the patient does not tolerate CL, has atopic or allergic conjiunctivitis, or has no motivation to wear CL? Patients who have advanced KC in one eye only and need a CL only in that eye are particularly unmotivated to wear CL.

29.8 Improving Vision in KC Patients

Phakic Toric Intraocular Lenses (pIOLs) These are an additional option for the correction of ametropia in stable KC. If the KC is not stable then the treatment should not be offered unless CXL is also performed. Phakic IOLs may be used to correct myopia and regular astigmatism [136–138].

Advantages: reversibility and preservation of accommodation.

Limitations: cannot correct for irregular astigmatism. Higher order aberrations are increased in KC and limit the amount of improvement in quality of vision that can be gained. In addition the pupillary axis is not aligned with the visual axis.

Disadvantages: loss of endothelial cells over time, cataract formation, pupil ovalization, lens rotation or decentration, photic phenomena and retinal detachment in isolated cases [136].

Improvement of UCVA with reduction in myopia and astigmatism has been reported with a variety of pIOL types such as; anterior chamber pIOLs, iris fixated IOLs and posterior chamber pIOLs [136–139]. If cataract is present then cataract extraction should be offered with implantation of a toric IOL [140, 141].

29.9 Intrastromal Corneal Ring Segments for the Treatment of KC

Intrastromal corneal rings segments (ICRS) are mainly crescent shape PMMA rings and have been used since the beginning of the nineties for correction of low myopia. They have been approved since 1996 (Intacs) by the FDA for the correction of myopia up to −3.5 D with no more than 1 D cylinder of astigmatism and are, used in

Europe for the correction of myopia up to −4.5 D [142, 143]. Parallel to the development of Intacs, Paulo Ferrara from Brazil developed the Ferrara ring initially for the treatment of myopia but later for the treatment of KC as well. In 2004 Intacs were approved by the FDA for the treatment of KC in cases where the VA is unsatisfactory with spectacle correction and the patient is CL intolerant [142].

ICRS are inserted into a circumferential channel created in the corneal stroma. A small incision is first made up to 70–80% of corneal thickness as measured by ultrasound pachymetry. The incision acts as an entry point through which the tunnels are created either mechanically, using surgical dissection, or with the use of femtosecond laser. The stromal rings are then fed into the created channel.

1. **Intacs:** Hexagonal in cross-section each segment is 150°of arcin length with a 7 mm optical zone. Variable thicknesses are available from 250 to 450 μm in 50 μm steps (Figs. 29.4 and 29.5). **Intacs SK** (SK for severe keratoconus) has a noval cross-section, 6 mm optical zone, 400–450 μm thickness and is produced in variable lengths from 90 to 150°. Both are produced by AJL in Spain.
2. **Ferrara Rings**: Pyramidal in cross-section with a flat base of 600 μm, these are available with either a 5 mm or 6 mm optical zone, variable thickness of 150–350 μm in 50 μm increments and a length of 90°, 120°, 160°, 210°or 340°of arc. Ferrara rings are yellow in order to reduce halos and glare. They are also produced by AJL in Spain. **Kerarings** are similar to Ferrara rings but produced by Mediphacosin Brazil and are available in lengths up to 355°. Both companies

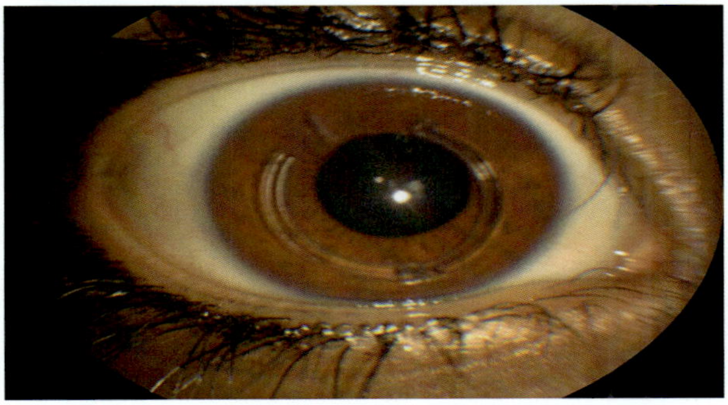

Fig. 29.4 Intacs in a kissing position they behave like a single 300° single ring

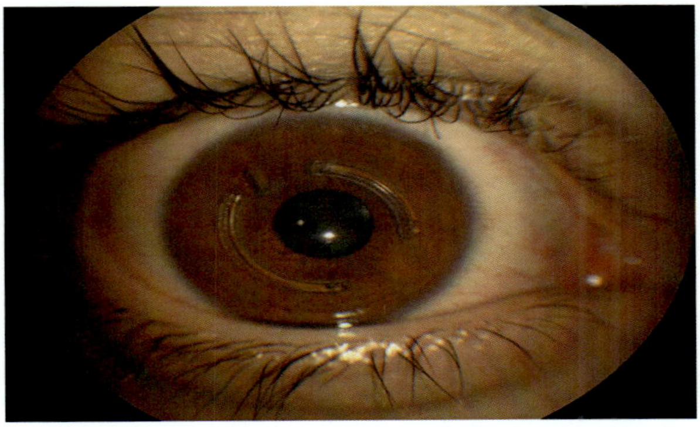

Fig. 29.5 Different arc length Intacs SK

also produce a variable thickness ring which progressively increases in thickness from the site of insertion and reaches the maximal thickness at the distal part of the ring (tunnel).

3. **Barbara Rings:** Semicircular with a flat base, these are available in a variety of diameters and thicknesses. The main distinguishing feature of this ring is that it gradually increases in thickness from the insertion site reaches the maximal ring thickness at the centre of the ring (tunnel) parallel to the maximal corneal steepness, then decreases in thickness at the distal end (Fig. 29.6), it is practically a customized ring.
4. **MyoRing** Unlike the up-mentioned segments, this is a full 360°PMMA round ring available in 5 and 6 mm diameter. It is flexible and available in variable thicknesses from200 to 400 µm in 20 µm increments. It is inserted into a pocket created by a special automatic keratome or using femtosecond laser at a depth of 300 µm. Developed by Albert Daxer, marketed by Dipotex (Austria).

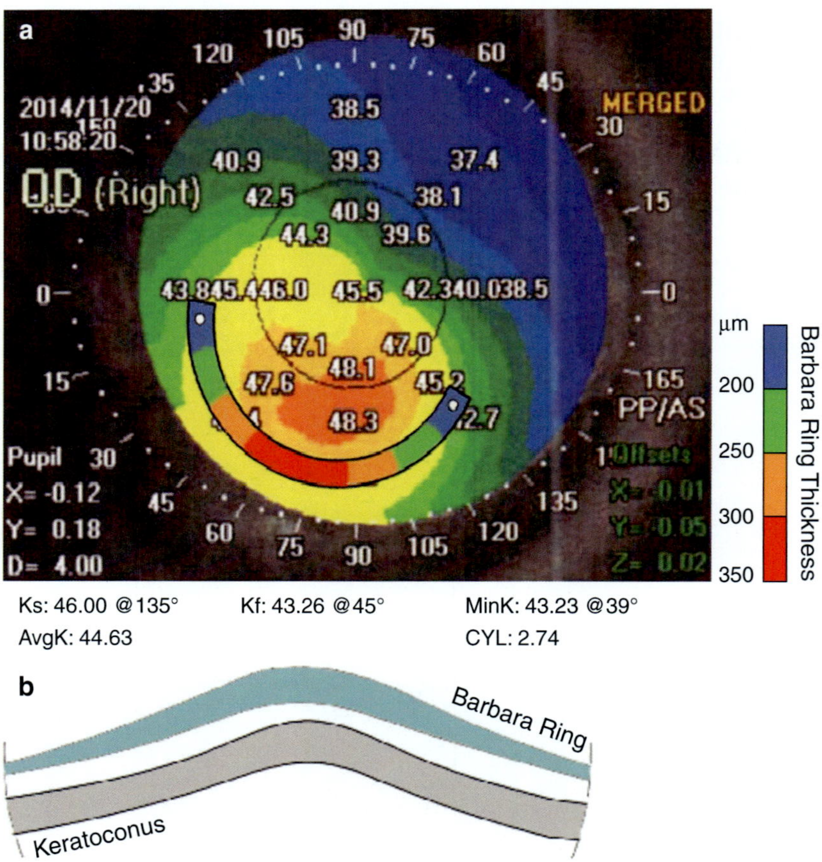

Fig. 29.6 (**a**, **b**) Barbara ring, shows how the ring is customized so that the thicker part lies over the steepest part of the KC. (**b**) The corneal protrusion in keratoconus increases gradually toward the steepest point of the cornea. The Barbara Ring is customized ring that thickens gradually and the area of maximal thickness parallels the steepest area of the cornea

The ICRS flatten the central cornea in myopic eyes and regularize the irregular cornea in KC, Ireduce regular and irregular astigmatism [142] (Figs. 29.7, 29.8, and 29.9). The degree of effect increases proportionally to the thickness of the ring and inversely to the optical zone diameter [144, 145].

The results ICRS have been shown to improve UCVA and BSCVA, reduce myopia and regular or irregular astigmatism, reduce keratometry readings reduce higher order aberrations (HOA), regularize corneal topography and increase CL tolerability [142, 146–161].

Rabinovitz in his review on Intacs for treating KC states: "Most studies to date show an average of 2 to 3D of flattening accompanied by 2–3 lines of gain in best-corrected vision. However, the range is large and variable ranging from 2 lines of loss of BCVA to a gain of 8 lines in BCVA". Seventy to eighty percent of patients treated noted an improvement in best-corrected and uncorrected vision [162].

ICRS also produce similar positive out comes in ectasia secondary to LASIK, [163–169], post PRK ectasia [170], in pellucid marginal degeneration [171] and in the correction of astigmatism [172].

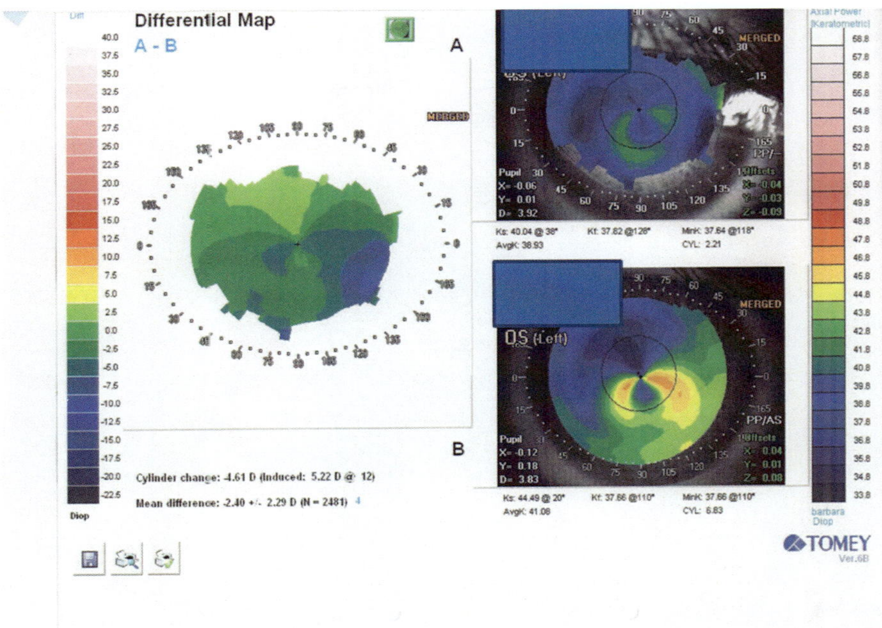

Fig. 29.7 Differential map after ICRS showing flattening of the cornea, TMS 5, Tomey, Japan

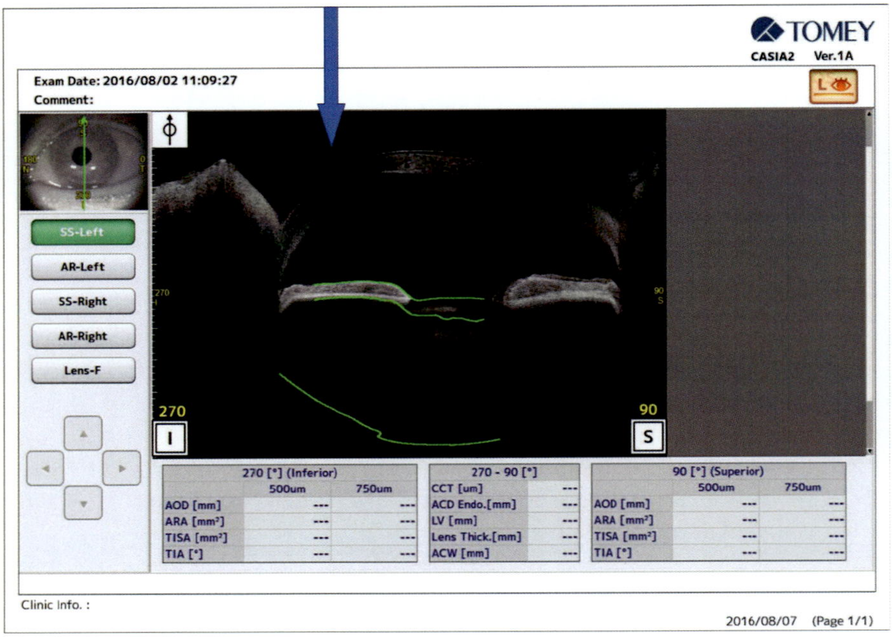

Fig. 29.8 Pellucid Marginal Degeneration note he thinning and the protrusion of the inferior part of the cornea (see arrow) CASIA2, Tomey, Japan

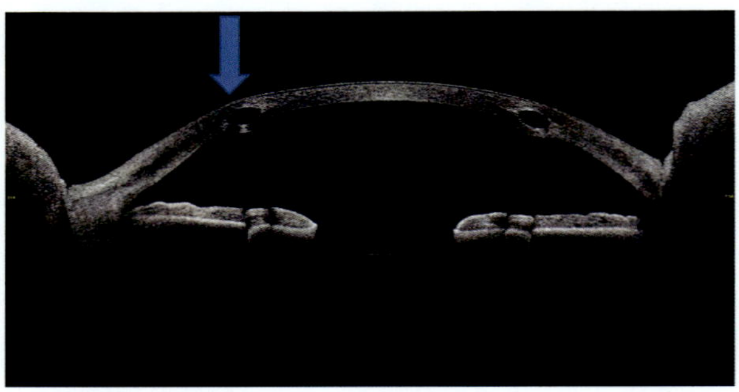

Fig. 29.9 Intacs SK in the same case of Fig. 29.3 showing how the Intacs SK ring segment flattens the cornea at the ring position. CASIA 2,Tomey, Japan

ICRS provide similar or even superior results to PKP in the second eye of KC patients with fewer post-operative complications [173, 174] (Figs. 29.10a–c and 29.11a, b).

ICRS positively enhance the biomechanical properties of the cornea by inducing central flattening and peripheral steepening over the rings and help to redistribute stress [175].

ICRS used in conjunction with CXL may produce an additive effect. The optimal sequence is to perform ICRS first followed immediately by CXL, however they can also be implanted after CXL if required [176–178]. Implanting the ICRS first has proven to be more effective in reducing Kmax values, spherical equivalent and cylinder compared to performing cross-linking first [179].

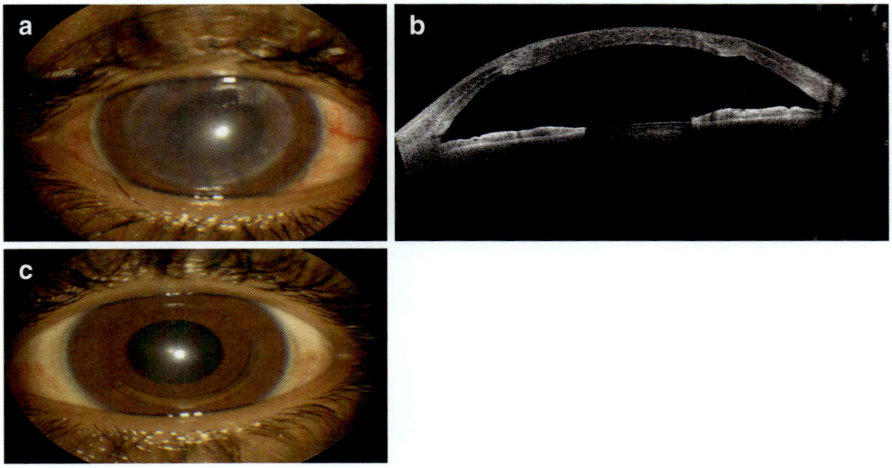

Fig. 29.10 (**a**) Cloudy cornea after PKP, episode of rejection. (**b**) OCT of the cornea in Fig. 29.11a. CASIA2, Tomey, Japan (**c**) Intacs segment in the fellow eye of the patient in Fig. 29.11a

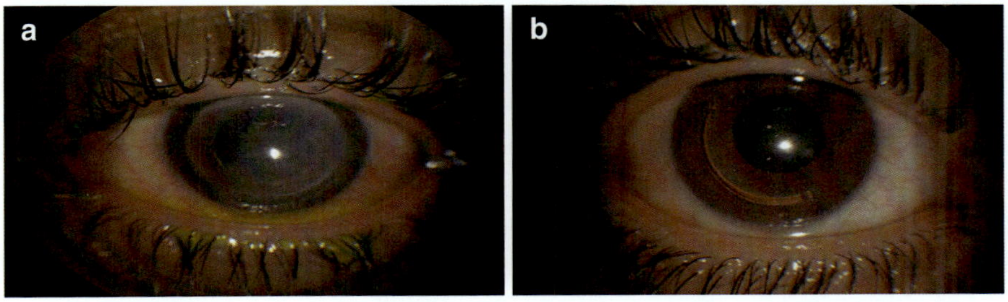

Fig. 29.11 (**a**) Bullous keratopathy after PKP. (**b**) Intacs segment in the fellow eye of the patient in Fig. 29.12a

The more advanced the KC the greater the effect of the ICRS on corneal shape, however the lesser the functional improvement in VA achieved and vice versa. This is what I have deduced from my own experience over more than 16 years of implanting ICRS. Alio et al. reports the opposite effect with less improvement in VA in lower grades of KC [180, 181].

The aim of ICRS implantation in KC is not to be free of glasses or CL but to enable the patient to achieve a functional level of VA with glasses or to better tolerate a CL such as a soft K instead of a RGP CL. In some cases a functional and satisfactory UCVA can be achieved with no need for glasses and this is often the case in non-advanced KC but less so in advanced cases. ICRS can also be helpful in preventing or delaying the need for PKP or DALK.

G. Ferrara et al. reported recently on ICRS use in pediatric patients. The mean age of patients was 13 ± 2.1 years (range 8–16 years). Significant corneal flattening was achieved after ring implantation with improvement in UDVA and CDVA, without any post-operative complications being reported [182].

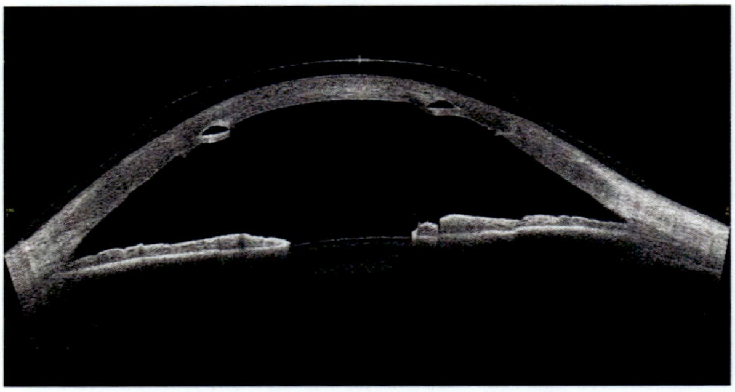

Fig. 29.12 Ferrara Rings and a soft K CL after PKP, CASIA 2, Tomey, Japan

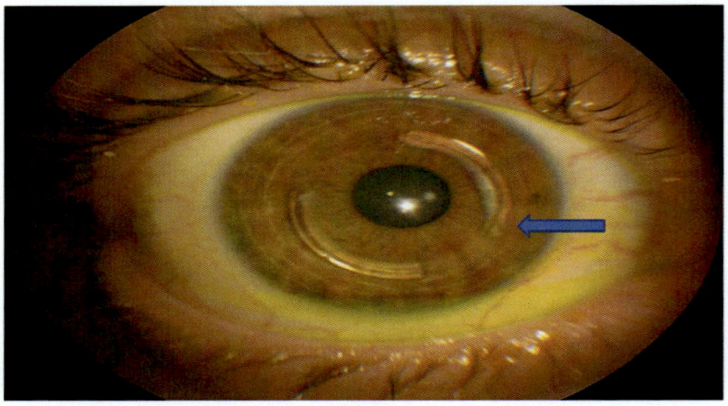

Fig. 29.13 Extrusion of ICRS. See the staining by fluorescein, arrow

Similar improvements in VA and corneal flattening have been reported after MyoRing implantation for KC which also led to cone stabilization and increased corneal thickness [158–161].

Once the cornea has been regularized by insertion of the ICRS with reduction in regular and irregular astigmatism and the creation of a favorable biomechanical effect on the cornea, additional treatments can then be added to improve the VA such as PRK, phakic IOLs or CXL. Various combinations of these treatments have been reported to produce favorable results [183–189].

ICRS has been compared to DALK in the treatment of advanced KC. Both techniques were shown to improve UCVA, BCVA and K readings however DALK provided the greatest improvement in VA and refractive error. The authors concluded that ICRS implantation may be an alternative treatment to DALK providing satisfactory outcomes but with less visual impact [190].

ICRS implantation can be helpful in reducing astigmatism in post-PKP and post-DALK eyes [191–194] (Fig. 29.12).

The complications of ICRS These include post-operative keratitis, pannus formation, extrusion and ICRS migration. None of these complications are sight threatening but in most cases the ICRS needs to be removed [162, 195, 196]. Extrusion is the most common complication which may be a result of eye rubbing or superficial implantation of the ring (Figs. 29.13 and 29.14). Both mechanical

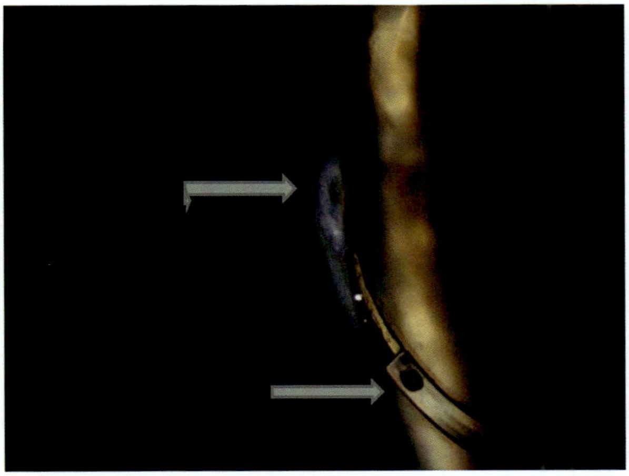

Fig. 29.14 Cutting of the ring segment and reinsertion after extrusion, may preserve the positive effect instead of the removal which will reverse the effect of the ISCR. See the location of the extrusion upper arrow and the new proximal position of the ring segment lower arrow

and femtosecond laser-assisted techniques resulted in a more superficial ICRS placement than predicted. The actual placement depth is often only 55–66% of that intended but can range from 40% to 80% [197–200]. Intraoperative complications are more common with mechanical implantation than femtosecond laser-assisted. These include superficial or asymmetric channel formation and perforation which can be superficial or into the anterior chamber. Intraoperative complication rates decrease with increasing experience of the surgeon. Complications associated with femtosecond laser –assisted implantation include incomplete channel formation, endothelial perforation and incorrect entry of the channel. Visual and refractive results are not significantly different between the two surgical techniques [195, 201].

29.10 Ring Position and Nomograms

Many combinations of ICRS can be implanted:

1. Two symmetrical segments.
2. Two asymmetrical segments.
3. One segment.
4. Variable thickness of the same ring: thin at the insertion site and then progressively thickens (Ferrara and Keraring types).
5. Variable thickness of the same ring: thin at the insertion site, gradually increases in thickness before then decreasing again at the distal part (Barbara Ring).

The location of the incision determines the placement of the ICRS, which then subsequently affects the corneal shape. These decisions are made according to the surgeon's evaluation of the individual case.

The following factors should be considered when choosing the ring: grade of KC, type of KC, the degree of myopia and astigmatism, and the Q value with the aim to bring this value as close as possible to the physiological value (−0.23). Some surgeons also take into consideration the angle of the coma [142, 202].

29.11 Limitations of the Nomograms

The refractive effect of ring segments depends on the biomechanical interactions between the ring segment and the stromal tunnel, which are still poorly understood. The same apparent pattern of KC can result indifferent refractive errors. Nomograms are based on a combination of empirical data and the subjective analysis of the surgeon. There is a need for new mathematical and scientific based biomechanical models of KC to assist in calculating the optimal design and location for ICRS implantation. Various nomograms have been proposed by the ring manufacturers.

Jorge Alio in Spain is leading a project collecting data on ICRS implantation incorporating pre- and post-operative data which is then evaluated using neural networking in the hope of defining new nomograms for ICRS.

29.11.1 Do ICRS Halt the Progression of KC?

Long-term stability has been reported following Intacs implantation in eyes with progressive KC. In one study 92.9% of eyes did not show signs of progression post-operatively indicating that Intacs implantation may have a therapeutic effect on KC progression [203]. Long-term stability of KC has also been reported using femtosecond laser assisted Ferrara ring implantation in a young group of KC patients with a high potential for progression [204]. However not all studies report such positive results. Implantation of Intacs and Ferrara Rings in 18 eyes was found to significantly improve the visual, refractive, and topographic parameters in the short term, but regression was later noted after 5 years and it was felt that ICRS did not significantly influence progression in this group of young KC [205]. This study did however include much smaller numbers than the previous two in which stability was reported.

29.12 Photorefractive Keratectomy (PRK)

PRK was first reported by Jes Mortensen and is a safe means of reducing astigmatism in KC [206, 207]. Tam be reported long-term satisfaction rates of at least 57%

(16 of 28 treated eyes) over a median follow-up period of 7 years after PRK [208]. Safety and efficacy of PRK in form fruste KC has also been reported [209, 210].

CXL can be used as a stabilizing procedure to give PRK an additional protective value in KC patients. Several reports have confirmed the predictability, efficacy, stability and safety of PRK combined with CXL, particularly if no more than 50 μ are ablated [211–213].

Simultaneous PRK followed by CXL seems to be a promising treatment capable of offering functional vision in patients with KC [211]. Same-day simultaneous topography-guided PRK and CXL aiming for partial correction of myopia and astigmatism with maximal ablation depth of 50 μ (the **Athens protocol**) appears to be superior to sequential CXL with later PRK in the visual rehabilitation of progressing KC over a mean follow-up period of 36 ± 18 months (range: 24–68 months) [214].

In a case report on a patient suffering from bilateral KC treated using the Athens protocol in one eye and followed for 5 years, a regression of over 10 D in keratometry was observed in the treated eye accompanied by regularization of corneal shape and improvement in VA. The untreated eye had a greater than 12 D increase in keratometry [215]. The use of mitomycin C for the prevention of corneal haze in combined PRK and CXL remains controversial [213].

The Athens protocol is reported as an effective mean of stabilizing the cornea in KC, improving corneal contour, reducing irregular astigmatism and offering a better quality of vision. By normalizing the corneal surface and stabilizing the cornea it not only treats the symptoms but also the cause of KC [216].

29.13 Summary

The effect of KC on functional vision and quality of life is often worse than one would expect. It is typically diagnosed during the peak years for education, income-earning, and child-rearing [17]. Treatment algorithms are similar whether the patient is adult or a child and depend on the stage of the disease, except that CXL should be performed earlier in children and follow-up intervals kept shorter due to a faster rate progression.

ICRS should be offered to KC patients as a safe and reversible means of improving VA, PRK combined with CXL, or phakic IOLs are additional means for improving VA and quality of vision. Keratoplasty should be considered only as a last resort.

Table 29.1 summarizes a practical approach to the keratoconic patient.

Treatment selection should be based on an informed discussion with the patient. The surgeon should take the effort to understand the patients expectations and individual needs and incorporate these into a personalized treatment protocol.

Table 29.1 Guidelines for the management of Keratoconus

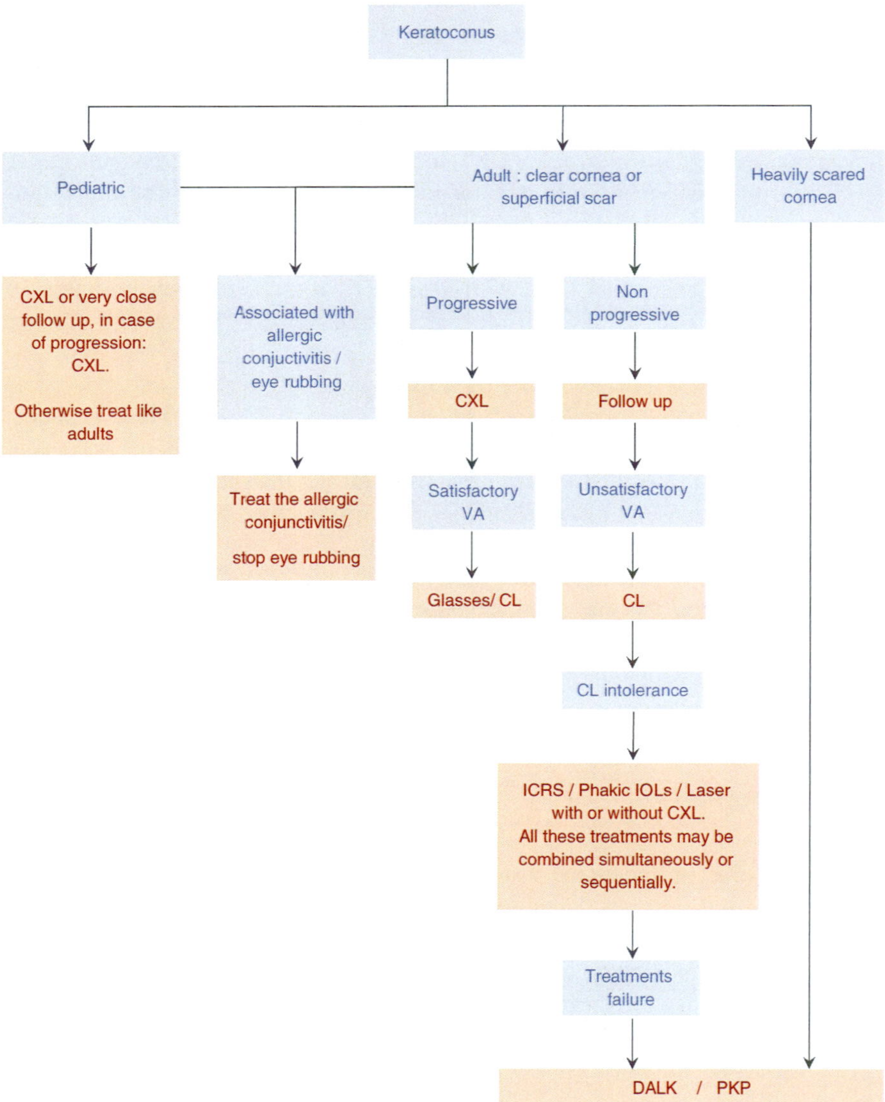

References

1. Parker JS, van Dijk K, Melles GRJ. Treatment options for advanced keratoconus: a review. Surv Ophthalmol. 2015;60:459–80.
2. Reinhart WJ, Musch DC, Jacobs DS, Lee WB, Kaufman SC, Shtein RM. Deep anterior lamellar keratoplasty as an alternative to penetrating keratoplasty. Ophthalmology [Internet]. 2011 [cited 2017 Mar 19];118(1):209–18. Available from: http://www.ncbi.nlm. nih.gov/pubmed/21199711.

3. Henein C, Nanavaty MA. Systematic review comparing penetrating keratoplasty and deep anterior lamellar keratoplasty for management of keratoconus. Contact Lens Anterior Eye [Internet]. 2017 [cited 2017 Mar 19];40(1):3–14. Available from: http://www.ncbi.nlm.nih.gov/pubmed/27802912.
4. Williams KA, Lowe M, Bartlett C, Kelly T-L, Coster DJ, et al. Risk factors for human corneal graft failure within the australian corneal graft registry. Transplantation [Internet]. 2008 [cited 2017 Nov 25];86(12):1720–4. Available from: http://www.ncbi.nlm.nih.gov/pubmed/19104411
5. Al-Mohaimeed MM. Penetrating keratoplasty for keratoconus: visual and graft survival outcomes. Int J Health Sci (Qassim) [Internet]. 2013 [cited 2016 Nov 26];7(1):67–74. Available from: http://www.ncbi.nlm.nih.gov/pubmed/23559907.
6. Troutman RCSC. Relaxing incision for control of postoperative astigmatism following keratoplasty. Ophthalmic Surg. 1980;11:117–20.
7. Troutman RC, Gaster RN. Surgical advances and results of keratoconus. Am J Ophthalmol [Internet]. 1980 [cited 2017 Nov 4];90(2):131–6. Available from: http://www.ncbi.nlm.nih.gov/pubmed/6999909.
8. Feizi S, Zare M, Feizi S, Zare M. Current approaches for management of postpenetrating keratoplasty astigmatism. J Ophthalmol [Internet]. 2011[cited 2016 Nov 26];2011:708736. Available from: http://www.ncbi.nlm.nih.gov/pubmed/21811668.
9. de Toledo JA, de la Paz MF, Barraquer RI, Barraquer J. Long-term progression of astigmatism after penetrating keratoplasty for keratoconus: evidence of late recurrence. Cornea [Internet]. 2003 [cited 2017 Dec 16];22(4):317–23. Available from: http://www.ncbi.nlm.nih.gov/pubmed/12792474
10. Patel SV, Malta JB, Banitt MR, Mian SI, Sugar A, Elner VM, et al. Recurrent ectasia in corneal grafts and outcomes of repeat keratoplasty for keratoconus. Br J Ophthalmol [Internet]. 2009 [cited 2017 Dec 16];93(2):191–7. Available from: http://www.ncbi.nlm.nih.gov/pubmed/19019928.
11. Barbara R, Barbara A. Recurrent keratoconus. Int J Keratoconus Ectatic Corneal Dis Int J Kerat Ect Cor Dis [Internet]. [Cited 2017 Mar 26];22(22):65–6865. Available from: http://www.jaypeejournals.com/eJournals/ShowText.aspx?ID=5070&Type=FREE&TYP=TOP&IN=_eJournals/images/JPLOGO.gif&IID=391&isPDF=YES.
12. Bergmanson JPG, Goosey JD, Patel CK, Mathew JH. Recurrence or re-emergence of keratoconus – what is the evidence telling us? Literature review and two case reports. Ocul Surf [Internet]. 2014 [cited 2017 Dec 16];12(4):267–72. Available from: http://www.ncbi.nlm.nih.gov/pubmed/25284772.
13. Ertan A, Muftuoglu O. Keratoconus clinical findings according to different age and gender groups. Cornea [Internet]. 2008 [cited 2017 Sep 22];27(10):1109–13. Available from: http://www.ncbi.nlm.nih.gov/pubmed/19034122.
14. Pearson AR, Soneji B, Sarvananthan N, Sandford-Smith JH. Does ethnic origin influence the incidence or severity of keratoconus? Eye [Internet]. 2000 [cited 2017 Jul 12];14(4):625–8. Available from: http://www.ncbi.nlm.nih.gov/pubmed/11040911.
15. Georgiou T, Funnell CL, Cassels-Brown A, O'Conor R. Influence of ethnic origin on the incidence of keratoconus and associated atopic disease in Asians and white patients. Eye (Lond) [Internet]. 2004 [cited 2016 Aug 13];18(4):379–83. Available from: http://www.ncbi.nlm.nih.gov/pubmed/15069434.
16. Slim EA, Jarade EF, Charanek BM, Antoun JS, Hemade AI, Awada SH, et al. Acute corneal hydrops mimicking infectious keratitis as initial presentation of keratoconus in a 10-year-old child. Case Rep Ophthalmol Med [Internet]. 2015 [cited 2017 Nov 4];2015:1–4. Available from: http://www.hindawi.com/journals/criopm/2015/308348/
17. Rehany U, Rumelt S. Corneal hydrops associated with vernal conjunctivitis as a presenting sign of keratoconus in children. Ophthalmology [Internet]. 1995 [cited 2017 Nov 4];102(12):2046–9. Available from: http://www.ncbi.nlm.nih.gov/pubmed/9098316.
18. Kaimbo WKD. Corneal hydrops associated with vernal conjunctivitis as a presenting sign of keratoconus in a Congolese child. Bull Soc Belge Ophtalmol [Internet]. 2002. [Cited 2017 Nov 4];(283):29–33. Available from: http://www.ncbi.nlm.nih.gov/pubmed/12058484.

19. Al Suhaibani AH, Al-Rajhi AA, Al-Motowa S, Wagoner MD. Inverse relationship between age and severity and sequelae of acute corneal hydrops associated with keratoconus. Br J Ophthalmol [Internet]. 2007 [cited 2017 Sep 22];91(7):984–5. Available from: http://www.ncbi.nlm.nih.gov/pubmed/17576720.
20. Reeves SW, Stinnett S, Adelman RA, Afshari NA. Risk factors for progression to penetrating keratoplasty in patients with keratoconus. Am J Ophthalmol [Internet]. 2005 [cited 2017 Sep 22];140(4):607. e1-607.e6. Available from: http://www.ncbi.nlm.nih.gov/pubmed/16226512
21. Wagner H, Barr JT, Zadnik K, Group the CLE of K (CLEK) S. Collaborative longitudinal evaluation of keratoconus (clek) study: methods and findings to date. Cont Lens Anterior Eye [Internet]. 2007 [cited 2017 Nov 19];30(4):223–32. Available from: http://www.ncbi.nlm.nih.gov/pubmed/17481941.
22. Chatzis N, Hafezi F. Progression of keratoconus and efficacy of corneal collagen cross-linking in children and adolescents. J Refract Surg [Internet]. 2012 [cited 2017 Jul 2];28(11):753–8. Available from: http://www.healio.com/doiresolver?doi=10.3928/1081597X-20121011-01.
23. Wollensak G, Spoerl EST. Riboflavin/ultraviolet-A-induced collagen crosslinking for the treatment of keratoconus. Am J Ophthalmol. 2003;135:620–7.
24. Raiskup F, Theuring A, Pillunat LE, Spoerl E. Corneal collagen crosslinking with riboflavin and ultraviolet-A light in progressive keratoconus: ten-year results. J Cart Refract Surg. 2015;41:41–6.
25. Kumar Kodavoor S, Arsiwala AZ, Ramamurthy D. One-year clinical study on efficacy of corneal cross-linking in indian children with progressive keratoconus. Cornea [Internet]. 2014 [cited 2017 Jul 2];33(9):919–22. Available from: http://www.ncbi.nlm.nih.gov/pubmed/25055145.
26. Bakshi E, Barkana Y, Goldich Y, Isaac Avni DZ. No titlecorneal cross-linking for progressive keratoconus in children: our experience. Int J Keratoconus Ectatic Corneal Dis. 2012;1(1):53–6.
27. Barbara R, Pikkel J, Garzozi H, Barbara A. Collagen cross-linking and keratoconus in pediatric patients. Int J Keratoconus Ectatic Corneal Dis Int J Keratoco Ectatic Corneal Dis [Internet]. [cited 2017 Mar 26]. 11(11):57–6057. Available from: http://www.jaypeejournals.com/eJournals/ShowText.aspx?ID=2674&Type=FREE&TYP=TOP&IN=_eJournals/images/JPLOGO.gif&IID=211&isPDF=YES.
28. Arora R, Gupta D, Goyal JL, Jain P. Results of corneal collagen cross-linking in pediatric patients. J Refract Surg [Internet]. 2012 [cited 2017 Sep 22];28(11):759–62. Available from: http://www.ncbi.nlm.nih.gov/pubmed/23347368.
29. Hanna R, Berkwitz E, Jamyl Habib Castillo BT. Collagen cross-linking for the treatment of keratoconus in pediatric patients. [Cited 2017 Mar 26]; Available from: http://www.jaypeejournals.com/eJournals/ShowText.aspx?ID=8430&Type=FREE&TYP=TOP&IN=_eJournals/images/JPLOGO.gif&IID=651&isPDF=YES.
30. Vinciguerra P, Albé E, Frueh BE, Trazza S, Epstein D. Two-year corneal cross-linking results in patients younger than 18 years with documented progressive keratoconus. Am J Ophthalmol [Internet]. 2012 [cited 2017 Sep 22];154(3):520–6. Available from: http://www.ncbi.nlm.nih.gov/pubmed/22633357.
31. Magli A, Forte R, Tortori A, Capasso L, Marsico G, Piozzi E. Epithelium-off corneal collagen cross-linking versus transepithelial cross-linking for pediatric keratoconus. Cornea [Internet]. 2013 [cited 2017 Sep 22];32(5):597–601. Available from: http://www.ncbi.nlm.nih.gov/pubmed/23132450.
32. Luca Buzzonetti MD, Gianni Petrocelli M. No title transepithelial corneal cross-linking in pediatric patients: early results. J Refract Surg. 2012;28(November):763–7.
33. Badawi AE. Accelerated corneal collagen cross-linking in pediatric keratoconus: one year study. Saudi J Ophthalmol Off J Saudi Ophthalmol Soc. 2017[Internet] [cited 2017 Nov 1];31(1):11–8. Available from: http://www.ncbi.nlm.nih.gov/pubmed/28337057.
34. Krachmer JH, Feder RS, Belin MW. Keratoconus and related noninflammatory corneal thinning disorders. Surv Ophthalmol [Internet]. [Cited 2017 Mar 19];28(4):293–322. Available from: http://www.ncbi.nlm.nih.gov/pubmed/6230745.

35. Gautam V, Chaudhary M, Sharma AK, Shrestha GS, Rai PG. Topographic corneal changes in children with vernal keratoconjunctivitis: a report from Kathmandu, Nepal. Contact Lens Anterior Eye [Internet]. 2015 [cited 2017 Nov 4];38(6):461–5. Available from: http://linkinghub.elsevier.com/retrieve/pii/S1367048415300035.
36. Bawazeer AM, Hodge WG, Lorimer B. Atopy and keratoconus: a multivariate analysis. Br J Ophthalmol [Internet]. 2000 [cited 2016 Aug 13];84(8):834–6. Available from: http://www.ncbi.nlm.nih.gov/pubmed/10906086.
37. McMonnies CW, Boneham GC. Keratoconus, allergy, itch, eye-rubbing and hand-dominance. Clin Exp Optom [Internet]. 2003 [cited 2016 Aug 13];86(6):376–84. Available from: http://doi.wiley.com/10.1111/j.1444-0938.2003.tb03082.x.
38. Hawkes E, Nanavaty MA. Eye rubbing and keratoconus : a literature review. Int J Keratoconus Ectatic Corneal Dis. 2014;3(3):118–21.
39. Gatinel D. Eye rubbing, a sine qua non for keratoconus? Int J Keratoconus Ectatic Corneal Dis. 2016;5(1):6–12.
40. Elizabeth Hawkes MAN. Eye rubbing and keratoconus: a literature review. Cor Dis. 2014;3(3):118–21.
41. CW McMonnies. Cornea. Mechanisms of rubbing-related corneal trauma in keratoconus. Cornea. 2009;28(6):607–l.
42. McConnies CW. Eye rubbing type and prevalence including contact lens "removal-relief" rubbing. Clin Exp Optom [Internet]. 2016 [cited 2017 Sep 30];99(4):366–72. Available from http://www.ncbi.nlm.nih.gov/pubmed/27306478.
43. Pucci N, Novembre E, Cianferoni A, Lombardi E, Bernardini R, Caputo R, et al. Efficacy and safety of cyclosporine eyedrops in vernal keratoconjunctivitis. Ann Allergy Asthma Immunol [Internet]. 2002 [cited 2017 Nov 8];89(3):298–303. Available from: http://www.ncbi.nlm.nih.gov/pubmed/12269651.
44. Tesse R, Spadavecchia L, Fanelli P, Rizzo G, Procoli U, Brunetti L, et al. Treatment of severe vernal keratoconjunctivitis with 1% topical cyclosporine in an Italian cohort of 197 children. Pediatr Allergy Immunol [Internet]. 2010 [cited 2017 Nov 8];21(2p1):330–5. Available from: http://www.ncbi.nlm.nih.gov/pubmed/19840298.
45. Leonardi A. Management of vernal keratoconjunctivitis. Ophthalmol Ther [Internet]. 2013 [cited 2017 Sep 30];2(2):73–88. Available from: http://www.ncbi.nlm.nih.gov/pubmed/25135808.
46. Sangwan VS, Jain V, Vemuganti GK, Murthy SI. Vernal keratoconjunctivitis with limbal stem cell deficiency. Cornea [Internet]. 2011 [cited 2017 Sep 22];30(5):491–6. Available from: http://www.ncbi.nlm.nih.gov/pubmed/21598432.
47. Cameron JA, Al-Rajhi AA, Badr IA. Corneal ectasia in vernal keratoconjunctivitis. Ophthalmology [Internet]. 1989 [cited 2017 Sep 22];96(11):1615–23. Available from: http://www.ncbi.nlm.nih.gov/pubmed/2616147.
48. Gomes JAP, Tan D, Rapuano CJ, Belin MW, Ambrósio R, Guell JL, et al. Global consensus on keratoconus and ectatic diseases the group of panelists for the global delphi panel of keratoconus and ectatic diseases. Cornea. 2015 [Cited 2017 Jul 2];34(4):359–69. Available from: http://www.corneasociety.org/sites/default/files/global_consensus_on_keratoconus_and_ectatic.1.pdf.
49. Sykakis E, Karim R, Evans JR, Bunce C, Amissah-Arthur KN, Patwary S, et al. Corneal collagen cross-linking for treating keratoconus. In: Hamada S, editor. Cochrane database of systematic reviews [Internet]. Chichester: Wiley; 2015 [cited 2017 Jul 2]. p. CD010621. Available from: http://www.ncbi.nlm.nih.gov/pubmed/25803325.
50. Galvis V, Tello A, Ortiz AI, Escaf LC. Patient selection for corneal collagen cross-linking: an updated review. Clin Ophthalmol [Internet]. 2017 [cited 2017 Jul 2];11:657–68. Available from: http://www.ncbi.nlm.nih.gov/pubmed/28435217.
51. Wang Q, Savini G, Hoffer KJ, Xu Z, Feng Y, Wen D, et al. A comprehensive assessment of the precision and agreement of anterior corneal power measurements obtained using 8 different devices. Wedrich A, editor. PLoS One [Internet]. 2012 [cited 2017 Jul 5];7(9):e45607. Available from: http://www.ncbi.nlm.nih.gov/pubmed/23049823.

52. Shetty R, Arora V, Jayadev C, Nuijts RMMA, Kumar M, Puttaiah NK, et al. Repeatability and agreement of three scheimpflug-based imaging systems for measuring anterior segment parameters in Keratoconus. Investig Ophthalmol Vis Sci. 2014;55(8):5263.
53. Mehravaran S, Asgari S, Bigdeli S, Shahnazi A, Hashemi H. Keratometry with five different techniques: a study of device repeatability and inter-device agreement. Int Ophthalmol [Internet]. 2014 [cited 2017 Jul 5];34(4):869–75. http://www.ncbi.nlm.nih.gov/pubmed/24562593.
54. Hashemi H, Yekta A, Khabazkhoob M. Effect of keratoconus grades on repeatability of keratometry readings: comparison of 5 devices. J Cataract Refract Surg [Internet]. 2015 [cited 2017 Jul 5];41(5):1065–72. Available from: http://www.ncbi.nlm.nih.gov/pubmed/26049838.
55. Wollensak G. Crosslinking treatment of progressive keratoconus: new hope. Curr Opin Ophthalmol. 2006;17(4):356–60.
56. Raiskup F, Spoerl E. Corneal cross-linking with hypo-osmolar riboflavin solution in thin keratoconic corneas. Am J Ophthalmol. 2011;152(1):28–32.
57. Hafezi F, Mrochen M, Iseli HP, Seiler T. Collagen crosslinking with ultraviolet-A and hypoosmolar riboflavin solution in thin corneas. J Cataract Refract Surg [Internet]. 2009 [cited 2017 Mar 3];35(4):621–4. Available from: http://linkinghub.elsevier.com/retrieve/pii/S0886335009000625.
58. Kymionis G, Diakonis V, Coskunseven E, Jankov M, Yoo S, Pallikaris I. Customized pachymetric guided epithelial debridement for corneal collagen cross linking. BMC Ophthalmol. 2009;9(1):10.
59. Koller T, Mrochen M, Seiler T. Complication and failure rates after corneal crosslinking. J Cataract Refract Surg. 2009;35(8):1358–62.
60. Raiskup F, Hoyer A, Spoerl E. Permanent corneal haze after riboflavin-UVA-induced cross-linking in keratoconus. J Refract Surg [Internet]. 2009 [cited 2017 Jul 15];25(9):S824–8. Available from: http://www.ncbi.nlm.nih.gov/pubmed/19772259.
61. Pollhammer M, Cursiefen C. Bacterial keratitis early after corneal crosslinking with riboflavin and ultraviolet-A. J Cataract Refract Surg. 2009;35(3):588–9.
62. Sharma N, Maharana P, Singh G, Titiyal JS. < i> Pseudomonas</i> keratitis after collagen crosslinking for keratoconus: case report and review of literature. J Cataract Refract Surg. 2010;36(3):517–20.
63. Rama P, Di Matteo F, Matuska S, Paganoni G, Spinelli A. < i> Acanthamoeba</i> keratitis with perforation after corneal crosslinking and bandage contact lens use. J Cataract Refract Surg. 2009;35(4):788–91.
64. Demirci G, Ozdamar A. Case of corneal perforation as a complication after uneventful cxl without Infection. Int J Keratoconus Ectatic Corneal Dis J Kerat Ect Cor Dis [Internet]. [Cited 2017 Mar 26];22(33). Available from: http://www.jaypeejournals.com/eJournals/ShowText.aspx?ID=5598&Type=FREE&TYP=TOP&IN=_eJournals/images/JPLOGO.gif&IID=425&isPDF=YES.
65. Al-Qarni A, AlHarbi M. Herpetic keratitis after corneal collagen cross-linking with riboflavin and ultraviolet-A for keratoconus. Middle East Afr J Ophthalmol [Internet]. 2015 [cited 2017 Jul 15];22(3):389–92. Available from: http://www.ncbi.nlm.nih.gov/pubmed/26180483.
66. Goldich Y, Uri Elbaz DSR. Anterior uveitis after collagen cross-linking for keratoconus. Int J Kerat Ect Cor Dis. 2015;4(3):110–4.
67. Kymionis GD, Grentzelos MA, Kounis GA, Diakonis VF, Limnopoulou AN, Panagopoulou SI. Combined transepithelial phototherapeutic keratectomy and corneal collagen cross-linking for progressive keratoconus. Ophthalmology [Internet]. 2012 [cited 2012 Oct 27];119(9):1777–84. Available from: http://www.ncbi.nlm.nih.gov/pubmed/22683058.
68. Comparison of combined transepithelial phototherapeutic keratectomy and mechanical debridement during corneal cross-linking. J Refract Surg @BULLET [Internet]. 2017;[Cited 2017 May 19];33(4). Available from: https://www.healio.com/ophthalmology/journals/jrs/2017-4-33-4/%7Bb57dd521-f228-4280-9b88-5d1c1ca2ee8a%7D/comparison-of-combined-transepithelial-phototherapeutic-keratectomy-and-mechanical-debridement-during-corneal-cross-linking.pdf.

69. Wollensak G, Iomdina E. Biomechanical and histological changes after corneal crosslinking with and without epithelial debridement. J Cataract Refract Surg. 2009;35(3):540–6.
70. Raiskup F, Hillen M. Corneal cross-linking can halt the progression of keratoconus, but what is the best approach. Int J Keratoconus Ectatic Corneal Dis. 4(2):47–51.
71. Caporossi A, Mazzotta C, Baiocchi S, Caporossi T, Paradiso AL. Transepithelial corneal collagen crosslinking for keratoconus: qualitative investigation by in vivo HRT II confocal analysis. Eur J Ophthalmol [Internet]. 2012 [cited 2012 Oct 27];22(Suppl 7):S81–8. Available from: http://www.ncbi.nlm.nih.gov/pubmed/22344471.
72. Barbara R, Abdelaziz L, Barua A, Garzozi H, Barbara A. Collagen corneal cross-linking and the epithelium. Int J Keratoconus Ectatic Corneal Dis Ep Int J Kerat Ect Cor Dis. 11(33):179–84.
73. Lombardo M, Pucci G, Barberi R, Lombardo G. Interaction of ultraviolet light with the cornea: clinical implications for corneal crosslinking. J Cataract Refract Surg. 2015;41.
74. Leccisotti A, Islam T. Transepithelial corneal collagen cross-linking in keratoconus. J Refract Surg (Thorofare, NJ 1995). 2010;26(12):942.
75. Stojanovic A, Chen X, Jin N, Zhang T, Sten SF. Safety and efficacy of epithelium-on corneal collagen cross-linking using a multifactorial approach to achieve proper stromal riboflavin saturation. J Cataract Refract Surg. 2012;38(2):283–91.
76. Filippello M, Stagni E, O'Brart D. Transepithelial corneal collagen crosslinking: bilateral study. J Cataract Refract Surg. 2012;283–91.
77. Cruzat A, Shukla AN, Arafat SN, Alageel S, Colon C, Chodosh J, et al. Ex vivo study of transepithelial corneal cross-linking. J Refract Surg [Internet]. 2017 [cited 2017 Mar 15];33(3):171–7. Available from: http://www.ncbi.nlm.nih.gov/pubmed/28264131.
78. Gore DM, O'Brart D, French P, Dunsby C, Allan BD. Transepithelial riboflavin absorption in an ex vivo rabbit corneal model. Investig Opthalmology Vis Sci [Internet]. 2015 [cited 2017 Mar 18];56(8):5006. Available from: http://www.ncbi.nlm.nih.gov/pubmed/26230765.
79. Kaya V, Utine CA, Yilmaz OF. Efficacy of corneal collagen cross-linking using a custom epithelial debridement technique in thin corneas: a confocal microscopy study. J Refract Surg [Internet]. 2011 [cited 2017 Mar 3];27(6):444–50. Available from: http://www.ncbi.nlm.nih.gov/pubmed/21162472.
80. Samaras K, O'brart DP, Doutch J, Hayes S, Marshall J, Meek KM. Effect of epithelial retention and removal on riboflavin absorption in porcine corneas. J Refract Surg [Internet]. 2009 [cited 2017 Mar 3];25(9):771–5. Available from: http://www.healio.com/doiresolver?doi=10.3928/1081597X-20090813-03.
81. Vinciguerra P, Randleman JB, Romano V, Legrottaglie EF, Rosetta P, Camesasca FI, et al. Transepithelial iontophoresis corneal collagen cross-linking for progressive keratoconus: initial clinical outcomes. J Refract Surg [Internet]. 2014 [cited 2017 Mar 3];30(11):746–53. Available from: http://www.ncbi.nlm.nih.gov/pubmed/25375847.
82. Vinciguerra P, Romano V, Rosetta P, Legrottaglie EF, Kubrak-Kisza M, Azzolini C, et al. Iontophoresis-assisted corneal collagen cross-linking with epithelial debridement: preliminary results. Biomed Res Int [Internet]. 2016 [cited 2017 Mar 3];2016:1–5. Available from: http://www.hindawi.com/journals/bmri/2016/3720517/.
83. Bikbova G, Bikbov M. Transepithelial corneal collagen cross-linking by iontophoresis of riboflavin. Acta Ophthalmol [Internet]. 2014 [cited 2017 Mar 3];92(1):e30–4. Available from: http://www.ncbi.nlm.nih.gov/pubmed/23848196.
84. Cantemir A, Alexa A-I, Galan BG, Anton N, Ciuntu RE, Danielescu C, et al. Iontophoretic collagen cross-linking versus epithelium-off collagen cross-linking for early stage of progressive keratoconus – 3 years follow-up study. Acta Ophthalmol [Internet]. 2017 [cited 2017 Nov 22];95(7):e649–55. Available from: http://www.ncbi.nlm.nih.gov/pubmed/29110439.
85. Aldahlawi NH, Hayes S, O'Brart DPS, O'Brart ND, Meek KM. An investigation into corneal enzymatic resistance following epithelium-off and epithelium-on corneal cross-linking protocols. Exp Eye Res [Internet]. 2016 [cited 2017 Mar 3];153:141–51. Available from: http://linkinghub.elsevier.com/retrieve/pii/S0014483516303529.

86. Buzzonetti L, Petrocelli G, Valente P, Iarossi G, Ardia R, Petroni S. Iontophoretic transepithelial corneal cross-linking to halt keratoconus in pediatric cases: 15-month follow-up. Cornea. 2015;34(5):512–5.
87. Gore DM, O'Brart DP, French P, Dunsby C, Allan BD, Meek KM. A comparison of different corneal iontophoresis protocols for promoting transepithelial riboflavin penetration. Investig Opthalmol Vis Sci [Internet]. 2015 [cited 2017 Mar 3];56(13):7908. Available from: http://iovs.arvojournals.org/article.aspx?doi=10.1167/iovs.15-17569.
88. Cassagne M, Laurent C, Rodrigues M, Galinier A, Spoerl E, Galiacy SD, et al. Iontophoresis transcorneal delivery technique for transepithelial corneal collagen crosslinking with riboflavin in a rabbit model. Investig Opthalmol Vis Sci [Internet]. 2016 [cited 2017 Mar 18];57(2):594. Available from: http://www.ncbi.nlm.nih.gov/pubmed/24644053.
89. Wernli J, Schumacher S, Spoerl E, Mrochen M, C B, S GR. The efficacy of corneal cross-linking shows a sudden decrease with very high intensity UV light and short treatment. Time Investig Opthalmol Vis Sci [Internet]. 2013 [cited 2017 Mar 7];54(2):1176. Available from: http://iovs.arvojournals.org/article.aspx?doi=10.1167/iovs.12-11409.
90. Schumacher S, Oeftiger L, Mrochen M. Equivalence of biomechanical changes induced by rapid and standard corneal cross-linking, using riboflavin and ultraviolet radiation. Investig Opthalmol Vis Sci [Internet]. 2011 [cited 2017 Mar 7];52(12):9048. Available from: http://www.ncbi.nlm.nih.gov/pubmed/22025568.
91. Lin J-T, Cheng D-C. Modeling the efficacy profiles of UV-light activated corneal collagen crosslinking. PLoS One [Internet]. 2017 [cited 2017 May 14];12(4):e0175002. Available from: http://www.ncbi.nlm.nih.gov/pubmed/28384251.
92. Krueger RR, Herekar S, Spoerl E. First proposed efficacy study of high versus standard irradiance and fractionated riboflavin/ultraviolet a cross-linking with equivalent energy exposure. Eye Contact Lens Sci Clin Pract [Internet]. 2014 [cited 2017 Mar 15];40(6):353–7. Available from: http://www.ncbi.nlm.nih.gov/pubmed/25365552.
93. Hammer A, Richoz O, Mosquera SA, Tabibian D, Hoogewoud F, Hafezi F. Corneal biomechanical properties at different corneal cross-linking (CXL) irradiances. Investig Opthalmol Vis Sci [Internet]. 2014 [cited 2017 Mar 15];55(5):2881. Available from: http://www.ncbi.nlm.nih.gov/pubmed/24677109.
94. Tomita M, Mita M, Huseynova T. Accelerated versus conventional corneal collagen crosslinking. J Cataract Refract Surg [Internet]. 2014 [cited 2017 Mar 7];40(6):1013–20. Available from: http://www.ncbi.nlm.nih.gov/pubmed/24857442.
95. Alnawaiseh M, Rosentreter A, Böhm MRR, Eveslage M, Eter N, Zumhagen L. Accelerated (18 mW/cm^2) corneal collagen cross-linking for progressive keratoconus. Cornea. 2015;34(11):1427–31.
96. Hashemi H, Fotouhi A, Miraftab M, Bahrmandy H, Seyedian MA, Amanzadeh K, et al. Short-term comparison of accelerated and standard methods of corneal collagen crosslinking. J Cataract Refract Surg. 2015;41(3):533.
97. Razmjoo H, Peyman A, Rahimi A, Modrek H. Cornea collagen cross-linking for keratoconus: a comparison between accelerated and conventional methods. Adv Biomed Res [Internet]. 2017 [cited 2017 Mar 18];6(1):10. Available from: http://www.ncbi.nlm.nih.gov/pubmed/28299302.
98. Elbaz U, Shen C, Lichtinger A, Zauberman NA, Goldich Y, Chan CC, et al. Accelerated (9-mW/cm2) corneal collagen crosslinking for keratoconus—A 1-year follow-up. Cornea [Internet]. 2014 [cited 2017 Mar 15];33(8):769–73. Available from: http://www.ncbi.nlm.nih.gov/pubmed/24937167.
99. Marino GK, Torricelli AAM, Giacomin N, Santhiago MR, Espindola R, Netto MV. Accelerated corneal collagen cross-linking for postoperative LASIK ectasia: two-year outcomes. J Refract Surg [Internet]. 2015 [cited 2017 Mar 15];31(6):380–4. Available from: http://www.ncbi.nlm.nih.gov/pubmed/26046704.
100. Bozkurt E, Ozgurhan EB, Akcay BIS, Kurt T, Yildirim Y, Günaydin ZK, et al. Refractive, topographic, and aberrometric results at 2-year follow-up for accelerated corneal cross-link

for progressive keratoconus. J Ophthalmol. 2017[Internet] [cited 2017 Mar 18];2017:1–6. Available from: http://www.ncbi.nlm.nih.gov/pubmed/28197339.

101. Piñero DP, Artola A, Ruiz-Fortes P, Soto-Negro R, Pérez-Cambrodi RJ. Clinical outcomes at 1 year following corneal ectasia treatment with accelerated transepithelial cross-linking. Int J Keratoco Ectatic Corneal Dis. 2016;(3):93–6.
102. Henriquez MA, Rodríguez AM, Izquierdo L. Accelerated epi-on versus standard epi-off corneal collagen cross-linking for progressive keratoconus in pediatric patients. Cornea [Internet]. 2017 [cited 2017 Nov 3];36(12):1503–8. Available from: http://www.ncbi.nlm.nih.gov/pubmed/28938381.
103. Ozgurhan EB, Kara N, Cankaya KI, Kurt T, Demirok A. Accelerated corneal cross-linking in pediatric patients with keratoconus: 24-month outcomes. J Refract Surg [Internet]. 2014 [cited 2017 Mar 18];30(12):843–9. Available from: http://www.ncbi.nlm.nih.gov/pubmed/25437484.
104. Zhang X, Sun L, Chen Y, Li M, Tian M, Zhou X. One-year outcomes of pachymetry and epithelium thicknesses after accelerated (45 mW/cm(2)) transepithelial corneal collagen cross-linking for keratoconus patients. Sci Rep [Internet]. 2016 [cited 2017 Jul 12];6:32692. Available from: http://www.ncbi.nlm.nih.gov/pubmed/27597655.
105. Kymionis GD, Tsoulnaras KI, Grentzelos MA, Liakopoulos DA, Tsakalis NG, Blazaki SV, et al. Evaluation of corneal stromal demarcation line depth following standard and a modified-accelerated collagen cross-linking protocol. Am J Ophthalmol [Internet]. 2014 [cited 2017 Mar 3];158(4):671–5. e1. Available from: http://www.ncbi.nlm.nih.gov/pubmed/25034113.
106. Brittingham S, Tappeiner C, Frueh BE. Corneal cross-linking in keratoconus using the standard and rapid treatment protocol: differences in demarcation line and 12-month outcomes. Invest Ophthalmol Vis Sci. 2014;55(12):8371–6. doi:10. Invest Ophthalmol Vis Sci [Internet]. 2014 Dec 23 [cited 2017 Mar 15];55(12):8371–6. Available from http://iovs.arvojournals.org/Article.aspx?doi=10.1167/iovs.14-15444.
107. Ozgurhan EB, Sezgin Akcay BI, Yildirim Y, Karatas G, Kurt T, Demirok A. Evaluation of corneal stromal demarcation line after two different protocols of accelerated corneal collagen cross-linking procedures using anterior segment optical coherence tomography and confocal microscopy. J Ophthalmol. 2014;2014:981893.
108. Badawi A. Corneal endothelial changes after accelerated corneal collagen cross-linking in keratoconus and postLASIK ectasia. Clin Ophthalmol [Internet]. 2016 [cited 2017 Mar 15];10:1891–8. Available from: http://www.ncbi.nlm.nih.gov/pubmed/27757009.
109. Cingü AK, Sogutlu-Sari E, Çınar Y, Şahin M, Türkçü FM, Yüksel H, et al. Transient corneal endothelial changes following accelerated collagen cross-linking for the treatment of progressive keratoconus. Cutan Ocul Toxicol [Internet]. 2014 [cited 2017 Mar 15];33(2):127–31. Available from: http://www.ncbi.nlm.nih.gov/pubmed/23859485.
110. Medeiros CS, Giacomin NT, Bueno RL, Ghanem RC, Moraes HV, Santhiago MR. Accelerated corneal collagen crosslinking: technique, efficacy, safety, and applications. J Cataract Refract Surg [Internet]. 2016 [cited 2017 Mar 7];42(12):1826–35. Available from: http://linkinghub.elsevier.com/retrieve/pii/S0886335016305132.
111. Richoz O, Hammer A, Tabibian D, Gatzioufas Z, Hafezi F. The biomechanical effect of corneal collagen cross-linking (CXL) with riboflavin and UV-A is oxygen dependent. Transl Vis Sci Technol. 2013[Internet] [cited 2017 Mar 4];2(7):6. Available from: http://www.ncbi.nlm.nih.gov/pubmed/24349884.
112. Santhiago MR. Accelerated corneal cross-linking: we must acquire knowledge as fast. J Refract Surg [Internet]. 2016 [cited 2017 Mar 12];32(6):362–3. Available from: http://www.healio.com/doiresolver?doi=10.3928/1081597X-20160519-01.
113. Turkcu UO, Yuksel N, Novruzlu S, Yalinbas D, Bilgihan A, Bilgihan K. Protein oxidation levels after different corneal collagen cross-linking methods. Cornea [Internet]. 2016 [cited 2017 Jul 8];35(3):388–91. Available from: http://www.ncbi.nlm.nih.gov/pubmed/26751992.
114. Yuksel N, Ozel-Turkcu U, Yalinbas D, Novruzlu S, Bilgihan A, Bilgihan K. Comparison of aqueous humor nitric oxide levels after different corneal collagen cross-linking methods.

Curr Eye Res. 2016[Internet] [cited 2017 Jul 8];41(12):1539–42. Available from: http://www.ncbi.nlm.nih.gov/pubmed/27216990.

115. Mazzotta C, Traversi C, Paradiso AL, Latronico ME, Rechichi M. Pulsed light accelerated crosslinking versus continuous light accelerated crosslinking: one-year results. J Ophthalmol [Internet]. 2014 [cited 2017 Jul 8];2014:604731. Available from: http://www.ncbi.nlm.nih.gov/pubmed/25165576.
116. Mazzotta C, Traversi C, Caragiuli S, Rechichi M. Pulsed vs continuous light accelerated corneal collagen crosslinking: in vivo qualitative investigation by confocal microscopy and corneal OCT. Eye (Lond). 2014;28(10):1179.
117. Moramarco A, Iovieno A, Sartori A, Fontana L. Corneal stromal demarcation line after accelerated crosslinking using continuous and pulsed light. J Cataract Refract Surg. 2015[Internet] [cited 2017 Mar 4];41(11):2546–51. Available from: http://www.ncbi.nlm.nih.gov/pubmed/26703505.
118. Mazzotta C, Baiocchi S, Bagaglia SA, Fruschelli M, Meduri A, Rechichi M. Accelerated 15 mW pulsed-light crosslinking to treat progressive keratoconus: Two-year clinical results. J Cataract Refract Surg. 2017[Internet] [cited 2017 Nov 4];43(8):1081–8. Available from. http://www.ncbi.nlm.nih.gov/pubmed/28917411.
119. Choi M, Kim J, Kim EK, Seo KY, Kim T. Comparison of the conventional dresden protocol and accelerated protocol with higher ultraviolet intensity in corneal collagen cross-linking for keratoconus. Cornea [Internet]. 2017 [cited 2017 Mar 18];36:523. Available from: http://www.ncbi.nlm.nih.gov/pubmed/28230557.
120. Toker E, Çerman E, Özcan DÖ, Seferoğlu ÖB. Efficacy of different accelerated corneal crosslinking protocols for progressive keratoconus. J Cataract Refract Surg [Internet]. 2017 [cited 2017 Nov 2];43(8):1089–99. Available from: http://www.ncbi.nlm.nih.gov/pubmed/28917412.
121. Yıldırım Y, Olcucu O, Gunaydin ZK, Ağca A, Ozgurhan EB, Alagoz C, et al. Comparison of accelerated corneal collagen cross-linking types for treating keratoconus. Curr Eye Res [Internet]. 2017 [Cited 2017 Jul 12];42(7):1–5. Available from: https://www.tandfonline.com/doi/full/10.1080/02713683.2017.1284241.
122. Greenstein SA, Fry KL, Hersh PS. In vivo biomechanical changes after corneal collagen cross-linking for keratoconus and corneal ectasia: 1-year analysis of a randomized, controlled, clinical trial. Cornea [Internet]. 2012 [cited 2017 Nov 4];31(1):21–5. Available from: http://www.ncbi.nlm.nih.gov/pubmed/21993470.
123. Kymionis GD, Tsoulnaras KI, Grentzelos MA, Liakoppoulos DA, et al. Evaluation of corneal stromal demarcation line depth following standard and a modified-accelerated collagen cross-linking protocol. Am J Ophthalmol [Internet]. 2014 [Cited 2017 Nov 22];158(4):671–5.e1. Available from: http://www.sciencedirect.com/science/article/pii/S0002939414003961.
124. Kling S, Hafezi F. Biomechanical stiffening: slow low-irradiance corneal crosslinking versus the standard Dresden protocol. J Cataract Refract Surg [Internet]. 2017 [cited 2017 Nov 2];43(7):975–9. Available from: http://www.ncbi.nlm.nih.gov/pubmed/28823446.
125. Seiler TG, Fischinger I, Koller T, Zapp D, Frueh BE, Seiler T. Customized corneal cross-linking: one-year results. Am J Ophthalmol [Internet]. 2016 [cited 2017 May 19];166:14–21. Available from: http://www.ncbi.nlm.nih.gov/pubmed/26944278.
126. Mazzotta C, Moramarco A, Traversi C, Baiocchi S, Iovieno A, Fontana L. Accelerated corneal collagen cross-linking using topography-guided UV-A energy emission: preliminary clinical and morphological outcomes. J Ophthalmol [Internet]. 2016 [cited 2017 May 19];2016:1–10. Available from: https://www.hindawi.com/journals/joph/2016/2031031/.
127. Cassagne M, Pierné K, Galiacy SD, Asfaux-Marfaing M-P, Fournié P, Malecaze F. Customized topography-guided corneal collagen cross-linking for keratoconus. J Refract Surg. 2017[Internet] [cited 2017 Nov 14];33(5):290–7. Available from: http://www.ncbi.nlm.nih.gov/pubmed/28486719.
128. Nordström M, Schiller M, Fredriksson A, Behndig A. Refractive improvements and safety with topography-guided corneal crosslinking for keratoconus: 1-year results. Br J Ophthalmol

[Internet]. 2017 [cited 2017 Nov 14];101(7):920–5. Available from: http://www.ncbi.nlm.nih.gov/pubmed/27899371.
129. Seiler T, Hafezi F. Corneal cross-linking-induced stromal demarcation line. Cornea. 2006;25(9):1057–9.
130. Kymionis GD, Grentzelos MA, Plaka AD, Tsoulnaras KI, Diakonis VF, Liakopoulos DA, et al. Correlation of the corneal collagen cross-linking demarcation line using confocal microscopy and anterior segment optical coherence tomography in keratoconic patients. Am J Ophthalmol [Internet]. 2014 [cited 2017 Mar 3];157(1):110–5. e1. Available from: http://linkinghub.elsevier.com/retrieve/pii/S000293941300617X.
131. Spadea L, Tonti E, Vingolo EM. Corneal stromal demarcation line after collagen cross-linking in corneal ectatic diseases: a review of the literature. Clin Ophthalmol [Internet]. 2016 [cited 2017 Apr 12];10:1303–10. Available from: http://www.ncbi.nlm.nih.gov/pubmed/27695286.
132. Tian M, Ma P, Zhou W, Feng J, Mu G. Outcomes of corneal crosslinking for central and paracentral keratoconus. Medicine (Baltimore) [Internet]. 2017 [cited 2017 Mar 18];96(10):e6247. Available from: http://www.ncbi.nlm.nih.gov/pubmed/28272223.
133. Raiskup F, Spoerl E. Corneal crosslinking with riboflavin and ultraviolet A. I. Principles. Ocul Surf [Internet]. 2013 [cited 2017 Jul 7];11(2):65–74. Available from: http://www.ncbi.nlm.nih.gov/pubmed/23583042.
134. Rathi VM, Mandathara PS, Dumpati S. Contact lens in keratoconus. Indian J Ophthalmol [Internet]. 2013 [cited 2017 Jun 3];61(8):410–5. Available from: http://www.ncbi.nlm.nih.gov/pubmed/23925325.
135. Moodaley L, Liu C, Woodward EG, O'Brart D, Muir MK, Buckley R. Excimer laser superficial keratectomy for proud nebulae in keratoconus. Br J Ophthalmol [Internet]. 1994 [cited 2017 Jun 3];78(6):454–7. Available from: http://www.ncbi.nlm.nih.gov/pubmed/8060928.
136. Jorge L, PS-Díez A. Phakic intraocular lenses in keratoconus. Int J Keratoconus Ectatic Corneal Dis Int J Kerat Ect Cor Dis. 2015;44(33):103–6.
137. Budo C, Bartels MC, van Rij G. Implantation of Artisan toric phakic intraocular lenses for the correction of astigmatism and spherical errors in patients with keratoconus. J Refract Surg. 2005;21:218–22.
138. Kato N, Toda I, Hori-Komai Y, Sakai C, Arai H, Tsubota K. Phakic intraocular lens for keratoconus. Ophthalmology [Internet]. 2011 [cited 2017 Mar 26];118(3):605–5. e2. Available from: http://www.ncbi.nlm.nih.gov/pubmed/21376252.
139. Gupta S. Implantable contact lenses in keratoconus. Int J Keratoconus Ectatic Corneal Dis Keratoconus Int J Kerat Ect Cor Dis [Internet]. 2016;55(11):17–2017. Available from: http://www.jaypeejournals.com/eJournals/ShowText.aspx?ID=9480&Type=FREE&TYP=TOP&IN=_eJournals/images/JPLOGO.gif&IID=723&isPDF=YES.
140. Levy J, Pitchkhadze A, Lifshitz T. Treatment of stable keratoconus by cataract surgery with toric IOL implantation. Int J Kerat Ect Cor Dis. 2012;1(2):128–30.
141. Parikakis EA, Chatziralli IP, Peponis VG, David G, Chalkiadakis S, Mitropoulos PG. Toric intraocular lens implantation for correction of astigmatism in cataract patients with corneal ectasia. Case Rep Ophthalmol [Internet]. 2013 [cited 2017 Nov 29];4(3):219–28. Available from: http://www.ncbi.nlm.nih.gov/pubmed/24348406.
142. Barbara A. Textbook on keratoconus, new insights. 2012.
143. Nosé W, Neves RA, Burris TE, Schanzlin DJ, Belfort Júnior R. Intrastromal corneal ring: 12-month sighted myopic eyes. J Refract Surg. 1996;12(1):20–8.
144. Zare MA, Hashemi H, Salari MR. Intracorneal ring segment implantation for the management of keratoconus: safety and efficacy. J Cataract Refract Surg. 2007;33(11):1886–91.
145. Burris TE, Ayer CT, Evensen DA, Davenport JM. Effects of intrastromal corneal ring size and thickness on corneal flattening in human eyes. Refract Surg. 1991;7(1):46–50.
146. Siganos CS, Kymionis GD, Kartakis N, Theodorakis MA, Astyrakakis N, Pallikaris IG. Management of keratoconus with Intacs. Am J Ophthalmol. 2003;135(1):64–70.
147. Colin JVS. Implantation of Intacs and a refractive intraocular lens to correct keratoconus. J Cataract Refract Surg. 2003;29:832–4.

148. Colin J. European clinical evaluation: use of Intacs prescription inserts for the treatment of keratoconus. J Cataract Refract Surg. 2006;32:747–55.
149. Kymionis GD, Bouzoukis DI, Portaliou DMPI. New Intacs SK implantation in patients with post-laser in situ keratomileusis corneal ectasia. Cornea. 2010;29(2):214–6.
150. Shetty R, Narayana KM, Mathew K, Anand D, Mhaske P, Shetty B. Safety and efficacy of Intacs in Indian eyes with keratoconus: an initial report. Indian J Ophthalmol. 2009;57(2):115–9.
151. Salgado-Borges JM, Costa-Ferreira C, Monteiro M, Guilherme-Monteiro J, Torquetti L, Ferrara P, et al. Refractive, tomographic and biomechanical outcomes after implantation of ferrara ICRS in keratoconus patients.
152. Siganos D, Ferrara P, Chatzinikolas K, Bessis N, Papastergiou G. Ferrara intrastromal corneal rings for the correction of keratoconus. J Cataract Refract Surg. 2002;28(11):1947–51.
153. Peris-Martinez C, Menezo Rozalen JL. Keratoconic corneas after ferrara rings implantation: histopathological findings. Acta Ophthalmol. 2008;86:0.
154. Barbara A, Barbara R. Long-term follow-up of ferrara rings segments for the treatment of keratoconus. Int J Kerat Ect Cor Dis [Internet]. 2013 [cited 2017 Dec 13];2(1):34–9. Available from: http://www.jaypeejournals.com/eJournals/ShowText.aspx?ID=4549&Type=FREE&TYP=TOP&IN=_eJournals/images/JPLOGO.gif&IID=354&isPDF=YES.
155. El Dib RP, de Freitas D. A systematic review of Ferrara's ring in the treatment of keratoconus. J Refract Surg. (Thorofare, NJ 1995. 2008;24(9):865.
156. Leonardo Torquetti J, Torquetti L, Ferrara G, Ferrara P. Predictors of clinical outcomes after intrastromal corneal ring segments implantation. Int J Keratoco Ectatic Corneal Dis. 2012;1(1):26–30.
157. Coskunseven E, Kymionis GD, Tsiklis NS, Atun S, Arslan E, Jankov MR, et al. One-year results of intrastromal corneal ring segment implantation (KeraRing) using femtosecond laser in patients with keratoconus. Am J Ophthalmol. 2008;145(5):775.
158. Daxer B, Mahmood H, Daxer A. MyoRing treatment for keratoconus: DIOPTEX PocketMaker vs Ziemer LDV for corneal pocket creation. Int J Keratoconus Ectatic Corneal Dis Int J Kerat Ect Cor Dis. 11(33):151–2.
159. Daxer A. MyoRing treatment of keratoconus. Int J Kerat Ect Cor Dis. 2015;4(2):76–83.
160. Daxer A. Corneal thickness after myoring implantation for keratoconus. Int J Keratoconus Ectatic Corneal Dis Int J Kerat Ect Cor Dis. 2014;33(11):15–9.
161. Daxer A. MyoRing for central and noncentral keratoconus. Int J Keratoconus Ectatic Corneal Dis Noncentral Keratoconus Int J Kerat Ect Cor Dis [Internet]. 2012 [Cited 2017 Apr 10];11(22):117–9. Available from: http://www.jaypeejournals.com/eJournals/ShowText.aspx?ID=3338&Type=FREE&TYP=TOP&IN=_eJournals/images/JPLOGO.gif&IID=258&isPDF=YES.
162. Ys R. Intacs for keratoconus. Ophthalmol Clin. 2006;46(3):91–103.
163. Brenner LF, Alió JL, Vega-Estrada A, Baviera J, Beltrán J, Cobo-Soriano R. Indications for intrastromal corneal ring segments in ectasia after laser in situ keratomileusis. J Cataract Refract Surg. 2012;38:2117.
164. Suiter BG, Twa MD, Ruckhofer JSD. A comparison of visual acuity, predictability, and visual function outcomes after intracorneal ring segments and laser in situ keratomileusis. Trans Am Ophthalmol Soc. 2000;98:51–5.
165. Carrasquillo KG, Rand J, Talamo J. Intacs for keratoconus and post-LASIK ectasia: mechanical versus femtosecond laser-assisted channel creation. Cornea. 2007;26(9):956–62.
166. Sharma M, Boxer WBS, et al. Comparison of single-segment and double-segment Intacs for keratoconus and post-LASIK ectasia. Am J Ophthalmol. 2006;141(5):891–5.
167. Tan BU, Purcell TL, Torres LF, Schanzlin DJ. New surgical approaches to the management of keratoconus and post-LASIK ectasia. Trans Am Ophthalmol Soc. 2006;104:212.
168. Kymionis GD, Siganos CS, Kounis G, Astyrakakis N, Kalyvianaki MI, Pallikaris IG. Management of post-LASIK corneal ectasia with Intacs inserts: one-year results. Arch Ophthalmol. 2003;121(3):322.

169. Kymionis GD, Tsiklis NS, Pallikaris AI, Kounis G, Diakonis VF, Astyrakakis N, et al. Long-term follow-up of Intacs for post-LASIK corneal ectasia. Ophthalmology. 2006;113:1909–17.
170. Ramez Barbara J, Barbara R, Zadok D, Pikkel J, Marcovich A, Garzozi H, et al. Collagen corneal cross-linking followed by intac implantation in a case of post-PRK ectasia. Int J Keratoco Ectatic Corneal Dis [Internet]. 2012 [cited 2017 Mar 26];1(1):68–72. Available from: http://www.jaypeejournals.com/eJournals/ShowText.aspx?ID=2677&Type=FREE&TYP=TOP&IN=_eJournals/images/JPLOGO.gif&IID=211&isPDF=YES.
171. Barbara A, Shehadeh-Masha'our R, Zvi F, Garzozi H. Management of pellucid marginal degeneration with intracorneal ring segments. J Refract Surg. 2005;21:296–8.
172. Ruckhofer J, Stoiber J, Twa MD, Grabner G. Correction of astigmatism with short arc-length intrastromal corneal ring segments: preliminary results. Ophthalmology. 2003;110(3):516–24.
173. Rodríguez LA, Guillén PB, Benavides MA, Garcia L, Porras D, Daqui-Garay RM. Penetrating keratoplasty versus intrastromal corneal ring segments to correct bilateral corneal ectasia: preliminary study. J Cataract Refract Surg. 2007;33(3):488–96.
174. Barbara R, Barbara A. Intrastromal corneal ring segments with and without collagen corneal crosslinking vs penetrating keratoplasty for the treatment of keratoconus. Int J Kerat Ect Cor Dis [Internet]. 2014 [cited 2017 Mar 26];3(2):88–94. Available from: http://www.jaypeejournals.com/ejournals/ShowText.aspx?ID=6724&Type=FREE&TYP=TOP&IN=_eJournals/images/JPLOGO.gif&IID=506&isPDF=YES.
175. Dauwe C, Touboul D, Roberts CJ, Mahmoud AM, Kérautret J, Fournier P, et al. Biomechanical and morphological corneal response to placement of intrastromal corneal ring segments for keratoconus. J Cataract Refract Surg. 2009;35(10):1761–7.
176. Barbara R, Garzozi H, Barbara A. Combined intacs SK and collagen corneal crosslinking for the treatment of keratoconus. Int J Keratoconus Ectatic Corneal Dis pages. 2012;1(2):109–16.
177. Coskunseven E, Jankov MR, Hafezi F, Atun S, Arslan E, Kymionis GD. Effect of treatment sequence in combined intrastromal corneal rings and corneal collagen crosslinking for keratoconus. J Cataract Refract Surg. 2009;35(12):2084–91.
178. Ertan A, Karacal H, Kamburoğlu G. Refractive and topographic results of transepithelial cross-linking treatment in eyes with intacs. Cornea [Internet]. 2009;28(7):719–23. Available from: http://www.ncbi.nlm.nih.gov/pubmed/19574920.
179. Nicula C, Pop RN, Nicula D V. Comparative results in a combined procedure of intrastromal corneal rings implantation and cross-linking in patients with keratoconus: a retrospective study. Ophthalmol Ther [Internet]. 2017 [Cited 2017 Nov 4];313–21. Available from: http://www.ncbi.nlm.nih.gov/pubmed/29086187.
180. Alió JL, Vega-Estrada A, Sanz-Díez P, Peña-García P, Durán-García ML, Maldonado M. Keratoconus management guidelines. Int J Keratoconus Ectatic Corneal Dis. 2015;4(1):1–39.
181. Piñero DP, Alio JL. Intracorneal ring segments in ectatic corneal disease – a review. Clin Exp Ophthalmol. 2010;38(2):154–67.
182. Intrastromal corneal ring segments in children with keratoconus. Int J Keratoconus Ectatic Corneal Dis Int J Kerat Ect Cor Dis [Internet]. 2017;66(22):45–8. Available from: http://www.jaypeejournals.com/eJournals/ShowText.aspx?ID=13121&Type=FREE&TYP=TOP&IN=_eJournals/images/JPLOGO.gif&IID=1022&Value=26&isPDF=YES
183. Al-Tuwairqi W, Sinjab MM. Intracorneal ring segments implantation followed by same-day topography-guided PRK and corneal collagen CXL in low to moderate keratoconus. J Refract Surg. 2013;29(1):59–63.
184. Coskunseven E, Jankov MR, Grentzelos MA, Plaka AD, Limnopoulou AN, Kymionis GD. Topography-guided transepithelial PRK after intracorneal ring segments implantation and corneal collagen CXL in a three-step procedure for keratoconus. J Refract Surg. 2013;29(1):54–8.
185. Al-Tuwairqi W, Sinjab MM. Intracorneal ring segments implantation followed by same-day Topography-guided PRK and corneal collagen CXL in low to moderate keratoconus. J

Refract Surg [Internet]. 2013 [cited 2016 Aug 13];29(1):59–64. Available from: http://www.healio.com/doiresolver?doi=10.3928/1081597X-20121228-04.
186. Adel Barbara RB. How to improve visual acuity after intrastromal corneal ring segments? implantation for keratoconus and post-LASIK ectasia. Int J Keratoconus Ectatic Corneal Dis Int J Kerat Ect Cor Dis [Internet]. [Cited 2017 Mar 26];33(22):69–75. Available from: http://www.jaypeejournals.com/eJournals/ShowText.aspx?ID=6721&Type=FREE&TYP=TOP&IN=~/eJournals/images/JPLOGO.gif&IID=506&isPDF=YES.
187. El-Raggal TM, Abdel Fattah AA. Sequential intacs and verisyse phakic intraocular lens for refractive improvement in keratoconic eyes. J Cataract Refract Surg. 2007;33(6):966–70.
188. Kamburoglu G, Ertan A, Bahadir M. Implantation of Artisan toric phakic intraocular lens following intacs in a patient with keratoconus. J Cataract Refract Surg. 2007;33:528–30.
189. Moshirfar MF, Carlton R, Meyer JJ, Neuffer MC, Espandar L, Mifflin M. Simultaneous and sequential implantation of intacs and verisyse phakic intraocular lens for refractive improvement in keratectasia. Cornea. 2011;30(2):158–63.
190. Özertürk Y, Sari ES, Kubaloglu A, Koytak A, Piñero D, Akyol S, et al. J Cataract Refract Surg [Internet]. 2012 [cited 2017 Nov 5];38(2):324–32. Available from: http://www.ncbi.nlm.nih.gov/pubmed/22322167.
191. Lisa C, García-Fernández M, Madrid-Costa D, Torquetti L, Merayo-Lloves J, Alfonso JF. Femtosecond laser–assisted intrastromal corneal ring segment implantation for high astigmatism correction after penetrating keratoplasty. J Cataract Refract Surg [Internet]. 2013 [cited 2016 Nov 26];39(11):1660–7. Available from: http://linkinghub.elsevier.com/retrieve/pii/S0886335013008742.
192. Arantes JCD, Coscarelli S, Ferrara P, Araújo LPN, Ávila M, Torquetti L. Intrastromal corneal ring segments for astigmatism correction after deep anterior lamellar keratoplasty. J Ophthalmol [Internet]. 2017 [cited 2017 Nov 4];2017:8689017. Available from: http://www.ncbi.nlm.nih.gov/pubmed/28951784.
193. Arriola-Villalobos P, Díaz-Valle D, Güell JL, Iradier-Urrutia MT, Jiménez-Alfaro I, Cuiña-Sardiña R, et al. Intrastromal corneal ring segment implantation for high astigmatism after penetrating keratoplasty. J Cataract Refract Surg [Internet]. 2009 [cited 2016 Nov 26];35(11):1878–84. Available from: http://linkinghub.elsevier.com/retrieve/pii/S0886335009007652.
194. Coscarelli S, Ferrara G, Alfonso JF, Ferrara P, Merayo-Lloves J, Araújo LPN, et al. Intrastromal corneal ring segment implantation to correct astigmatism after penetrating keratoplasty. J Cataract Refract Surg [Internet]. 2012 [cited 2016 Nov 26];38(6):1006–13. Available from: http://linkinghub.elsevier.com/retrieve/pii/S0886335012003690.
195. Coskunseven E, Kymionis GD, Tsiklis NS, Atun S, Arslan E, Siganos CS, et al. Complications of intrastromal corneal ring segment implantation using a femtosecond laser for channel creation: a survey of 850 eyes with keratoconus. Acta Ophthalmol [Internet]. 2011 [cited 2017 Nov 4];89(1):54–7. Available from http://www.ncbi.nlm.nih.gov/pubmed/19681760.
196. Barbara A, Barbara R. Intacs intracorneal ring segments complications in patients suffering from keratoconus. Int J Keratoconus Ectatic Corneal Dis J Kerat Ect Cor Dis. 22(33):121–8.
197. Sadigh AL, Aali TA, Sadeghi A. Outcome of intrastromal corneal ring segment relative to depth of insertion evaluated with scheimpflug image. J Curr Ophthalmol [Internet]. 2016 [cited 2017 Nov 5];27:25–31. Available from: www.sciencedirect.com.
198. Barbara R, Barbara A, Naftali M. Depth evaluation of intended vs actual intacs intrastromal ring segments using optical coherence tomography. Eye [Internet]. 2016 [cited 2017 Nov 5];30(1):102–10. Available from: http://www.ncbi.nlm.nih.gov/pubmed/26493037.
199. Gorgun E, Kucumen RB, Yenerel NM, Ciftci F. Assessment of intrastromal corneal ring segment position with anterior segment optical coherence tomography. Ophthal Surg Lasers Imaging [Internet]. 2012 [cited 2017 Dec 15];43(3):214–21. Available from: http://www.ncbi.nlm.nih.gov/pubmed/22390964.
200. Kouassi FX, Buestel C, Raman B, Melinte D, Touboul D, Gallois A, et al. Comparison of the depth predictability of intra corneal ring segment implantation by mechanical versus femto-

second laser-assisted techniques using optical coherence tomography (OCT Visante ({\textregistered})). J Fr Ophtalmol. 2011;94–9.

201. Kubaloglu A, Sari ES, Cinar Y, Cingu K, Koytak A, Coşkun E, et al. Comparison of mechanical and femtosecond laser tunnel creation for intrastromal corneal ring segment implantation in keratoconus: prospective randomized clinical trial. J Cataract Refract Surg [Internet]. 2010 [cited 2017 Dec 15];36(9):1556–61. Available from: http://www.sciencedirect.com/science/article/pii/S0886335010008497.
202. Torquetti L, Sandes J, Ferrara G, Ferrara P. Ferrara intrastromal corneal ring segments. Barbara A, editor. Int J Keratoconus Ectatic Corneal Dis [Internet]. 2016 [cited 2017 Mar 26];5(3):114–27. Available from: http://www.jaypeejournals.com/eJournals/ShowText.aspx?ID=10529&Type=FREE&TYP=TOP&IN=~/eJournals/images/JPLOGO.gif&IID=807&isPDF=YES.
203. Bedi R, Touboul D, Pinsard L, Colin J. Refractive and topographic stability of intacs in eyes with progressive keratoconus: five-year follow-up. J Refract Surg [Internet]. 2012 [cited 2017 Dec 15];28(6):392–6. Available from: http://www.healio.com/doiresolver?doi=10.3928/1081597X-20120509-01.
204. Fernández-Vega Cueto L, Lisa C, Madrid-Costa D, Merayo-Lloves J, Alfonso JF. Long-term follow-up of intrastromal corneal ring segments in paracentral keratoconus with coincident corneal keratometric, comatic, and refractive axes: stability of the procedure. J Ophthalmol [Internet]. 2017 [cited 2017 Dec 15];2017:4058026. Available from: http://www.ncbi.nlm.nih.gov/pubmed/28948045.
205. Vega-Estrada A, Alió JL, Plaza-Puche AB. Keratoconus progression after intrastromal corneal ring segment implantation in young patients: five-year follow-up. J Cataract Refract Surg [Internet]. 2015 [cited 2017 Sep 20];41(6):1145–52. Available from: http://www.ncbi.nlm.nih.gov/pubmed/26189375.
206. Mortensen J, Ohrstrom A. Excimer laser photorefractive keratectomy for treatment of keratoconus. J Refract Surg. 1994;10:368–74.
207. Mortensen J, Carlsson K, Öhrstrom A. Excimer laser surgery for keratoconus. J Cataract Refract Surg. 1998;24(7):893–8.
208. Tambe DS, Ivarsen A, Hjortdal J. Photorefractive keratectomy in keratoconus. Case Rep Ophthalmol [Internet]. 2015 [cited 2017 Mar 26];6(2):260–8. Available from: http://www.ncbi.nlm.nih.gov/pubmed/26327912.
209. Koller T, Iseli HP, Donitzky C, Papadopoulos N, Seiler T, et al. Topography-guided surface ablation for forme fruste keratoconus. Ophthalmology. 2006;113(12):2198–202.
210. Alpins N, Stamatelatos G. Customized photoastigmatic refractive keratectomy using combined topographic and refractive data for myopia and astigmatism in eyes with forme fruste and mild keratoconus. J Cataract Refract Surg. 2007;33(4):591–602.
211. Kymionis GD, Kontadakis GA, Kounis GA, Portaliou DM, Karavitaki AE, Magarakis M, et al. Simultaneous topography-guided PRK followed by corneal collagen cross-linking for keratoconus. J Refract Surg. 2009;25(9):807.
212. Kanellopoulos AJ. Short and long term complications of combined topography guided PRK and CXL (the Athens Protocol) in 412 keratoconus eyes (2–7 years follow-up). Investigative Ophth & Vis Sci. 2011;52:5202.
213. Kankariya V, Kymionis G, Kontadakis G, Yoo S. Update on simultaneous topo-guided photorefractive keratectomy immediately followed by corneal collagen cross-linking for treatment of progressive keratoconus. Int J Keratoconus Ectatic Corneal Dis Ect Cor Dis. 11(33).
214. Kanellopoulos AJ. Comparison of sequential vs same-day simultaneous collagen cross-linking and topography-guided PRK for treatment of keratoconus. J Refract Surg [Internet]. 2009 [cited 2017 May 19];25(9):S812–8. Available from: http://www.ncbi.nlm.nih.gov/pubmed/19772257.
215. Siqueira JA, Dias LC, Siqueira R, Valbon B, Santos R, Dawson D, et al. Long-term improvement after the athens protocol for advanced keratoconus with significant ectasia progression

in the fellow eye long- term improvement after the athens protocol for advanced keratoconus with significant ectasia progression in the fellow. Int J Keratoconus Ectatic Corneal Dis Eye J Kerat Ect Cor Dis [Internet]. [cited 2017 Mar 26];22(33):1025–68. Available from: http://www.jaypeejournals.com/eJournals/ShowText.aspx?ID=5599&Type=FREE&TYP=TOP&IN=_eJournals/images/JPLOGO.gif&IID=425&isPDF=YES.

216. Shah S, Mohan S, Rajan M, John B, Badlani V. Our experience with Athens protocol -simultaneous topo-guided photorefractive keratectomy followed by corneal collagen cross linking for keratoconus. Int J Res Med Sci Int J Res Med Sci Shah S Int J Res Med Sci [Internet]. 2016 [cited 2017 May 19];44(77):2639–44. Available from: www.msjonline.org.

Chapter 30
Should Pellucid Marginal Degeneration Be Managed Differently Than Keratoconus?

Mayank A. Nanavaty and Ahmed Shalaby Bardan

30.1 Introduction

Pellucid marginal degeneration (PMD) is a bilateral, peripheral corneal ectatic disorder characterized by a band of thinning 1–2 mm in width, typically in the inferior cornea, extending from the 4 to the 8 o'clock position. The area of thinning is usually found 1–2 mm central to the inferior limbus. Atypical cases of PMD with thinning extending beyond the inferior 4 clock hours occur [1], as do cases in which the thinning is confined to a superior location [2, 3]. Unilateral cases have also been reported [4, 5].

Schlaeppi [6] chose the name pellucid, meaning clear, to describe the thinning disorder. These corneas are generally clear an avascular, with no iron ring, infiltrate, or lipid deposition. Stromal scars have been described at the level of Descemet's membrane extending into the mid stroma, located at the superior aspect of thinned area. Cameron reported such scars in 39% of PMD patients [7]. Subtle Descemet's folds, which are occasionally seen concentric to the inferior limbus, may disappear with external pressure. Whilst the cornea can become quite thin, rupture rarely occurs [8–10]. Acute hydrops can occur and the result is edema, scarring and vascularization of the inferior cornea.

Maguire et al. [11], have described the corneal contour in PMD as a typical crab-claw illustrating the shift in astigmatism from the superior to the inferior corneal. However, the crab-claw appearance on a power map can also be seen with inferior keratoconus. The topographic appearance is also described as 'kissing birds' (Figs. 30.1 and 30.2). Corneal topography may reveal corneal contour abnormali-

M. A. Nanavaty (✉)
Brighton & Sussex Medical School, University of Sussex, Brighton, UK

Sussex Eye Hospital, Brighton & Sussex University Hospitals NHS Trust, Brighton, UK
e-mail: mayank.nanavaty@bsuh.nhs.uk

A. Shalaby Bardan
Brighton & Sussex Medical School, University of Sussex, Brighton, UK

A. Barbara (ed.), *Controversies in the Management of Keratoconus*,
https://doi.org/10.1007/978-3-319-98032-4_30

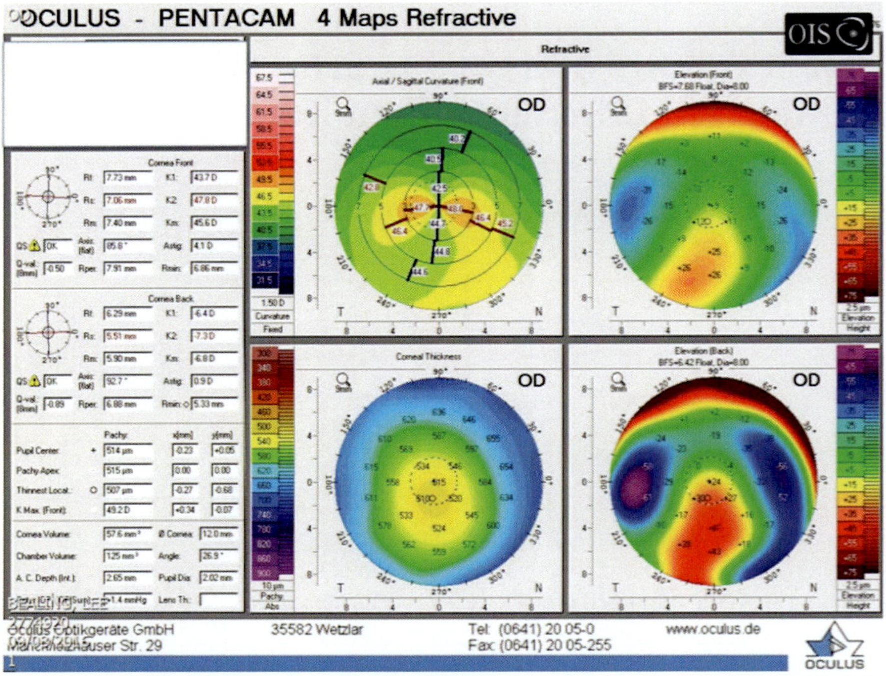

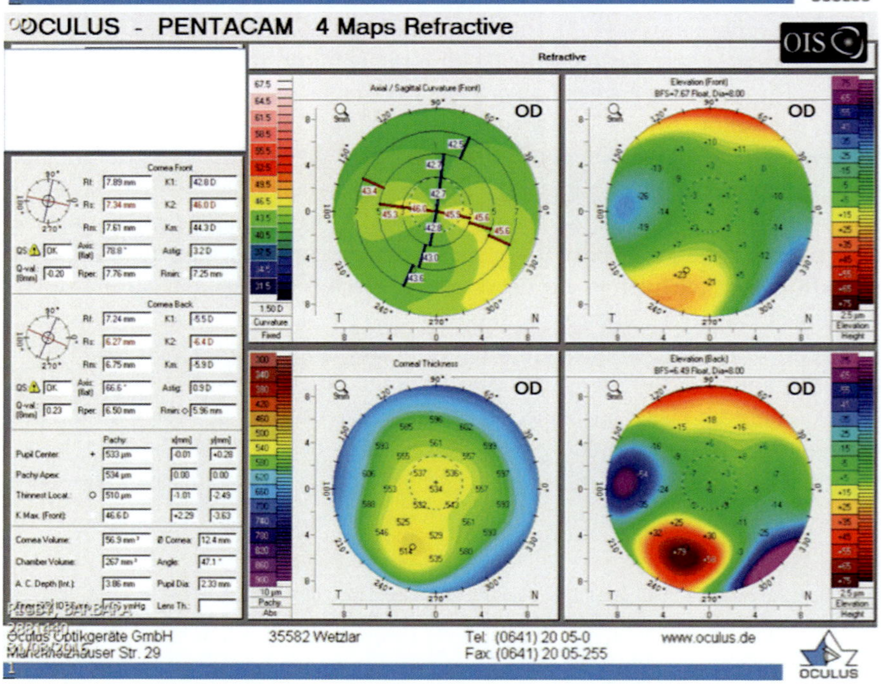

Figs. 30.1 and 30.2 Topographic examples of pellucid marginal degeneration

ties in asymptomatic family members of a PMD patient even when the slit lamp examination is normal [12].

Patients with this condition usually present for treatment between the second and fifth decades of life with complaints of blurred vision resulting from irregular astigmatism. There is no racial or gender predisposition.

30.2 Distinguishing Pellucid Marginal Degeneration from Keratoconus and Other Peripheral Thinning of Cornea

In contrast to keratoconus, maximal corneal protrusion typically occurs just superior to, rather than within, the area of thinning. The result is a corneal contour, which is resembles a 'beer belly'. The protruding cornea is of normal thickness. The abnormal corneal contour induces a shift in the axis of astigmatism from against-the-rule, superiorly, to with–the-rule, near the point of maximal protrusion. PMD and keratoconus can occur in the same eye [13]. Members of the same family may have both the disease.

PMD can be distinguished from other peripheral thinning disorders found in the differential diagnosis.

30.2.1 Keratoconus

The findings typical of keratoocus, specifically, protusion within the area of corneal thinning, striae, and Fleischer's ring, are not seen in PMD.

30.2.2 Terrien's Marginal Degeneration

Terrien's marginal degeneration can cause high astigmatism in a similar age group. However in contrast to PMD, this disorder has a male predilection. It commonly affects the cornea, superiorly as well as inferiorly, with vascularization and lipid deposition. When corneal protrusion occurs in Terrien's degeneration, it is usually within the area of thinning.

30.2.3 Mooren's Ulcer

Mooren's ulcer is usually unilateral and is associated with marked inflammation and pain, an epithelial defect in the area of ulceration, undermining of the central edge of the ulcer, and vascularisation up to the peripheral edge. Corneal changes in

Mooren's ulcer are not confined to the inferior or superior cornea. Finally, idiopathic furrow degeneration, while bilateral and non-inflammatory, occurs in the elderly within a corneal arcus.

30.3 Management of Pellucid Marginal Degeneration in Comparison to Keratoconus

30.3.1 Non-surgical Management Options

Like keratoconus, spectacles usually fail to adequately correct the high irregular astigmatism associate with typical cases of PMD. Large diameter, rigid gas-permeable contact lenses can be tried. However, because of the contour abnormality, a stable long-term fit can be difficult to achieve. The hybrid lenses have been used successfully in PMD [14]. The newer generation of scleral lenses made from gas permeable plastic may also be of benefit [15, 16].

30.3.2 Surgical Management Options

Corneal crosslinking is the treatment of choice to halt any documented progression (same as in keratoconus). If there is no progression, various surgical options can be offered to patients with PMD for visual rehabilitation as described below.

30.3.2.1 If Progressing: Corneal Collagen Cross-Linking CXL

The use of corneal collagen crosslinking to stabilize the cornea and stop progression can be used for PMD is same as in keratoconus. In literature there is no distinct definition of parameters of progression specific for PMD. So similar parameters as in keratoconus can be used. Consider CXL in any patient with PMD diagnosed at an early age before 20. Any case of PMD with documented progression based on maximum keratometry, pachymetry or significant change in topography and refractive parameters can be a suitable candidate to offer corneal crosslinking.

The criteria where corneal crosslinking may not be suitable in PMD cases are same as in keratoconus cases, such as: corneal thickness <400 m at thinnest location, maximum keratomtery >60 D, previous herpes keratitis, severe autoimmune conditions, etc.

30.3.2.2 Non-progressing But for Visual Rehabilitation

Early to Moderate Cases

A more conservative tissue-saving approach to early and moderate PMD involves reinforcement of ectatic corneal stroma with intrastromal ring segments, such as Intacs and Ferrara rings (same as in keratoconus management). Initially developed for mild myopia and demonstrated to be effective in keratoconus [17], these inserts can be used to minimize regular and irregular astigmatism by supporting weakened collagen fibrils. The segments are usually implanted through a temporal incision, one inferiorly and second superiorly [18–21]. The inferior 0.25 or 0.45 mm segment is inserted through the thinnest part of the cornea or just above it providing reinforcement and a barrier minimizing irregular astigmatism induced by the ectatic band just below it. Dissecting the channels for the inserts through such thin tissue is prone to error, and femtosecond laser has been successfully used to precisely place the channels. Overall, this reversible procedure may provide a safe approach to stabilize progressively degenerating corneas.

If the Area of Thinning Is <2 mm

Wedge resection or crescentic lamellar or penetrating keratoplasty can be performed. Maclean et al. [22] report that full excision of thinned tissue is often possible with mean residual astigmatism of 1.4 D. but long term astigmatic drift increases it to 2.1 D over 55–138 months.

If the Area of Thinning Is >2–3 mm

Large eccentric keratolasty can be performed. However, the risk of rejection and graft vascularization is higher because of the close proximity of the graft to the limbus. A better alternative may be a total lamellar keratopalsty followed by a smaller, central penetrating keratoplasty. Duran et al. [23] have also described a technique for crescent resection of the thin peripheral area to treat pellucid marginal degeneration. A combination technique described by Rasheed and Rabinowitz [24] for advanced PMD includes a simultaneous inferior lamellar keratoplasty with a central full-thickness penetrating keratoplasty. A lamellar graft, which is then trephined, initially reinforces inferior ectatic cornea and a 7.5 mm graft is sutured centrally. Simultaneous technique allows for relatively rapid visual rehabilitation, and reinforcement of inferior cornea helps minimize astigmatism.

In Keratoconus

If all the conservative options fail to achieve visual rehabilitation, then the penetrating keratoplasty and deep anterior lamellar keratoplasty remain the most popular choice amongst corneal surgeons.

30.4 Summary

PMD is a challenging condition especially when the patient present in an advanced state with high irregular astigmatism, extreme inferior thinning and loss of best corrected visual acuity even by the conservative methods like scleral gas permeable contact lenses. The surgical options described above need high surgical skills and experience and all have their own merits and demerits. There is always a risk of recurrence of the condition in the lower edge of the corneal graft. Therefore, appropriate bespoke titration of management options is necessary for individual patients.

Financial Interests The author does not have any financial or proprietary interest in any product or procedure mentioned in this chapter

References

1. Rao SK, Fogla R, Padmanabhan P, Sitalakshmi G. Corneal topography in atypical pellucid marginal degeneration. Cornea. 1999;18(3):265–72.
2. Bower KS, Dhaliwal DK, Barnhorst DA Jr, Warnicke J. Pellucid marginal degeneration with superior corneal thinning. Cornea. 1997;16(4):483–5.
3. Cameron JA, Mahmood MA. Superior corneal thinning with pellucid marginal corneal degeneration. Am J Ophthalmol. 1990;109(4):486–7.
4. Basak SK, Hazra TK, Bhattacharya D, Sinha TK. Unilateral pellucid marginal degeneration. Indian J Ophthalmol. 2000;48(3):233–4.
5. Wagenhorst BB. Unilateral pellucid marginal degeneration in an elderly patient. Br J Ophthalmol. 1996;80(10):927–8.
6. V S. La dystrophie marginale infericure pellucide de la cornee. Probl Actuels Ophthalmol. 1957;1:672–7.
7. Cameron JA. Deep corneal scarring in pellucid marginal corneal degeneration. Cornea. 1992;11(4):309–10.
8. Akpek EK, Altan-Yaycioglu R, Gottsch JD, Stark WJ. Spontaneous corneal perforation in a patient with unusual unilateral pellucid marginal degeneration. J Cataract Refract Surg. 2001;27(10):1698–700.
9. Lucarelli MJ, Gendelman DS, Talamo JH. Hydrops and spontaneous perforation in pellucid marginal corneal degeneration. Cornea. 1997;16(2):232–4.
10. Orlin SE, Sulewski ME. Spontaneous corneal perforation in pellucid marginal degeneration. CLAO J. 1998;24(3):186–7.
11. Maguire LJ, Klyce SD, McDonald MB, Kaufman HE. Corneal topography of pellucid marginal degeneration. Ophthalmology. 1987;94(5):519–24.

12. Santo RM, Bechara SJ, Kara-Jose N. Corneal topography in asymptomatic family members of a patient with pellucid marginal degeneration. Am J Ophthalmol. 1999;127(2):205–7.
13. Kayazawa F, Nishimura K, Kodama Y, et al. Keratoconus with pellucid marginal corneal degeneration. Arch Ophthalmol. 1984;102(6):895–6.
14. Astin CL. The long-term use of the SoftPerm lens on pellucid marginal corneal degeneration. CLAO J. 1994;20(4):258–60.
15. Pullum KW, Buckley RJ. A study of 530 patients referred for rigid gas permeable scleral contact lens assessment Cornea. 1997;16(6):612–22.
16. Biswas S, Brahma A, Tromans C, Ridgway A. Management of pellucid marginal corneal degeneration. Eye (Lond). 2000;14(Pt 4):629–34.
17. Colin J, Cochener B, Savary G, Malet F. Correcting keratoconus with intracorneal rings. J Cataract Refract Surg. 2000;26(8):1117–22.
18. Akaishi L, Tzelikis PF, Raber IM. Ferrara intracorneal ring implantation and cataract surgery for the correction of pellucid marginal corneal degeneration. J Cataract Refract Surg. 2004;30(11):2427–30.
19. Kymionis GD, Aslanides IM, Siganos CS, Pallikaris IG. Intacs for early pellucid marginal degeneration. J Cataract Refract Surg. 2004;30(1):230–3.
20. Mularoni A, Torreggiani A, di Biase A, et al. Conservative treatment of early and moderate pellucid marginal degeneration: a new refractive approach with intracorneal rings. Ophthalmology. 2005;112(4):660–6
21. Ertan A, Bahadir M. Intrastromal ring segment insertion using a femtosecond laser to correct pellucid marginal corneal degeneration. J Cataract Refract Surg. 2006;32(10):1710–6.
22. MacLean H, Robinson LP, Wechsler AW. Long-term results of corneal wedge excision for pellucid marginal degeneration. Eye (Lond). 1997;11(Pt 5):613–7.
23. Duran JA, Rodriguez-Ares MT, Torres D. Crescentic resection for the treatment of pellucid corneal marginal degeneration. Ophthalmic Surg. 1991;22(3):153–6.
24. Rasheed K, Rabinowitz YS. Surgical treatment of advanced pellucid marginal degeneration. Ophthalmology. 2000;107(10):1836–40.

Index

A. Barbara (ed.), *Controversies in the Management of Keratoconus*,
https://doi.org/10.1007/978-3-319-98032-4